MW01268359

The Cannabinoids: Chemical, Pharmacologic, and Therapeutic Aspects

Academic Press Rapid Manuscript Reproduction

The Cannabinoids: Chemical, Pharmacologic, and Therapeutic Aspects

Edited by

STIG AGURELL

Astra Lakemedel AB
Sodertalje, Sweden
and
Department of Pharmacology
Karolinska Institute
Stockholm, Sweden

WILLIAM L. DEWEY

Department of Pharmacology
Medical College of Virginia
Virginia Commonwealth University
Richmond, Virginia

ROBERT E. WILLETTE

Duo Research
Annapolis, Maryland

1984

ACADEMIC PRESS, INC.
(Harcourt Brace Jovanovich, Publishers)

ORLANDO SAN DIEGO SAN FRANCISCO NEW YORK LONDON
TORONTO MONTREAL SYDNEY TOKYO SÃO PAULO

ACADEMIC PRESS, INC.
Orlando, Florida 32887

United Kingdom Edition published by
ACADEMIC PRESS, INC. (LONDON) LTD.
24/28 Oval Road, London NW1 7DX

Library of Congress Cataloging in Publication Data
Main entry under title:

The cannabinoids : chemical, pharmacologic, and therapeutic aspects.

Includes index.
1. Cannabinoids--Congresses. 2. Tetrahydrocannabinol--Congresses. I. Agurell, Stig. II. Dewey, William L. III. Willette, Robert.
RM666.C266C36 1983 615'.7827 83-24444
ISBN 0-12-044620-0 (alk. paper)

PRINTED IN THE UNITED STATES OF AMERICA

84 85 86 87 9 8 7 6 5 4 3 2 1

CONTENTS

Section I. CLINICAL ASPECTS

Section II. CHEMICAL ASPECTS

Section III. METABOLIC AND PHARMACOKINETIC ASPECTS

Section IV. REPRODUCTIVE ASPECTS

Section VI. CELLULAR ASPECTS

CONTRIBUTORS

Numbers in parentheses indicate the pages on which the authors' contributions begin.

Stig Agurell (165, 211, 219, 239), *Astra Lakemedel AB, Sodertalje, Sweden; and Department of Pharmacology, Karolinska Institute, Stockholm, Sweden*

Mary D. Albert (359, 385), *Department of Biology, Boston College, Chestnut Hill, Massachusetts*

Ramona G. Almirez (471), *Department of Pharmacology, Uniformed Services, University of the Health Sciences, Bethesda, Maryland; and Department of Obstetrics and Gynecology, University of Texas Health Science Center, San Antonio, Texas*

S. Andersson (219), *Department of Pharmacology, Karolinska Institute, Stockholm, Sweden; and Astra Lakemedel AB, Sodertalje, Sweden*

M. Asberg (239), *Department of Psychiatry, Karolinska Hospital, Stockholm, Sweden*

Ricardo H. Asch (471), *Department of Pharmacology, Uniformed Services, University of the Health Sciences, Bethesda, Maryland; and Department of Obstetrics and Gynecology, University of Texas Health Science Center, San Antonio, Texas*

Robert L. Balster (545), *Department of Pharmacology, Medical College of Virginia, Virginia Commonwealth University, Richmond, Virginia*

Andrzej Bartke (411), *Department of Pharmacology, University of Texas Health Science Center, San Antonio, Texas*

Richard J. Bastiani (263), *Syva Company, Palo Alto, California*

J. A. Bedford (871), *Research Institute of Pharmaceutical Sciences, School of Pharmacy, University of Mississippi, University, Mississippi*

D. A. Benigni (871), *The Research Institute of Pharmaceutical Sciences, School of Pharmacy, University of Mississippi, University, Mississippi*

Vickie Berger (441), *Department of Biology, Bucknell University, Lewisburg, Pennsylvania*

M. Binder (709), *Institut für Physiologische Chemie der Ruhr-Universität, Bochum, Germany*

Lynne Bird (441), *Department of Biology, Bucknell University, Lewisburg, Pennsylvania*

R. Dean Blevins (319, 327, 751, 891), *Department of Biological Sciences, Health Science Division, East Tennessee State University, Johnson City, Tennessee*

Alan S. Bloom (575, 591), *Department of Pharmacology and Toxicology, Medical College of Wisconsin, Milwaukee, Wisconsin*

E. G. Boeren[1] (89), *Research Institute of Pharmaceutical Sciences, School of Pharmacy, The University of Mississippi, University, Mississippi*

E. Bohnenberger (709), *Biologishes Institut II der Universität Freiburg, Freiburg, Germany*

A. Breuer (777), *Hebrew University Pharmacy School, Jerusalem, Israel*

Dolores Brine (185), *Research Triangle Institute, Research Triangle Park, North Carolina*

Maureen Bronson (309), *College of Physicians and Surgeons, Columbia University, New York, New York; and Laboratorie de Toxicologie Cellulaire, Paris, France*

Sumner Burstein (729), *Department of Biochemistry, University of Massachusetts Medical School, Worcester, Massachusetts*

L. W. Cadwell (97), *Research Triangle Institute, Research Triangle Park, North Carolina*

E. A. Carlini (777), *Department of Psychobiology, Excola Paulista de Medicina, São Paulo, Brazil*

Paul Consroe (829), *Department of Pharmacology and Toxicology, College of Pharmacy, University of Arizona, Tucson, Arizona*

Lisa H. Conti (649), *Department of Psychology, University of Vermont, Burlington, Vermont*

C. E. Cook (135), *Research Triangle Institute, Research Triangle Park, North Carolina*

S. Gail Craddock (47), *Department of Health and Human Services, Public Health Service, Alcohol, Drug Abuse, and Mental Health Administration, Rockville, Maryland*

Susan L. Dalterio (411), *Department of Pharmacology, University of Texas Health Science Center, San Antonio, Texas*

Ken H. Davis, Jr. (97), *Research Triangle Institute, Research Triangle Park, North Carolina*

William L. Dewey (523, 545), *Department of Pharmacology, Medical College of Virginia, Virginia Commonwealth University, Richmond, Virginia*

Stephanie DiGuiseppi (111), *Department of Psychiatry, University of North Carolina, School of Medicine, Chapel Hill, North Carolina*

S. Dikstein (777), *Hebrew University Pharmacy School, Jerusalem, Israel*

Edward F. Domino (245), *Department of Psychiatry and Pharmacology, University of Michigan, Ann Arbor, Michigan*

[1] Present address: Packard-Becker B. V., Subsidiary of Ambac International Corporation, Delft, The Netherlands.

Laurence E. Domino[2] (245), *Department of Psychiatry and Pharmacology, University of Michigan, Ann Arbor, Michigan*

Steven E. Domino[3] (245), *Department of Psychiatry and Pharmacology, University of Michigan, Ann Arbor, Michigan*

Michael P. Dumic (891), *Department of Biological Sciences, Health Science Division, East Tennessee State University, Johnson City, Tennessee*

H. Edery (777), *Israel Institute for Biological Research, Sackler School of Medicine, Tel Aviv University, New Ziona, Israel*

Hala N. ElSohly (89), *Research Institute of Pharmaceutical Sciences School of Pharmacy, The University of Mississippi, University, Mississippi*

M. A. ElSohly (89, 871), *Research Institute of Pharmaceutical Sciences, School of Pharmacy, University of Mississippi, University, Mississippi*

John W. Everett (497), *Departments of Obstetrics and Gynecology and Anatomy, Duke University Medical Center, Durham, North Carolina*

Kenneth E. Ferslew[4] (281), *Department of Pharmacology and Therapeutics, Section of Toxicology, Louisiana State University School of Medicine, Shreveport, Louisiana*

Barbara Schneiderman Fish (829), *Department of Pharmacology and Toxicology, College of Pharmacy, University of Arizona, Tucson, Arizona*

Karl P. Flora (859), *Pharmaceutical Resources Branch, Developmental Therapeutics Program, Division of Cancer Treatment, National Cancer Institute, Bethesda, Maryland*

Robert D. Ford (545), *Department of Pharmacology, University of Maryland Dental School, Baltimore, Maryland*

I. Franke (709), *Institut für Physiologische Chemie der Ruhr-Universität, Bochum, Germany*

G. I. Fujimoto (401), *Department of Biochemistry, Albert Einstein College of Medicine, Bronx, New York; and The Rockefeller University, New York, New York*

Hampton K. Gillespie (165, 219), *Veterans Administration Medical Center, Palo Alto, California*

Harold M. Ginzburg (47), *Department of Health and Human Services, Alcohol, Drug Abuse, and Mental Health Administration, Rockville, Maryland*

James Glass (47), *Department of Health and Human Services, Public Health Service, Alcohol, Drug Abuse, and Mental Health Administration, Rockville, Maryland*

Mari S. Golub (657), *California Primate Research Center, Davis, California*

M. A. Gonzalez-Castillo (739), *Departments of Pharmacology and Biochemistry, University of Puerto Rico School of Medicine, San Juan, Puerto Rico*

[2] Present address: Department of Psychiatry, University of Michigan, Ann Arbor, Michigan.

[3] Present address: Vanderbilt University Medical School, Nashville, Tennessee.

[4] Present address: Department of Pharmacology, East Tennessee State University, School of Medicine, Johnson City, Tennessee.

Gail P. Goo (657), *California Primate Research Center, Davis, California*
Charles N. Gutierrez (319, 327), *Division of Microbiology, Veterans Administration, Mountain Home, Tennessee*
M. M. Halldin (211), *Department of Pharmacognosy, Faculty of Pharmacy, Uppsala, Sweden*
Jack Harclerode (441), *Department of Biology, Bucknell University, Lewisburg, Pennsylvania*
Harold F. Hardman (635), *Department of Pharmacology and Toxicology, Medical College of Wisconsin, Milwaukee, Wisconsin*
E. C. Harland (871), *The Research Institute of Pharmaceutical Sciences, School of Pharmacy, University of Mississippi, University, Mississippi*
Louis S. Harris (523, 545), *Department of Pharmacology, Medical College of Virginia, Virginia Commonwealth University, Richmond, Virginia*
D. J. Harvey (291), *University Department of Pharmacology, Oxford, United Kingdom*
Richard L. Hawks (123), *Division of Research, National Institute on Drug Abuse, Rockville, Maryland*
R. T. Henrich (345), *Department of Pediatrics, College of Physicians and Surgeons, Columbia University, New York, New York*
Cecilia J. Hillard (591), *Department of Pharmacology and Toxicology, Medical College of Wisconsin, Milwaukee, Wisconsin*
Leo E. Hollister (3, 165, 211, 219), *Veterans Administration Medical Center, Palo Alto, California*
Michael J. Hosko (635), *Department of Pharmacology and Toxicology, Medical College of Wisconsin, Milwaukee, Wisconsin*
John F. Howes (881), *SISA Pharmaceutical Laboratories, Inc., Cambridge, Massachusetts*
Robert Hubbard (47), *Department of Health and Human Servics, Public Health Service, Alcohol, Drug Abuse, and Mental Health Administration, Rockville, Maryland*
Claude L. Hughes, Jr. (487, 497), *Departments of Obstetrics and Gynecology and Anatomy, Duke University Medical Center, Durham, North Carolina*
Sheila A. Hunter (729), *Department of Biochemistry, University of Massachusetts Medical School, Worcester, Massachusetts*
Syed Husain (453), *Department of Pharmacology, University of North Dakota, School of Medicine, Grand Forks, North Dakota*
J. Stanford Hutcheson (111), *Department of Psychiatry, University of North Carolina, School of Medicine, Chapel Hill, North Carolina*
Marietta R. Issidorides (671), *Department of Psychiatry, University of Athens, Athens, Greece*
S. L. Kanter (211), *Veterans Administration Medical Center, Palo Alto, California*
Ralph Karler (845), *Department of Pharmacology, University of Utah, School of Medicine, Salt Lake City, Utah*

L. C. Krey (401), *Department of Biochemistry, Albert Einstein College of Medicine, Bronx, New York; and The Rockefeller University, New York, New York*

Michael W. Lame (453), *Department of Pharmacology, University of North Dakota, School of Medicine, Grand Forks, North Dakota*

N. Lander (777), *Hebrew University Pharmacy School, Jerusalem, Israel*

Colette Latour (309), *College of Physicians and Surgeons, Columbia University, New York, New York; and Laboratorie de Toxicologie Cellulaire, Paris, France*

K. Leander (239), *Department of Organic Chemistry, University of Stockholm, Stockholm, Sweden*

J. Roberto Leite (777), *Department of Psychobiology, Excola Paulista de Medicina, São Paulo, Brazil*

J. T. A. Leuschner (291), *University Department of Pharmacology, Oxford, United Kingdom*

Jan Erik Lindgren (219, 165), *Astra Lakemedel AB, Sodertalje, Sweden; and Department of Pharmacology, Karolinska Institute, Stockholm, Sweden*

L. Macedonia (401), *Department of Biochemistry, Albert Einstein College of Medicine, Bronx, New York; and The Rockefeller University, New York, New York*

Paul G. Mahlberg (79), *Department of Biology, Indiana University, Bloomington, Indiana*

Barbara R. Manno (281), *Department of Pharmacology, Section of Toxicology, Louisiana State University and School of Medicine, Shreveport, Louisiana*

Joseph E. Manno (281), *Department of Pharmacology, Section of Toxicology, Louisiana State University and School of Medicine, Shreveport, Louisiana*

Billy R. Martin (523), *Department of Pharmacology, Medical College of Virginia, Virginia Commonwealth University, Richmond, Virginia*

Lawrence E. McCarthy (859), *Department of Pharmacology, Dartmouth Medical School, Hanover, New Hampshire*

I. A. McDaniel, Jr. (97), *Research Triangle Institute, Research Triangle Park, North Carolina*

R. Mechoulam (775), *Hebrew University, Jerusalem, Israel*

Loren L. Miller (21), *Burroughs Wellcome Company, Research Triangle Park, North Carolina*

S. P. Montgomery (815), *Department of Psychology, The University of Texas at El Paso, El Paso, Texas*

P. L. Moody (97), *Research Triangle Institute, Research Triangle Park, North Carolina*

Robert Mooney (441), *Department of Biology, Bucknell University, Lewisburg, Pennsylvania*

A. Morishima (345), *Department of Pediatrics, College of Physicians and Surgeons, Columbia University, New York, New York*

D. E. Moss (815), *Department of Psychology, The University of Texas at El Paso, El Paso, Texas*

J. C. Murphy (871), *Research Institute of Pharmaceutical Sciences, School of Pharmacy, University of Mississippi, University, Mississippi*

Richard E. Musty (563, 649, 795), *Department of Psychology, University of Vermont, Burlington, Vermont*

Gabriel G. Nahas (309), *College of Physicians and Surgeons, Columbia University, New York, New York; and Laboratorie de Toxicologie Cellulaire, Paris, France*

T. Nogawa (345), *Department of Pediatrics, College of Physicians and Surgeons, Columbia University, New York, New York*

Agneta Ohlsson (165, 219), *Astra Lakemedel AB, Sodertalje, Sweden; and Department of Pharmacology, Karolinska Institute, Stockholm, Sweden*

W. D. M. Paton (291), *University Department of Pharmacology, Oxford, United Kingdom*

Mario Perez-Reyes (111, 185, 227), *Department of Psychiatry, University of North Carolina, School of Medicine, Chapel Hill, North Carolina*

C. G. Pitt (135), *Research Triangle Institute, Research Triangle Park, North Carolina*

G. Porath (777), *Israel Institute for Biological Research, Sackler School of Medicine, Tel Aviv University, New Ziona, Israel*

Raj K. Razdan (63), *SISA Institute for Research, Inc., Cambridge, Massachusetts*

Benjamin M. Rigor (603), *Department of Anesthesiology, University of Louisiana, School of Medicine, Louisville, Kentucky*

John A. Rosecrans (545), *Department of Pharmacology, Medical College of Virginia, Virginia Commonwealth University, Richmond, Virgina*

J. Rosenfeld (151), *Department of Pathology, McMaster University, Hamilton, Ontario, Canada*

B. M. Sadler (185, 227), *Research Triangle Institute, Research Triangle Park, North Carolina*

A. A. Salo (815), *Department of Psychology, The University of Texas at El Paso, El Paso, Texas*

H. Sanderman, Jr. (709), *Biologisches Institut II der Universität Freiburg, Freiburg, Germany*

J. Santos-Martinez (739), *Department of Physiology and Pharmacology, School of Medicine, Universidad Central de Csribe, Cayey, Puerto Rico*

E. N. Sassenrath (657), *California Primate Research Center, Davis, California*

Heather Sawyer (441), *Department of Biology, Bucknell University, Lewisburg, Pennsylvania*

Pamela M. Scher (471), *Department of Pharmacology, Uniformed Services, University of the Health Sciences, Bethesda, Maryland; and Department of Obsterics and Gynecology, University of Texas Health Science Center, San Antonio, Texas*

V. H. Schindler (135), *Research Triangle Institute, Research Triangle Park, North Carolina*

William T. Schmeling (635), *Department of Pharmacology and Toxicology, Medical College of Wisconsin, Milwaukee, Wisconsin*

B. Schmidt (709), *Institut für Physiologische Chemie der Ruhr-Universität, Bochum, Germany*

Avital Schurr (603), *Department of Anesthesiology, University of Louisiana, School of Medicine, Louisville, Kentucky*

H. H. Seltzman (135), *Research Triangle Institute, Research Triangle Park, North Carolina*

William Semple (563), *Department of Psychology, University of Vermont, Burlington, Vermont*

B. Shalita (777), *Hebrew University Pharmacy School, Jerusalem, Israel*

M. S. Shelton (751), *Department of Biological Sciences, Health Sciences Division, East Tennessee State University, Johnson City, Tennessee*

O. Shinohara (345), *Department of Pediatrics, College of Physicians and Surgeons, Columbia University, New York, New York*

Carol Grace Smith (471), *Department of Pharmacology, Uniformed Services, University of the Health Sciences, Bethesda, Maryland; and Department of Obstetrics and Gynecology, University of Texas Heath Science Center, San Antonio, Texas*

Richard Smith (441), *Department of Biology, Bucknell University, Lewisburg, Pennsylvania*

Jolane Solomon (359, 385), *Department of Biology, Boston College, Chestnut Hill, Massachusetts*

M. Srebnik (777), *Hebrew University Pharmacy School, Jerusalem, Israel*

Richard W. Steger (411, 815), *Department of Pharmacology, University of Texas Health Science Center, San Antonio, Texas*

C. R. Tallent (135), *Research Triangle Institute, Research Triangle Park, North Carolina*

Harold Taylor (185), *Research Triangle Institute, Research Triangle Park, North Carolina*

S. K. Tilak (427), *Department of Zoology, University of Toronto, Toronto, Ontario, Canada*

E. Toro-Goyco (739), *Departments of Pharmacology and Biochemistry, University of Puerto Rico School of Medicine, San Juan, Puerto Rico*

Stuart A. Turkanis (845), *Department of Pharmacology, University of Utah, School of Medicine, Salt Lake City, Utah*

Carlton E. Turner[5] (89), *Research Institute of Pharmaceutical Sciences School of Pharmacy, University of Mississippi, University, Mississippi*

Jocelyn C. Turner (79), *Department of Biology, Indiana University, Bloomington, Indiana*

[5] Present address: Office of Drug Abuse Policy, White House, Washington, D. C.

Lee Tyrey (487, 497), *Departments of Obstetrics and Gynecology and Anatomy, Duke University Medical Center, Durham, North Carolina*

B. Rao Vishnuvajjala (859), *Pharmaceutical Resources Branch, Developmental Therapeutics Program, Division of Cancer Treatment, National Cancer Institute, Bethesda, Maryland*

M. E. Wall (185, 227), *Research Triangle Institute, Research Triangle Park, North Carolina*

C. W. Waller (871), *The Research Institute of Pharmaceutical Sciences, School of Pharmacy, University of Mississippi, University, Mississippi*

C. Warick (135), *Research Triangle Institute, Research Triangle Park, North Carolina*

M. Widman (211), *Department of Pharmacognosy, Faculty of Pharmacy, Uppsala, Sweden*

D. M. Wilkison (621), *Department of Pharmacology and Toxicology, Medical College of Wisconsin, Milwaukee, Wisconsin*

D. R. Wing (291), *University Department of Pharmacology, Oxford, United Kingdom*

F. J. Witteler (709), *Institut für Physiologische Chemie der Ruhr-Universität, Bochum, Germany*

I. Zamir (777), *Hebrew University Pharmacy School, Jerusalem, Israel*

A. M. Zimmerman (427), *Department of Zoology, University of Toronto, Toronto, Ontario, Canada*

PREFACE

Books and review articles on the scientific aspects of marijuana and its constituents have appeared as early as ninety years ago. Investigations and subsequent reporting of work in this important area of research were sporadic prior to the identification of delta-9-tetrahydrocannabinol as the active constituent of marijuana in the 1960s. The latter half of that decade and the majority of the 1970s were characterized by continued advances in our understanding of the chemistry, metabolism, distribution, pharmacological effects, and toxicity of marijuana, its active ingredients, their metabolites and analogs. A number of scientific meetings were convened during these years to give scientists from around the world the opportunity to exchange results and ideas for future experimentation. Proceedings from meetings held in Savannah, Georgia, in 1974, in Helsinki, Finland, in 1975, and in Rheims, France, in 1978, as well as other books and review articles have been especially useful to scientists investigating these interesting compounds.

The last meeting on cannabis and its constituents, open to an international group of scientists, was held in 1978. The number of publications on the effects of cannabis and its constituents that appeared since that time were fewer than the number that appeared in the same time period in the middle 1970s. This observation and other indicators suggested that there had been a significant decrease in the number of scientists investigating these interesting compounds. Investigations of the potential therapeutic uses of cannabinoids were one exception to this trend. In an effort to revitalize interest in investigations into the basic science aspects of the cannabinoids, some two hundred scientists, who had published in this field and many of whom had participated in the earlier meetings, were asked to attend a meeting on cannabinoids and to alert colleagues to do the same. We had indicated that our intent was to meet to present current scientific advances without the controversial issues of legality or morality of the use or abuse of these drugs. The meeting was held in Louisville, Kentucky, in August 1982, immediately after the combined meeting of The American Society for Pharmacology and Experimental Therapeutics and The Society of Toxicology. We thank the council of ASPET and especially Ms. Kay Croker, its executive officer, for helping us to convene this meeting in conjunction with their annual meeting. We are especially thankful to Dr. William Waddell, Chairman of the Department of Pharmacology at The University of Louisville, and his committee who made the arrangements for the meeting comfortable and stimulating. We are very appreciative of Astra CNS Research whose financial support made the meeting possible.

The majority of the chapters in this book have been written by scientists who made the meeting a large success by presenting their excellent scientific data. A few scientists who were not able to attend the meeting have made contributions to this volume and a few of those who presented information at the meeting choose not to submit a manuscript. Each manuscript has been reviewed by at least two reviewers. The quality of the papers is not consistent, but the editors hope that each reader will find considerable useful information that will stimulate him or her to pursue investigations into the effects of these important and widely used chemical agents.

Section I CLINICAL ASPECTS

HEALTH ASPECTS OF CANNABIS USE

Leo E. Hollister

Veterans Administration Medical Center and
Stanford University School of Medicine
Palo Alto, California

I. INTRODUCTION

This topic is extremely broad and embraces both the adverse consequences of chronic use of cannabis as well as the potential application of cannabinoids or their homologs as therapeutic agents. Each year the National Institute on Drug Abuse issues a review, "Marijuana and Health", directed to the United States Congress (1). These comprehensive reviews are more detailed than that which can be presented here. Short reviews of the subject have also been published in the past few years (2,3).

II. ADVERSE EFFECTS ON HEALTH

A. General Considerations

The ambiguity currently surrounding the health hazards of cannabis may be attributed to a number of factors besides those which ordinarily prevail. First, it has been difficult either to prove or to disprove health hazards in man from animal studies. When such studies of cannabis reveal possible harmful effects, the doses used are often large although drug administration is generally short. Second, use of cannabis by humans is still mainly by young persons in the best of health. Fortunately, the pattern of use is more often one of intermittent rather than regular use, the doses of drug usually being relatively small. This factor might lead to an underestimate of the potential impact of cannabis on health. Third, canna-

ISBN 0-12-044620-0

bis is often used in combination with tobacco and alcohol, as well as with a variety of other illicit drugs. Thus, potential health hazards from cannabis may be difficult to distinguish from those concomitantly used drugs. Finally, the whole issue of cannabis use is so laden with emotion that serious investigations of the health hazards of the drug have been colored by the prejudices of the experimenter, either for or against the drug as a potential hazard of health.

B. Chronic Use of Cannabis

The acute effects of cannabis, taken by a variety of routes, have been well described (4,5). The effects of chronic use of cannabis are more to the point when considering the issues of its status as a possible social drug. Three large-scale field trials of cannabis users have been implemented, but the results of these trials have done little to allay apprehensions about the possible ill effects of chronic use. Once again, objections have been made about the small samples used, the sampling techniques and the adequacy of the studies performed.

If field studies fail to provide evidence of harm from prolonged use of cannabis, it is unlikely that experimental studies will do better, and such has been the case.

Experimental studies suggest that tolerance develops rapidly, that a mild withdrawal reaction may occur, and that some acute effects may be reversed (for instance, a slow heart rate with chronic use rather than a rapid one as seen with acute use). Other effects of chronic cannabis use are related in a specific publication of the New York Academy of Sciences on Chronic Cannabis Use (6). On the whole, we must rely heavily on experiments of nature to determine possible adverse effects.

C. Psychopathology

Cannabis may directly produce an acute panic reaction,a toxic delirium, or an acute paranoid state. Whether it can directly evoke depressive or schizophrenic states, or whether it can lead to sociopathy or even to the "amotivational syndrome" is much less certain. The existence of a specific cannabis psychosis, postulated for many years, is still not established. The fact that users of cannabis may have higher levels of various types of psychopathology does not infer a causal relationship. Indeed, the evidence rather suggest that virtually every diagnosable psychiatric illness among cannabis users began before the first use of the drug. Use of alcohol and tobacco, as well as sexual experience and "acting-out" behavior, usually antedated the use of cannabis (7). Thus, it seems likely that psychopathology may predispose to cannabis use rather than the other way around.

It would seem reasonable to assume that cannabis might unmask latent psychiatric disorders and that this action probably accounts for the great variety that have been described following its use. On the other hand, evidence for a specific type of psychosis associated with its use is still elusive. Needless to say, use of cannabis should be discouraged (as would probably be the case with most socially used psychoactive drugs) in any patient with a history of prior emotional disorder (8).

Whether chronic use of cannabis changes the basic personality of the user so that they become less impelled to work and to strive for success has been a vexing question. As with other questions concerning cannabis use, it is difficult to separate consequences from possible causes of drug use. It has been postulated that the apparent loss of motivation seen in some cannabis users is really a manifestation of a concurrent depression, for which cannabis may have been a self-prescribed treatment (9).

If this syndrome is so difficult to prove, why does concern about it persist? Mainly because of clinical observations. One cannot help being impressed by the fact that promising youngsters change their goals in life drastically after entering the illicit drug culture, usually by way of cannabis. While it is clearly impossible to be certain that these changes were caused by the drug (one might equally argue that the use of drug followed the decision to change life style), the consequences are often sad. With cannabis as with most other pleasures, moderation is the key word. Moderate use of the drug does not seem to be associated with this outcome, but when drug use becomes a preoccupation, trouble may be in the offing.

D. Brain Damage

The startling report of cerebral atrophy in ten young men who were chronic users of cannabis aroused a great deal of controversy (10). Two studies using computerized tomography have effectively refuted the original claim of brain atrophy (11,12).

A model in monkeys chronically smoking cannabis produced EEG abnormalities from deep electrodes and postmortem histopathological alterations of the brain. EEG abnormalitiesand ultrastructural changes were reported in animals chronically exposed to amount of cannabis consistent with human use (13).

Thus, the issue of brain damage is not totally resolved, although the original observation of brain atrophy seems to have been disproven. The issue is of tremendous importance and probably can only be settled by some suitable animal model, as studies in man are confounded by too many other variables.

E. Tolerance/Dependence

The demonstration of tolerance in man was delayed by ethical restrictions on the amount of exposure permissible to human subjects. For instance, in an early study subjects were exposed only to a test oral dose of 20 mg of delta-9-tetrahydrocannabinol (THC) and then given the same dose or placebo repeated at bedtime for four more days followed by the same THC dose as a challenge on the fifth day. Using such small doses and relatively infrequent intervals, it was impossible to show tolerance to the psychic effects of the drug, although tolerance to the tachycardia and dizziness produced by the drug was evident (14).

Definite evidence of tolerance to the effects of THC in man was adduced only when it became permissible to use comparably large doses over longer periods of time. Subjects in one 30-day study were given high oral doses (70 to 210 mg/day) of THC around the clock. Tachycardia actually became bradycardia and a progressive loss of "high" was noted (15). Similar tolerance to cannabis smoking was observed in a 64-day study in which at least one cigarette daily had to be smoked with smoking as desired later in the same day. Additionally, in this study tolerance developed to the respiratory depressant effect of THC (16).

In man, mild withdrawal reaction was uncovered after abrupt cessation of doses of 30 mg of THC given every 4 hours orally for 10 to 20 days. Subjects became irritable, had sleep disturbances, and had decreased appetite. Nausea, vomiting and occasionally diarrhea were encountered. Sweating, salivation and tremors were autonomic signs (15). Relatively few reports of spontaneous withdrawal reactions from suddenly stopping cannabis use have appeared, despite the extraordinary amount of drug consumed. Five young persons experienced restlessness, abdominal cramps, nausea, sweating, increased pulse rate and muscle aches when their supplies of cannabis were cut off. Symptoms persisted for one to three days (60). The rarity of reports of these reactions may reflect the fact that they are mild and seldom is a user completely cut off from additional drug.

F. Lung Problems

Virtually all users of cannabis in North America take the drug by smoking. As inhaling any foreign material into the lung may have adverse consequences, as is well proven by tobacco, this mode of administration of cannabis might also be suspect.

Young, healthy volunteers in a chronic smoking experiment had pulmonary function tests before and after 47 to 59 days of daily smoking of approximately five marijuana cigarettes a day. Decreases were found in forced expiratory volume in one second, in maximal mid-expiratory flow rate, in plethysomographic specific airway conductance, and diffusing capacity. Thus, very heavy marijuana smoking for six to eight weeks caused mild but significant airway obstruction (17).

Quite possibly such dramatic early changes are not progressive with continued smoking (18). Compared with tobacco, cannabis smoking yields more residue ("tar") but the amount of smoke inhaled is very likely to be considerably less. The study in which five cigarettes daily were consumed represented heavy use of the drug, compared with 20 to 40 tobacco cigarettes which might be consumed by a heavy tobacco smoker. The issue of damage to lungs from cannabis is also confounded by the fact that many cannabis users also use tobacco. As yet, it is far easier to find pulmonary cripples from the abuse of tobacco than it is to find any evidence of clinically important pulmonary insufficiency from smoking of cannabis.

G. Cardiovascular Problems

Tachycardia, orthostatic hypotension and increased blood concentrations of carboxyhemoglobin from cannabis smoking would undoubtedly have deleterious effects on persons with heart disease due to arteriosclerosis of the coronary arteries or congestive heart failure. A direct test of the effects of marijuana smoking in exercise-induced angina proved this harmful effect of the drug. Smoking one cigarette containing 19 mg of THC decreased the exercise time until angina by only 9%. Thus, smoking marijuana increased myocardial oxygen demand and decreased myocardial oxygen delivery (19).

Clearly, smoking of any kind is bad for patients with angina, but the particular effect of cannabis in increasing heart rate makes this drug especially bad for such patients. Fortunately, few angina patients are devotees of cannabis.

H. Endocrine and Metabolic Effects

Changes in male sex hormones have been a source of controversy every since the first report of a decreased serum testosterone level. Decreased levels were associated with morphological abnormalities in sperm and with decreased sexual functioning (20). One possible cause for the lowered serum testosterone levels might be an impairment of synthesis of testosterone in the testis (21). Another possibility might be an increased conversion of testosterone peripherally to estrogens, a factor that might be pertinent to other endocrine side effects.

Data on the effects of cannabis on the female reproductive system are sparse. Preliminary unpublished data indicate that women who use cannabis four times a week or more have more anovulatory menstrual cycles than do non-users of the same age. Animal work tends to support this observation. THC administered to rats suppressed the cyclic surge of LH secretion and ovulation (22).

The endocrine changes may be of relatively little consequence in adults, but they could be of major importance in the prepubertal male who may use cannabis. If the pattern of hormonal changes that induces puberty is altered by cannabis use, then permanent alterations in bodily and psychosexual development could ensue. Should use of cannabis in early adolescence delay physical growth, could this lead to adverse psychosocial consequences? The questions are not academic, as recent surveys of cannabis use indicate that some boys (and girls) may be exposed to it even as early as the pre-pubertal years.

I. Pregnancy and Fetal Development

This is another area of great uncertainty about the meaning of data. Virtually every drug that has been studied for dysmorphogenic effects has been found to have them, if the doses are high enough or if enough species are tested or if treatment is prolonged. The placenta is no barrier to the passage of most drugs, so the assumption should be made that they will reach the fetus if taken during pregnancy.

Studies in primates, still unpublished, indicate that "reproductive efficiency" is reduced when one or both parents have been treated chronically with cannabis, that is, the number of completed pregnancies per mating is reduced. Only variable and nonspecific abnormalities have been found in the aborted offspring, and these were not much different from the findings in spontaneously aborted offspring.

It is still good practice in areas of ignorance, such as the effects of drugs on fetal development, to be prudent. The current admonition against using cannabis during pregnancy is based more on ignorance than on definite proof of harm. While no clinical association has yet been made between cannabis use during pregnancy and fetal abnormalities, such events are likely to be rare at best and could easily be missed. The belated recognition of the harmful effects on the fetus of smoking tobacco and drinking alcoholic beverages indicates that the same caution with cannabis is wise.

J. Miscellaneous Problems

1. Cell Metabolism. Virtually all the changes reported have been *in vitro* and tend to indicate both slowing of the cell cycle as well as increased mitotic activity (22,23). These conflicting findings are difficult to relate to clinical findings.

2. Chromosomal Abnormalities. A slight increase (3.4% versus 1.2%) of chromosomal abnormalities was reported in marijuana users as compared with non-users (24). Theclinical significance of such changes is unknown.

3. Immunity. Impaired cellular immunity was reported early on in chronic users of marijuana, but later studies have failed to confirm this observation (25,26). Once again, the clinical significance of such impairment is questionable.

4. Contaminants. Contamination of cannabis withinsecticides, fungi, bacteria and insects is entirely possible, given the conditions of its growth. A few cases of pulmonary disease have resulted from such contamination, althoughthe frequency is rare.

5. Possible Accumulation of Drug. Being highly lipophilic, THC should be expected to be sequestered in fatty tissues. Metabolites of the drug are excreted in urine long after exposure to the last dose. The excretion of these metabolites is not associated with any cannabis-like effects, however. Nor has any recognized health hazard been attributed to such accumulation.

K. Summary of Adverse Reactions

It has been remarked facetiously that the most adverse consequence of cannabis use is getting caught up in the criminal justice system because of such use. That observation may still be true. Yet, it is reasonable to assume that drug-taking, especially by young persons, may seriously interfere with their maturation process. Further, evidence from all drugs, both social as well as therapeutic, indicates that side effects of consequence are inevitable. One will have to make risk-benefit judgements in the case of cannabis just as one does with other drugs.

III. THERAPEUTIC ASPECTS

The therapeutic aspects of cannabis have been the subject of two reviews in recent years (27,28). In this review, we shall consider some potential uses of cannabis currently under investigation, somewhat in order of their importance and promise.

A. Antiemetic for Patients in Cancer Chemotherapy

Nausea and vomiting which accompanies the use of cancer chemotherapeutic agents is extremely difficult to treat with ordinary antiemetic drugs, such as prochlorperazine. This drug, as well as many others, acts specifically at chemoreceptor trigger zones in the medulla sensitive to chemical stimuli that induce vomiting, e.g. apomorphine. For reasons still not clear, the vomiting induced by anticancer drugs does not always respond to such antiemetics even though it is chemically induced.

The first serious trial of THC as an antiemetic was a controlled comparison of this drug with placebo in 20 patients undergoing cancer chemotherapy. Doses of 15 mg of THC every four hours were given orally as gelatin capsules in which THC was dissolved in sesame oil. Doses were started two hours before chemotherapy and repeated two and six hours later. Results were outstanding. Fourteen of 20 patients in whom an evaluation could be made had an antiemetic effect from THC while none was observed from placebo during 22 courses (29).

These favorable findings have been largely, but not totally, confirmed. An open study in 53 patients refractory to other treatments, revealed that ten had complete control of vomiting by THC administered prior to chemotherapy and for 24 hours after, 28 had 50% or more reduction in vomiting, and only 15 had no therapeutic effect. Four patients were dropped from the study because of adverse effects (30). A controlled crossover trial comparing doses of 15 mg of THC versus 10 mg of prochlorperazine in 84 patients was done by he original group who proposed THC as treatment. Response was complete to THC in 36 of 79 courses but to prochlorperazine in only 16 or 78 courses. Of 25 patients who received both drugs, 20 preferred THC. However, of the 36 courses of THC that resulted in a complete antiemetic response, 32 were associated with a "high" (31). Additional controlled studies have confirmed the antiemetic efficacy. One hundred sixteen patients were randomized to receive 15 mg of THC, 10 mg of prochlorperazine or placebo. Many patients given THC found it to be unpleasant (32). Fifteen patients were treated with courses of either THC or placebo, patients acting as their own controls. The THC regimen produced more relief of nausea and vomiting than placebo in 14 of these 15 patients who had received high-dose methotrexate (33). Plasma concentrations of greater than 10 mg/ml of THC were associated with best results. A crossover controlled trial of THC, thiethylperazine and metoclopramide found no difference in the antiemetic effect of the three agents. Adverse effects of THC were sufficiently greater than those of the other two drugs to question its utility (34). A comparison of THC, prochlorperazine and placebo found the latter two treatments not to differ, THC being superior to either (35).

Nabilone, a synthetic homolog of THC developed in 1972, has been tested for antiemetic activity. One hundred thirteen patients were treated in a crossover study with either nabilone or prochlorperazine. Response rates were significantly greater with nabilone therapy, but side effects were also more common (36). This drug has not succeeded in totally eliminating the objectionable mental effects of cannabinoids. Two other synthetic THC homologs, levonantradol and BRL 4664 have been found in open studies to have antiemetic effects (37,38). It remains to be seen whether any of these synthetics will be appreciably better than THC itself. In the meantime, extremely promising results have been obtained with intravenous doses, somewhat larger than usually given, of metoclopramide. A comparison of this drug with prochlorperazine and placebo showed it to be more effective than either, the only disturbing side effect being sedation (39). Using doses of 1 mg/kg of metoclopramide intravenously before and several times after treatment with cisplatin (perhaps the most emetic anticancer drug), protection was "total" in 48% of courses and "major" in another 23% (40).

Thus, the present situation is that while THC and some of its homologs are undoubtedly antiemetics, they have drawbacks, particularly the mental effects so desired by social users. The advent of newer antiemetics with few mental effects, such as metoclopramide and maybe domperidone, may make the issue moot.

B. Glaucoma

A survey of possible ocular effects of cannabis was added to a multifaceted study of the effects of chronic smoking of large amounts of the drug. Decreases of intraocular pressure up to 45% were found in nine of 11 subjects after 30 minutes of smoking (41). This effect lasted for four to five hours after smoking a single cigarette. Its magnitude was unrelated to the total number of cigarettes smoked. Thus, it appeared that a maximal effect was produced by the amount of THC absorbed from a single cigarette containing 19 mg of THC. In patients with ocular hypertension or glaucoma, seven of 11 patients showed a fall in intraocular pressure of 30%. The effect is real, for it has been confirmed. Intravenous injection of THC in doses of 22 mcg/kg and 44 mcg/kg produced an average fall in intraocular pressure of 37%, with some decreases as much as 51% (42). Similar experiments in rabbits, using several routes of administration have also confirmed the reduction in pressure.

Smoking cannabis or taking it intravenously are hardly reasonable recommendations to make for patients with glaucoma, many of whom are elderly. If the drug could beadministered topically, however, any impediments to its use would be overcome. Thus far, all experiments have been done in rabbits, a traditional animal model for studying topical eye medications. The problem of high lipid solubility of THC has been overcome by developing mineral oil as the vehicle for instillation in the eye. The degree of lowering of pressure is at least as great as with the conventional eye drops, such as pilocarpine, and the duration of effect is often longer. A minimal systemic absorption of the drug occurs when it is applied to the conjunctivae, but it is of no consequence in producing mental effects. Besides THC, other cannabinoids, such as cannabinol or THC metabolites, such as 8alpha- and 8beta,11-dihydroxy-delta-9-THC have shown this effect in rabbits (43,44). As these agents have no mental effects, they are of considerable interest for this purpose.

An extract prepared from the non-psychoactive components of cannabis has been used alone and in combination with timolol eye-drops with success. The effects of the two agents are additive and are said to be effective when other measures have failed. The composition of this extract is still uncertain (45). A synthetic THC homolog, BW 146Y, was given orally to treat glaucomatous patients. Although intraocular pressures were reduced, mild orthostatic hypotension and subjective effects were noted (46).

The outlook for this exploitation of cannabinoids in treatment is still promising. It will take a considerable amount of further developmental work to be sure that whichever cannabinoid is selected for clinical use will be lastingly effective and well tolerated. Nonetheless, the potential benefit will be great, for glaucoma treatment still does not prevent blindness as often as it might. Further, the effects of cannabinoids may be additive with those of other drugs, so that the overall benefit to patients may be greater than is currently possible.

C. Analgesia

THC in single oral doses of 10 and 20 mg was compared with codeine (60 and 120 mg)in patients with cancer pain. The larger THC dose was comparable to both doses of codeine, but the smaller dose, which was better tolerated, was less effective than either dose of codeine (47). When the THC was given intravenously in doses of 44 mcg/kg to patients undergoing dental extraction, an analgesic effect was demonstrated. It was not as good as that achieved by doses of 157mcg/kg of diazepam intravenously. Anxiety and dysphoria were produced in these patients, several of whom actually preferred the placebo to the dose of 22 mcg/kg of THC (48).

In the chronic spinal dog model, THC, nantradol and nabilone shared some properties with morphine. They increased the latency of the skin twitch reflex and suppressed withdrawal abstinence. These actions were not antagonized by naltrexone, suggesting that they are not mediated through opiate receptors (49). A single clinical study compared intramuscular levonantradol and placebo in postoperative pain and confirmed a significant analgesic action. However, no dose-response was observed and the number of side effects were rather high (50.

Considering the present array of very effective new analgesics of the agonist-antagonist type, as well as the prospect of others that may be even more selective on specific opiate receptors, it seems unlikely that any THC homolog will prove to be the analgesic of choice. But it is really too early to be sure.

D. Muscle Relaxant

The aroma of cannabis smoke is often found around wards housing patients with spinal cord injuries. Part of the streetlore is that cannabis helps to relieve the involuntary muscle spasms that can be so painful and disabling in this condition. Some confirmation of a muscle relaxant, or antispastic, action of THC came from an experiment in which oral doses of 5 of 10 mg of THC were compared with placebo. The 10 mg dose of THC reduced spasticity by clinical measurement

(51). A single small study such as this can only point to the need for more study of this potential use of THC, or possibly of some of its homologs. Presently used muscle relaxants, such as diazepam, cyclobenzaprine, baclofen and dantrolene have major limitations.

E. Anticonvulsant

Anticonvulsant activity was one of the first therapeutic uses suggested for cannabis and was documented experimentally many years ago (52). Subsequently, a great many studies in various animal species have validated this action.

Despite all these various lines of evidence supporting an anticonvulsant action of various cannabinoids, clinical testing has been rare. A single case report of better control of seizures following regular marijuana smoking was not very convincing (53). A clinical trial in 15 patients not adequately controlled by anticonvulsants added cannabidiol in doses of 200 or 300 mg/day or placebo to their treatment. Control of seizures was somewhat better in those patients receiving cannabidiol (54). As this cannabinoid has little psychoactivity, it would be the obvious one to try in future clinical studies.

F. Miscellaneous Uses

1. Bronchial Asthma. Bronchodilation from marijuana smoke was discovered during a general study of the effects of the drug on respiration. Normal volunteer subjects were exposed to marijuana smoke calculated to deliver 85 mcg/kg or 32 mcg/kg. The high-dose group showed a fall of 38% in airway resistance and an increase of 44% in airway conductance (55). Ten stable asthmatic patients were treated in another study with aerosols of placebo-ethanol, of THC 200 mcg in ethanol, or of salbutamol 100 mcg. Forced expiratory volume in 1 second, forced vital capacity and peak flow rate were measured on each occasion. Salbutamol and THC significantly improved ventilatory function. Improvement was more rapid with salbutamol but the two treatments were equally effective at the end of one hour (56). Whether effective doses of THC delivered by aerosol would be small enough to avoid the mental effects is uncertain. The fact that THC increases airway conductance by a mechanism of action that may be different from the usual beta adrenergic stimulants makes further inquiry necessary.

2. Insomnia. Although early speculation had suggested that THC might differ from conventional hypnotics in not reducing rapid eye movement (REM) sleep, study of the drug in

the sleep laboratory showed that it did (57). Another sleep laboratory study showed that a dose of 20 mg of THC given orally decreased (REM) sleep. Abrupt discontinuation of THC after 4 to 6 nights of use produced a mild insomnia but no marked REM rebound. The lack of effect on REM rebound seen with low doses of THC was not apparent when very high doses (70 to 210 mg) were given orally. REM was reduced during treatment and marked REM rebound was observed after withdrawal (58).

These studies indicate that the sleep produced by THC does not differ much from that of most currently used hypnotics. The side effects of the drug before sleep induction as well as the hangover effects make the drug less acceptable than the currently popular benzodiazepines, such as flurazepam. As many other effective hypnotics are currently being developed, it seems unlikely that THC will find a place in treatment of insomnia.

3. Hypertension. THC itself occasionally produces orthostatic hypotension (5). The development of effective antihypertensive drugs has been one of the outstanding achievements of pharmacology over the past 30 years. The prospect of a new antihypertensive based on orthostatic hypotension, perhaps the least desirable mode of lowering blood pressure, is hardly very enticing (59). Further, it is by no means certain that the mental effects of any homolog of THC can be completely eliminated without losing many of the desired pharmacological actions as well. The issue seems hardly worth pursuing.

G. Prospects as a Therapeutic Agent

Cannabis and THC homologs should be treated like any other investigational new drug as the search for a clinical use in medicine goes on. We should expect neither less nor more in regard to safety and efficacy than we would from other new agents. At present, cannabis has not yet made its way back into the formularies. It is unlikely that it ever will. The ingenuity of pharmaceutical chemists in developing THC analogs may yet find a way to exploit some of these potential therapeutic uses without the side effects that make cannabis itself undesirable. Modern inquiry into this drug spans less than decades, which is hardly enough time to settle the issue.

IV. SUMMARY

Both the adverse consequences of social use of cannabis as

well as the potential therapeutic use of cannabinoids or their homologs are still uncertain. It seems likely that adverse consequences will be fully documented and that therapeutic uses may be found. Only the former concern the chronic user of cannabis, who must still make a personal decision whether the risks outweigh the benefits from the drug.

REFERENCES

1. Petersen, R. C., Marijuana and health: 1980, NIDA Research monograph 31, U.S. Government Printing Office, Washington, D.C., 1980.
2. Nahas, G. G., Current status of marijuana research, Amer. Med. Assoc. 242:2775-2778 (1979).
3. Anonymous, AMA Council on Scientific Affairs, Marijuana. Its health hazards and therapeutic potentials, Amer. Med. Assoc. 246:1823-1827 (1981).
4. Isbell, H., Gorodetsky, C. W., Jasinski, D., Claussen, U., Spulak, F. V., and Korte, F., Effects of (-)-delta-9-tetrahydrocannabinol in man, Psychopharmacol. 11:184-188 (1967).
5. Hollister, L. E., Richards, R. K., and Gillespie, H. K., Comparison of tetrahydrocannabinol and synhexyl in man, Clin. Pharmacol. and Ther. 9:783-791 (1968).
6. Dornbush, R. L., Freidman, A. F., and Fink, M. (eds.), "Chronic Cannabis Use", Ann. N. Y. Acad. 282:1-430 (1976).
7. Halikas, J. A., Goodwin, D. W., and Guze, S. B., Marijuana use and psychiatric illness, Arch. Gen. Psych. 27:162-165 (1972).
8. Abruzzi, W., Drug-induced psychosis, Inter. Addictions 121:183-193 (1977).
9. Kupfer, D. J., Detre, T., Koral, J., and Fajans, P., A comment on the "amotivational syndrom" in marijuana smokers, Amer. J. Psych. 130:1319-1321 (1973).
10. Campbell, A. M. C., Evans, M., Thompson, J. L. G., and Williams, M. R., Cerebral Atrophy in young cannabis smokers, Lancet, 1219 (1971).
11. Kuehnle, J., Mendelson, J. H., David, K. R., and New, P. F. J. , Computed tomographic examination of heavy marijuana smokers, Amer. Med. Assoc. 237:1231-1232 (1977).
12. Co, B. T. , Goodwin, D. W. , Gado, M., Mikhael, M., and Hill, S. Y., Absence of cerebral atrophy in chronic cannabis users of computerized transaxial tomography, J. Amer. Med. Assoc. 237:1229-1230 (1977).
13. Harper, J. W., Heath, R. G., and Myers, W., Effects of cannabis sativa on ultrastructure of the synapse on mon-

key brain, Neurosci. Res. 3:87-93 (1977).

14. Hollister, L. E., and Tinklenbert, J. R., Subchronic oral doses of marijuana extract, Psychopharmacol. 29:247-252 (1973).
15. Jones, R. and Benowitz, N., The 30-day trip: Clinical studies of cannabis tolerance and dependence, in "Pharmacology of Marijuana", (M. C. Braude and S. Szara, eds.), Raven Press, New York, pp. 627-645 (1976).
16. Belleville, J. W., Gasser, J. C., and Miyake, T., Tolerance to the respiratory effects of marijuana in man, Pharmacol. Exper. Ther. 1997:326-331 (1976).
17. Tashkin, D. P., Shapiro, B. J., Lee, Y. E., and Harper, C. E., Subacute effects of heavy marijuana smoking on pulmonary function in healthy men, New England J. Med. 294-125-129 (1976).
18. Vachon, L., The smoke in marijuana smoking, New England J. Med. 294:160-161 (1976).
19. Aronow, W. S., and Cassidy, J., Effect of marijuana and place-marijuana smoking on angina pectoris, New England J. Med. 291(2):65-67 (1974).
20. Kolodny, R. C., Masters, W. H., Kolodner, R. M., and Toro, G., Depression of plasma testosterone levels after chronic intensive marijuana use, New England J. Med. 290:872-874 (1974).
21. Goldstein, H., Harclerode, J., and Nyquist, S. E., Effects of chronic administration of delta-9-tetrahydrocannabinol and cannabidiol on rat testicular esterase isozymes, Life Sciences 20:951-954 (1977).
22. Ayalon, D., and Tsafriri, A., Suppression of the cyclic surge of luteinizing hormone secretion and of ovulation in the rat by delta-1-tetrahydrocannabinol, Nature 243:470-471 (1973).
22. Leuchtenberger, C., and Leuchtenberger, R., Correlated cytological and cytochemical studies of the effects of fresh smoke from marijuana cigarettes on growth and DN metabolism of animal and human lung culture, in "Pharmacology of Marijuana", (M. C. Braude and S. Szara, eds.) pp. 595-612. Raven Press, New York, 1976.
23. Zimmerman, A. M., and McClean, D. K., in "Drugs and Cell Cycle (Zimmerman, Padilla and Cameron, eds.) p. 67, Academic Press, New York, 1973.
24. Stercherer, M. A., Kunysz, T. J., and Allen, M. A., Chromosome breakage in users of marijuana, Amer. J. Obst. Gyn. 118:106-113 (1974).
25. Nahas, G. G., Suciv-Foca, N., Armand, J-P., and Morishima, A., Inhibition of cellular mediated immunity in Marijuana smokers, Science 183:419-420 (1974).
26. Lau, R. J., Tubergen, D. G., Barr, Jr., M., Domino, E. F., Benowitz, W. and Jones, R. T., Phytohemagglutinin-

induced lymphocyte transformation in humans receiving delta-9-tetrahydrocannabinol, Science 192:805-807 (1976).
27. Cohen, S., and Stillman, R. C., (eds.), "The Therapeutic Potential of Marijuana", p. 515, Plenum Press, New York (1976).
28. Lemberger, L., Potential therapeutic usefulness of marijuana, Ann. Rev. Pharmacol. on Toxicol. 20:151-172 (1980).
29. Sallan, S. E., Zinberg, N. E., and Frei, E., Antiemetic effect of delta-9-tetrahydrocannabinol in patients receiving cancer chemotherapy, New England J. Med. 293:795-797 (1975).
30. Lucas, Jr., V. S., and Laszlo, J., Tetrahydrocannabinol for refractory vomiting induced by cancer chemotherapy, Amer. Med. Assoc. 243:1241-1243 (1980).
31. Sallan, S. E., Cronin, C., Zelen, M., and Zinberg, N. E., Antiemetics in patients receiving chemotherapy for cancer. A randomized comparison of delta-9-tetrahydrocannabinol and prochlorperazine, New England Med. 302:135-136 (1980).
32. Frytak, S., Moertel, C. G., O'Fallon, J. R., Rubin, J., Creagar, E. T., O'Donnell, M. J., Schott, A. J., and Schwartas, N. W., Delta-9-tetrahydrocannabinol as an antiemetic in patients receiving cancer chemotherapy. A comparison with prochlorperazine and placebo, Ann. Internal Med. 91:825-830 (1979).
33. Chang, A. S., Shiling, D. J., Stillman, R. C., Goldberg, N. H., Seipp, C. A., Barofsly, D., Simon, R. M., and Rosenberg, S. A., Delta-9-tetrahydrocannabinol as an antiemetic in cancer patients receiving high-dose methotrexate. A prospective, randomized evaluation, Annals. int. Med. 91:819-824 (1979).
34. Colls, B. M., Ferry, D. G., and Gray, A. J., The antiemetic activity of tetrahydrocannabinol versus metoclopramide and thiethylperazine in patients undergoing cancer chemotherapy, New Zealand Med. J. 91:449-451 (1980).
35. Orr, L. L., McKernan, J. F., and Bloome, B., Antiemetic effect of tetrahydrocannabinol: compared with placebo and prochlorperazine in chemotherapy-associated nausea and emesis, Arch. Int. Med. 140:1431-1433 (1980).
36. Herman, T. S., Einhorn, L. H., Jones, S. E., Nagy, C., Chester, A. B., Dean, J. C., Furnas, B., Williams, S. D., Leigh, S. A., Dorr, R. T., and Moon, T. E., Superiority of nabilone over prochlorperazine as an antiemetic in patients receiving cancer chemotherapy, New England J. Med. 300:1295-1297 (1979).
37. Cronin, C. M., Sallan, S. E., Gelber, R., Lucas, V. S., and Laszlo, J., Antiemetic effect of intramuscular levonantradol in patients receiving anti-cancer chemotherapy,

J. Clin. Pharmacol. 21:43S-50S (1981).
38. Stagret, M., Bron, D., Rosencweig, M., and Kenis, Y., Clinical studies with a THC analog (BRL 4664) in the prevention of cisplatin-induced vomiting, J. Clin. Pharmacol. 21:60S-63S (1981).
39. Gralla, R. J., Itri, L. M., Pisko, S. E., Squillante, A. E., Kelsen, D. P., Braunn, Jr., D. W., Bordin, L. A., Braunn, T. J., and Young, C. W., Antiemetic efficacy of high-dose metoclopramine: randomized trials with placebo and prochlorperazine in patients with chemotherapy-induced nausea and vomiting, New England J. Med. 303:905-909 (1981).
40. Strum, S. B., McDermed, J. E., Opfell, E. W., and Riech, L. P., Intravenous metoclopramide. An effective antiemetic in cancer chemotherapy, J. Amer. Med. Assoc. 247:2683-2686 (1982).
41. Hepler, R. S., and Frank, I. M., Marijuana smoking and intraocular pressure, J. Amer. Med. Assoc. 217:1392 (1971).
42. Cooler, P. and Gregg, J. M., Effect of delta-9-tetrahydrocannabinol on intraocular pressure in humans, Southern Med. J. 70:951-954 (1977).
43. Green, K., Marijuana and the eye, Invest. Opthalmol. 14:261-263 (1975).
44. Green, K., Wynn, H., and Bowman, K. A., A comparison of topical cannabinoids on intraocular pressure, Exper. Eye Res. 27:239-246 (1978).
45. West. M. E., and Lockhart, A. B., The enhanced effect of the combination of cannasol and timolol and pilocarpine inn intraocular pressure, West Indian Med. J. 29:280 (1980).
46. Tiedemann, J. S., Shields, M. P., and Weber, P. A., Effect of synthetic cannabinoids on elevated intraocular pressure, Opthalmology 88:270-277 (1981).
47. Noyes, R., Brunk, S. F., Aver, D. H., and Canter, A., The analgesic properties of delta-9-tetrahydrocannabinol and codeine, Clin. Pharmacol. Ther. 18:84-89 (1975).
48. Raft, D., Gregg, J., Ghia, J., and Harris, L., Effects of intravenous tetrahydrocannabinol on experimental and surgical pain: psychological correlates of the analgesic response, Clin. Pharmacol. Ther. 21:26-33 (1977).
49. Gilbert, P. E., A comparison of THC, nantradol, nabilone, and morphine in the chronic spinal dog, J. Clin. Pharmacol. 21:311S-319S (1981).
50. Jain, A. K., Ryan, J. E., McMahon, F. G., and Smith, G., Evaluation of intra-muscular levonantradol in acute postoperative pain, J. Clin. Pharmacol. 21:320S-326S (1981).
51. Petro, D. J., and Ellenberger, C. E., Treatment of human spasticity with delta-9-tetrahydrocannabinol, J. Clin.

Pharmacol. 21:413S-416S (1981).
52. Loewe, S., and Goodman, L. S., Anticonvulsive action of marijuanna-active substances, Fed. Proc. 6:352 (1947).
53. Consroe, P. F., Wood, G. C. and Guchsbaum, H., Anticonvulsant nature of marijuana smoking, J. Amer. Med. Assoc. 234:306-307 (1975).
54. Carlini, E. A., and Cunnha, J. A., Hypnotic and antiepileptic effects of cannabidiol, J. Clin. Pharmacol. 21:417S-427S (1981).
55. Vachon, L., Fitzgerald, M. X., Solliday, N. H., Gould, I. A., and Gaensler, E.A., Single-dose effect of marijuana smoke. Bronchial dynamics and respiratory-center sensitivity in normal subjects, New England Med. 288:985-989 (1973).
56. Williams, S. J., Hartley, J. P. R., and Graham, J. D. P., Bronchodilator effect of delta-1-tetrahydrocannabinol administered by aerosol to asthmatic patients, Thorak 31:720-723 (1976).
57. Pivir, R. T., Zarcone, J., Dement, W. C., and Hollister, L. E., Delta-9-tetrahydrocannabinol and synhexyl:effects on human sleep patterns, Clin. Pharmacol. Ther. 13:426-425 (1972).
58. Feinberg, I., Jones, R., and Walker, J., Effects of marijuana tetrahydrocannabinol on electroencephalographic sleep patterns, Clin. Pharmacol. Ther. 19:782-794 (1976).
59. Anonymous Editorial, Cannabis and the cardiovascular system, Brit. Med. J. 1:450-451 (1978).
60. Besusan, S. D., Marijuana withdrawal symptoms, Brit, Med. J. July:112 (1971).

MARIJUANA: ACUTE EFFECTS ON HUMAN MEMORY

Loren L. Miller

Burroughs Wellcome Co.
Research Triangle Park, North Carolina

I. INTRODUCTION

The single, most consistently reported, behavioral effect of cannabinoids in humans is an alteration in memory functioning (1). Interest in the effects of cannabis on memory stemmed from anecdotal reports of the effects of cannabis on mood and thinking. In 1845, the French psychiatrist de Tours Moreau (2) provided an elegant characterization of the effects of hashish on human mental functioning. Moreau stated that one of the more prominent effects of hashish was a "gradual weakening of the power to direct thoughts at will". Ideas extraneous to the focus of an individual's attention appeared to enter the mind producing a loosening of associations. Other early investigators such as Bromberg (3) and Ames (4) employing less potent cannabis preparations than those used by Moreau and his followers also noted fragmentation of thought and confusion on attempting to remember recent occurrences.

Objective substantiation of some of these observations has been gained in studies employing known doses of delta-9-tetrahydrocannabinol (THC). Tinklenberg et al. (5) found that orally administered THC (20, 40, 60 mg) impaired immediate memory for digits recalled in forward or reverse order with peak impairment at 1.5 and 3.5 hours, respectively. Memory impairment was intermittent and not dependent on dose. The transient nature of the memory loss was reminiscent of the waxing and waning effect following marijuana intoxication described by Clark et al. (6). Oral THC has also been found to induce "temporal disintegration," which is defined as a difficulty in retaining, coordinating and serially indexing those memories, perceptions, and expectations that are rele-

ISBN 0-12-044620-0

vant to the attainment of some goal (7,8). The measure of temporal disintegration was the Goal Directed Serial Alternation Test (GDSA) that required a subject to subtract and add numbers from each other until some specified number was reached. The dose-related disruption found on this task was thought to be related to impaired time perception. Also, the inability to temporally coordinate recent memories with intentions might account for disorganized speech patterns found by Weil and Zinberg (9) following marijuana intoxication. Since words and phrases are hierarchically ordered in a goal directed fashion, speech may become disorganized under the drug and a person is likely to lose his train of thought. While the GDSA has proven to be an interesting measure with which to assess the effects of cannabinoids, Abel (10) has questioned its reliability. Studies by Rafaelsen et al. (11) and Tinklenberg et al. (12) have found some difficulty in replicating their original findings with the GDSA. This lack of replicability appears to be due in part to limited within drug session employment of the GDSA task that resulted in an abbreviated sampling of the behavior in question.

In order to determine a specific locus of action of marijuana on memory, it has been suggested that testable models of human memory be employed so that any selective impairment due to intoxication might be determined (1,13). One such model has been proposed by Shiffrin and Atkinson (14). The model is based on psychological evidence as well as neurophysiological and anatomical observations which suggest that memory might be best conceptualized as a two component process containing a short-term and long-term storage component. The model illustrated in Figure 1 consists of three basic aspects: a sensory information in an unaltered form for a few milliseconds while analysis, identification, and encoding take place. The short-term memory store is an individual's working memory. It is responsible for holding the trace of the external stimulus and at the same time matching the memory trace of the stimulus with a previously encoded representative of the stimulus from the long-term storage component. The short-term store and long-term store differ in terms of both information capacity and duration. Only a small number of items can be maintained in the short-term store at any given time. Maintenance of memory can be achieved by various control processes including rehearsal, imagery, or use of mnemonics. When information resides in short-term storage for a reasonable period of time, it is automatically transferred to long-term memory. The long-term store is a permanent repository for information.

A number of studies have investigated the actions of marijuana on different stages of memory employing this model. The experimental paradigm usually consists of a free recall task involving lists of words. The dependent variable is the prob-

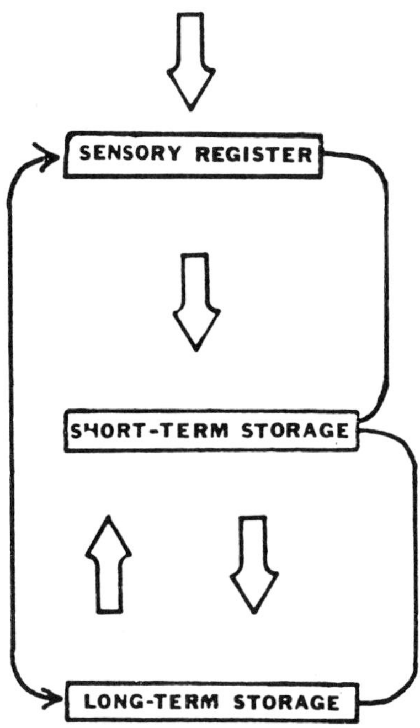

FIGURE 1. Structure of the memory system.

ability of recall or number of words recalled as a function of position of word in a list or its "serial position". A bimodal U-shaped function relating probability of recall to serial position of an item can be plotted. Since the beginning and end of the serial position curve respond differently to a range of experimental variables, the positions are thought to represent output from different storage mechanisms. The probability of recall for both early and late items is higher than for middle items. These two effects are termed, respectively, the primacy and recency effects.

A study by Darley et al. (15) demonstrated the effects of orally administered THC (20 mg) on the different stages of memory proposed by this model. Subjects were presented with 10 lists of 20 words, each of which was followed by an immediate recall test. Immediately following the last list, half the subjects ingested a 20 mg dose of THC, the other half placebo. One hour later, subjects were given a delayed recall and recognition test. Then, the whole sequence of list presentation, immediated, delayed recall, and recognition was repeated. The results indicated that if THC was administered after list presentation but before delayed recall, no effects were noted which were different from placebo, suggesting that retrieval processes were not influenced (see Figure 2).

When THC was administered prior to list presentation, performance during immediate recall testing was depressed except for those items in the terminal list positions, suggesting that some aspect of long-term storage was disrupted. However, items appeared to enter the sensory register and short-term store equally well (see Figure 2). Since the memory of THC-treated subjects was lower for both delayed recall and recognition, it was suggested that transfer of information from short-term to long-term memory did not take place. One possible reason for the lack of transfer is that subjects did not rehearse incoming information, a process necessary for transfer to occur (16). However, Darley and Tinklenberg (13) found that drugged subjects still displayed impaired recall when amount of rehearsal was fixed in both groups. It was felt

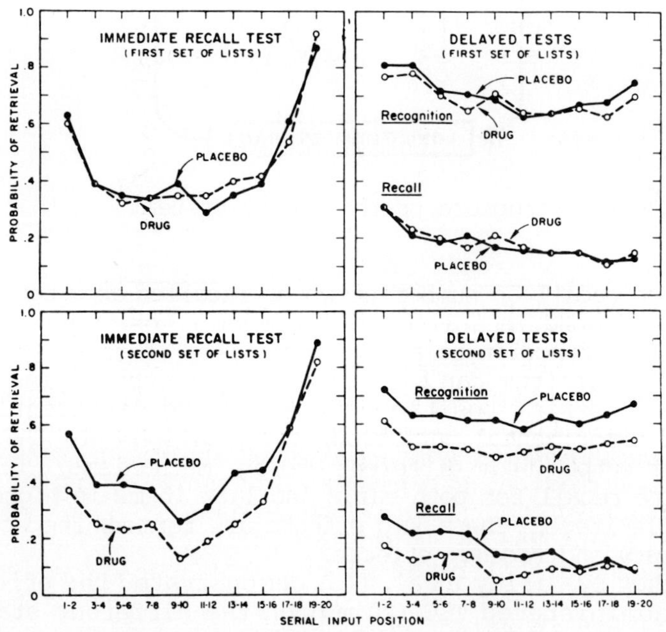

FIGURE 2. The probability of immediate recall (left panel) and delayed recall and recognition (right panel) as a function of the serial input position of items. Separate functions are plotted for drug and placebo groups. The top panel comprises free recall and recognition data when encoding took place prior to drug ingestion, the bottom panel following drug ingestion.

that there was a reduced level of attention to list items probably because of increased competition during the intoxicated state from the subjects' own thoughts, which might have accounted for the inadequate transfer. Another possibility was that items residing in the short-term store were lost more quickly and this resulted in the transfer deficit.

Although the results of the Darley et al. study suggested that storage of information rather than retrieval of information was affected by THC or marijuana intoxication, this view is still open to speculation. The lack of definitiveness has arisen because of methodological and theoretical considerations. These issues are discussed in a later portion of this paper.

Research efforts in our laboratory concerning the effects of marijuana on memory have centered mainly on assessing the actions of the drug on free recall. This paradigm was employed because of its strong theoretical underpinnings and because of the consistency with which marijuana produces reliable effects across studies using this technique. The research to be described took place over a period of 4 years in an effort to define and analyze the effects of marijuana on human memory.

II. METHODS AND RESULTS

A. Smoking Technique and Volunteer Characteristics

Recruitment of volunteers took place mainly in a large university community. Most were upper level undergraduates along with some medical, dental and graduate students; all were males. Other volunteers were also recruited who were not students at the time of study, but all had at least one year of college. All participants were run through ascreening battery including a physical examination, psychiatric interview, MMPI, medical history and laboratory tests including liver function tests, urinalysis and EKG. We found we rejected about 25-30% of our interviewees on the basis of laboratory tests or physical examinations and very few on psychological bases. The medical history included a drug taking inventory in which volunteers were required togivea detailed history of drug use. At the time of the inventory all volunteers were made aware of federal confidentiality requirements and that no names would appear on any hospital records. We found that almost all had some experience with harder drugs especially amphetamines and hallucinogens at some time or another. We attempted to recruit moderate users of marijuana whose use ranged from a few times a week to a few times per month. Most fell into this category because most were in school. Our choices were also limited to those not currently using other drugs except for tobacco and occasional alcohol use. Very heavy marijuana users were also excluded. The volunteers who were eventually selected were used in repeated studies. All had extensive practice with a variety of cognitive tasks during the course of our research. This eliminated a lot of novelty from the situation and they knew what to expect as soon as they entered the experimental situation.

All of our studies were conducted with smoked marijuana. The cigarettes were obtained from the National Institute on Drug Abuse (NIDA) and varied in THC content. We originally employed a standardized procedure. Volunteers were presented with a single cigarette, instructed to inhale deeply, hold the smoke in their lungs for 10-15 sec. before taking the next puff. Puff inspiration was supervised and timed by an observer. Smoking took between 7 and 10 min. and volunteers were required to smoke as much of the butt as possible. Volunteers were run individually and testing was performed in a quiet comfortable room.

The smoking procedure was altered after an initial study when it was discovered that the standardized procedure was not to the liking of our participants. It was considered to be overly regimented, less enjoyable and somewhat irritating to the throat. Also, participants did not like to smoke alone. Again, it was deemed less enjoyable. All enjoyed the social aspects of smoking. So we opted to smoke in small groups of 3-6 and employed an ad lib smoking procedure. Approximately half the volunteers were assigned to placebo and half to a marijuana condition. Volunteers were instructed to smoke in any manner they desired but again told to consume as much of the cigarette as possible. These changes in procedure proved effective in keeping them motivated, coming to experiments, and made for a more enjoyable experience especially since a number of experimental procedures were considered tedious.

B. Experiments on Memory

In most of the memory studies to be described, three basic measures were usually employed. These included (1) subjective measures of intoxication consisting of ratings of potency of marijuana and the pleasantness of theexperience witheach being rated on a 1-100 point scale, (2) a physiological measure, pulse rate, which was expressed in terms of beats per minute (BPM) and (3) memory measures which usually consisted of number of words correctly recalled on a free recall test and hit and false alarm rates on a recognition memory task. A recognition memory task differs from free recall in that

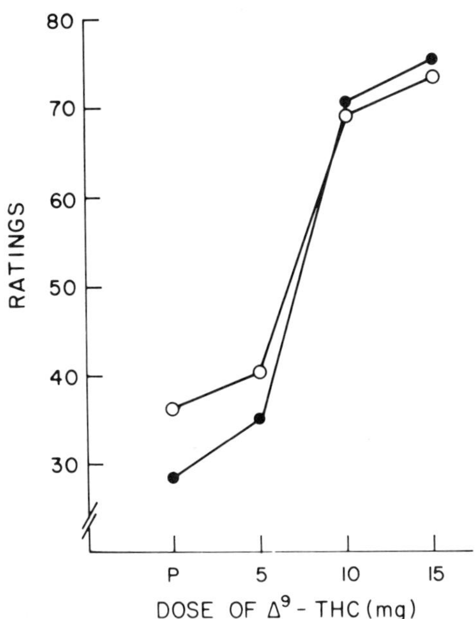

FIGURE 3. Mean potency (open circles) and pleasantness (closed circles) ratings as a function of dosage of THC contained in marijuana. P = placebo.

recognition simply involves the identification of previously presented information which is presented in the context of old material (i.e., a subject is given a list of words, some of which he was presented with and some which are new, or "distractors", and told to pick out the items he remembers having seen on the original recall list). In free recall previously presented information must be reproduced.

In an initial study (17), dose-response data for each of these measures was obtained. The design was performed with each volunteer being run as his own control under 4 drug conditions, 0, 5, 10 and 14 mg THC contained in the marijuana cigarettes. A total of 16 volunteers were run on four different occasions. Although the design was not a complete Latin square, both dosage and word lists were counterbalanced across sessions. In any session, four subjects were allowed to hear 8 different word lists 40 items in length. Four of the word lists were presented at a 2 sec rate and four at a 4 sec rate. Immediate and delayed recall tests (delayed recall occurred 20 minutes after the last list) were given. New word lists were employed in each session. Each of the four volunteers received one of the above doses of marijuana in any session. Potency, pleasantness ratings and pulse rate were also measured 10-15 minutes following smoking. The results are presented in Figures 3,4,5, and 6. Potency and pleasantness ratings rose with dosage of THC contained inthe marijuana with the biggest jump in ratings occuring at the 10 mg dose. Pulse rate was also elevated following intoxication with both the peak effect of the drug and duration of action varying directly with dosage.

Both immediate and delayed free recall were reduced in a dose-related manner following intoxication with marijuana for both presentation rates. Delayed recognition tests indicated that the distribution of hit and false alarm rates did not vary as a function of dosage. These results indicated that although recall was reduced following intoxication, subjects were familiar enough with previously presented items so that recognition was accurate. The recognition data did not support those of Darley and Tinklenberg (13) or Zeidenberg et al. (18) but paralleled results reported by Dornbush (19).

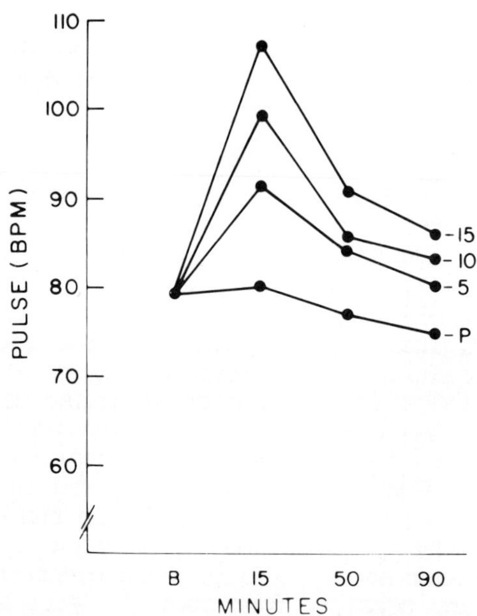

FIGURE 4. Mean pulse rate changes over time as a function of dosage of THC contained in marijuana. P = placebo; B = baseline.

In a number of studies determining the effects of marijuana on recall/recognition, recognition memory has been little influenced whereas recall deficits are universally reported following marijuana intoxication. In those cases where some recognition changes are noted, it is usually the result of an increase in false alarm rates (identifying a newly presented item as being previously seen). Hit rates (identifying an old item correctly) are usually unaffected by marijuana. These false alarm rates rather than reflecting a true memory loss may be considered intrusive type errors. Marijuana has been found in several studies to increase intrusion errors (1). In a free recall task, this usually involves the introduction of intra or extra list word associations during the free recall of words, or the introduction of unrelated extraneous material during prose recall. Thus, some of the memory loss produced by cannabinoids may be a result of increased imagery or thought flow due to the intrusion of irrelevant associations.

Intrusions are often reflected in conversational speech following intoxication. An analysis of speech samples indicates that marijuana produces more free verbalizations and associations, vivid imagery and a decreased awareness of a listener (9). The distortions in speech do not appear to

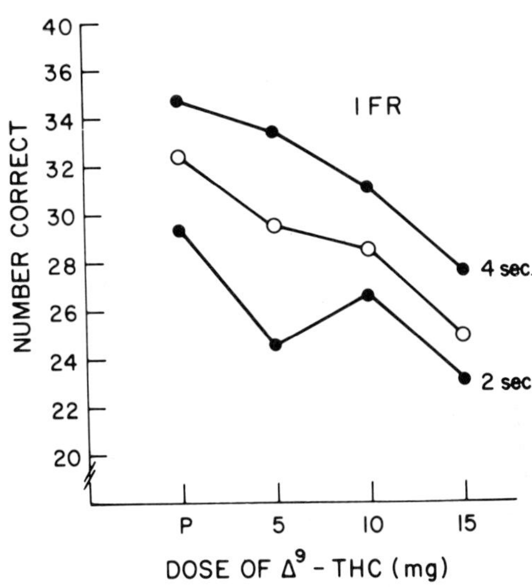

FIGURE 5. Mean number of words correctly recalled on the immediate free recall test (IFR) as a function of dosage of THC contained in marijuana and presentation rate. P = placebo. Open circles represent the combined means.

occur at a syntaxical level. However, the intoxicated subject displays lapses in memory for what was said as well as a tendency to be tangential. Other studies have shown that marijuana intoxication resulted in increased latency of verbal response, produced fewer syllables per phrase and a prolongation of syllables suggesting a deficit in information processing and a decreased ability to focus verbal communication (18,20). Intrusions as a consequence of marijuana intoxication are a robust phenomena when measured.

The next study we initiated was similar in scope to the previous study except that we employed a single marijuana dose (14 mg THC and a between subjects design). Thirty-four volunteers were randomly assigned to either a placebo or marijuana condition and were presented with 20 fifteen item word lists. After each list a recall test was given and following lists 10 and 20 a delayed recall test was administered which consisted of having subjects write down all the words they could remember from the previous lists. One of the lists was repeated at positions 1, 6, 11 and 16, but subjects were not informed of this prior to testing. This latter procedure was originally employed by Hebb (21) in studies of the human memory trace.

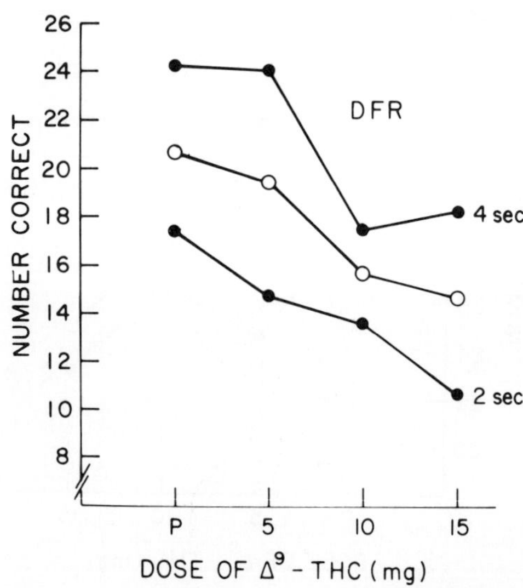

FIGURE 6. Mean number of words correctly recalled on the delayed free recall test (DFR) as a function of dosage of THC contained in marijuana and presentation rate. P = placebo. Open circles represent the combined means.

Repeating the same list allowed us to assess the effect of marijuana on memory consolidation over trials while presentation of the different lists enabled us to determine whether practice on lists within a session would produce an attenuation of the effect of marijuana over time. A recognition memory test was also presented following the second delayed free recall test. The basic results are presented in Figures 7 and 8. In the first graph, it should be noted that marijuana reduced recall on each of the non-repeated lists and practice over 16 lists did not attenuate the effect of the drug. Recall on the repeated lists was also reduced following drug, but the number of items gained on each presentation trial was about the same. This suggests one major effect of the drug is on initial formation of a memory trace, but with repeated presentation the amount of information gained on subsequent trials is similar. The serial position curves which reflect number of words recalled as a function of input serial position are presented in Figure 8. For immediate free recall (IFR), a U-shaped serial position curve was found for both drug and placebo conditions. The marijuana group displayed a deficit in recall at all positions with a greater reduction occurring in the middle portion of all positions with a greater reduction occurring in the middle portion of the list. The serial position results departed slightly from those reported by Abel (16) and Darley et al. (13) in that little effect of marijuana on terminal list items was shown in their

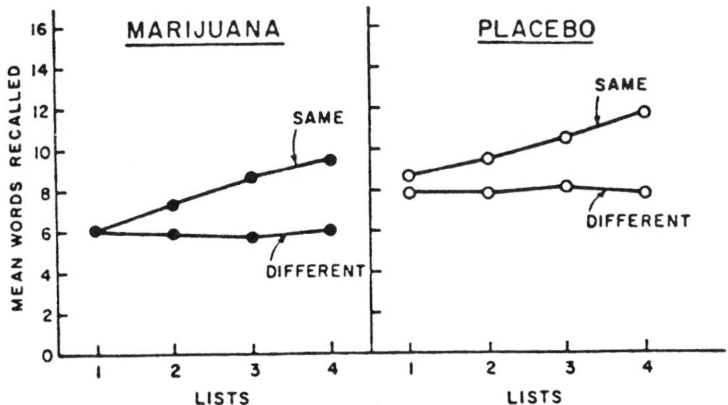

FIGURE 7. Mean number of words recalled over repeated (same) and nonrepeated (different) lists. Recall for 16 nonrepeated lists is presented in blocks of four lists.

studies. On the delayed free recall test (DFR), differences between the two groups still existed although floor effects appeared to occur. A negative recency effect was also noted. This refers to the inferior recall of terminal list items which were recalled well on the immediate free recall test (22).

On the recognition memory test, false alarm rates were moderately elevated while hit rates were relatively equal in both groups. A signal detection analysis applied to this data indicated that neither 'd', an unbiased indicator of memory strength nor B, a measure of the criterion which an individual chooses to make a response, were affected by marijuana. Again, memory trace strength as measured by a recognition memory test was not altered.

Intrusion errors were elevated on both the IFR and DFR tests. On the immediate free recall test, internal intrusions, which consisted of the introduction of words during recall that were contained in lists presented prior to a given IFR, were not significantly elevated in the marijuana condition in comparison to the placebo condition. However, more external intrusions consisting of words not presented in any list occurred following marijuana intoxication.

Long term retention was estimated by determining whether items recalled on the IFR test would also be recalled on the DFR test. Two conditional probability scores were calculated for each subject. The first score consisted of the proportion of items recalled on the DFR test given correct recall on the IFR test (R2/R1). A second probability score consisting of the proportion of items recalled on the DFR test given that recall did <u>not</u> occur on the IFR test (R2/R1). Items on the repeated lists were not included in this analysis. No differences were found between marijuana and placebo groups in the magnitude of these two scores. R2/R1 was higher than R2/N1 for both groups indicating that if an item was recalled on the IFR test it was more likely to be recalled in the DFR than if it was not recalled on the IFR test. However, the R2/R1 probability was quite low, 0.26 for the placebo group and 0.23 for the marijuana group. If a high proportion of items recalled in the IFR test were being retained, the R2/R1 score would be closer to 1. The R2/N1 scores were approximately 0.03 for both groups indicating that if an item was not recalled initially it was very unlikely to occur on the DFR test.

Summarizing our memory results to this point, it was found that (1) recall but not recognition memory was reduced following intoxication with marijuana, (2) the recall deficit was dose related, (3) the incidence of intrusion errors increased following intoxication, and (4) long-term retention levels under drug are equivalent to those found for placebo when levels of initial recall are taken into account.

In another study, (23,24) the effect of marijuana on the recall of prose material was investigated. This was of particular interest since an earlier study suggested that memory for narrative material was particularly sensitive to the effects of marijuana (25). This study also sought to determine the effect of cueing on memory impairments produced by the drug, or more specifically, whether the use of retrieval cues would reverse the recall deficits. Failure to recall an item during intoxication does not necessarily mean that an item is no longer available in memory, but may simply mean that an item is not accessible (26). Finally, the effect of marijuana on possible state dependent learning was measured.

The design was conducted in two phases. On day 1, volunteers (n = 40) smoked a single one gram cigarette containing 0.94% THC or a placebo cigarette. Following smoking each volunteer heard and at the same time read a brief narrative of approximately 200 words. The narrative was presented twice. It contained a total of 24 basic facts and volunteers were instructed to recall as many of the facts as possible. On day 2, half of the volunteers in the drug group were switched to placebo while the other half continued on drug. The placebo group was also split with half volunteers continuing on placebo and half on drug. The drug dosage remained the same on both days. Following treatment on day 2, volunteers performed the following tasks: (1) recalled the story presented on day 1, (2) were presented with 24 questions concerning the story each of which could be answered with a simple phrase from the

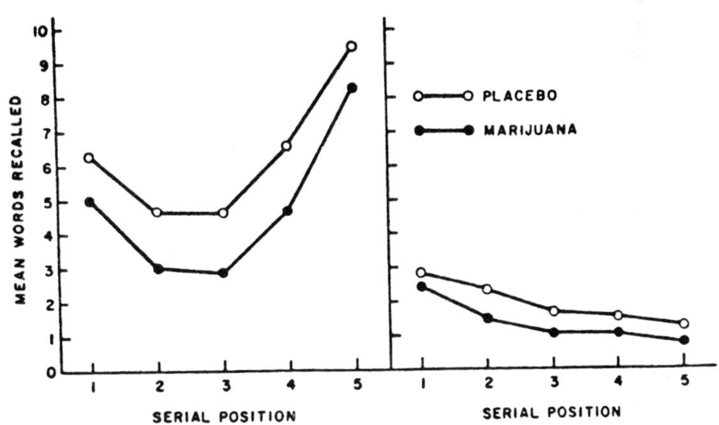

FIGURE 8. Mean number of words recalled for immediate free recall (left panel) and delayed free recall (right panel) as a function of serial input position of items on nonrepeated lists.

story (these questions served as retrieval cues), (3) were presented with a new story which had to be recalled, and (4) presented with 24 questions concerning the new story. The basic dependent variables in this study were number of memory units recalled during free and cued recall on both days, serial position curves, and recall as a function of change in drug state.

The recall results were presented on Table I and in Figures 9 and 10. It can be seen from Table I that on day 1 free recall was significantly reduced following intoxication. Statistically the results were overpowering. Of the 20 subjects in the marijuana group only one did as well as any individual in the placebo group. Serial position curves also developed for free recall on day 1 and these are presented in the left half of Figure 9. A significant primacy effect was found (recall is higher for initially presented items) but the recency effect was not as pronounced as is usually found in the recall of word lists.

On day 2, recall of the old story remained low in groups receiving marijuana on day 1, but retention deficits from day 1 to day 2 were low. Retrieval cues did reverse the recall deficits in all groups but no cued recall advantage was found for the marijuana groups receiving drug on day 1 or day 2. Marijuana was also found to affect retrieval on day 2 of information encoded in either the placebo or drug state on day 1. This was determined by calculating the two conditional probability scores discussed previously. The first consisted of the proportion of correct items recalled on the retention test given correct recall on the immediate test on day 1 (R2/R1). The second consisted of the proportion of items recalled on the retention test given that recall did not occur on day 1 (R2/N1). It was found that R2/R1 probability was

TABLE I. Mean Number of Prose Units Recalled Under Each Recall Condition (+/- S.E.M.)

Group	Day 1	Day 2 (old story)		Day 2 (new story)	
	FR	FR	CR	FR	CR
M-P	6.8 (4.4)	6.3 (3.3)	9.2 (4.0)	12.1 (3.3)	14.8 (3.6)
M-M	7.3 (2.3)	5.8 (2.4)	8.6 (2.0)	9.6 (3.0)	12.8 (3.1)
P-M	11.6 (3.0)	8.5 (3.3)	12.0 (3.1)	9.6 (4.3)	12.9 (4.5)
P-P	12.4 (4.3)	11.5 (3.2)	14.5 (3.6)	15.5 (4.6)	17.5 (4.9)

significantly reduced following intoxication on day 2, meaning that the recall of items on day 2 which were originally recalled on day 1 was significantly reduced by marijuana. The R2/N1 probability was not affected. Thus, retrieval of initially recalled items was reduced by marijuana but not by placebo.

Another interesting finding concerned the effect of marijuana on state dependent learning (see Figure 10). On day 2, recall of the story presented on day 1 was not related to the change in drug state which occurred on day 2. However, recall of the new story was subject to some transfer deficit and this was related to the serial position of items. It appears from Figure 10 that the P-P group displays a significant amount of positive transfer or learning to learn going from recall of story 1 to recall of story 2. However, the M-P group displays a significant reduction in recall in comparison to group P-P, although the two placebo groups should display equivalent recall of the new story.

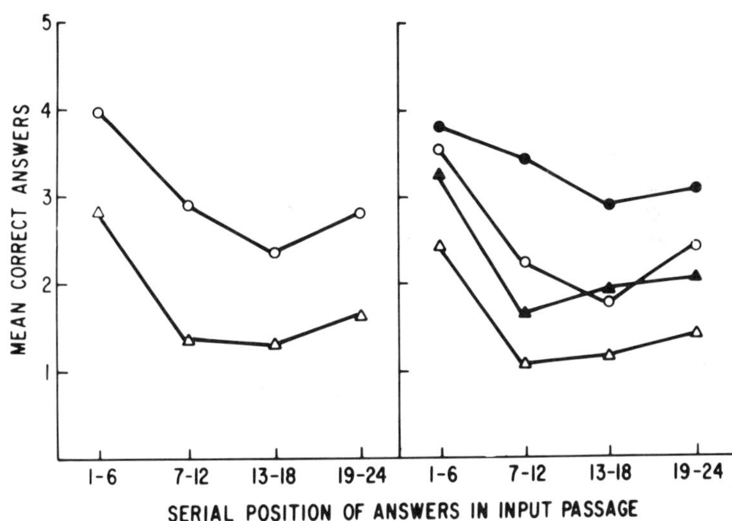

FIGURE 9. Mean number of correct answers as a function of serial position of answers in the input passage (old story). Circles = placebo; triangles = marijuana; closed = cued; open = uncued. The left side of the figure represents immediate free recall by marijuana and placebo groups on day 1. The right side of the figure represents cued and uncued recall of the old story as a function of drug state on day 1.

The mechanism by which marijuana reduces free recall remains elusive. We thought that one way in which the drug altered recall was to interfere with a volunteer's ability to organize the material prior to the recall test. By organization is meant that volunteers recalling word lists tend to develop word groups in a list and as recall trials continue, words are added to these groupings. The question was whether marijuana reduced recall by interfering with subjective organization. The next study addressed this question.

Another purpose of this study was to compare the effect of marijuana on the recall of verbal and pictorial memory. Marijuana has been reported to facilitate both visual and mental imagery (4,27). Since imagery has been posited to be an important component in the encoding of certain types of visual materials especially pictures, it was of interest to test the effect of marijuana on memory for material which might be encoded differently from words.

In this study, 28 volunteers were recruited with each being run as his own drug control in two phases with each being separated by a week. A single one gram cigarette containing 14 mg THC was smoked. Two lists of common objects

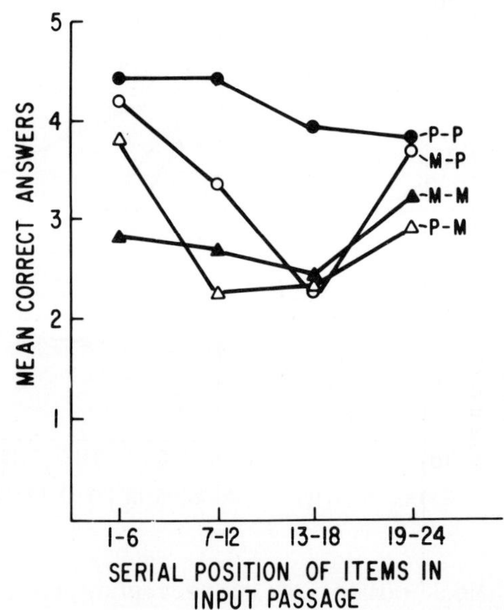

FIGURE 10. Mean number of correct answers as a function of serial position of answers in the input passage (new story) and change in drug state. Cued and uncued recall scores are combined.

were constructed. One list consisted of words typed on slides while the other consisted of simple black line drawings. During the initial session half of the volunteers received placebo and half marijuana. Following smoking half the volunteers were presented with words at a 3 second rate for 5 trials. An immediate free recall test following each trial. Then, the pictures were presented for five trials with a recall test following each trial. The other half of the volunteers experienced pictures first followed by words. One week after the initial session, another session was run with volunteers receiving drug in the first session now receiving placebo and vice versa. Pulse rate measures and potency and pleasantness ratings were also taken.

The results are presented in the Figures 11 and 12. First, there was little overall difference in the recall of pictures and words except on trial 1 where pictures were superior. Marijuana reduced the recall of both, but there was a differential effect of drug on words and pictures as a function of recall trials. Recall of words was initially reduced under drug but as training continued improvement in recall occurred

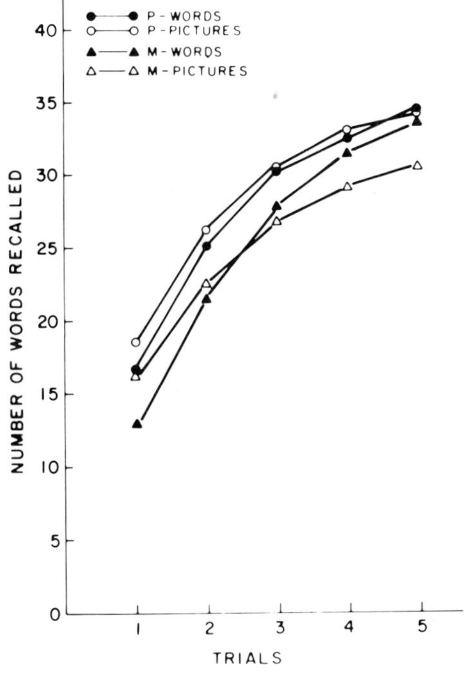

FIGURE 11. Mean number of pictures and words recalled as a function of trials.

so that by trial 5, both treatment conditions were equal. With pictures, however, a divergence in performance took place so that under marijuana performance remained inferior throughout acquisition in comparison to placebo.

In this study, a volunteer's ability to organize material for recall was measured. Previous studies have shown that as recall increases over trials, organization becomes more consistent. Four different measures of subjective organization were calculated. 1) Tulvings (26) - subjective organization measure (SO). This measure is an index of the frequency with which pairs of words recalled on trial N are also recalled together and in the same order on trial N + 1 (an intertrial repetition). 2) SO_2 - Tulvings SO measure was modified so that items recalled together on trial N and N + 1 were considered to be intertrial repetitions regardless of order. 3) SO-OR - this measure considered only those items which were adjacent to each other during list presentation and recall and represents to the extent to which a volunteer reproduced the serial organization of the list as presented for learning. 4) Deviation Ratio - this measure consists of the number of intertrial repetitions minus chance performance divided by the total number of intertrial repetitions possible. This measure corrects for chance occurrence of clustering. The results of these analyses are presented in Figure 12. They indicated (1) as recall improved, all measures of subjective organization increased and were highly correllated with recall, (2) subjective organization did not differ for pictures and words, and (3) although recall was significantly reduced following intoxication, measures of subjective organization were not affected by marijuana. Thus, recall was reduced by the drug but evidently this effect was not mediated by any alteration in organizational capacity as measured by consistency in recall from trial to trial. However, it should be noted that subjective organization measures do not tap into qualitative aspects of organization and that other measures of organization could still be affected by the drug.

One findings of the study which proved to be rather revealing occurred when a factor analysis was applied to the difference scores (placebo-marijuana) for pulse rate, memory and subjective ratings. Three different factors emerged from this analysis, Factorl, labeled pulse rate accounted for 40.02% of the variance of the factor matrix while two other factors, memory and subjective ratings accounted for 34.70% and 25.28% of the variance, respectively. This means that the effects of marijuana on measures of pulse rate, memory, and subjective ratings are statistically independent of each other. If changes in subjective ratings, pulse rate and memory were related to each other, they would load on the same factor. These results pose some difficulty for attempting to

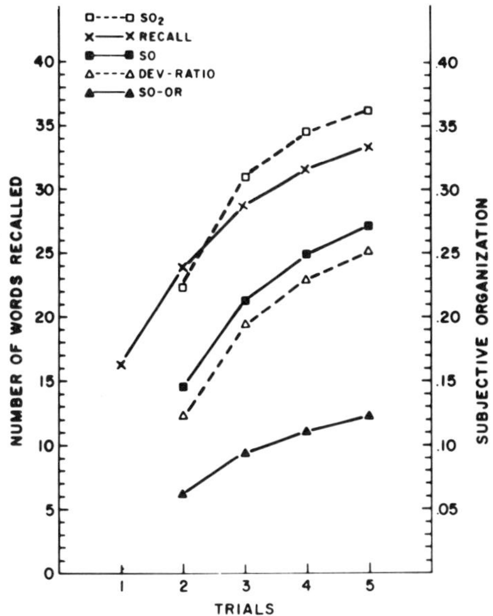

FIGURE 12. Mean number of items recalled (collapsed across recall and treatment conditions) and measures of subjective organization as a function of trials. See text for explanation of various measures of subjective organization.

predict on the basis of either physiological changes or subjective estimates of how "high" an individual describes himself as being, changes in recall ability. Whether this is generalizable to other types of drug-induced behavioral change remains to be seen.

While the studies conducted to date in our laboratory indicate that a persistent effect of marijuana is to reduce the free recall of variety of stimulus materials, the mechanism by which the drug produces its effect on storage and retrieval processes is not as yet apparent. The finding that recall rather than recognition is reduced may suggest that while the intoxicated subject's ability to retrieve information from memory is impaired, material appears to be encoded well enough for recognition to occur. However, recall may be more difficult for the intoxicated individual than recognition, not because these tasks involve different types of memory processing, but because of the way in which these two type of tasks are set up. Recall involves a large or open ended set of alternatives while recognition usually involves a binary choice. Since marijuana has been reported to distort temporal judgment, recall may be difficult for the intoxicated individual because of an inability to restrict his search set to temporally recent items. This may account in part for the increase in intrusion errors found under the drug. Recognition automatically restricts this search set. Thus, the intoxicated subject may be deficient in retrieving unique items of information on the basis of contextual cues which would normally permit a differentiation between items searched for and competing irrelevant items. However, with continued practice, intoxicated subjects do encode and retrieve repeatedly presented material although retrieval of unique information from episodic memory remains impaired.

It has been assumed in the literature on marijuana and memory, based mainly on the serial position curve results, that storage rather than retrieval is influenced by the drug. However, theoretical and methodological difficulties suggest that the hypothesis is open to speculation.

First, the results of our studies suggest that recognition memory is little affected by cannabinoids. Two factor memory theory postulates that recognition memory is a measure of storage while recall is a measure of both storage and retrieval (28). According to Kintsch (29), recognition involves "checking the familiarity or response strength of an item, but recall involves an additional process of search and retrieval." Whereas deficits in recall and recognition could be interpreted as being due to a storage problem, a deficit in recall but not recognition could be interpreted as a retrieval failure. Tulving and Pearlstone (30) have drawn a distinction between what is in memory and what can be retrieved -- i.e., availability vs. accessibility. Recall is an insensitive indicator of what is available in memory (31), whereas a recognition test can often detect the availability of previously learned information when recall (accessibility) fails to do so (32). Viewed in the above context, a plausible interpretation of cannabinoid disruption of recall but not recognition is that cannabinoids disrupt accessibility of information acquired during cannabinoid intoxication.

On a methodological level, one possible reason retrieval deficits have not been shown is that a retrieval deficit is measured usually in terms of a delayed recall test. Ona delayed recall test, the amount of information remaining in the memory is reduced substantially in comparison to an immediate free recall test. Therefore, the amount of information available for recall is lessened and recall levels are generally very low -- "the floor effect" (see the right panel in Figure 8). The assessment of drug-induced recall deficits is difficult when the baseline level of recall is very low. On the other hand, the Miller et al. (23) prose study indicated that recall of prose was reduced 24 hours following intoxication. In that particular study, recall level was 90% of baseline prior to the delayed recall test.

III. MARIJUANA AND MEMORY - AN INTEGRATIVE ASSESSMENT

Recently, a method for analyzing impaired memory, termed the "restricted reminding technique", has been developed (33). This method provides for the assessment and simultaneous analysis of storage, retention and retrieval during a verbal memory task. In the restricted reminding task, an individual must recall information spontaneously without presentation. The usual free recall paradigm analysis of memory is confounded because of interference produced by the immediate recall of items which were recently presented. According to Bushke and Fuld (33), an item can be considered to be in long-term memory only when it is recalled without repeated presentation. Recall is assessed independently of confounding due to continued presentation of stimuli on each trial.

The data to be described are strikingly similar (in pattern of effects on memory but not magnitude) to those found with patients experiencing amnesia due to herpes simplex encephalitis (34), Korsakoff syndrome (35,36), or Alzheimer's disease (37). Herpes simplex and Alzheimer's disease are thought to affect the limbic system via disruption of muscarinic limbic pathways (34, 38,39), while Korsakoff syndrome may be due to lesions in the hippocampus, mamilliary bodies and/or dorsalmedial nucleus of the thalamus (40).

The task employed was a free recall task in which words in a list are presented individually until recall of the word occurs once. Following initial recall, words are not presented again so that eventually recall trials occur without any further presentation of items. All words are recalled on each trial. Buschke has argued that storage and retrieval of items in memory cannot be evaluated when all items are presented before every recall attempt because immediate recall of items does not demonstrate that an item resides in long-term memory (33). The dependent variables in this paradigm are long-term storage, which consists of the number of items encoded on a given trial, while retrieval consists of the number of items recalled on each trial that are considered to be in long-term storage.

Miller et al.(41), employing the restricted reminding technique, ran 16 male volunteers in a crossover design with each receiving both smoked marijuana (10.5 mg THC) or placebo in successive sessions separated by one week. In each session, a different 30-item word list was employed with words being presented at a 3-second rate. Recall testing occurred for 12 trials. The results of this study are presented in Figures 13 and 14. Only the most salient features will be emphasized.

In Fig. 13, it can be seen that the number of items eventually encoded under marijuana and placebo were essentially the same although it took more recall trials for the same number of items to be encoded under drug. However, retrieval of items from long-term storage was significantly impaired under drug and this was due to the fact that more memory lapses or recall failures took place following intoxication. That is, intoxicated subjects displayed an inconsistency in recall. For example, under marijuana an encoded word might be retrieved on a given trial following which a 3 to 4 trial lapse in recall would occur before the word would be recalled again. In Fig. 14, it can be seen that intrusion error rates were significantly elevated in the drug condition in comparison to placebo. Intrusions consisted of the number of different extra list words which were emitted. What intoxicated subjects tended to do was commit an intrusion error, encode the word and repeat it on the majority of recall trials or if they committed one error, they might drop that word and substitute another. Thus, extraneous words from long-term memory were introduced which may have interfered with recall.

These data suggest that the mechanism of impaired recall in the intoxicated individual may be in his capacity to integrate material in some meaningful fashion for recall to occur. Buschke suggests that when items of information are consis-

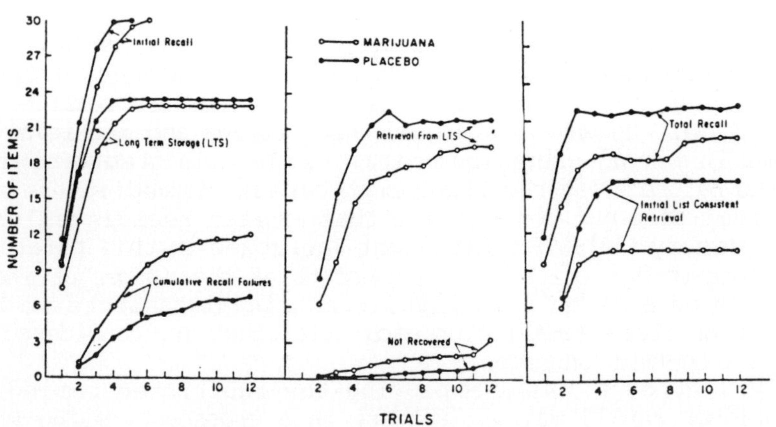

FIGURE 13. Analysis of free recall by restricted reminding for placebo and marijuana.

tently retrieved in memory they are integrated with the retrieval of other items in the list. Thus, items in memory are encoded within a given context. Information about a target item and its relationship to other words in the semantic system provides a basis of organization. That is, the learner imposes structure on information already in long-term memory. Marijuana may affect an individual's capacity to make use of information in his semantic memory to employ efficient recall strategies. Thus, the depth to which information is processed following cannabis intoxication may be an important mechanism by which recall is impaired. Intrusion errors may be seen as being secondary to organizing and integrating deficiencies since information from long-term memory which is the basis for semantic organization intrudes on the recall process.

These data are consistent with the interpretation of Adam (42) for the effect of anesthetic gases on memory processes. These agents may make memory traces temporarily inaccessible, a form of anterograde amnesia. Impaired retrieval of information occurs because encoding processes are not consistent with efficient retrieval.

In conclusion, the deleterious effect of cannabis on free recall memory are a reliable and consistent finding. The pattern of memory deficits are similar to those found in neurally compromised patients with memory disorders thought to be mediated by cholinergic limbic dysfunction. These memory deficiencies are characterized by: 1) lapses in recall, 2) inconsistent retrieval of information, and 3) memory intrusions.

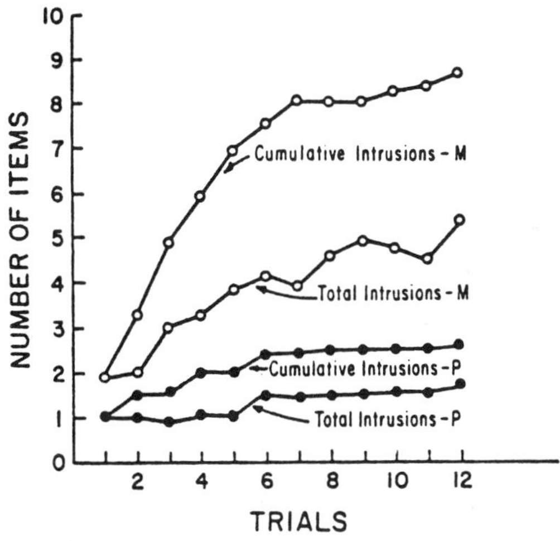

FIGURE 14. Total number of intrusion errors and cumulative intrusion errors for placebo and marijuana conditions.

REFERENCES

1. Miller, L. L., Marijuana and human cognition: a review of laboratory investigations, in "The Therapeutic Potential of Marijuana", (S. Cohen and R. C. Stillman, eds.). Plenum Press, New York, (1976).
2. Moreau, J. J., Duhachish et de l'alienation mentale: Etudes psychologious 34, Pacis: Libraire de Roxten, Maison Paris, 1845.
3. Bomberg, W., Marijuana intoxication, Amer. J. Psych. 91:303-330, (1934).
4. Ames, F. A., A clinical and metabolic study of acute intoxication with cannabis sativa and its role in the model psychoses, J. Mental Sci. 104:972-999 (1958).
5. Tinklenberg, J.R., Kopell, B. S., Melges, F. T., and Hollister, L. E., Marijuana and alcohol: time production and memory functions, Arch. Gen. Psych. 27:812-815 (1972).
6. Clark, L. D., Hughes, R., and Nakashima, E. N., Behavioral effects of marijuana: experimental studies, Arch. Gen. Psych. 23:193-198 (1970).
7. Melges, F. T., Tinklenberg, J. R., Hollister, L. E., and Gillespie, H. K., Marijuana and temporal disintegration, Science 168:1118-1120 (1970).
8. Melges, F. T., Tinklenberg, J. R., Hollister, L. E., and Gillespie, H. K., Marijuana and temporal span of awareness, Arch. Gen. Psych. 24:564-567 (1971).
9. Weil, A. T., and Zinberg, N. E., Acute effects of marijuana on speech, Nature 222:434-437 (1969).
10. Abel, E. L., Marijuana, learning and memory, in "International Review of Neurobiology", (C. Pfeiffer and J. Smythies, eds.). Academic Press, New York, 1975.
11. Rafaelsen, L., Christup, A., Bech, P., and Rafaelesen, O. J., Effects on cannabis and alcohol on psychological tests, Nature 242:117-118, (1973).
12. Tinklenbert, J. R., Kopell, B. S., Melges, F. T., and Hollister, L. E., Marijuana and alcohol: time production and memory functions, Arch. Gen. Psych. 27:812-815, (1972).
13. Darley, C. F., and Tinklenberg, J. R., Marijuana and memory, in "Marijuana: effects on human behavior", (L. L. Miller, ed.). Academic Press, New York, 1974.
14. Shiffrin, W., and Atkinson, R. E., Storage and retrieval processes in long-term memory, Psychol. Rev. 76:179-193, (1969).
15. Darley, C. F., Tinklenberg, J. R., Roth, W. T., Hollister, L. E., and Atkinson, R. C., Influence of Marijuana

on storage and retrieval processes in memory, Memory and Cognition 1:196-200, (1973).
16. Abel, E. L., Marijuana and memory: acquisition or retrieval? Science 173:1038-1040, (1971).
17. Miller, L. L., and Cornett, T. L., Marijuana: dose effects on pulse rate, subjective estimates of intoxication, free recall and recognition memory, Pharmacol. Biochem. Behav. 9:573-577, (1976).
18. Zeidenberg, P., Clark, W. C., Jaffe, J., Anderson, W. W., Chin, S., and Malitz, S., Effect of oral administration of delta-9-tetrahydrocannabinol on memory, speech and perception of thermal stimulation: results with four normal human volunteer subjects, Preliminary report, Compreh. Psych. 14:549-556, (1973).
19. Dornbush, R. L., Marijuana and memory: effects of smoking on storage, Trans. Acad. Sci. 234:94-100 (1971).
20. Paul, M. I., and Carson, I. M., Marijuana and communication, Lancet 270-271 (1973).
21. Hebb, D. O., Distinctive features of learning in the higher animal, in "Brain Mechanisms and Learning", (J. B. Delafresnaye, ed.). Oxford University Press, New York (1961).
22. Watkins, M. J., and Watkins, O. L., Processing of recency items for free recall, J. Exper. Psych. 102:488-493, (1974).
23. Miller, L. L., McFarland, D., Cornett, T. L., and Brightwell, D., Marijuana and memory impairment: effect on free recall and recognition memory, Pharmacol. Biochem. Behav. 7:99-103 (1977).
24. Miller, L. L., McFarland, D. J., Cornett, T. L., Brightwell, D. R., and Wikler, A., Marijuana: effects on free recall and subjective organization of pictures and words, Psychopharmacology 55:257-262 (1977).
25. Miller, L., Drew, W. G., and Kiplinger, G. F., Effects of marijuana on recall of narrative material and Stroop-colour word performance, Nature 237:172-173 (1972).
26. Tulving, E., Subjective organization in free recall of "unrelated" words, Psychol. Rev. 69:344-345 (1962).
27. Tart, C. T., Marijuana intoxication: common experiences, Nature 226:701-704 (1970).
28. McCormack, P. D., Recognition memory: How complex a retrieval system? Can. J. Psychol. 26:19-41 (1972).
29. Kintsch, W., Models for free recall and recognition, in "Models of Human Memory", (D. A. Norman, ed.). Academic Press, New York, 1970.
30. Tulving, E., and Pearlstone, (1966).
31. Hulicka, I. M., and Weiss, R. L., Age differences in retention as a function of learning, J. Consulting Psychol. 29:125-129, (1965).

32. Harwood, E., and Naylor, G. F. K., Recall and recognition in elderly and young subjects, Australian J. Psych. 21:251-257 (1969).
33. Buschke, H., Retrieval in verbal learning, Trans. Acad. Sci. 236:721-729 (1974).
34. Peters, B. H., and Levin, H. S., Memory enhancement after physostigmine treatment in the amnesic syndrome, Arch. Neurol. 34:215-219 (1977).
35. Kovner, R., Mattis, S., Goldmeier, E., and Davis L., Korsakoff amnesic syndrome: the result of simultaneous deficits in several independent processes, Brain and Language 12:23-32 (1981).
36. Fuld, P. A., Storage, retention and retrieval in Korsakoff's syndrome, Neuropsychologica 14:225-236 (1976).
37. Davis, K. L. et al., Cholinomimetic agents and human memory: clinical studies in Alzheimer's disease and scopolamine dementia. Pharmacological strategies in aging and dementia and the cholinergic hypothesis, in "Strategy for the Development of an Effective Treatment for Senile Dementia", (T. Cook and S. Gershon, eds.). Mark Powley Associates, Inc., New Canann, Conn., 1981.
38. Davies, P., and Maloney, A. J. F., Selective loss of central cholinergic neurons in Alzheimers disease, Lancet 2:1043 (1976).
39. Whitehouse, P. J., Price, D. ., Struble, R. G., Clark, A. W., Gayle,J. T., and DeLong, M. R., Alzheimer's disease and senile dementia: loss with neurons in the basal forebrain, Science 215:1237-1239 (1982).
40. Meissner, W. W., Learning and memory in the Korsakoff syndrome, Internat. J. Neuropsych. 4:6-20 (1968).
41. Miller, L. L., Cornett, T., and McFarland, D., Marijuana: an analysis of storage and retrieval deficits in memory with the technique of restricted reminding, Pharmacol. Biochem. Behav. 8:327-332 (1978).
42. Adam, N., Disruption of memory functions associated with general anesthetics in "Functional disorders of memory", (J. F. Kihlstrom and F. J. Evans, eds.). Lawrence Erlbaum Press, Hillsdale, New Jersey, 1979.
43. Miller, L., Cornett, T., Brightwell, D., McFarland, D., and Drew, W. G., Marijuana: effects on storage and retrieval of prose material, Psychopharmacology 51:311-316 (1977).
44. Buschke, H., Retrieval in verbal learning, Trans. Acad. Sci. 236:721-729 (1974).

CHARACTERISTICS, BEHAVIORS, AND OUTCOMES FOR MARIJUANA USERS SEEKING TREATMENT IN DRUG ABUSE TREATMENT PROGRAM

Harold M. Ginzburg

Division of Research
National Institute on Drug Abuse
Rockville, Maryland

S. Gail Craddock
Robert Hubbard
James Glass

Research Triangle Institute
Research Triangle Park, North Carolina

I. INTRODUCTION

The Institute of Medicine report "Marijuana and Health" (1), the National Institute on Drug Abuse research monograph "Marijuana Research Findings: 1980" (2), and the National Academy of Science Committee on Substance Abuse and Habitual Behavior report, "An Analysis of Marijuana Policy" (3), concur in the finding that marijuana is not a harmless drug. Cannabinoids have the capacity to reduce the effective functioning of individuals under its influence. Prolonged or excessive use may cause serious harmful biological and social effects in many users. The "Marijuana and Health" report concludes:

> The scientific evidence published to date indicates that marijuana has a broad range of psychological and biological effects, some of which, at least under certain conditions, are harmful to human health. Unfortunately, the available information does not tell us how serious this risk may be.

ISBN 0-12-044620-0

Use of marijuana is widespread. The present government estimates are that 53 million Americans have tried marijuana at least once, 31 million have used it during the past year, and about 22 million have used it during the past month (4).

Further findings of the most recent National Household Survey (4), are that two-thirds (68.2 percent) of young adults (age 18-25), three-in-ten (30.9 percent) youth (age 12-17), and one-fifth (19.6 percent) of older adults (older than 26) report ever having used marijuana. There is a relationship between marijuana use and age-cohort. Experience increases four-fold between respondents age 12-13 (8 percent) and 14-15 (32 percent); a majority (51 percent) of youth age 16-17 report using marijuana. Young adults age 18-21 and 22-25 have the highest experience rates of all age subgroups (69 percent and 68 percent, respectively). Marijuana experience is less common among older adults; although almost one-half (48 percent) of those age 26-34 report ever using marijuana, only 10 percent of those age 35 and older report having ever done so.

More males than females, regardless of age, have ever used marijuana. Three-quarters of young adult males, compared to 61 percent of young adult females have ever used the drug. One-fourth (26 percent) of older males, compared to 14 percent of same age females have experience using marijuana. Among youth, 34 percent of males and 28 percent of females report ever using marijuana.

Use of both alcohol and marijuana is well documented in the Research Triangle Institute Adolescent Drinking Behavior study (5). Only 14 percent of abstainers ever used marijuana while 82 percent of the heaviest category of drinkers of beverage alcohol have ever used marijuana.

Lifetime prevalence and recency of use during calendar year 1979 are presented for the three age groups in Table IA. These data are compared with the results of the High School Survey (6) in Table 1B for the years 1979, 1980, and 1981. The older the age group, the less likely that an individual will have used or experimented with marijuana in the month prior to being interviewed. While there are many individuals who report using marijuana at varying frequencies and with other psychoactive substances, there are no general population estimates for the adverse effects of cannabinoids alone or in combination with other drugs. The "Adolescent Drinking Behavior" study has demonstrated a correlation between frequent marijuana use and increased absences from school, decreased school performance, and reports of increased difficulties with police, parents, and friends. Severe adverse effects have been studied indirectly through examination of post-mortem body fluids in driver-victims of fatal motor vehicle accidents (7), or by road-side screening for sobriety (8). However,

TABLE IA. Lifetime Prevalence and Recency of Use by Age at Time of Interview

Age[a]	N	Ever Used	Past Month	Past Year, Not Past Month	Not Past Year	Never Used
Youth (12-17)	2165	30.9%	16.7%	7.4%	6.7%	69.1%
Young Adults (18-25)	2044	68.2%	35.6%	11.5%	21.4%	31.8%
Older Adults (over 25)	3015	19.6%	6.0%	3.0%	10.6%	80.4%

TABLE IB. High School Seniors[b]

	Ever Used	Past Year	Last 30 Days	Daily in Past 30 Days
Class of 1979 (n = 15,550)	60.4%	50.8%	36.5%	10.3%
Class of 1980 (n = 15,900)	60.3%	48.8%	33.7%	9.1%
Class of 1981 (n = 17,500)	59.5%	46.1%	31.6%	7.0%

[a]National Household Survey, 1979 (4).
[b]Survey of High School Seniors, 1981 (5).

mildly impaired individuals or unidentified severely impaired individuals may not be studied if they:

- do not seek assistance voluntarily
- are not <u>forced</u> to seek assistance
- or are treated for a drug-related problem, <u>but</u> the problem is not identified as related to marijuana use.

Because of these problems there is a concern about identifying appropriate treatment resources for individuals with problems related to marijuana use. In the past traditional drug abuse treatment programs were oriented more toward opioid users. Consequently, marijuana users may not have been referred to drug abuse treatment programs; if they were, effective treatment resources may not have been available. Thus, it is now important to ask if appropriate and effective treatment is being rendered to individuals who principally abuse marijuana.

This paper describes a twice weekly, or greater, use of marijuana subgroup by its demographic characteristics and performance in either drug free outpatient or therapeutic community treatment programs. This is a special group of persons whose marijuana use has affected their functioning to the extent that treatment was considered necessary. We examine their special characteristics and why their marijuana use has become problematic. Finally, we look at the treatment services provided to these individuals and how treatment has helped them.

II. METHODS

The Treatment Outcome Prospective Study (TOPS) examined a national sample of drug abuse treatment programs receiving federal and/or state monies to support their service programs. More than 11,000 clients entering more than 50 treatment units in ten cities during the calendar years 1979-1981 participated in TOPS. Of these 11,000 clients:

- 5,324 clients entered outpatient methadone maintenance or detoxification treatment programs,
- 2,879 clients entered drug freeoutpatienttreatment programs (DFOP),
- 2,800 clients entered therapeutic communities (TC).

Clients entering a detoxification or outpatient methadone programs typically had a significant history of use of heroin or other opioids. Clients with marijuana as a primary drug problem, or reported marijuana use without regular (weekly or greater) use of narcotics were most likely to be seen in either of the drug-free environments. Self-reported use patterns and perceived drug-related problems are used to define the subgroups discussed below. The data presented are not representative of all marijuana users; they are the subgroup of clients entering the participating DFOP and TCprograms during 1979-1981 with a drug use pattern of marijuana useat least twice weekly for the year prior to admission to treatment. This pattern twice weekly or greater use, was selected as a minimum criteria to establish a pattern of regular use. Any client using marijuana and any other opioid or non-opioid on a weekly or greater basis is excluded from this analysis. This set of criteria were met by 736 (25.5 percent) of the DFOP clients and 250 (8.9 percent) of the TC clients.

There is a very high association between alcohol and marijuana consumption (84 percent for DFOP clients and 69 percent for TC clients) and, therefore, those who used beverage alcohol were included in the data analyses as long as their pattern of marijuana use was at least twice weekly.

III. RESULTS

In the following section we present descriptive data on the characteristics and behaviors of clients in the year prior to entering TOPS programs and on the treatment servicesand treatment outcomes during the first three months in treatment.

A. Admission Characteristics

Table II profiles the admission characteristics of the full DFOP and TC cohorts and their respective twice weekly marijuana subgroups. Approximately two-thirds of all admissions to both DFOP and TC's during each of three calendar years studied (1979, 1980, 1981) used marijuana at least weekly; more that half of these (approximately 40 percent of the total number of admissions) used it on a daily basis. These are greater frequency rates than for beverage alcohol (63 percent for at least weekly use for both modalities; 20 percent daily use for DFOP's and 30 percent daily use for TC's).

Clients in this sample are younger than the average age of others admitted to their respective treatment programs. The subgroups are less likely to have had a previous treatment experience but they have a higher referral rate from the criminal justice system as compared to their respective cohorts.

Almost three-quarter (70 percent) of all DFOP admissions seem to consume moderate to heavy amounts of alcohol, and the study sample differs little (74 percent) from this rate. Admissions to TC's also demonstrate little differences in drinking patterns from their respective cohorts. (Alcohol consumption patterns are a composite score of quantity/frequency of ounces of absolute alcohol).

Overall, the twice weekly marijuana users report fewer drug-related problems than their respective samples. Fifty-percent of DFOP cohort reported, three or more drug-related problems, while only one-third of the twice weekly marijuana group reported three or more problems. While 60% of the entire TC cohort reported three drug-related problems, only

TABLE II. Description of Twice Weekly Marjuana User Subgroups and Their RespectiveEntire Cohorts for Calendar Years 1979, 1980 and 1981

	DRUG FREE OUTPATIENT		THERAPEUTIC COMMUNITY	
	Twice Weekly Marijuana Users (n = 736)	Entire Cohort (n = 2879)	Twice Weekly Marijuana Users (n = 250)	Entire Cohort (n = 2800)
SEX/AGE				
Male Under 21	31.1%	18.1%	29.2%	13.7%
Male 21-30	35.2	34.2	39.6	42.1
Male Over 30	12.2	14.8	21.2	21.6
Female Under 21	9.5	9.2	3.2	5.4
Female 21-30	8.7	17.3	5.2	13.6
Female Over 30	2.7	6.5	1.6	3.6
RACE/ETHNICITY				
White	80.0%	79.6%	60.4%	52.6%
Black	10.5	10.4	33.2	39.9
Hispanic	8.6	8.5	6.0	6.6
Other	0.9	1.6	0.4	0.9

PRIOR TREATMENT EXPERIENCES				
None	75.1%	65.8%	57.6%	47.2%
1 Or 2	16.0	19.7	25.6	27.4
3 or More	8.9	14.5	16.8	25.4
SOURCE OF REFERRAL				
Self	17.9%	19.4%	24.1%	24.0%
Family or Friends	22.8	31.1	14.1	31.2
Criminal Justice	34.2	20.6	39.4	19.0
Other	25.0	28.9	22.5	25.8
DRINKING TYPE				
Non-Drinker	12.1%	16.3%	28.8%	31.0%
Infrequent/Light	13.9	13.5	8.0	9.3
Moderate	39.7	34.5	22.8	17.9
Heavy	34.2	35.7	40.4	41.9
DRUG RELATED PROBLEMS (Multiple Responses)				
Medical	22.0%	34.3%	20.0%	42.2%
Psychological	30.5	51.2	36.3	51.7
Family	45.8	56.0	48.8	66.9
Legal	38.2	33.6	31.0	48.6
Job	32.1	35.0	31.2	46.6
Financial	35.3	44.6	34.7	56.9
DRUG RELATED PROBLEMS				
None	22.4%	19.0%	33.3%	17.1%
1 or 2	41.2	30.9	27.3	19.7
3 or 4	28.1	32.0	25.3	32.0
5 or 6	8.3	18.2	14.1	31.2

TABLE II. - Continued

DEPRESSIVE SYMPTOMS				
None	49.2%	38.3%	44.8%	36.8%
Felt Depressed	12.3	14.1	18.8	19.7
Suicidal Ideation	31.6	34.2	25.2	29.8
Suicidal Attempt	7.0	13.4	11.2	13.8
PREDATORY ILLEGAL ACTS				
None	67.5%	66.2%	57.0%	44.1%
1 to 10 Acts	26.9	25.4	30.0	30.0
11 or More Acts	5.6	8.3	13.0	25.9
WEEKS OF FULL TIME WORK IN YEAR PRIOR TO ADMISSION				
None	30.3%	32.0%	38.9%	41.7%
1 to 13	19.1	18.2	18.4	17.3
14 to 39	24.5	24.3	29.3	26.2
40 to 52	26.1	25.5	13.4	14.9
DRUG USE NETWORK				
Low Involvement	51.9%	44.4%	59.6%	35.6%
Mod. Involvement	24.0	24.5	22.0	25.4
High Involvement	24.0	31.1	18.4	39.0

40% of the twice weekly marijuana group reported three or more. Except for legal and employment problems among DFOP clients, the twice weekly marijuana users reported problems of all types less frequently than the entire cohort.

Depressive symptoms, though, present in more than half the twice weekly marijuana subgroups. Predatory illegal acts are reported somewhat less frequently than in the complete cohorts.

Pre-treatment employment rates were not substantively different between the study samples and all admissions in their respective cohorts. A drug use network composite score reflects peer use of drugs and involvement in illegal drug sales, and there appears to be less of this type of activity in the twice weekly marijuana users, particularly in the TC group.

B. Intreatment Performance

Client intreatment performance is examined on four outcome variables:

- Retention in treatment
- Marijuana use
- Self-reported drug-related problems
- Depression

These four outcome variables were examined in an attempt to determine treatment effectiveness. Table III presents retention data for both marijuana samples and their respective cohorts. The median time in treatment was 11 weeks for all DFOP and 12 weeks for TC clients, and one week less (10 and 11, respectively) for their subgroups. More than one-third of the DFOP and one-quarter of the TC clients terminated treatment in less than one month. Less than one-third of the DFOP and slightly more than one-third of the TC clients remained in treatment more than six months.

The outcome variables of marijuana use, drug related problems and depression indicators for the twice weekly or greater marijuana users remaining in treatment at least three months in either DFOP or TC are presented in Table IV.

For those remaining in programs, the treatment experience appears to decrease undesirable behavior while in treatment. Table IV appears to indicate that, as expected, TC treatment has an impact on reducing marijuana use. TC's are restricted, often closed environments; DFOP's are not as restrictive. Almost one-half of the clients in DFOP continue their level of pretreatment use of marijuana while they remain in treatment.

TABLE III. Retention Data on the Twice Weekly Marijuana User Subgroups and Their Respective Entire Cohorts for Calendar Years, 1979, 1980 and 1981

RETENTION IN TREATMENT (Time in weeks)	DRUG FREE OUTPATIENT		THERAPEUTIC COMMUNITY	
	Twice Weekly Marijuana Users (n = 736)	Entire Cohort (n = 2879)	Twice Weekly Marijuana Users (n = 250)	Entire Cohort (n = 2800)
Median Time in Treatment	10 Weeks	11 Weeks	11 Weeks	12 Weeks
One Week or Less	17.3%	18.9%	10.4%	9.9%
2 - 4 Weeks	15.8	14.9	16.8	18.7
5 - 8 Weeks	10.2	8.8	8.8	8.5
9 - 13 Weeks	19.6	20.4	21.2	22.3
14 - 26 Weeks	5.4	7.3	6.4	6.5
27 - 39 Weeks	21.3	19.3	22.4	21.1
40 - 52 Weeks	3.8	3.7	7.2	6.6
Over 52 Weeks	6.7	6.7	6.8	6.5

TABLE IV. Changes in Marijuana Use, Drug Related Problems, and Depression between the Year Prior to Treatment and the First Three Months in Treatment for the Marijuana Subgroups

	Outpatient Drug Free (N = 200)	Therapeutic Community (N = 94)
Marijuana Use:		
No/Low Use	0.0%	0.0%
Continuing Problem	47.5%	2.1%
Some Reduction	29.0%	4.3%
Large Reduction	23.5%	93.6%
Drug Related Problems:		
No Problem	17.4%	20.7%
No Reduction	25.4%	18.5%
Some Reduction	36.8%	29.3%
Large Reduction	20.4%	31.5%
Depression:		
No Problem	44.9%	42.9%
Reduced Depression	32.3%	37.4%
Continued or Increased Depression	4.0%	8.8%
Continued or Increased Suicidal Tendencies	18.7%	11.0%

There is more than a fifty percent reduction in drug-related problems during the first three months in treatment for both DFOP (57 percent) and TC (61 percent) twice weekly or greater marijuana users. DFOP and TC (TC in all categories) had fewer problems in the year prior to admission than their respective cohorts (Table IV).

Self-reported depression is shown to decrease during the first three months in treatment in both DFOP (32 percent) and TC (34 percent) marijuana user groups. However, reports of depression were given by 4 percent and 9 percent, respectively, of the clients remaining in each program. Of even greater clinical importance, continued or increased suicidal tendencies were reported by 19 percent of the DFOP clients and 11 percent in the TC clients.

IV. DISCUSSION

Though there are some key differences between the twice weekly marijuana users and their respective treatment populations, what is most striking is that the marijuana subgroup is substantively not very different in its behavior and demographic characteristics. Whether or not this group resumes the use of other drugs, progresses to using other psychoactive drugs or continues in a marijuana abuse pattern remains unknown until the 90 day, one year and two year post treatment interviews are completed and the data analyzed in 1983.

The twice weekly marijuana users appear to represent a unique subpopulation in the treatment system. While marijuana use per se may not be their primary difficulty, their drug use appears to be the reason for their admission to a drug abuse treatment program. Those that do remain in treatment appear to have significant changes in their drug taking behavior, their drug-related problems and their levels of depression during treatment. Clinically, most of these individuals would be considered to have improved during exposure to treatment. It is difficult to assess what has happened to their counterparts that have terminated from treatment after a nominal period of time. However, the results of the post treatment interviews will provide some insights into the behaviors of those who did terminate treatment prematurely.

Based on the data presented in this paper, no statements of casual relationships can be made although some apparent associations may be commented upon. Whether the regular marijuana user preceded or succeeded the initialdysfunctional activities is uncertain at this time. However, it was the marijuana user, per se, that would have been sufficient for referral for therapeutic intervention. Marijuana user, by itself, is an unusual reason for referral to a drug abuse treatment program. Few individuals use marijuana without using other psychoactive substances used, even if the only other psychoactive substance used on a regular basis is beverage alcohol. Criminal behavior, depressive symtomatology and other dysfunctional behaviors are usually involved in the referral to treatment (as with other types of drug users). Treatment programs must discern whether marijuana use is the primary problem or merely a labelling mechanism for referral to a drug abuse treatment program. If it is a label, its decreased use will not necessarily result in a more functional individual, just one not using drugs.

REFERENCES

1. Institute of Medicine, "Marijuana and Health". National Academy Press, Washington, D.C., 1982.
2. Petersen,R.(ed.), "Marijuana Findings: 1980". National Institute on Drug Abuse Research Monograph Series No. 31, DHHS Publication No. (ADM) 80-1001, Washington, D.C., 1980.
3. National Academy of Science Committee on Substance Abuse and Habitual Behavior, "An Analysis of Marijuana Policy". National Academy of Science Press, Washington, D.C., 1982.
4. Fishburne, P. M., Abelson, H. I., and Cisin, I, "National Survey on Drug Abuse: Main Findings 1979". National Institute on Drug Abuse, Rockville, Md., 1980.
5. Rachal, J. V., Guess, L. L., Hubbard, R. L., Maisto, S. A., Cavanaugh, E. R., Waddell, R., and Benrud, C. H., "Adolescent drinking behavior", Volume I, Research Triangle Institute Report, Research Triangle Park, N.C., 1980.
6. Johnston, L. D., Bachman, J. G., and O'Malley, P. M., "Highlights from Student Drug Use in America, 1975 - 1981", DHHS Publication No. (ADM) 82-1208, Washington, D.C., 1981.
7. Sterling-Smith, R. S., A special study of drivers most responsible in fatal accidents. Summary for Management Report, Contract No. DOT-HS-310-3-595, April, 1976.
8. Reeve, V. C., Incidence of marijuana in a California impaired driver population. State of California, Department of Justice, Division of Law Enforcement Investigative Branch, Sacramento, 1979.
9. Craddock, S. G., Hubbard, R. L., Bray, R. M., Cavanaugh, E. R., and Rachal, J. V., Client Characteristics, Behaviors and Intreatment Outcomes--1980 TOPS Admission Cohort, Research Triangle Institute Report, Research Triangle Park, N.C., 1982.

Section II CHEMICAL ASPECTS

CHEMISTRY AND STRUCTURE-ACTIVITY RELATIONSHIPS OF CANNABINOIDS: AN OVERVIEW

Raj K. Razdan*

SISA Institute for Research, Inc.
Cambridge, Massachusetts

I. INTRODUCTION

In the past 20 years the general increase in the illicit use of marijuana, the steady lowering of the age at which young people first experiment with the substance, and the increasing number of high school students who use it on a daily basis, have given cause for grave concern to society. Thus marijuana has become the subject of intense socio-political controversy. However, the recent use of marijuana and its active constituent, tetrahydrocannibinol, for the treatment of glaucoma and as an antinauseant in patients undergoing cancer chemotherapy, has revived public interest in its therapeutic potential.

The present article gives an overview of the synthesis of (-)-delta-1-3,4-trans-tetrahydrocannabinol (THC) and its metabolites in man and the known SAR in cannabinoids.

The term 'cannabinoids' is used for the typical C_{21}-groups of compounds present in Cannabis Sativa L. (family Moraceae) and includes their analogs and transformation products (10,11,18).

As shown in Figure 1, two different numbering systems, dibenzopyran and monoterpenoid, are generally used for cannabinoids. In the present article the monoterpenoid numbering system is used.

(-)-3,4-Trans-delta-1-THC, (1) the main pharmacologically active constituent of marijuana, is a resin which is optically

---

*Supportedby NIDA grant No.DA-00574-08 and NINCDSgrant No. NS-15346.

ISBN 0-12-044620-0

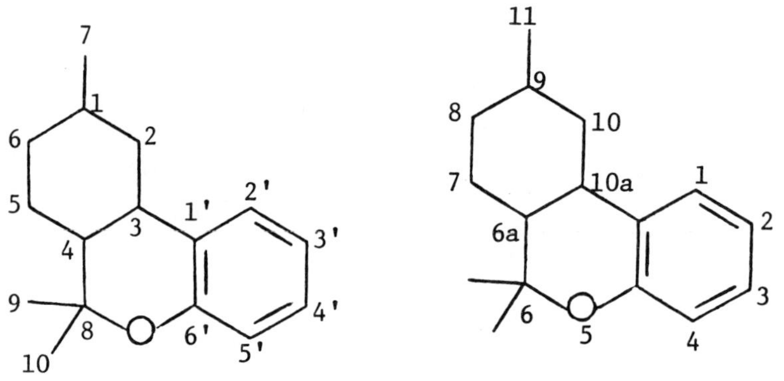

Monoterpenoid

Dibenzopyran

FIGURE 1. Numbering systems used in cannabinoids.

active and is generally referred to as delta-1-THC. It is also known as delta-9-THC based on the dibenzopyran numbering system. The other physiologically active isomer is delta-6-THC (2; alternate name delta-8-THC) and is found only in a few varieties of the plant. The isomers with a 3,4-cis ring junction are cis-delta-1-THC (3) and (cis-delta-6-THC (4), both of which have been synthesized, but only 3 has been found in the plant so far. On theoretical grounds the trans compounds (1 and 2) are expected to be more thermodyamically stable compared to the cis compounds 3 and 4. In the trans series, delta-6-THC (2) is more stable than delta-1-THC (1), since 1 is easily isomerized to (2) on treatment with acids. The main interest pharmacologically, therefore, centers on the thermodynamically less stable trans-delta-1-THC (1) and its various derivatives and metabolites. This has posed many synthetic problems, because during chemical reactions the more stable derivatives of trans-delta-6-THC (2) are mostly found.

II. SYNTHESIS

With this background let us now examine the various syntheses for (-)-delta-1- and delta-6-THCs (1 and 2). The various approaches to sterospecific syntheses are shown in Fig. 2.

Since the structure of delta-1-THC is not complex, the basic strategy can be envisioned as joining of the aromatic

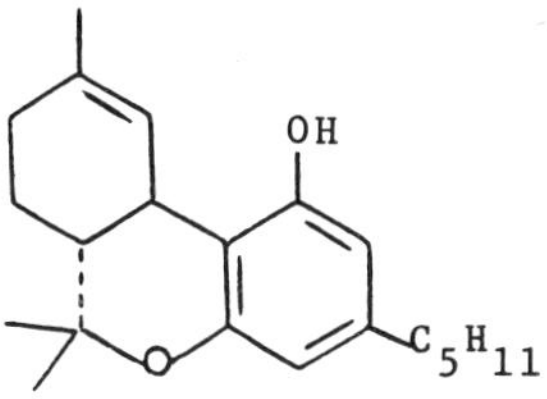

OH C_5H_{11}

Δ^1 - THC

1

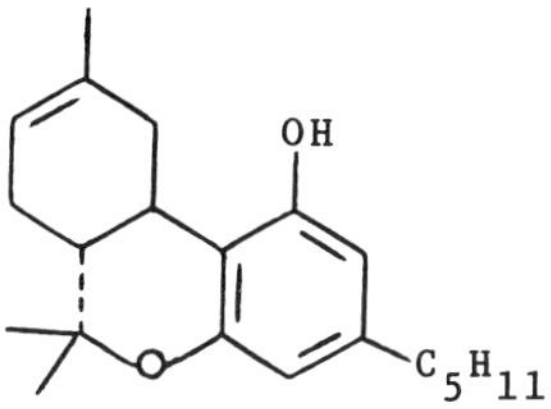

OH C_5H_{11}

Δ^6 - THC

2

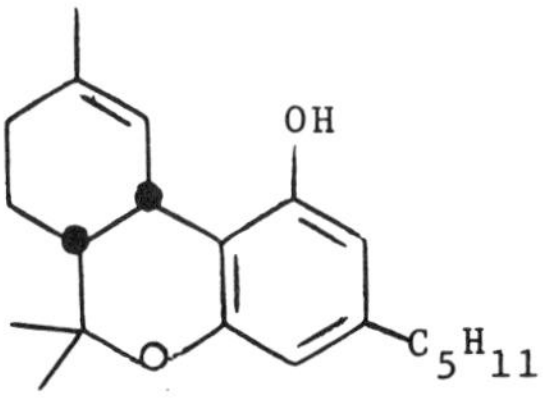

OH C_5H_{11}

cis - Δ^1 - THC

3

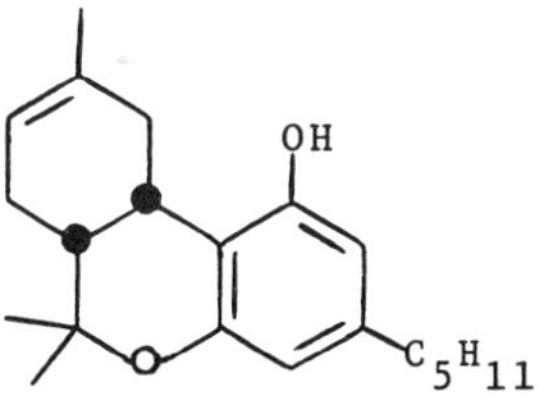

OH C_5H_{11}

cis - Δ^6 - THC

4

and the alicyclic parts of the molecule by condensation of olivetol with an optically active monoterpene. Mainly, it is the selection of the monoterpene and the reaction conditions which dictate or control the position of the double bond in the delta-1- or delta-6-position in the final product.

A. From Verbenol

In 1967, Mechoulam, et al., described a synthesis of (−)-delta-6-THC (2) from verbenol, a pinane derivative, and olivetol in the presence of acid catalysts (12). They visualized that the attack by olivetol will be favored from the side opposite the bulky dimethyl-methylene bridge in verbenol and will thus provide stereochemical control of the reaction to give mainly trans products. The final conversion of delta-6-

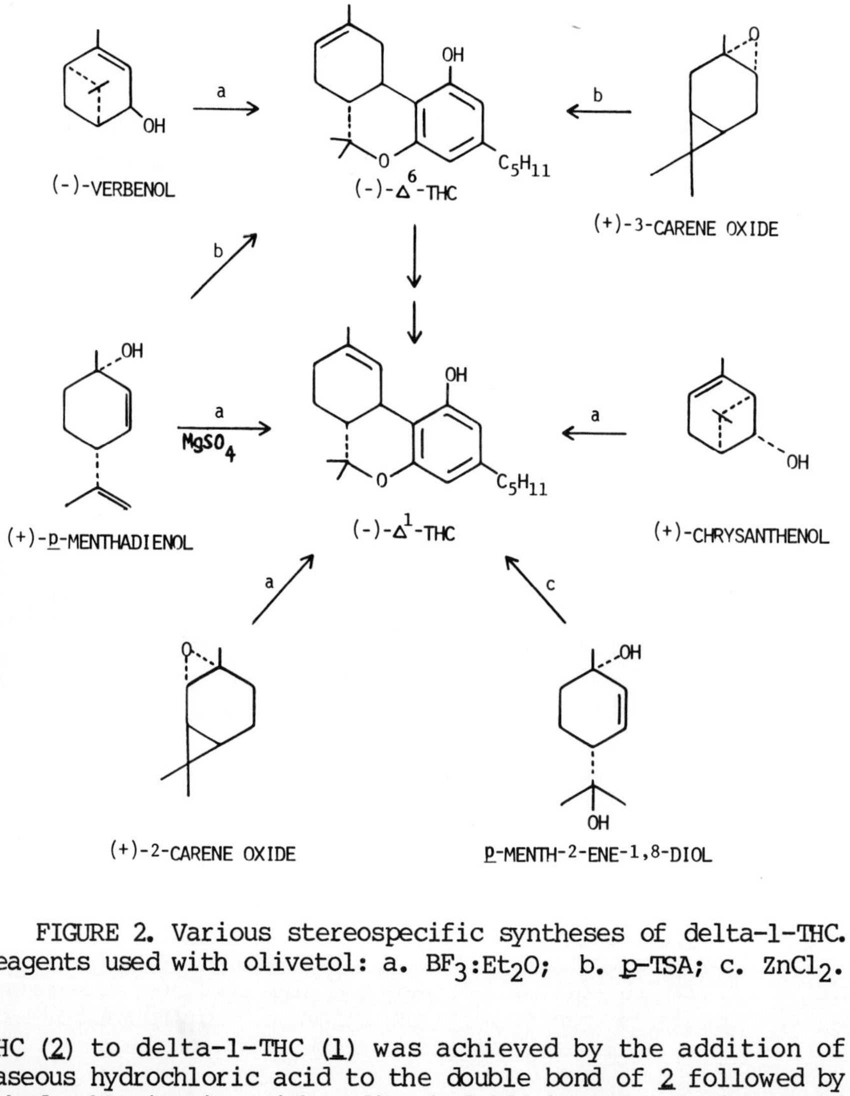

FIGURE 2. Various stereospecific syntheses of delta-1-THC. Reagents used with olivetol: a. BF_3:Et_2O; b. p-TSA; c. $ZnCl_2$.

THC (2) to delta-1-THC (1) was achieved by the addition of gaseous hydrochloric acid to the double bond of 2 followed by dehydrochlorination with sodium hydride in THF. A mixture of 1 and 2 was thus obtained which was separated by careful chromatography. Following the same sequence of reactions the unnatural (+)-delta-6- and (+)-delta-1-THC were similarly prepared from (+)-verbenol.

B. From Chrysanthenol

It is apparent that the mechanism of the verbenol route is

likely to involve a common allylic cation, since both _cis_- and _trans_-verbenols give the same products. However, on mechanistic grounds Razdan, et al., reasoned that by virtue of the position of the double bond, verbenol can lead only to delta-6-THC since the double bond has to migrate into that position during the ring opening of the cyclobutane ring (19). On the other hand, on the basis of similar arguments, they thought chrysanthenol should lead directly to delta-1-THC. This was indeed found to be the case albeit the yield was moderate (19).

C. From p-Menthadienol

A facile entry into cannabinoids utilizing (+)-_p_-menthadienol was demonstrated by Petrzilka, et al., in 1967 (15). By condensing the olivetol in the presence of weak and strong acids they obtained (-)-cannabidiol and (-)-delta-6-THC (_2_) respectively. Presumably _2_ was being formed _via_ the intermediates cannabidiol > delta-1-THC > delta-6-THC, since both cannabidiol and delta-1-THC are known to give delta-6-THC in nearly quantitative yields on treatment with _p_-TSA. The delta-6-THC obtained by this procedure was accompanied by many by-products typical of all THC syntheses, and was purified by very careful column chromatography. It was converted to delta-1-THC by the usual procedure of addition and elimination of HCl but these authors improved the yield (claimed 100%) of delta-1-THC in the dehydrochlorination step.

Because of the commercial availability of the starting terpene, (+)-_cis/trans_-_p_-methadienol, this route was further developed by Razdan and co-workers (20) for the preparation of kilogram quantities of _1_ and _2_ at Arthur D. Little, Inc., Cambridge, MA, for the National Institute of Mental Health. They reported that the dehydrochlorination procedure was very sensitive to reaction conditions and showed (glc) that under the best conditions a mixture of 95% _1_ and 5% (-)-delta-1-THC (7) was always obtained. This new THC was completely characterized by isolation from this mixture by chromatography on silver nitrate-silica gel(21).

Razdan, et al., developed a modification of Petrzilka's cannabinoid synthesis utilizing BF_3-Et_2O/CH_2Cl_2 in the presence of $MgSO_4$ as the dehydrating agent (22). By this process delta-1-THC (_1_) of very high optical purity was formed in a simple one-step synthesis in 50% yield (glc) and was isolated in 31% yield after a simple and quick column chromatography (22). The purity of delta-1-THC was > 96% by glc and, in contrast to Petrzilka's process, no delta-6-THC (_2_) is formed under the new conditions. Furthermore, by a slight change in the reaction conditions of the new process, (-)-cannabidiol was obtained on a preparative scale.

D. From Carene Oxides

In 1970, Razdan and Handrick reported an entry into cannabinoids from carene derivatives (23). Treatment of (+)-trans-2-carene oxide and olivetol in the presence of acids gave mainly a mixture of (-)-trans- (1) and (-)-cis-delta-1-THC (3), from which the former was isolated by preparative gas chromatography. As expected, other transformation products such as iso-THCs were also formed during this reaction but no cannabidiol was detected. These results were interpreted as suggesting that the mechanism is different from the p-menthadienol route and that trans- and cis-delta-1-THCs are first formed which are then converted into their transformation products.

Recently, Montero has reported in a thesis that (+)-3-carene oxide and olivetol give delta-6-THC (2) and the corresponding diadduct, on refluxing in benzene with p-TSA (13).

E. From p-Menth-2-ene-1,8-diol

Handrick, et al., (Fig. 2) have recently used another readily available monoterpene p-menth-2-ene-1,8-diol (4) in the synthesis of (-)-delta-1-THC (1) (7). This synthon was selected to facilitate the ring formation at C-8 by the presence of a hydroxyl group rather than a double bond as in p-menthadienol. A variety of catalysts were studied and the best yield of 1 with the least amount of by-products was found to be with anhydrous $ZnCl_2/CH_2Cl_2$. The material was purified by preparative high pressure liquid chromatography (HPLC). Although the quality of 1 was excellent the isolated yield provided no advantage over the p-methadienol route.

Of all the procedures described above, as stated earlier, Petrzilka's process as developed by Razdan and co-workers (20) is presently used in the large scale preparation of delta-1-THC. Modification of Petrzilka's process ($BF_3 \cdot Et_2O/MgSO_4$) by Razdan, et al., (22) has also been developed (24) to produce a 50 g lot of 1 of very high purity. The purification is simplified by using preparative HPLC, thus avoiding large scale column chromatography. At present, this method is being scaled up by the National Cancer Institute.

III. METABOLITES OF TETRAHYDROCANNABINOLS

Extensive literature (1,10,11,28) has appeared in recent years describing the various metabolites of THC isomers isolated from *in vivo* or *in vitro* studies. These have been

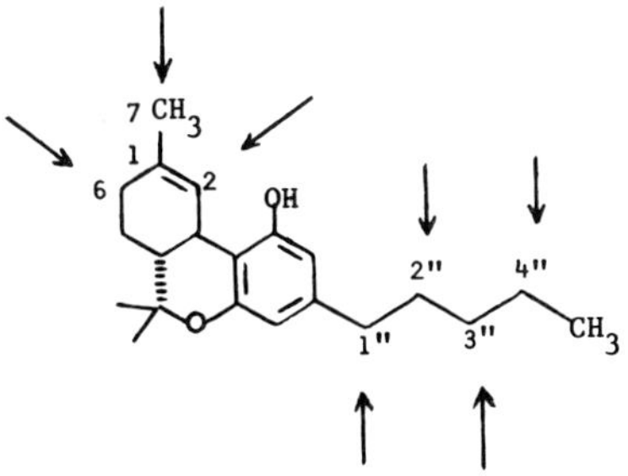

Δ^1 - THC

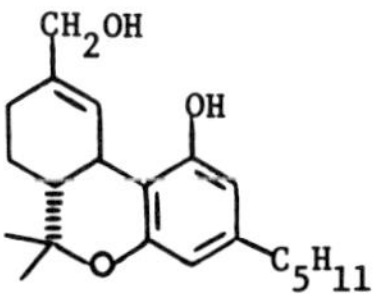

5

equiactive with Δ^1 - THC

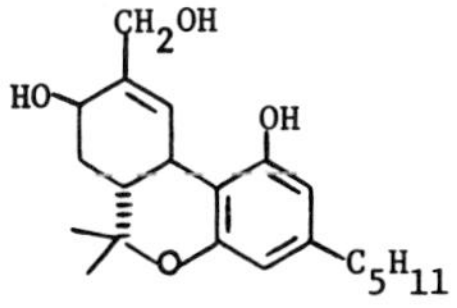

6

a 6 α, inactive

b 6 β ?

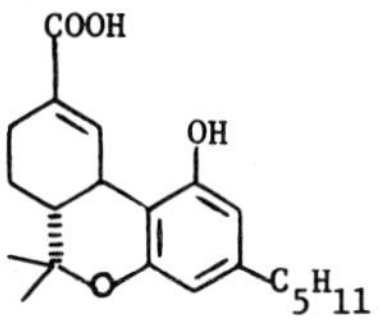

7

inactive

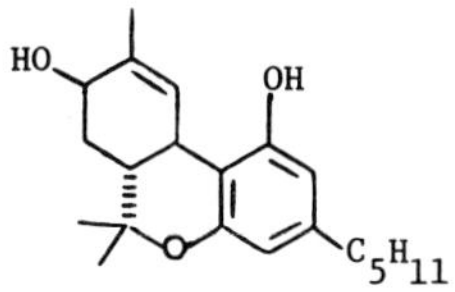

8

a 6α , 1/10th activity

b 6β , 1/4th activity

FIGURE 3. Sites of metabolism and the known metabolites of delta-1-THC in man.

carried out on a wide variety of animal species and in some cases different animal organ homogenates have been utilized. Important sites of metabolism of delta-1- and delta-6-THC and the metabolites of delta-1-THC so far identified in man (27) are shown in Figure 3. The hydroxylation at the 7-position appears to be the major initial point of attack in nearly every species tested, including man. This metabolite, 7-hydroxy-delta-1-THC, is pharmacologically equiactive with delta-1-THC, and still others are active to different degrees. This has complicated the understanding of marijuana activity in man. The problems associated with the synthesis of these metabolites in the delta-1-series are somewhat similar to those encountered in the synthesis of delta-1-THC itself as has already been discussed in the introduction. Thus a number of synthetic procedures which work satisfactorily in the delta-6 series prove to be inadequate in the delta-1 series. For the purpose of this review only the synthesis of delta-1-THC metabolites identified in man are discussed.

For the synthesis of 7-hydroxy-delta-1-THC (5), Pitt, et al., (16) have developed a regioselective route utilizing a base-induced epoxide-allylic alcohol rearrangement followed by SN' displacement (Figure 4). Delta-1-THC acetate was con-

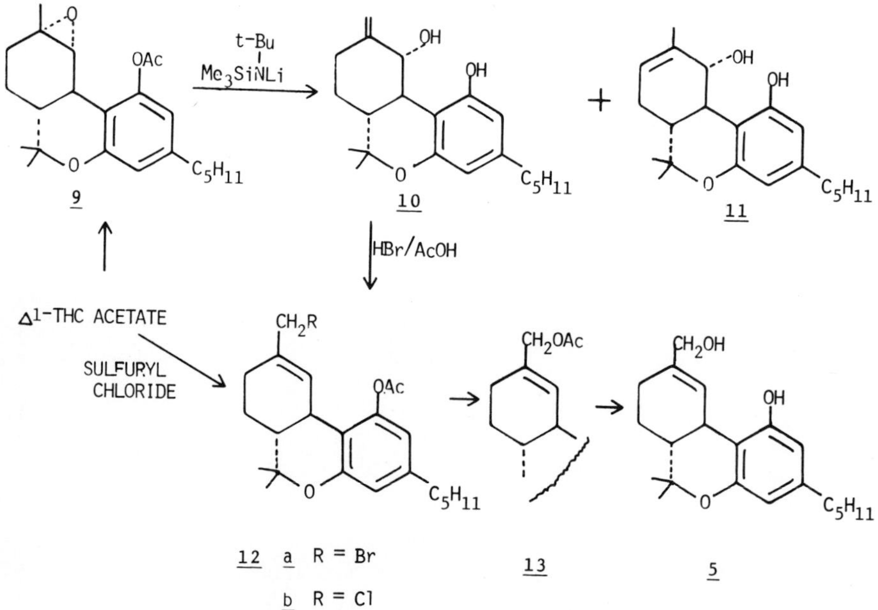

FIGURE 4. Synthesis of 7-hydroxy-delta-1-THC.

verted to the known alpha-epoxide 9 which was isomerized to a mixture of 10 and 11 containing mainly 10. Treatment with 5% HBr/AcOH formed 12a which on acetolysis with tetramethylammonium acetate in acetone followed by reduction with $LiAlH_4$ afforded the desired metabolite 5 in 20% yield. Alternatively, treatment of delta-1-THC acetate with sulfuryl chloride (17) gave a mixture containing 12b, which with silver acetate in acetic acid followed by hydrolysis with base, formed 5, albeit in poor yield (5%). Another metabolite 6-beta-hydroxy-delta-1-THC (8b) was also isolated (14%) from this synthesis.

Pitt, et al., also synthesized the carboxy metabolite 7 by selective acetylation of the phenolic hydroxyl group 5, oxidation (MnO_2,CH_3CN) to the aldehyde, and further oxidation with MnO_2 in methanol containing acetone cyanohydrin (16).

In a different approach, Razdan, et al., (25) (Figure 5) oxidized the exocyclic double bond of (-)-delta-1-THC (7) acetate (4) with m-chloroperbenzoic acid to the epoxide 15 which was hydrolyzed (basic conditions were used to avoid forming the delta-6-dehydration products) with 0.3N KOH/DMSO to form the triol 16. After acetylation, the diacetate alcohol 17 was

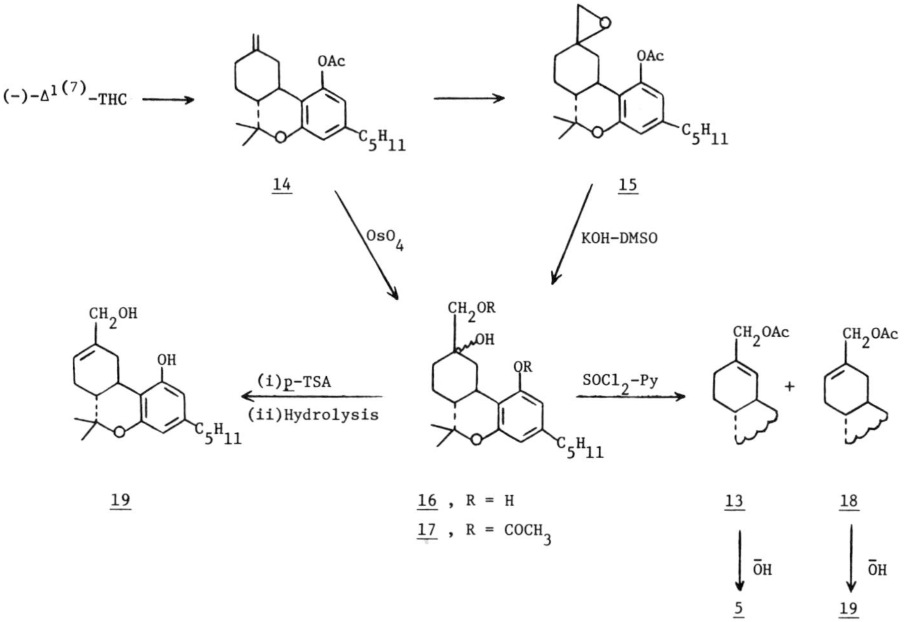

(-)-Δ1(7)-THC → 14 → 15

14 —OsO_4→ 16; 15 —KOH-DMSO→ 16

16 —(i) p-TSA, (ii) Hydrolysis→ 19

16 —$SOCl_2$-Py→ 13 + 18

13 —$\bar{O}H$→ 5; 18 —$\bar{O}H$→ 19

16, R = H
17, R = $COCH_3$

FIGURE 5. Synthesis of 7-hydroxy-delta-1-THC.

treated with $SOCl_2$/Py to give a mixture of the two metabolites as their diacetates 13 and 18. These were separated by HPLC and then hydrolyzed with base to yield 7-hydroxy-delta-1-THC (5). The overall yield of 5 from delta-1(7)-THC was 13%. Alternatively 17 was obtained from 14 by hydroxylation of the exocyclic double bond with OsO_4 in ether followed by acetylation. These syntheses were developed because delta-1(7)-THC became available in large quantities from the kilogram synthesis of delta-1-THC (20,21). The intermediate 17 also provided a facile route to the 7-hydroxy-delta-6-THC 19 (14). This was achieved by treatment with p-TSA followed by hydrolysis (overall yield, 75%).

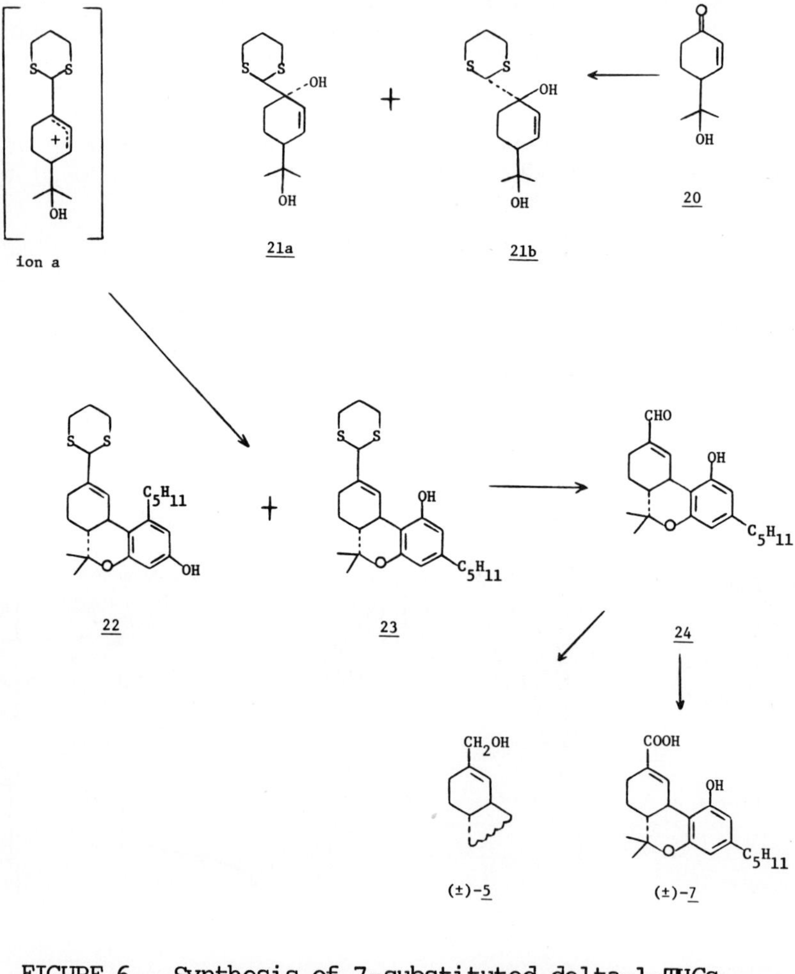

FIGURE 6. Synthesis of 7-substituted delta-1-THCs.

Uliss, et al., have recently reported a versatile route to 7-substituted delta-1-THC from the novel synthons 21a and 21b (26). This scheme (Figure 6) is based on the principal of reversal of reactivity of carbonyl compounds when masked as dithioacetals (i.e., umpolung). Interestingly, this route has resulted in the synthesis of delta-1 derivatives specifically, since, by introduction of the dithiane moiety into the THC structure, isomerization of the normally labile delta-1-unsaturation to the delta-6 isomer is effectively inhibited. The synthons 21a and 21b can be readily synthesized. Treatment with olivetol inthe presence of p-TSA gave amixture of delta-1-compounds 22 and 23 which was separated. The dithiane masking group in 3 was readily removed by HgO/BF_3-Et_2O togive the metabolite (+/−)-2 (3). This was converted by $LiAlH_4$ reduction to the metabolite (+/−)-5 or oxidized with MnO_2/CH_3OH containing acetone cyanohydrin, to the metabolite (+/−)-7 (16).

The SeO_2 oxidation of delta-1-THC acetate followed by $LiAlH_4$ reduction also gave 5 in very poor yield (1%) (2).

The 6-alpha- and 6-beta-hydroxy-delta-1-THCs (8a and 8b) are the two other metabolites which have been identified in man. The latter, 8b was directly prepared (Figure 7) by bro-

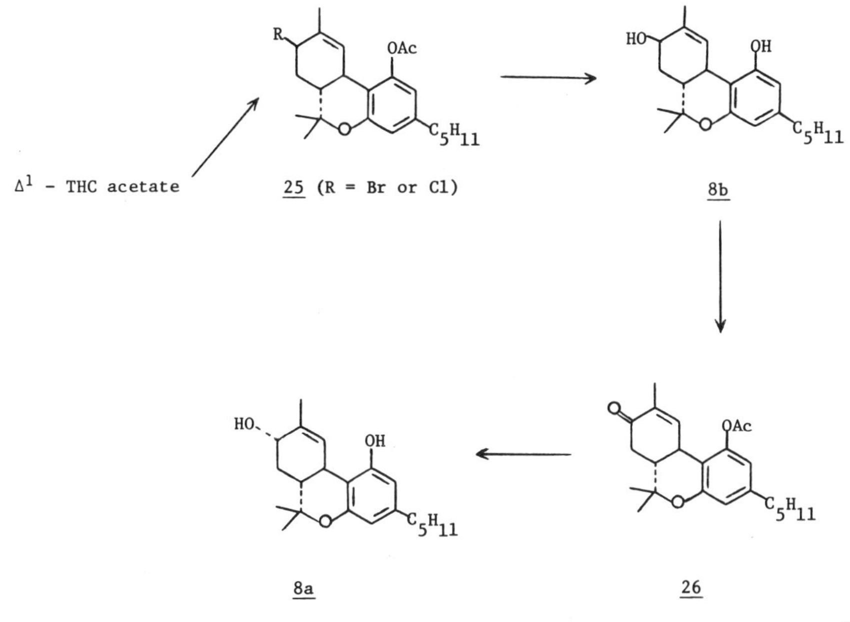

Δ^1 - THC acetate

25 (R = Br or Cl)

8b

8a

26

FIGURE 7. Synthesis of 6-beta-hydroxy-delta-1-THC.

mination of delta-1-THC acetate with N-bromosuccinimide (16) or sulfuryl chloride (17) followed by acetolysis and hydrolysis. The 6-alpha-metabolite 8a was prepared (16) from 8b by selective acetylation of the phenolic group and MnO_2 oxidation to 26 followed by $LiAlH_4$ reduction to 8a. It is interesting to note that 26 was also obtained by SeO_2 oxidation of delta-1-THC acetate.

The two dihydroxy metabolites 6a and 6b have been identified in humans (27) and were synthesized from the epoxide of delta-6-THC acetate (16). The sequence required epoxide-allylic alcohol rearrangement (BuLi), diacetylation, oxidation with OsO_4, acetylation of the primary 7-hydroxy group, dehydration ($SOCl_2$, pyridine) and finally saponification.

A few other metabolites from man have been observed by different workers but as yet none of them have been fully characterized.

Recent work from our laboratory has been directed to enlarge the scope of the versatile thioacetal route we reported (26) to 7-substituted delta-1-THCs from the snythons 21a and 21b (Figure 8). A practical synthesis of (+/-)-2'- and -3'-acetoxy olivetols was developed (5) and these were then converted to the corresponding metabolites (+/-)-2",7-dihydroxy-delta-1-THC, 27 (6) and (+/-)-3",7-dihydroxy-delta-1-THC, 28 (8), respectively, following essentially the sequence as shown in Figure 6. Until now, the metabolites with a functionalization both in the terpene portion and the aromatic side chain have not been synthesized. Thus they represent the first examples of such metabolites belonging to this class.

We have also found (Figure 8) that treatment of cannabidiol as its diacetate with N-bromosuccinimide gave the regiospecifically brominated compound 29 in >80% yield. Reaction with base including bicarbonate formed the novel delta-1-THC cannabinoid 30 (9). The 10-bromo-cannabidiol diacetate (29) is a key intermediate which has led to the synthesis of several 10-amino analogs of cannabidiol.

IV. SAR IN CANNABINOIDS

Based on CNS pharmacological profiles in laboratory animals the overall Structure-Activity Relationships (SAR) are summarized below:

1. Essentially a benzopyran structure with an aromatic hydroxyl group at 2'-position and an alkyl or alkoxyl group on the 4'-position are a requirement for activity.

2. The position and the environment around the aromatic hydroxyl group are very important for activity, viz.:

a. the OH at position C-2' is in itself necessary for CNS activity.
b. esterification of the phenol retains whereas etherification eliminates activity. Replacement of the OH by NH_2 retains while SH eliminates activity.
c. methyl substituents at C-2 in the alicyclic ring can significantly influence the CNS activity.

3. Substitution in the aromatic ring by electronegative groups, such as COOH or acetyl, eliminates activity, whereas alkyl and OH retain activity.

4. A minimum length of the aromatic side chain is a requirement for activity. Branching of the side chain, increases potency.

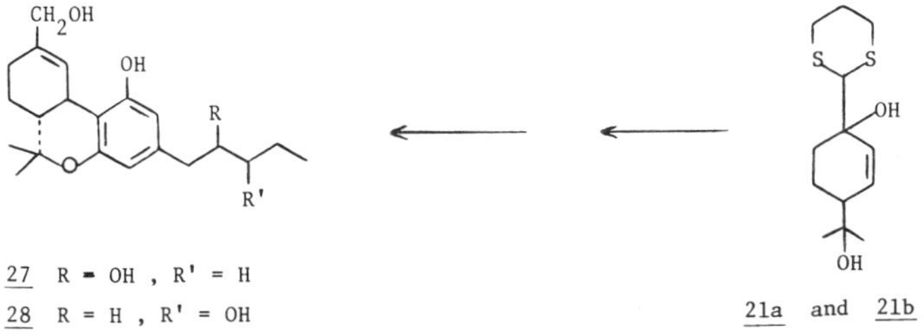

CH_2OH OH R R'

27 R = OH , R' = H
28 R = H , R' = OH

S S OH OH

21a and 21b

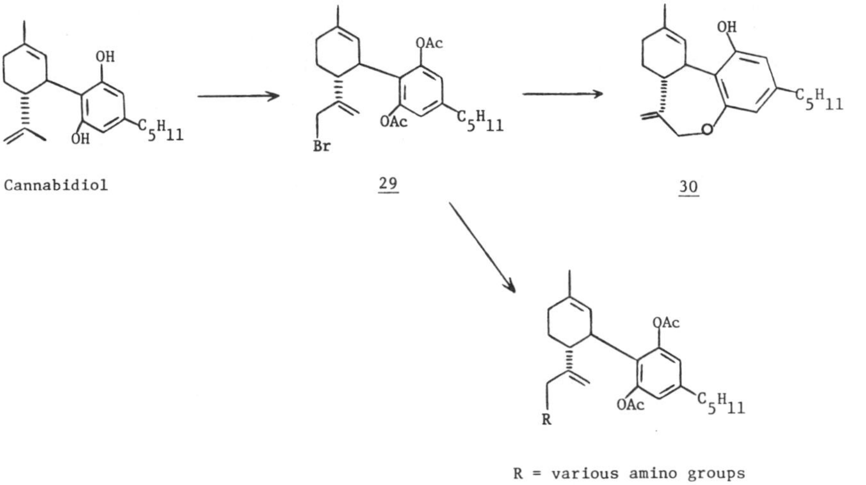

OH OH C_5H_{11}

Cannabidiol

OAc OAc C_5H_{11} Br

29

OH C_5H_{11}

30

OAc OAc C_5H_{11} R

R = various amino groups

FIGURE 8. Synthesis of various THC derivatives. In last structure, R = various amino groups.

5. The gem-dimethyl group in the pyran-ring is optimum for activity. Replacement of pyran O by N and ring expansion by one carbon can retain activity.

6. In the alicyclic ring the position of the double bond in delta-1-, -6-, or -3-THC retains activity. A 3,4-trans junction increases and a cis junction decreases activity. The natural THCs are active in the 3R,4R series only. A methyl at C-1 increases activity but metabolism to the 7-hydroxymethyl is not a pre-requisite for THC activity.

7. The alicylic ring can be substituted by a variety of nitrogen and sulfur-containing rings without loss of CNS activity. With the nitrogen and sulfur analogs, the optimum CNS activity is obtained when the heteroatom is in a phenethyl orientation, i.e., inserted in place by C-1 or C-5.

8. Planarity of the alicyclic ring is not a necessary criterion for activity.

9. In both carbocyclic and heterocyclic analogs, opening the pyran ring generally decreases activity.

REFERENCES

1. Burstein, S., in "Cannabinoid Analysis in Physiological Fluids", ACS Symposium Series 98, (J. A. Vinson, ed.). American Chemical Society, Washington, D. C., 1979.
2. Ben-Zvi, Z., Mechoulam, R., and Burstein, S., Synthesis of delta-1- and delta-1(6)-tetrahydrocannabinol metabolites, Tetrahedron Lett. 4495-4497 (1970).
3. Ben-Zvi, Z., Burstein, S., 7-oxo-delta-1-tetrahydrocannabinol: a novel metabolite of delta-1-tetrahydrocannabinol, Res. Commun. Pathol. Pharmacol. 8:223-2239 (1974).
4. Dev, S., and Prasad, R. S., Chemistry of ayurvedic crude drugs, Tetrahedron 32:1437-1441 (1976) and references cited therein.
5. Duffley, R. P., Handrick, G. R., Uliss, D. B., Lambert, G., Dalzell, H. C., and Razdan, R. K., Synthesis of 2'-and3'-acetoxyolivetols [5-(2- and 3-acetoxypentyl)-1,3-benzenediols]: Key intermediates in the synthesis of tetrahydrocannabinolderivatives, Synth.733-736 (1980).
6. Duffley, R. P., Lambert, G., Dalzell, H. C., and Razdan, R. K., Hashish: Synthesis of (+/-)-2',11-dihydroxy-delta-9-tetrahydrocannabinol (THC), a metabolite of delta-9-THC. Experientia 37:931-932 (1981).
7. Handrick, G. R., Uliss, D. B., Dalzell, H. C., and Razdan, R. K., Hashish: Synthesis of (-)-delta-9-tetrahydrocannabinol (THC) and its biologically potent metabolite 3'-hydroxy-delta-9-THC, Tetrahedron Lett. 681-684 (1979).

8. Handrick, G. R., Duffley, R. P., Lambert, G., Murphy, J. G., Dalzell, H. C., Howes, J. F., Razdan, R. K., Martin, B. R., Harris, L. S., and Dewey, W. L., 3'-Hydroxy- and (+/-)-3',11-dihydroxy-delta-9-tetrahydrocannabinol (THC); Biologically active metabolites of delta-9-THC, J. Med. Chem. 25:000 (1982).
9. Jorapur, V. S., Khalil, Z. H., Duffley, R. P., and Razdan, R. K., Hashish: Synthesis of a novel delta-9-tetrahydrocannabinol (THC) analog, Chem. Lett. 299-302 (1982).
10. Mechoulam, R. (ed.), "Marijuana, Chemistry, Pharmacology, Metabolism and Clinical Effects". Academic Press, New York, 1973.
11. Mechoulam, R., McCallum, N. K., and Burstein, S., Recent advances in the chemistry and biochemistry of cannabis, Chem. Rev. 76:75-112 (1976).
12. Mechoulam, R., Braun, P., and Gaoni, Y., Synthesis of delta-1-tetrahydrocannabinol and related cannabinoids, J. Amer. Chem. Soc. 94:6159-6165 (1972).
13. Montero, J. L., Ph. D. Thesis, Chromenes derivant de la phloroacetophenone; syntheses d'analogues et d'isosteres des cannabinoids. University of Lanqudoc, Montpelier, France; Chem. Abstr. 80:44430d (1976).
14. Nilsson, J. L. G., Nilsson, I. M., Agurell, S., Kermark, B. A., and Lagerlund, I, Metabolism of Cannabis XI: Synthesis of delta-7-tetrahydrocannabinol and 7-hydroxy-tetrahydrocannabinol, Acta Chem. Scand. 25:768-769 (1971).
15. Petrzilka,T., Haefliger, W., and Sikemeier, C., Synthese von haschisch-inhaltsstoffen, Helv. Chim. Acta. 52:1102-1134 91969).
16. Pitt, C. G., Fowler, M. S., Sathe, S., Sirivastava, S. C., and Williams, D. L., Synthesis of metabolites of delta-9-tetrahydrocannabinol, J. Am. Chem. Soc. 97:3798-3802 (1975).
17. Pitt, C. G., Hauser, F., Hawks, R. L., Sathe, S., and Wall, M. E., Synthesis of 11-hydroxy-delta-9-tetrahydrocannabinol, J. Amer. Chem. Soc. 94:8578-8579 (1972).
18. Razdan, R. K., in "Progress in Organic Chemistry", Vol. 8, (W. Carruthers, J. K. Sutherland, eds.). Butterworths, London, 1973.
19. Razdan, R. K., Handrick, G. R., and Dalzell, H. C., A one-step synthesis of (-)-delta-1-tetrahydrocannabinol from chrysanthenol, Experientia 31:16 (1975).
20. Razdan, R. K., Woodland, L. R., and Handrick, G. R., Large scale synthesis of (-)-trans-6a,10a-delta-8- and -delta-9-tetrahydrocannabinols, Arthur D.Little, Inc., Technical Report 3, to National Institute of Mental Health, Contract Ph-43-68-1339, January, 1972.

21. Razdan, R. K., Puttick, A. J., Zitko, B. A, and Handrick, G. R., Hashish VI: Conversion of (-)-delta-1(6)-tetrahydrocannabinol to (-)-delta-1(7)-tetrahydrocannabinol, Experientia 28:121-122 (1972).
22. Razdan, R. K., Dalzell, H. C., and Handrick, G. R., Hashish; a simple one-step synthesis of(-)-delta-1-tetrahydrocannabinol (THC) from p-mentha-2-,8-dien-1-ol and olivetol. J. Amer. Chem. Soc. 96:5860-5865 (1974).
23. Razdan, R. K., and Handrick, G. R., Hashish, A stereospecific synthesis of (-)-delta-1- and (-)-delta-1(6)-tetrahydrocannabinols, J. Amer. Chem. Soc. 92:6061-6062 (1970).
24. Razdan, R. K., Unpublished results from our laboratory.
25. Razdan, R. K., Uliss, D. B. and Dalzell, H. C., Hashish: Synthesis of 7-hydroxy-delta-1-tetrahydrocannabinol (THC); An important active metabolite of delta-1-THC in man, J. Amer. Chem. Soc. 95:2361-2362 (|973).
26. Uliss, D. B., Handrick, G. R., Dalzell, H. C., and Razdan, R. K., A terpenic synthon for delta-1-cannabinoids, J. Amer. Chem. Soc. 100:2929-2930 (1978).
27. Wall, M. E., Brine, D. R., Pitt, C. G., and Perez-Reyes, M., Identification of delta-9-tetrahydrocannabinol and metabolites in man, J. Amer. Chem. Soc. 94:8579-8581 (1972).
28. Wall, M. E., and Brine, D. R., in "Marihuana: Chemistry, Biochemistry and Cellular Effects" (G. G. Nahas, W. D. Paton, and J. E. Indanpaan-Heikkila, eds.). Springer-Verlag, New York, 1976.

SEPARATION OF ACID AND NEUTRAL CANNABINOIDS IN CANNABIS SATIVA L. USING HPLC*

Jocelyn C. Turner
Paul G. Mahlberg

Department of Biology
Indiana University
Bloomington, Indiana

I. INTRODUCTION

Chemobotanical studies in our laboratory on the site of cannabinoid synthesis in the *Cannabis* plant required a method for an accurate assessment of the cannabinoid profile. Previous methods primarily involved use of gas-liquid chromatography (GLC) (1,2). Because the majority of cannabinoids are present in the plant are found in the acid form, they cannot be directly detected by GLC due to thermal decarboxylation. High-performance liquid chromatography (HPLC) is able to detect directly both acidic and neutral cannabinoids. However, methods published to date were found to be inadequate for our use (3,4). The abundance of compounds in samples extraced from plant material made their analyses complex, and necessiated development of a more definitive method for determining cannabinoid profiles in plant samples.

II. MATERIALS AND METHODS

A. Plant Material

Compound leaves, with a 7.5 cm center leaflet, were collected for analysis from vegetative plants of a clone of a

*Supported by Dept. of Agriculture grant 53-32R6-1-84.

ISBN 0-12-044620-0

drug strain (152) routinely used in our investigations (5-8). The clone provides a source of genetically stable material on a year-round basis, and is grown in a greenhouse heated and cooled seasonally as required for the Indiana climate. Plants are maintained on a 20 hr day to insure vegetative growth.

B. Cannabinoid Extraction

Fresh leaf samples were extracted within 1 hr of being collected. After leaves had been extracted, they were dried in a 60°C oven for 24 hr and then weighed to determine dry weight. To extract cannabinoids, fresh leaf samples were placed in glass test tubes and approximately 1 ml "ChromAR" grade chloroform (Mallinckrodt) was added to each sample. After 1 hr, the extract was removed and filtered. The extraction procedure was repeated twice for a total of 3 times, and the combined filtrates for each sample were evaporated under a gentle stream of nitrogen. All steps were done at 4°C. Each sample was then resuspended in 100% ethanol containing two internal standards (eicosane and di-n-octyl phthalate), each at a concentration of 0.25 mg/ml.

C. High-performance Liquid Chromatography

Analyses were performed on a Hewlett-Packard 1084B HPLC equipped with a single-wavelength UV detector set at 254 nm. A reverse-phase Altex column (Ultrasil-octyl, 10 micron; 25 cm X 4.6mm ID) was used. The eluting solvents were acetonitrile (Burdick & Jackson, UV grade) and water. Water utilized was deionized, processed through a Lobar RP-8 size B (EM Reagents) column (9), and then filtered through a Gelman GA-6, 0.45 um filter on a Millipore all-glass filtering system. Samples were filtered with BAS Microfilters equipped with 1 mcm regenerated cellulose filters (Bioanalytical Systems, Inc.). For cannabinoid analysis, the instrument was programmed to pump a gradient starting with 25% acetonitrile at time 0 and reaching 85% acetonitrile at 35 min. Flow rate was 2 ml/min and oven temperature was 40°C. Sample size was generally 20 mcl.

D. Gas-liquid Chromatography

Analyses were performed on a Hewlett-Packard 5710A gas chromatograph equipped with a hydrogen flame ionization detector and a Hewlett-Packard 3380A integrator. Cannabinoid standards provided by NIDA were chromatographed and the integrator calibrated the columns using the internal standard method.

Glass columns (2 mm ID X 2.43 m) were cleaned, treated with 8% dimethyldichlorosilane in toluene, dried, and packed with 3% OV-1 or 3% OV-17 on 100/120 mesh Supelcoport. The inlet and detector temperatures were 250°C and 350°C, respectively. Nitrogen was used as the carrier gas with a flow rate of 20 ml/min. Samples injected consisted of 1 lambda aliquots and were analyzed on both the OV-1 and OV-17 columns. For the OV-1 column, a program of 200-240°C at 2°C/min with an additional 8 min isothermal period at 240°C was used. For the OV-17 column, the program was isothermal at 260°C for 15 min.

E. Heated Samples

Following analysis of fresh plant extracts by HPLC and GLC, samples were evaporated and heated, essentially using the method of Kanter et al. (10). Dry samples were placed in an oven at 200°C for 3 min. Samples were then removed, allowed to cool to room temperature and resuspended in ethanol to their original volume.

III. RESULTS AND DISCUSSION

A. HPLC Program

Initially, the method of Wheals and Smith was used to determine cannabinoid profiles in plant samples (3). Their HPLC method involved the use of methanol and 0.02 N sulfuric acid (80:20) at a flow rate of 2 ml/min. While this was quite adequate for separating cannabinoid standards (all neutral), the presence of additional extracted compounds made plant material more difficult to chromatograph. The Wheals and Smith isocratic method provided separation of cannabinoids in approximately 5 min, but plant samples contained a number of non-cannabinoid compounds that also chromatographed in the same region as the cannabinoids. Since it is desirable for our studies to analyze samples efficiently with little, if any, pretreatment, we therefore investigated other HPLC programs. We found that use of a gradient solvent system over a longer period of time could efficiently separate neutral cannabinoid standards (Fig. 1). At the same time, the gradient program allowed other plant compounds to chromatograph at retention times different from those of the cannabinoids, thus effectively separating cannabinoids from other plant compounds (Fig. 2). Therefore, our current method uses water and acetonitrile, beginning with 25% acetonitrile and progressing to 85% acetonitrile by 35 min.

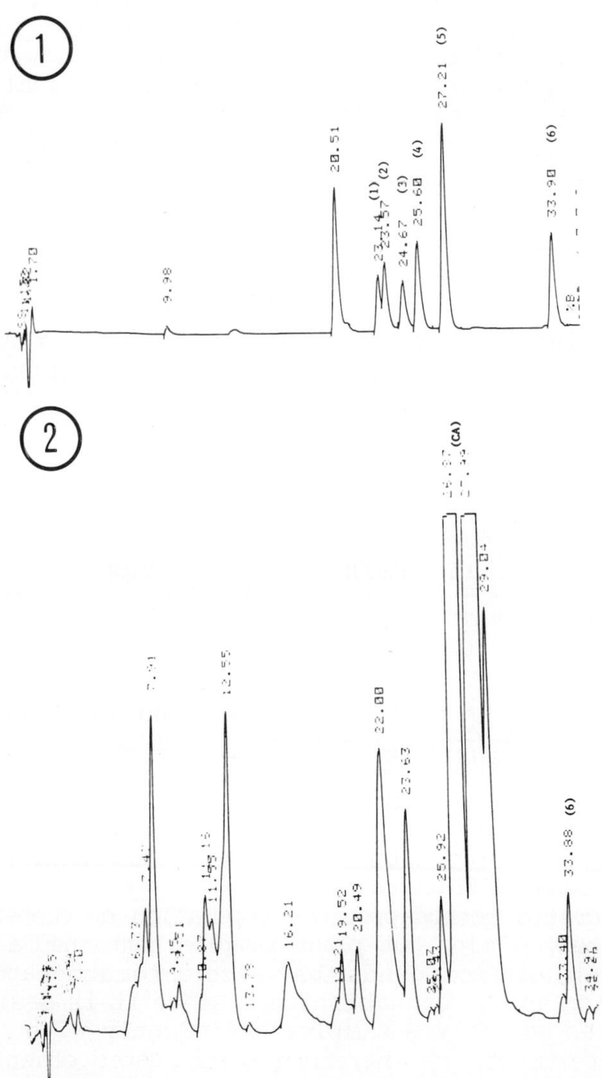

FIGURE 1. Chromatogram of a mixture of neutral cannabinoid standards. Water solvent at pH 2.7. Peaks: (1) CBD; (2) CBG; (3) CBN; (4) THC; (5) CBC; and (6) di-n-octyl phthalate (internal standard, IS). The peak at RT 20.51 is a second IS.

FIGURE 2. Chromatogram of plant extract (clone 152). Water solvent at pH 2.7. (CA) cannabinoid acids; (6) IS. No neutral cannabinoids were detected.

B. Solvent pH

The cannabinoids were chromatographed by the solvent gradient at unique retention times as compared to other plant components. Since acidic cannabinoids are the predominate form in living Cannabis plants, the separation of acid from neutral cannabinoids in plant material presented an additional problem. Large peaks of acidic cannabinoids occurred in the retention time region of the neutral forms, as determined from standards, and engulfed the small peaks of any neutral cannabinoids present (Fig. 2). Previous HPLC studies on marijuana had not encountered this problem since normal drying procedures had decarboxylated many of the acidic cannabinoids to the neutral form.

In order to detect and distinguish between acid and neutral cannabinoids, we changed the pH of the water solvent. It was found that an increase in water solvent pH resulted in a decrease in the retention time of cannabinoid acids (Figs. 3,4). To confirm the identity of the more rapidly eluted peaks as cannabinoid acids, the large peak area was collected from the HPLC using a fraction collector. Compounds present in the collected material were analyzed both by GLC and gas chromatography-mass spectrometry (GC/MS) and the presence of cannabinoids was confirmed (11). Cannabinoid acids cannot be directly detected by GLC or GC/MS due to thermal decarboxylation. It was assumed that the large moveable peaks were indeed acidic cannabinoids since cannabinoids were also confirmed in peaks at retention times corresponding to those found for neutral cannabinoid standards. Neutral cannabinoids were found to have stable retention times with regard to changes in solvent pH (Figs. 3,4). The other unknown peaks in the sample, also stable with regard to changes in solvent pH, were collected as separate fractions and found to contain no cannabinoids.

C. Heated Samples

Since cannabinoid acids decarboxylate upon being heated, this property was used to evaluate further the components of the peak determined to contain cannabinoid acids. Prior to heating, plant samples were anlayzed and the large cannabinoid acid peak was present (Fig. 5), while neutral cannabinoids were not detected. Acid cannabinoids represent the form primarily present in the living plant. The presence of neutral cannabinoids in plant samples analyzed by HPLC was found to reflect the method of sample preparation (12). A sample drying temperature of 60°C or prolonged drying at room temperature prior to extraction can result in decarboxylation of

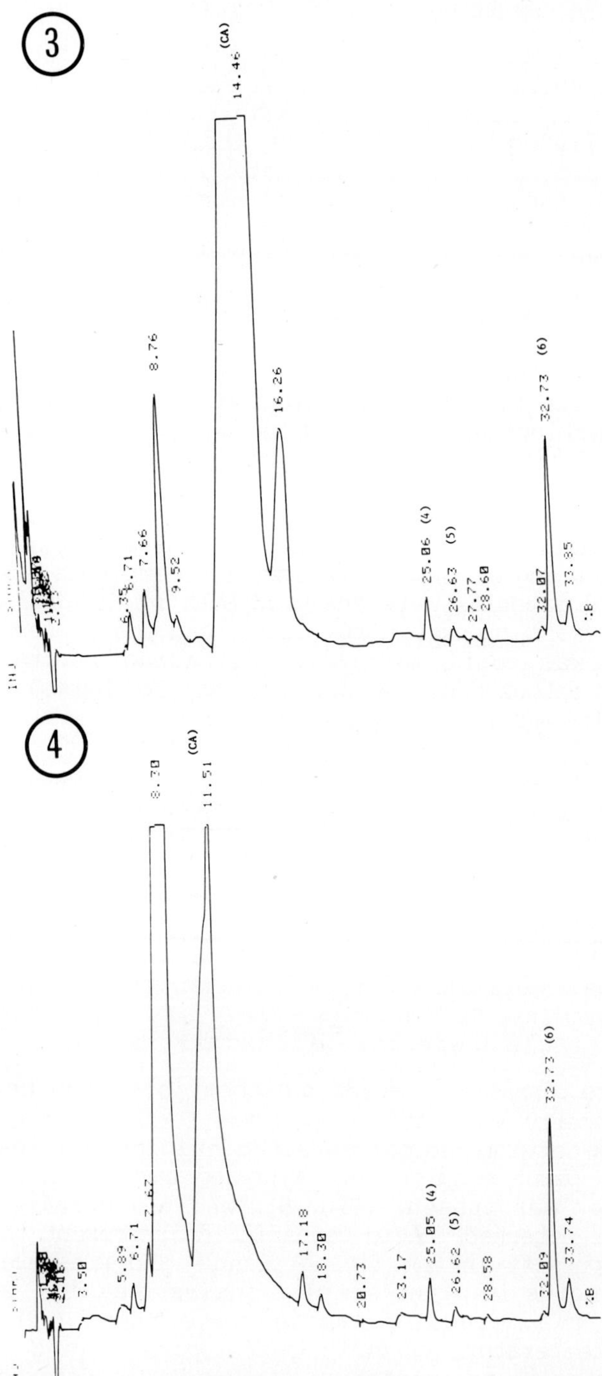
3
14.46 (CA)
8.76
16.26
32.73 (6)
6.35
6.71
7.66
9.52
25.06 (4)
26.63 (5)
27.77
28.60
32.07
33.85
4
8.70
11.51 (CA)
32.73 (6)
3.50
5.89
6.71
7.67
17.18
18.30
20.73
23.17
25.05 (4)
26.62 (5)
28.58
32.09
33.74

acid forms resulting in detectable levels of neutral cannabinoids in HPLC analyses (Figs. 3,4). After analyzing the unheated plant extract, it was then heated and reanalyzed. The large cannabinoid acid peak disappeared and significant amount of neutral cannabinoids were detected (Fig. 6). The fact that the large peaks previously determined to be cannabinoid acids disappeared after sample heating and neutral cannabinoid peaks appeared provides additional confirmation that the peaks were indeed cannabinoid acids. It also indicates that heating plant extracts to transform acid to neutral forms can be used as a procedure to quantify cannabinoids.

D. GLC Analyses

Plant samples were analyzed both by GLC and HPLC prior to heating the sample, and then again after the sample had been heated. Table I shows the quantities of cannabinoids detected. Using GLC, the amount of neutral cannabinoids detected in plant extracts and heated extracts was essentially the same. For GLC analyses, we routinely chromatograph samples on each of 2 columns. The OV-1 column separates cannabidiol (CBD) and cannabichromene (CBC) relatively well, provides excellent separation of delta-8-tetrahydrocannabinol (8-THC) and delta-9-THC (9-THC) and co-chromatographs cannabigerol (CBG) and cannabinol (CBN). The OV-17 column separates CBG distinctly from CBN, provides excellent separation of 8-THC and 9-THC, and separates CBD and CBC rather poorly. HPLC analysis in parallel with GLC reconfirms the presence of the above compounds in any given sample since CBD, CBN, and CBC are well separated. CBG chromatographs close to CBD and 8-THC cochromatographs with 9-THC. Since neutral cannabinoids may not be present in the living plant, plant extracts must be heated in order to quantitate the cannabinoid acids as decarboxylated neutral forms. While quantities compare well to those found for GLC analyses of the same sample (Table I), it is still unclear whether each cannabinoid acid, when decarboxylated by thermal treatment, is actually converted to its neutral form.

FIGURE 3. Chromatogram of plant extract (clone 152) dried at 60°C for 24 hr prior to extraction. Water solvent at pH 4.0. (CA) cannabinoid acids; (4) THC; (5) CBC; (6) IS.

FIGURE 4. Same sample analyzed in Fig. 3, but water solvent was at pH 6.0.

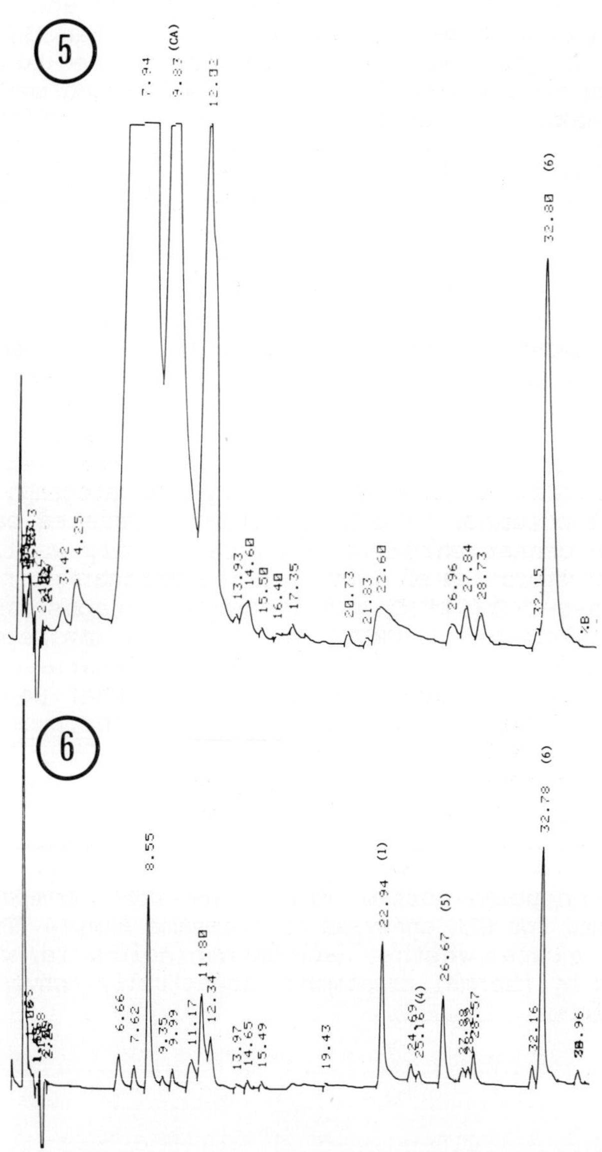

FIGURE 5. Chromatogram of plant extract (clone 152). Water solvent at pH 5.0. (CA) cannabinoid acids; (6) IS.

FIGURE 6. Same sample analyzed in Fig. 5, except that it was heated. (1) CBD; (4) THC; (5) CBC; (6) IS.

IV. COMMENTS AND CONCLUSIONS

Previously, accurate cannabinoid profiles of plant extracts only could be obtained by heating (10,13) or derivatization (2). The HPLC method we have developed provides efficient evaluaton of a plant sample with no pretreatment other than the actual extraction. We can definitively determine the presence of both acid and neutral cannabinoids, although individual cannabinoid acids have yet to be identified in our program. Also, while neutral cannabinoids are easily quantitated both GLC and HPLC, quantitation is not yet applicable with acidic cannabinoids. If the assumption is made that each cannabinoid acid decarboxylates directly to its neutral form on a one to one basis, then heating plant extracts would provide an easy method for quantification. However, the correctness of this assumption has yet to be demonstrated.

The ability to change cannabinoid acid retention times by adjusting solvent pH while neutral cannabinoid peaks remain stable has additional merits. For one, the peaks can be manipulated so as not to interfere with other compounds being chromatographed. Also, by rechromatographing the same sample but using a different solvent pH each time, cannabinoid acid peaks can be moved to reveal previously hidden peaks. In addition, the fact that the peak moves provides an indication of its identity as an acid cannabinoid. All other compounds found so far in chromatograms of Cannabis extracts are stable with changes in solvent pH.

TABLE I. GLC and HPLC Analyses of Cannabinoids Present in Fresh and Subsequently Heated Plant Extracts

		Total Cannabinoids (mg/100 mg dw)	
		Neutral	Acid
Fresh extract:	GLC	0.92	--[a]
	HPLC	ND[b]	CA[c]
Heated extract:	GLC	0.88	--
	HPLC	0.82	ND

[a]Cannabinoid acids are not detected by GLC.
[b]No neutral cannabinoids detected.
[c]Cannabinoid acids detected.

In summary, the acidic cannabinoids can be identified and isolated from plant materials by HPLC, as verified by GLC and GC-MS. A solvent gradient program, using the water solvent at pH 5.0, is now in routine use in our laboratory. The mobility of acid cannabinoids in contrast to neutral forms and other compounds was used to advantage to separate acid cannabinoids. Further studies are needed to identify individual cannabinoid acids, as well as to determine definitively whether cannabinoid acids are the only form present in living plants.

REFERENCES

1. Fetterman, P. S., Doorenbos, N. J., Keith, E. S., and Quimby, M. W., Experentia 27:988 (1971).
2. Turner, C. E., Hadley, K. W., Henry, J., and Mole, M. L., J. Pharm. Sci. 63:1872 (1974).
3. Wheals, B. B., and Smith, R. N., J. Chromatogr. 105:396 (1975).
4. Smith, R. N., J. Chromatogr. 115:101 (1975).
5. Turner, J. C., Hemphill, J. K., and Mahlberg, P. G., Amer. J. Bot. 64:687 (1977).
6. Turner, J. C., Hemphill, J. K., and Mahlberg, P. G., Amer. J. Bot. 65:1103 (1978).
7. Turner, J. C., Hemphill, J. K., and Mahlberg, P. G., Amer. J. Bot. 67:1397 (1980).
8. Lanyon, V. S., Turner, J. C., and Mahlberg, P. G., Bot. Gaz. 142:316 (1981).
9. Gurkin, M., and Ripphahn, J., Amer. Lab. 12:99 (1980).
10. Kanter, S. L., Musumeci, M. R., and Hollister, L. E., J. Chromatogr. 171:504 (1979).
11. Turner, J. C., and Mahlberg, P. G., J. Chromatogr. in press (1982).
12. Turner, J. C., and Mahlberg, P. G., Amer. J. Bot. Submitted (1982).
13. Kimura, M., and Okamoto, K., Experentia 26:819 (1970).

CONSTITUENTS OF CANNABIS SATIVA L. XXIIII: CANNABITETROL, A NEW POLYHYDROXYLATED CANNABINOID[1]

Hala N. ElSohly
Edward G. Boeren[2]
Carlton E. Turner[3]
Mamoud A. ElSohly

Research Institute of Pharmaceutical Sciences
School of Pharmacy
University of Miississippi
University, Mississippi

I. INTRODUCTION

Cannabis sativa L. contains many classes of chemical constituents, the most important of which are the cannabinoids. To date, 61 cannabinoids have been isolated from Cannabis (1). Cannabinoids were defined by Mechoulam and Gaoni (2) "as the group of C_{21} compounds typical of and present in Cannabis sativa, their carboxylic acids, analogs, and transformation products." The 61 cannabinoids can be broken down as follows:

a - Cannabigerol (CBG) type: 6 known
b - Cannabichromene (CBCtype: 4 known
c - Cannabidiol (CBD) type: 7 known
d - delta-9-Tetrahydrocannabinoltype: 9 known
e - delta-8-Tetrahydrocannabinoltype: 2 known
f - Cannabicyclol (CBL) type: 3 known
g - Cannabielsoin (CBE) type: 3 known

---

[1]Supported in part by NIDA contract No. 271-81-3803 and the Research Institute of Pharmaceutical Sciences.
[2]Current address: Packard-Becker B.V., Subsidiary of Ambac International Corporation, Delft, The Netherlands.
[3]Currently on leave.

ISBN 0-12-044620-0

h - Cannabinol (CBN) type: 6 known:
i - Cannabinodiol (CBND) type: 2 known
j - Cannabitriol (CBT) type: 6 known
k - Miscellaneous types: 9 known
l - Other cannabinoids: 4 known

This work will report the details for the isolation and tentative structure of a new polyhydroxylated cannabinoids which was named cannabitetrol (I), and will review the type of polyhydroxylated cannabinoids isolated from Cannabis, e.g., the cannabitriols (V-X), cannabiripsol (XI) and 8-hydroxy-iso-hexahydrocannabivarin (XII). (-)-Cannabirtiol or (-)-CBO (V), (+)-cannabitriol or (+)-CBO (VI), (+/-)-9,10dihydroxy-delta-6a(10a)-tetrahydrocannabinol (VII), (-)-10-ethoxy-9-hydroxy-delta-6a(10a)-tetrahydrocannabinol (IX) and cannabidiolic acid tetrahydrocannabitriol ester (ester at the 9-hydroxy group with cannabidiolic acid, CBDA-CBO) (X) make up the subclass of cannabinoids called cannabitriols.

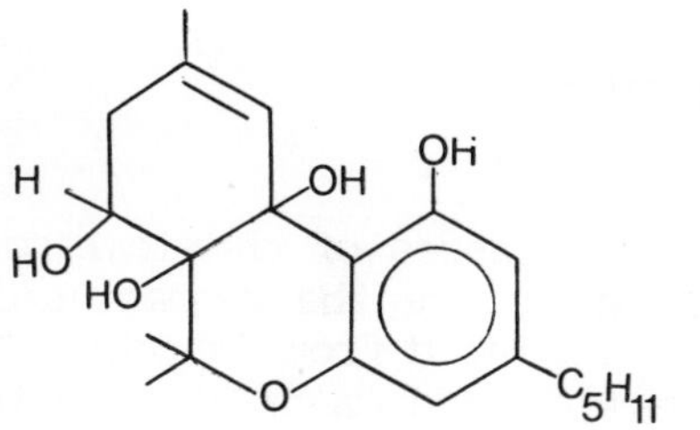

I

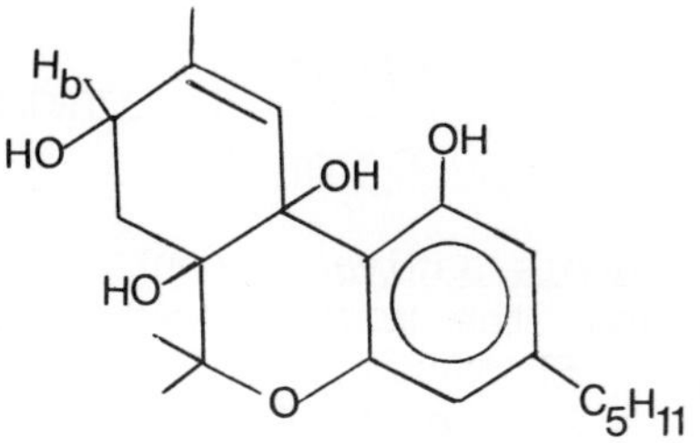

II

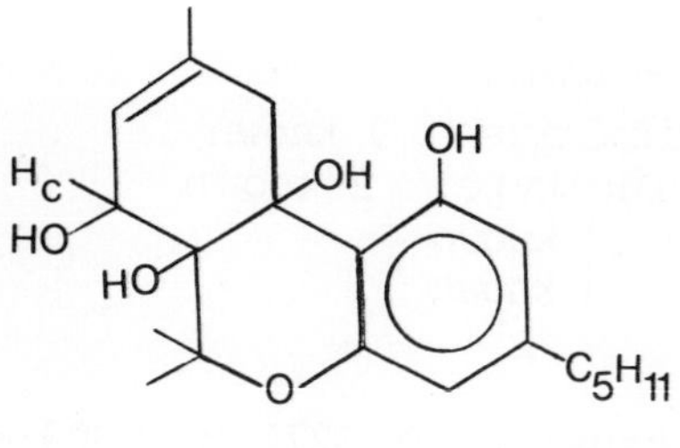

III

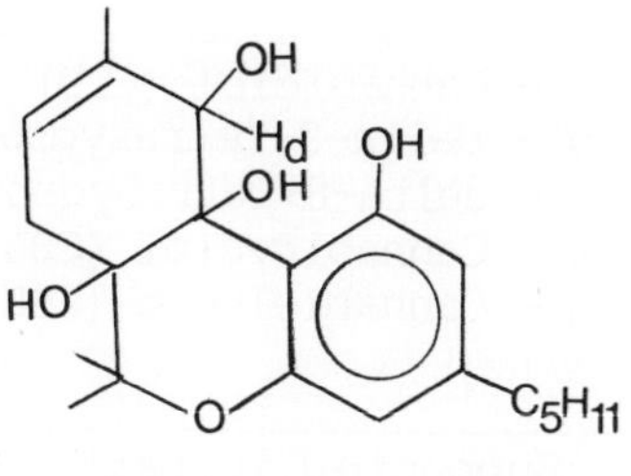

IV

The name cannabitriol was first proposed by Obata and Ishikawa in 1966 for a compound they isolated from Japanese hemp (3). This compound had a mp of 170-172° and gave a positive test with Gibb's reagent. Structural parameters were not such that Obta and Ishikawa proposed a structure. In 1976, Chan, et al., obtained (-)-cannabitriol from the benzene

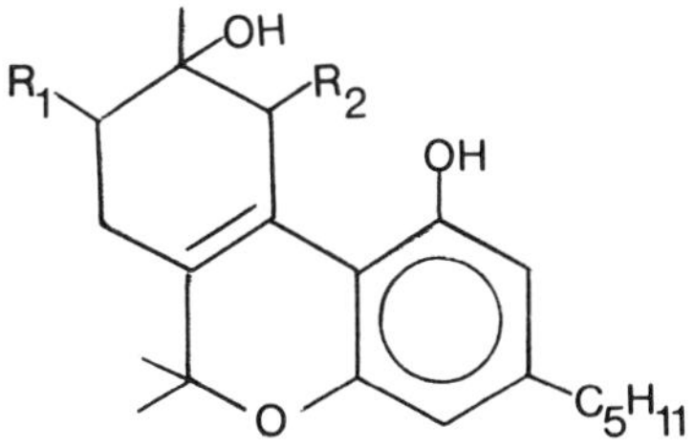

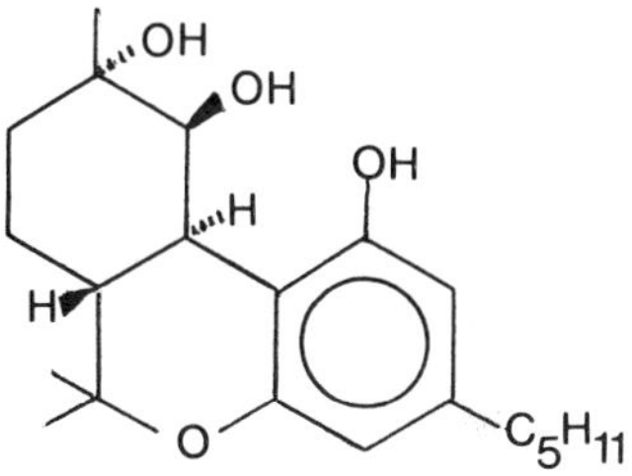

V	R_1=H	R_2=OH
VI	R_1=H	R_2=OH
VII	R_1=H	R_2=OH
VIII	R_1=H	R_2=OEt
IX	R_1=OH	R_2=H

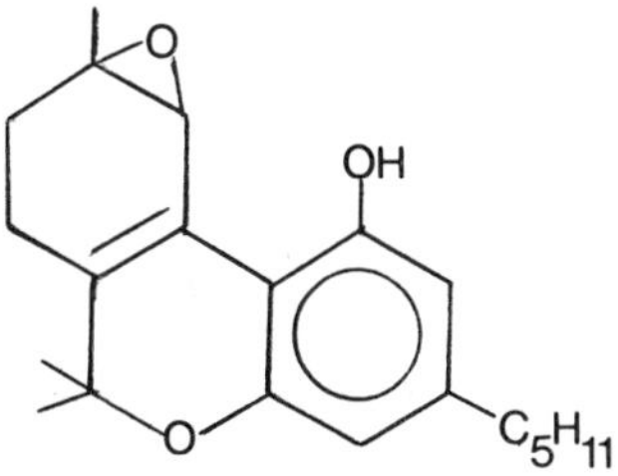

XI

XIII

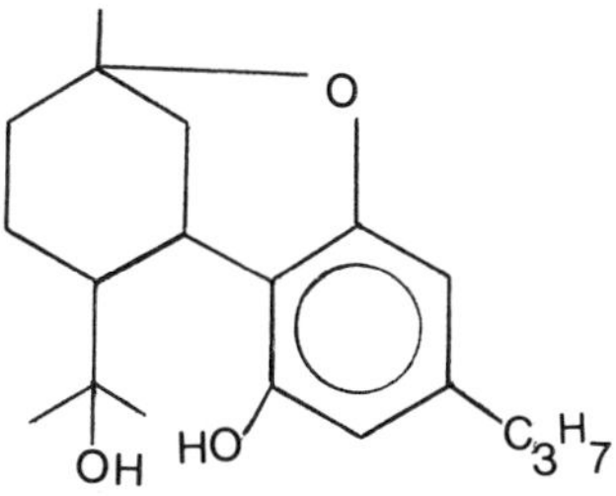

XII

extract of the dried leaves, twigs, and flowering tops of Jamaican ganja in a 0.025% yield (4). (+)-Cannabitriol was reported in 1977 by ElSohly, et al., from an ethanolic extract of Cannabis furnished by the National Institute on Drug Abuse (NIDA) (5).

The specific rotation reported for (-)-cannabitriol by Chan et al., was -107°; whereas (+)-cannabitriol had a specific rotation of $+7^{o}$ (4). This indicated that the isolated (+)-cannabitriol was a partially racemic mixture. (+/-)-8,9-dihydroxy-delta-6a(10a)-tetrahydrocannabinol (VII) and (+/-)-8,9-dihydroxy-delta-6a(10a)-tetrahydrocannabinol (IIX) were reported by ElSohly, et al., in 1978 (6). These compounds were obtained from a hexane extract of an Indian variant. (-)-10-Ethoxy-9-hydroxy-delta-6a(10a)-tetrahydrocannabinol (VIII) was isolated by ElSohly, et al., in 1977 from an ethanolic extract of Cannabis (5). The presence of the ethoxy group could suggest that this compound might be an artifact, especially since it was isolated from an ethanolic extract of Cannabis. The fact that VI and VIII were isolated from the same ethanolic extract indicated the possibility of a common epoxide intermediate (XIII) which would yield these two compounds upon reaction with water and ethanol, respectively.

Cannabidiolic acid-tetrahydrocannabitriol ester (X) was reported by Von Spulak, et al., in 1968 (7). The ester was obtained from a petroleum ether extract of hashish chromatographed on silca gel. This is the only reported ester of any cannabinoid occurring naturally. 8-Hydroxy-iso-hexahydrocannabivarin (XII) was isolated by Turner's group (9) from an ethanolic extract of an Indian variant and its structure was determined by synthesis.

Cannabiripsol (XI) was isolated from a hexane extract of South African Cannabis by Boeren, et al. (8). Purification was accomplished by chromatography with silica gel and polyamide, and the stereochemical assignment was based on synthesis.

The isolation and characterization of yet a new polyhydroxylated cannabinoid, cannabitetrol is the subject of this report.

II. EXPERIMENTAL

Optical rotation was carried out in 1 dm cell using a Perkin-Elmer model 141 polarimeter. Proton NMR spectra were recorded in $CDCl_3$ on a Brucker 300 MHz instrument and on a Varian EM-390 MHz instrument using TMS as internal standard. Mass spectra were obtained with a Varian MAT-711 and Finnigan 3200 GC/MS/DS instrument at 70 eV. IR spectra were taken on a Perkin-Elmer model 281B and uv spectra were recorded on a

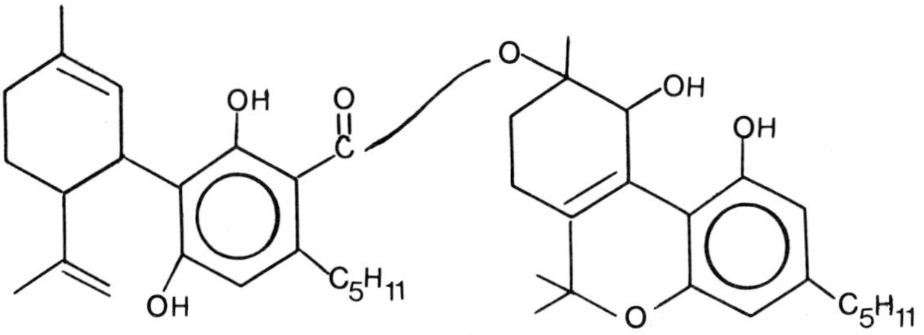

X

Beckman Acta III spectrometer. GC analyses were performed on a Beckman GC-45 and GC-72-5 gas chromatographs equipped with flame ionization detectors and operated isothermally at 210°, and at 191° for TMS-derivatives using 4-androstene-3,17-dione as internal standard. The inlet temperature was 240° and the detector temperature was 260°. Glass columns (2 mm i.d. x 2.4 m (6 ft.) were packed with 2% OV-17 on 100-120 mesh Chromosorb Q. Nitrogen was used as the carrier gas at a flow rate of 18-20 ml/min.

A. Plant Material

The leaves and small stems of Cannabis sativa L. grown in Mississippi from seeds of a Panamenian variant were used in this study. A Voucher specimen has been deposited in the Herbarium, Research Institute of Pharmaceutical Sciences, School of Pharmacy, University of Mississippi.

B. Isolation of Cannabitetrol

The dried plant material (7 kg) was extracted with ethanol (12 gallons x 6), and the ethanol extract evaporated to dryness (1.6 kg). A portion of the latter (700 g) was partitoned between chloroform (residue 378g) and water. Part of the chloroform extract (191 g) was dissolved in 1 liter n-hexane and then shaken with 3N NaOH (3 x 400 ml). The aqueous basic phase was acidified with 10% HCT and extracted with ether (35.2 g). A portion of the ether extract (17 g) was chromatographed on a polyamide column (320 g, 4.6 x 90 cm) packed in EtOH/H_2O (6:4). The polarity was decreased by gradually increasing the percentage of ethanol. Fraction #1 (6.4 g) eluted with 1.5 l of EtOH/H_2O (6:4) was again fractionated on a silica gel G column (600 g, 4.6 x 83 cm) using hexane/ether mixtures and 20 ml fractions were collected. Fractions #101-110 (151 mg) eluted with hexane/ether/6:4) were further purified by repeated chromatography on reversed phase Whatman KC_{18} plates to yield 40 mg of pure cannabitetrol (I) (yield

0.0045%). On silica gel G plate using hexane/EtOAC (7:3) (System I) and on reversed phase plate using $MeOH/H_2O$ (8:2) (System II) cannabitetrol showed one spot with R_f values of 0.48 and 0.21, respectively. GC analysis of the trimethyl silyl derivatives showed a RR_t of 0.25. This same compound was also obtained in this laboratory from a Mexican variant of Cannabis following a different isolation scheme.

C. Physical Characteristics

Cannabitetrol was obtained as a colorless oil; $[a]_D^{25}$ -51° (c 0.54, $CHCl_3$); IR($CHCl_3$) cm^{-1}; 3500-3100 (br,OH) 1630 and 1570, UV (MeOH): 282, 230 (sh) and 217 nm; MSL m/z (% rel. int.) 362 (6) for $C_{21}H_{30}O_5$, 344 (1), 329 (2), 301 (6), 274 (6), 260 (13), 259 (11), 245 (27) and 207 (100). NMR (($CDCl_3$, 300 MHz): 6.43 (s,1H), 6.38 (s,1H), 5.80 (br,s,1H), 2.50 (t,2H), 2.27 (dd, 1H,J=9Hz), 1.64 (s,3H), 1.39 (s,3H), 1.32 (s,3H), and 0.90 (t,3H).

D. Methylation

A few drops of a cold solution of diazomethane in ether was added to 1 mg of compound I and the reaction mixture was allowed to stand overnight at room temperature. GC/MS analysis of the material obtained after evaporation of the ether showed a molecular ion at m/z 376.

E. Acetylation

A solution of I (5 mg) in dry pyridine and acetic anhydride was stirred overnight at room temperature. The reaction mixture was poured over crushed ice and extracted with chloroform (3 x 5 ml); the $CHCl_3$ washed with $NaHCO_3$ solution (2 x 3 ml) and dried over anhydrous Na_2SO_4 and evaporated.

TLC of the reaction product, on precoated silica gel G and Whatman KC_{18} reversed phase plates, showed R_f values of 0.67 and 0.1 using Systems I and II, respectively. GC analysis gave a RR_t of 0.75. GC/MS analysis of the acetate showed a molecular ion at m/z 446.

III. DISCUSSION

An acidic polar fraction obtained from a Panamenian variant of Cannabis sativa L., revealed upon GC/MS analysis of its trimethyl silyl deriavative a new phenolic constituent with a relative retention time (RR_t) of 0.25 (RR_t of delta-9-THC is 0.22). This compound, named cannabitetrol (I), was isolated by repeated column and preparative chromatography, as an optically active colorless oil (40 mg). Mass spectral analysis of I showed a molecular ion at m/z 362 for $C_{21}H_{30}O_5$. The infrared spectrum showed strong hydroxyl absorption but no carbonyl bands, indicating that all oxygens in the molecule must be in the form of hydroxy groups and/or ether functions. The proton NMR spectrum was indicative of an olivetol moiety of a cannabinoid having the dibenzopyran type nucleus. The aromatic protons were observed at delta 6.43 (s,1H), and 6.38 (s,1H), thhe terminal methyl group of the pentyl side chain at 0.90 (t,3H) and the benzylic protons of the side chain at 2.50 (t,3H). In addition, peaks were found at 1.32 and 1.39 (s,3H eachh) for methyls on oxygenated carbon atoms and at 1.64 (s,3H) for a vinylic methyl group. A peak at 2.27 (dd,1H, J=9Hz and 3Hz) was assigned for a strongly shielded proton under a hydroxy group and another peak at 5.80 (s,1H) was assigned for an olefinic proton.

Methlylation of I with diazomethane resulted in a monomethyl ether, M^{+} m/z 376. However, acetylation (acetic anhydride/pyridine) provided a diacetate (MS: M^{+} m/z 446) indicating two acetylable hydoxyl groups, one aliphatic and one phenolic. These data indicated that the compound must be a cannabinoid with a dibenzopyran nucleus, one pheolic hydroxyl, one secondary hydroxyl and a trisubstituted double bond with a vinylic methyl. Considering these structure features and considering the molecular formula ($C_{21}H_{30}O_5$) the remaining two oxygen atoms must be in the form of tertiary hydroxy groups. These structure requirements could be accomodated by one of structures I-IV.

However, the NMR spectrum of cannabitetrol showed a doublet of a doublet at delta 2.27 (1H) and no other peaks were observed between 2.50 and 5.80. Therefore, the peak at 2.27 was assigned to the proton under the secondary hydroxy group. The multiplicity of this proton rules out the delta-8-type structures III and IV.

Additionally, this proton is not expected to appear at such a high field unless extremely shielded. Proton a (Structure I) and H_b (Structure II) couple with the neighbouring equatorial and axial protons resulting in a doublet of a doublet. Structure I is favored over structure II since proton H_a in structure I may be shielded by one of the geminal methyl groups or by the hydroxy group at C-6a. Therefore, the structure of the newly isolated compound was tentatively determined as 6a,7,10a-trihydroxy-delta-9-tetrahydrocannabinol, named cannabitetrol. Attempts for preparing a crystalline 3,5-dinitrobenzoyl ester derivative for x-ray crystallography failed.

We are in the process of isolating enough material for ^{13}C NMR data and to prepare crystalline derivative(s) for x-ray analysis. In addition, the biological activity of cannabitetrol will be investigated.

REFERENCES

1. Turner, C. E., ElSohly, M. A., and Boeren, E. G., Constituents of Cannabis sativa L. XVII. A review of the natural constituents, J. Nat. Products, 43:169 (1980).
2. Mechoulam, R., and Gaoni, Y., Recent advances in the chemistry of hashish, Fortsch. Chem. Org. Naturst. 25:175 (1967).
3. Obta, Y., and Ishikawa, Y., Studies of the constituents of hemp plant (Cannabis sativa L.). Part III. Isolaton of a Gibb's positive compound from Japanese hemp, Agr. Biol. Chem. 30:619 (1966).
4. Chan, W. R., Magnus, K. E., and Watson, H. A., The Structure of cannabitriol, Experientia, 32:283 (1976).
5. ElSohly, M. A., El-Feraly, F. S., and Turner, C. E., Isolation and Characterization of (+)-cannabitriol and (-)-10-ethoxy-9-hydroxy-delta-6a(10a)-tetrahydrocannabinol: Two new cannabinoids from Cannabis sativa L. extract, Lloydia 40:275 (1977).
6. ElSohly, M. A., Boeren, E. G., and Turner C. E., (+/-)-9,10-Dihydroxy-delta-6a(10a)-tetrahydrocannabinol and (+/-)-8,9-dihydroxy-delta-6a(10a)-tetrahydrocannabinol. Two new cannabinoids from Cannabis sativa L. Experientia 34:1127 (1978).
7. Von Spulak, F., Claussen, U., Fehlhaber, H. W., and Korte, F., Haschischh - XIX. Cannabidiol carbonsaure - tetrahydrocannabitriol ester ein neuer haschisch - inhaltsstoff, Tetrahedron, 24:5379 (1968).
8. Boeren, E. G., ElSohly, M. A., and Turner, C. E., Cannabiripsol: A novel Cannabis constituent, Experientia, 35:1278 (1979).
9. Turner, C. E., Mole, M. L., Hanus, L., and ElSohly H. N., Constituents of Cannabis sativa XIX. Isolation and structure elucidation of cannabiglendol, a novel cannabinoid from an Indian variant, J. Nat. Products 44:27 (1981).

SOME SMOKING CHARACTERISTICS OF MARIJUANA CIGARETTES*

K. H. Davis, Jr., I. A. McDaniel, Jr.
L. W Cadwell, P. L. Moody

Research Triangle Institute
Research Triangle Park, North Carolina

I. INTRODUCTION

The primary route of illicit consumption of Cannabis sativa L. is through the smoking of cigarettes made from the leaves and "tops" of the plant, which are commonly known as "marijuana". Marijuana cigarette smoking has been the subject of a number of research studies, and in recent times has received limited medical use for the relief of nausea associated with cancer chemotherapy and for the treatment of elevated intraoptic pressure associated with glaucoma.

We have been involved since 1974 in the manufacture, analysis and distribution of standardized machine-made marijuana cigarettes to clinical and basic research programs, and in the identification of factors affecting patient acceptability of these cigarettes. Lately, we have been particularly concerned with quantitating the cigarette smoking process with respect to delivery of delta-9-tetrahydrocannabinol (THC) in mainstream smoke, and with the determination of the effect on cannabinoid delivery of various measures employed to increase patient acceptability.

In earlier unpublished studies, we found that burning temperatures in two different potencies of standard marijuana cigarettes when smoked by human subjects were about 800°C. We also found that puffing conditions (40 mL/2-sec puff), approximating the standard puffing conditions established foruse with cigarette smoking machines in tobacco cigarette testing laboratories, would produce burning temperatures of about

*Supported by NIDA contract No. 271-81-3802.

ISBN 0-12-044620-0

800°C (1). Among other researchers Perez-Reyes et al. (2) and Kinzer et al. (3) measured similar puff volumes and puff durations in human subjects smoking marijuana cigarettes, although the puff frequencies measured by these researchers (approximately three puffs/min) were different from the one puff/min puff frequency built into most cigarette smoking machines. While such smoking conditions may not represent the smoking parameters of heavy marijuana smokers, they are representative of light to moderate smokers. Thus, smoke condensate collected from the smoking of standard marijuana cigarettes on a cigarette smoking machine should be representative of that ingested by light to moderate smokers, with respect to the cannabinoid profile, but not in quantitative terms. All except inexperienced smokers should receive heavier cannabinoid doses through cigarette smoking than are contained in these smoke condensates.

Investigational use of marijuana cigarettes has been complicated by lack of quantitative information about the delivery of THC in the mainstream smoke under various smoking conditions. In this study, a cigarette smoking machine was used to obtain mainstream smoke condensates in which the THC content was quantitated by use of GLC methodology with an internal standard. The data obtained provide an estimate of the lower limit of THC ingestion by marijuana smokers, as well as a measure of the total amount of THC produced in the smoke of marijuana cigarettes and the degree of destructive pyrolysis of THC. Changes in the rate of delivery of THC in the mainstream smoke of marijuana cigarettes with progressive burning were found and quantitated. The degrees of translation of THC into mainstream smoke for marijuana cigarettes of two different potencies were compared.

The popular cigarette rolling papers employed in "street" use of marijuana are less porous than the standard cigarette papers used in the manufacture of marijuana cigarettes. Possible differences in the performance of machine-made cigarettes rolled with standard papers as compared to those rolled with "street" papers in production of THC in the smoke were investigated.

Humidification of marijuana cigarettes prior to smoking is commonly used as a means of moderating their "harshness", as perceived by patients and research subjects. The effect of humidification on the production of THC into mainstream smoke was determined.

II. MATERIALS AND METHODS

A. Marijuana Cigarettes, 3.10% THC

Marijuana (leaf material and tops) grown by the University of Mississippi in 1980 were blended and treated with amounts of water calculated to raise the moisture content to ca. 18%. Cigarettes were manufactured on an AMF cigarette machine following removal of seeds, stems, and fines by sieving. Cigarettes were dried, analyzed for cannabinoid content, graded by hand, packed in metal cans, and stored at -20°C until needed. THC analysis values were obtained on a dry-weight basis.

B. Marijuana Cigarettes, 1.60% THC

Marijuana (leaf material) of 1978 and 1979 crop years, furnished by the University of Mississippi, was made into cigarettes as described above for 3.10% THC cigarettes.

C. Preparation of Cigarettes for Smoking Studies

In order to accommodate 70 mm "street" rolling papers, all cigarettes were cut from their original 85 mm length to 70 mm. For those cigarettes to be smoked with "street" papers, the original cigarette paper was removed without disturbing the plant material "rod" formed in manufacturing. The "street" paper was then put in place with the aid of a hand-held cigarette rolling device. Prior to smoking, all cigarettes were brought to 15-16% moisture content by humidification in a closed container over saturated aqueous sodium chloride solution for 16 hr. at room temperature.

D. Smoking Studies

A 15-port cigarette-smoking machine (non-commercial Liggett and Myers Tobacco Co., Inc. design, modification no. 4) was used for these studies. The smoke-condensate collection train consisted of a solvent bubbler trap charged with absolute ethanol upstream of a cylindrical smoke trap packed with sea sand (Fisher Chemical Co., Raleigh, NC). Prior to use, the sea sand was washed with organic solvents and water, then dried at 105°C. A flowmeter was placed in the suction line between the collection train and a small vacuum pump. This apparatus was operated with smoking parameters of 40 mL/2-sec puff, two puff/min/cigarette. In constant draft smoking machine runs, each cigarette was burned in a single, uninterrupted draft at a flow rate of 20 mL/sec.

For each smoking condition, at least four replicate 15-cigarette runs on the smoking machine were carried out. Cigarettes were ignited with a small Bunsen burner and extinguished in a container of dry ice at the end of smoking or after a predetermined number of puffs. The smoke condensate was collected from each run by washing the sand trap with absolute ethanol and combining the washings with the ethanol from the bubbler trap. Smoke condensate and cigarette butt fractions were preserved at -20°C for analysis.

E. GLC Analysis Procedures

Aliquots of smoke condensate solutions equivalent to about 2 mg THC were treated with 1 ml of a 3 mg/ml solution of

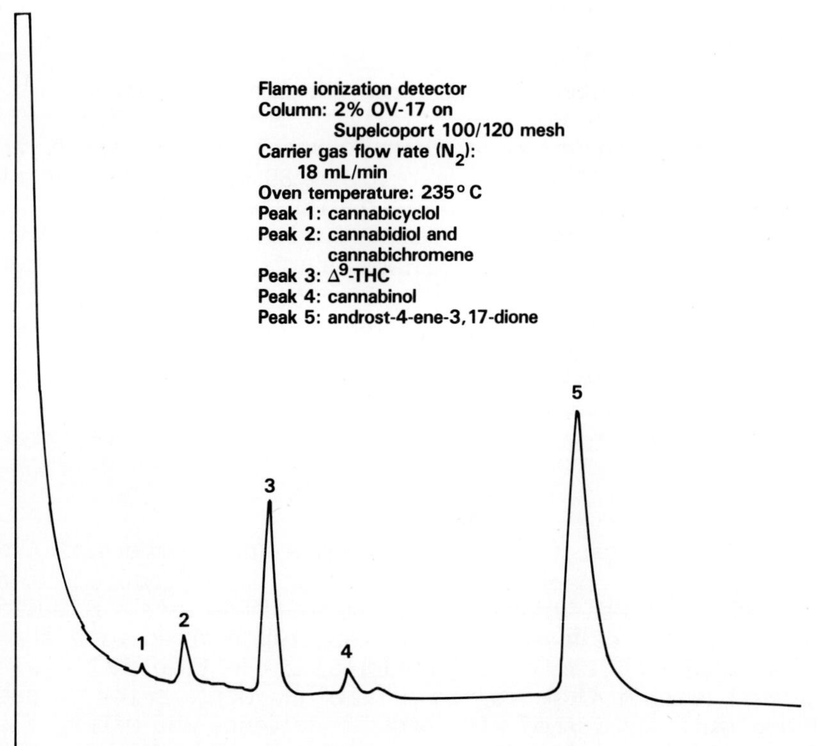

FIGURE 1. Gas-liquid chromatogram of marijuana smoke condensate.

androst-4-ene-3,17-dione (internal standard for GLC) in ethanol, evaporated nearly to dryness _in vacuo_ at room temperature, and restored with absolute ethanol to an approximate concentration of 0.3 mg/ml with respect to THC. Entire cigarette butt fractions from each smoking run were extracted for analysis by a modification of the procedure of Fetterman et al. (4). Each extract was treated with an amount of a 10 mg/ml solution of androst-4-ene-3,17-dione in ethanol equivalent to about 1.5 mg of the internal standard per 1 mg of THC present, evaporated nearly to dryness, and restored to a concentration of about 0.3 mg/ml with respect to THC. Marijuana cigarettes were extracted for analysis using both the Soxhlet extraction procedure of Davis et al. (5) and a modification of the procedure of Fetterman et al. (4).

Essentially the GLC procedure of Davis et al. (5) was used to analyze samples, prepared as described above, of smoke condensates, butt fractions and cigarettes on an automated GLC apparatus consisting of a Varian 2440 gas chromatograph (Walnut Creek, CA) with flame ionization detectors coupled to a Varian 8000 autosampler and a Spectraphysics 4100 computing integrator (Santa Clara, CA). A 1.83 m x 2 mm ID 2% OV-17 on Supelcoport 100/120 mesh (Supelco Inc., Bellefonte, PA) glass GLC column, operated at 225°C with a carrier gas (N_2) flow rate of 25 ml/min, was used. Samples for analysis were run _vs._ a calibration standard containing 0.3 mg/ml of THC and 0.45 mg/ml of androst-4-ene-3,17-dione, and all assay results were corrected for calibration changes. Volumes of 1 mclof each sample were injected for analysis.

F. Moisture Content Determinations

Cigarette moisture contents were determined from the weight loss ofcigarette samples dried at 105-112°C ina forced draft oven.

III. RESULTS

Smoke condensates from marijuana cigarette smoking studies were analyzed for THC content by use of automated GLC technology (see Figure 1). In a comparison of low porosity "street" cigarette papers with the medium porosity papers used in the manufacture of the standard cigarettes, six replicate smoking runs were made with each of the paper types. The amount of THC produced with each paper type, expressed as percent of the total THC present in the marijuana smoked, is shown in Table I. Popular low porosity "street" cigarette papers provide a

TABLE I. Effect of Low and Medium Porosity Papers on THC Production in Mainstream Smoke Condensate from Marijuana Cigarettes[1]

	Combustion replicates, % translation of Δ^9-THC into mainstream smoke						
	1	2	3	4	5	6	Mean ± S.E.[2]
	Intermittent Puff Mode[3]						
Medium porosity paper CORESTA value = ~ 50	16.4	19.2	15.3	17.6	12.1	21.7	17.0 ± 1.4
Low porosity paper CORESTA value = ~ 10	10.8	18.6	16.8	14.6	24.7	22.3	19.6 ± 1.5

[1]Marijuana cigarettes contained 1.60% Δ^9-THC (dry weight basis).

[2]Standard error.

[3]One 2 second puff per minute, 40 mL per puff, 15 cigarettes per replicate.

slight increase in the degree of translation of THC to mainstream smoke as compared with the standard medium porosity papers used in cigarette manufacturing. This difference was statistically insignificant.

In determining the effect of high and low moisture content on the delivery of THC, four replicate smoking runs were carried out with each of two batches of cigarettes, one at 8% moisture and one at 16% moisture. The results are shown in Table II. No difference was found in the THC content of the mainstream smoke of marijuana cigarettes burned at high moisture content or at low moisture content.

Cigarettes of 1.60 and 3.10% THC content were compared with respect to delivery of THC in the mainstream smoke. For each potency, the results from four replicate smoking runs are reported in Table III. No statistically significant difference was observed between the two cigarette potencies, which yielded in the mainstream smoke 19 and 16% respectively of the THC contained in the marijuana actually combusted.

In order to obtain an estimate of the total amount of THC produced by standard marijuana cigarettes, four replicate constant-draft smoking runs were carried out with each potency (1.60 and 3.10% THC). As shown in Table III, 69% of the THC present in the marijuana combusted was found in the smoke condensate.

An investigation into the rate with which THC was delivered into the mainstream smoke with progressive burning of the cigarette was carried out. Individual studies were done (four replicates each) in which smoking was terminated after 2, 5, 7 and 9 puffs respectively. The THC contents of the resulting smoke condensates are given in Table IV, and presented graphically in Figures 2 and 3. These data indicate an increasing

TABLE II. Effect of Low and High Moisture Content on THC Production in Mainstream Smoke Condensate from Marijuana Cigarettes[1]

	Combustion replicates, % translation of Δ^9-THC into mainstream smoke				
	1	2	3	4	Mean ± S.E.[2]
	Intermittent Puff Mode[3]				
Marijuana cigarettes, 15.5% moisture content	16.7	18.4	18.2	14.7	17.0 ± 0.9
Marijuana cigarettes, 8.2% moisture content	16.3	18.2	19.7	16.4	17.6 ± 0.8

[1]Marijuana cigarettes contained 1.60% Δ^9-THC (dry weight basis).

[2]Standard error.

[3]One 2 second puff per minute, 40 mL per puff, 15 cigarettes per replicate.

TABLE III. Comparison of THC Production in Smoke Condensate from Two Potencies of Marijuana Cigarettes

	Combustion replicates, % translation of Δ^9-THC into smoke						
	1	2	3	4	5	6	Mean ± S.E.[1]
	Constant Draft Mode[2]						
1.60% Δ^9-THC cigarettes	66.2	64.2	70.0	72.7	72.5	70.9	69.4 ± 1.4
3.10% Δ^9-THC cigarettes	71.2	67.9	71.1	66.3	–	–	69.1 ± 1.2
	Intermittent Puff Mode[3]						
1.60% Δ^9-THC cigarettes	16.2	21.8	19.5	18.4	–	–	19.0 ± 1.2
3.10% Δ^9-THC cigarettes	17.7	15.5	14.7	16.5	–	–	16.1 ± 0.6

[1]Standard error.

[2]Constant burn at flow rate of 1,200 mL per minute, 15 cigarettes per replicate.

[3]One 2 second puff per minute, 40 mL per puff, 15 cigarettes per replicate.

rate of production of THC with progressive smoking. The increase appears to be linear. The butt fractions from these smoking runs also were analyzed for THC content, with results as shown in Table IV and Figure 4. As compared to the calculated THC content based on the weight of the butt fractions, the THC assay values were lower than expected after 2 and 5 puffs (18.7 and 39.3% burned). However, after 7 and 9 puffs (67.6 and 80.3% burned), no difference was observed.

TABLE IV. Differential Production of THC in Mainstream Smoke Condensate for Marijuana Cigarettes[1]

Amount of cigarette burned (%)	Combustion replicates, Δ^9-THC content of butt fractions (mg)					Combustion replicates, translation into mainstream smoke, Δ^9-THC per gram burned (mg)				
	1	2	3	4	Mean ± S.E.[2]	1	2	3	4	Mean ± S.E.[2]
					Intermittent Puff Mode[3]					
18.7	89	80	95	99	90.8 ± 4.1	1.7	2.0	1.5	1.6	1.7 ± 0.1
39.3	68	70	77	82	74.2 ± 3.2	2.8	2.4	2.0	2.3	2.4 ± 0.2
67.6	36	41	50	46	43.2 ± 3.0	3.4	2.3	2.6	2.6	2.7 ± 0.2
80.3	23	24	23	30	25.0 ± 1.7	2.6	3.5	3.2	2.9	3.0 ± 0.2

[1]Marijuana cigarettes contained 1.60% Δ^9-THC (dry weight basis).

[2]Standard error.

[3]One 2 second puff per minute, 40 mL per puff, 15 cigarettes per replicate.

IV. DISCUSSION

Under smoking-machine conditions, which provide a reasonable approximation of the puff duration and puff volume of many marijuana cigarette smokers, the production of THC in mainstream smoke from standard marijuana cigarettes was determined. Under these puffing conditions, 16-19% of the THC contained in the marijuana actually combusted was found in the mainstream smoke condensate. This amount should be representative of the lower limit of ingestion by marijuana smokers. Under constant draft conditions in which the whole cigarette is consumed in a single puff, and under which virtually no smoke is lost as sidestream smoke, 69% translation of THC to mainstream smoke is obtained. This represents the maximum proportion of THC which could be obtained in the smoke from a marijuana cigarette. Some 31% of THC is not found upon analysis of the smoke condensate, and is presumed destroyedby pyrolysis.

In a series of progressive smoking experiments, smoking was interrupted after a certain number of puffs and the smoke condensate and butt fractions analyzed for THC. The rate of production of THC into the mainstream smoke increased in a linear fashion nearly three-fold from the beginning to the end

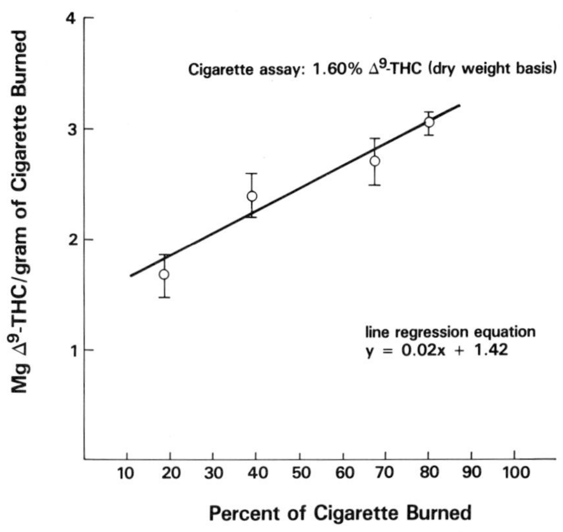

FIGURE 2. Differential production of THC: translation of THC into smoke vs. amount of cigarette (1.60% THC) burned.

of smoking. It therefore appears that smokers should receive increasingly greater amounts of THC per unit weight of marijuana burned as the cigarette is progressively consumed. The corresponding butt fractions showed a significant loss of THC during the early stages of smoking as compared to the expected THC content of the butts calculated on the basis of weight. During the latter stages of smoking, there was no significant difference between calculated and found THC contents of the butt fractions. It appears from those data that three phenomena occur in the burning marijuana cigarette which affect the initially uniform distribution of THC and its translation to smoke. First, there is initially a heavy destruction of THC by pyrolysis from the portion of the cigarette near the burning tip. Secon, the THC not destroyed by pyrolysis migrates away from the heat to concentrate in the cooler part of the cigarette. Once the initial migration has occurred and a moving equilibrium has been reached, further losses to pyrolysis are minimal. Third, there is also a continuous translation of THC to smoke, the rate of which increases sharply as cigarette. In order to verify these conclusions, the very

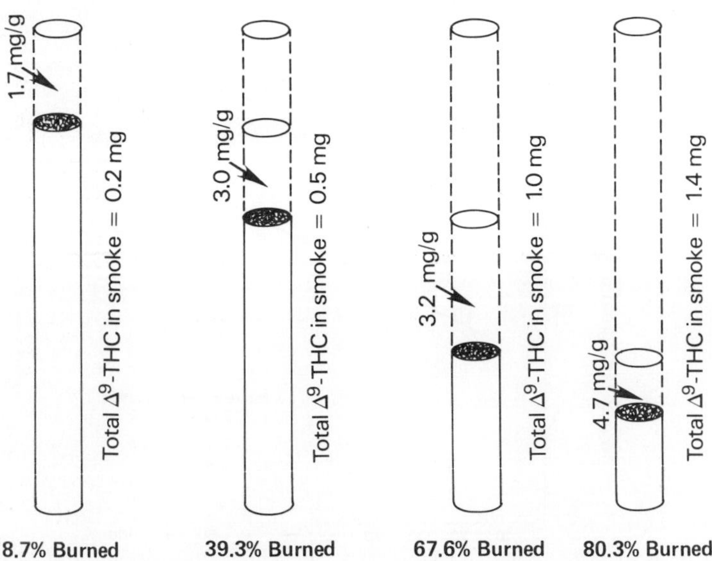

FIGURE 3. Differential production of THC in mainstream smoke condensate from marijuana cigarettes (1.60% THC) showing total THC translated to smoke and rate of production.

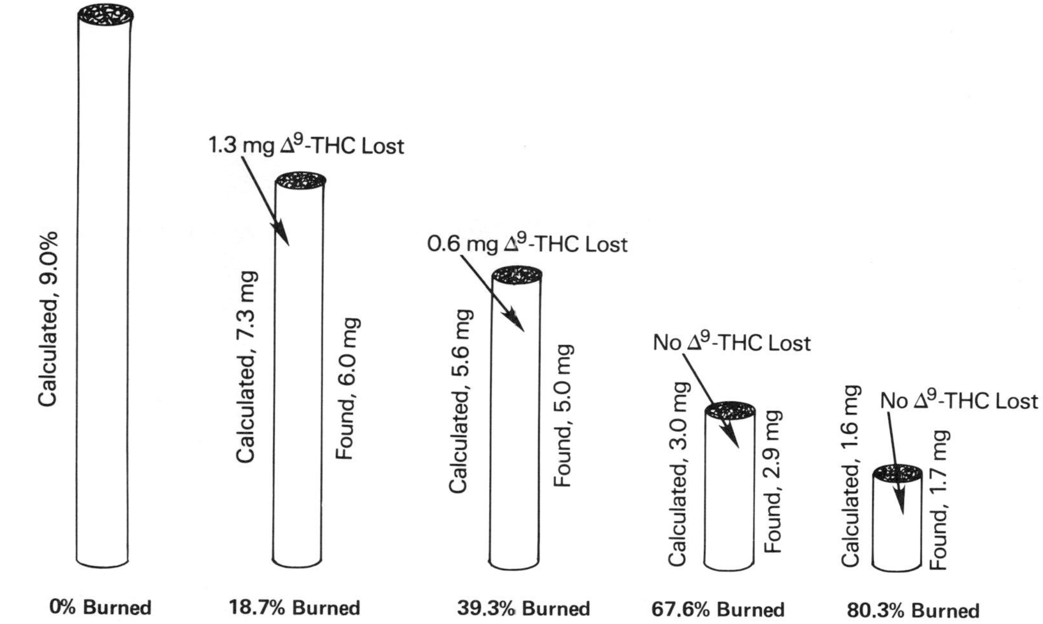

FIGURE 4. Differential loss of THC from marijuana cigarette butts showing calculated and found THC contents.

advancing heat drives the zone of THC concentration off of the interesting phenomena described herein will require more investigation.

Investigations into the effect of cigarette paper porosity on translation of THC to mainstream smoke indicate that there is no significant difference between popular "street" rolling papers of low porosity and standard medium porosity papers used in cigarette manufacture. Thus, the cigarette performance described above is representative of "street" rolling papers.

Humidification of marijuana cigarettes is a commonly used means of modifying their harshness upon smoking. The effect of high and low moisture content on the THC production of the standard cigarettes was investigated. No significant difference was found between the two conditions. Thus, neither humidification to increase acceptability to patients and research subjects nor accidental drying out of marijuana cigarettes alters their performance in the delivery of THC to mainstream smoke.

ACKNOWLEDGMENTS

We gratefully acknowledge Mr. V. L. Parker, Jr., and Mrs. B. A. Palazzolo for their assistance, and Drs. C. E. Cook, G. Barnett, R. L. Hawks and R. E. Willette for encouragement and helpful discussions.

REFERENCES

1. Ogg, C. L., Determination of particulate matter and alkaloids (as nicotine) in cigarette smoke, J. Assoc. Off. Analyt. Chem. 47:356-362 (1964).
2. Perez-Reyes, M., DiGuiseppi, S., David, K. H., Schindler, V. H., and Cook, C. E., Comparison of effects of marihuana cigarettes of three different potencies, Clin. Pharmacol. Ther. 31(5):617-624 (1982).
3. Kinzer, G. W., Foltz, R. L., Mitchell, R. I., Truitt, E. B. Jr., Fate of the cannabinoid components of marihuana during smoking, Bull. Narc. 26(3):41-54 (1974).
4. Fetterman, P. S., Keith, E. S., Waller, C. W., Guerrero, O., Doorenbos, N. J., and Quimby, M. W., Mississippi-grown Cannabis sativa L: preliminary observation on chemical definition of phenotype and variations in tetrahydrocannabinol content versus age, sex and plant part, J. Pharm. Sci. 60(8):1246-1249 (1971).

5. Davis, K. H., Jr., Martin, N. H., Pitt, C. G., Wildes, J. W., and Wall, M. E., The preparation of analysis of enriched and pure cannabinoids from marijuana and hashish, Lloydia 33(4):453-460 (1970).

AN AUTOMATED COMPUTER-BASED SYSTEM FOR THE STUDY OF MARIJUANA SMOKING DYNAMICS

J. Stanford Hutcheson
Mario Perez-Reyes*
Stephanie Di Guiseppi

Department of Psychiatry
University of North Carolina School of Medicine
Chapel Hill, North Carolina

I. INTRODUCTION

Tobacco cigarette smoking has been widely practiced by humans over the years, and therefore, much research regarding behavioral, pharmacological, and chemical properties of smoking has been conducted by the tobacco industry and various scientific disciplines (1). However, little information is available regarding the characteristics of marijuana cigarette smoking. Our studies involving marijuana cigarettes containing different THC dose levels prompted us to study smoking behavior and profiles of marijuana cigarette smokers (3). A variety of cigarette holders based on a differential pressure-flow technique, have been developed to study smoking behavior where filtertip tobacco cigarettes were used. Rawbone, et al., who studied inhalation and absorption of tobacco smoke used aa specially designed cigarette holder that contained a cellulose filter insert between the differential pressure ports based on the assumption that laminar flow through such a filter would produce a pressure drop that is linearly related to the flow of gas through the holder and cigarette (4). However, their study revealed that the pressure-flow relatioship of the cigarette holder was not truly linear, thereby suggesting that some turbulent flow was present. Filter tobacco cigarettes were used in the Rawbone study as has been the case

*Supported by NIDA contract No. 271-80-3705.

ISBN 0-12-044620-0

in most of the smoking behavior studies.

Marijuana cigarettes, unlike commercial filter cigarettes, are frequently loosely packed having a non-uniform density. This results in relatively lower draw resistnce and gas flow rates. Marijuana cigarettes also seem to produce considerably more resinous material and heavy particles than do filter cigarettes and would quickly clog a cellulose baffle located between pressure ports. Therefore, to study marijuana cigarette smoking dynamics, it is necessary to use a cigarette holder containing an orifice plate, which is unlikely to become restricted or clogged, and which is constructed of a material that is easy to clean. Such a holder should exhibit very low draw resistance, but the orifice plate will also produce turbulent flow which is no longer linearly related to the differential pressure across the baffel. Instead, the volume flow rate is proportional to the square root of the differential pressure (5,6). Much of the research regarding tobacco smoking dynamics has been conducted without the aid of a fast on-line computer. Most investigators had to rely on discrete electronic hardware to achieve some level of automated data acquisition and processing (2). The square root function associated with the orifice plate technique made this type of analysis more difficult and cumbersome. For real-time acquisition and analysis of marijuana cigarette volume flow rates involving the square root pressure-flow relationship, a fast laboratory computer (e.g., PDP-11/34) is necessary. The use of such a computer for on-line processing of the flow signal to obtain puff volume and related times parameters can easily provide the researcher with immediate smoking status information throughout the course of the experiment.

Research involving tobacco cigarette smoking behavior has demonstrated that an individual's smoking profile affects the level of the dose that is delivered to the smoker, which in turn, relates to how much is absorbed (4). Some investigators have attempted to measure inhalation and absorption of the cigarette smoke, and to analyze the inspired and expired gases (2,4). While these parameters are certainly of interest regarding marijuana smoking,, our primary interest and reason for developing a measurement system is to study puff volume profile and related parameters (i.e., puff duration, interpuff interval, etc.) during smoking, rather than the actual smoke volumes inhaled, and to determine if marijuana cigarettes with increased potencies affect an individual's smoking behavior. A puff volume transducer based on the orifice plate pressure-flow technique was designed for marijuana cigarette studies. Also, a computer program wss developed to acquire and process the signals from the transducer. The entire computerbased system was then calibrated and tested for linearity and accuracy.

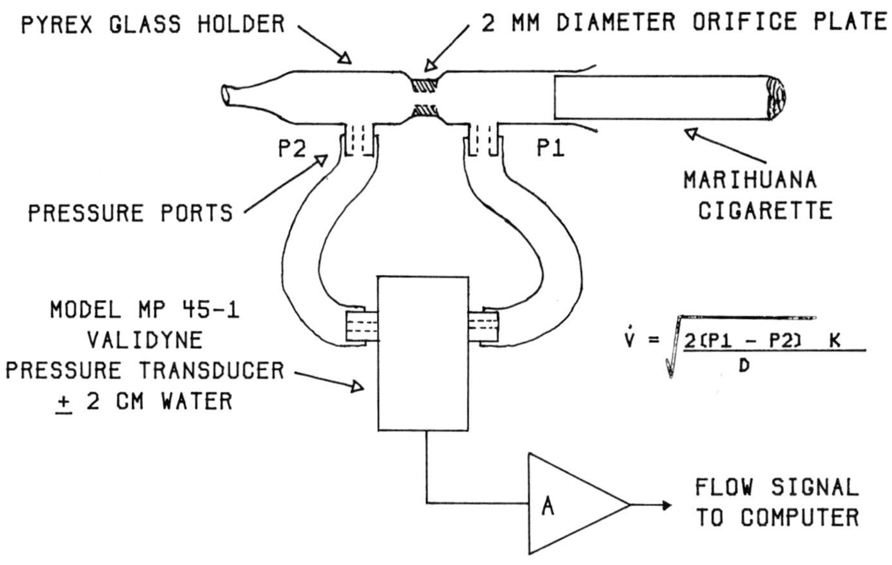

FIGURE 1. Schematic representing the smoking apparatus consisting of the puff volume transducer-holder, Validyne MP45-1 differential pressure transducer, and signal conditioning amplifier.

II. METHODS

A. Puff Volume Transducer

The design of our puff volume transducer, which also serves as the cigarette holder, is based on an application of Bernoulli's law to a simple physics principle - the Venturii flowmeter and is shown in Figure 1. A slight variation of this principle reveals that air, gas, or a fluid flowing through a pipe or tube having a relatively sharp reduction in internal cross sectional area at some point along its length, thereby creating a relatively small orifice, will develop a differential pressure across this constricted section that is proportional to the gas flowiing through the tube (5). Actually, the flow is linearly proportional to the square root of the differential pressure divided by the density of the gas according to the equation:

$$V = \frac{2(P1 - P2)}{D} K$$

where V is gas flow, P1-P2 is differential pressure, D is density of the gas, and K is a constant that takes into account the fixed cross sectional areas of the holder. The integral of this flow signal over time yields total volume through the tube. Therefore, our puff volume transducer is constructed from a pyrex glass tube having an internal diameter (7 mm) slightly less than the outer diameter of a cigarette. This material was selected because it will sustain the intense heat from a marijuana cigarette and also permit easy cleaning. The glass tube is configured to accomodate a cigarette and also permit also cleaning. The glass tube is conigured to accomodate a cigarette at one end and provide a mouth piece for the subject at the other end. An orifice plate located midway along the tube and containing a 2 mm diameter orifice creates the necessary reduction in area. Small pressure sensing ports are constructed in the side of the glass tube, with one located on each side of the baffle. The pressure differential due to flow then appears between these two ports.

The remainder of the smoking dynamics transducer aapparatus then consists of Validyne Model MP45-1 differential pressure transducer, having a sensitivity of +/- 20 mm (water), connected via Tygon tubing to each pressure port of the puff volume transducer. The signal from the pressure transducer is first amplified and low-pass filtered (10 Hz, 12dB per octave), and then routed to a laboratory mini-computer for processing by an on-line program.

B. System Configuration

A block diagram of the overall computer-based smoking dynamic system is shown in Figure 2. The smoking transducer is located in a shielded subject room, containing an exhaust fan for smoke evacuation, which is remotely located from the computer. The system is controlled by a video terminal located near the smoking apparatus, which also allows the experimenter to monitor calibration results and experiment parameters. An oscilloscope is used to monitor the analog flow signal in order to insure that the signal does not exceed the range of the computer's analog to digital converter. The smoking dynamics program runs on a Digital Equipment Corporation PDP-11/34 minicomputer and under the RT-11 operating system. The PDP-11/34 contains 32K words of memory, a 12-bit A to D converter, a 16-bit parallel 1/0 interface, and a real-

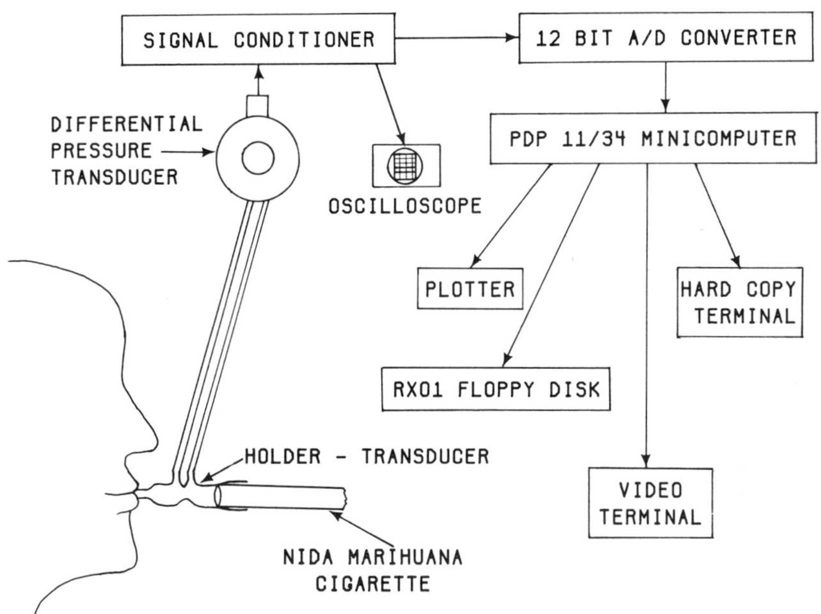

FIGURE 2. Block diagram showing the complete computer-based smoking dynamics system.

time programmable clock. Also, the configuration includes an RX01 floppy disk system for program and data storage, a hard-copy terminal for numerical printouts, and a Hewlett-Packard 7225B X-Y plotter for graphical representation of the data.

The smoking-dynamics on-line program processes the volume flow rate signal from the puff volume transducer in real-time on a puff-by-puff basis. It is written in FORTRAN and calls several assembly language modules that were specifically developed for smoking dynamics acquisition and analysis. A software flow-chart is shown in Figure 3. Basically, the program is arranged in four sections; 1) subject and experiment information entry, 2) calibration, 3) data acquisition and processing, and 4) data output and storage. The information input section of the program permits the experimenter to enter the subject's name, birth date, weight, etc. as well as the experiment information (e.g., type, data, data-set names, comments, etc.).

The calibration section allows the complete system to be calibrated by drawing known volumes of smoke through the cigarette and holder using a 50 ml syringe. A mechanical stop was installed on the syringe at the 50 ml volume mark to insure that each volume is the same. The average of five such volumes is used by the calibration routine to compute the scale factors. We averaged the 5 volumes to compensate for different flow rates. Following calibration, the calibration information is saved on disk for possible future use. Calibration prior to each experiment is important due to ambient

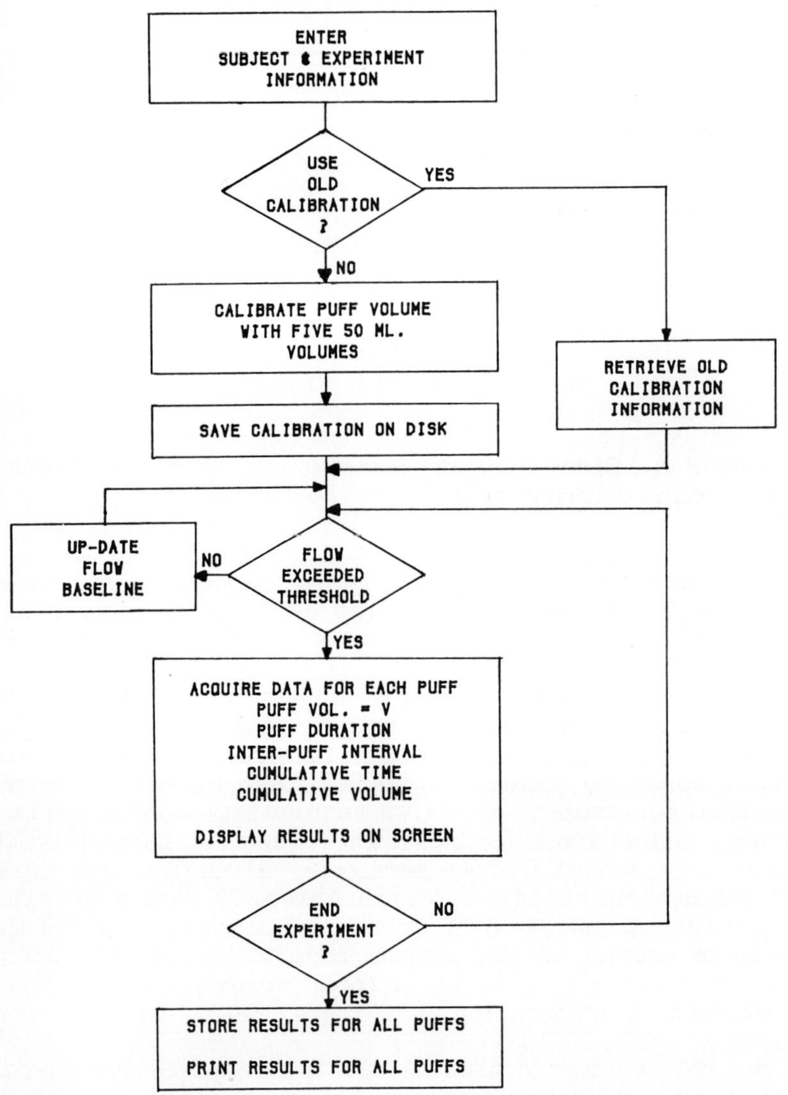

FIGURE 3. Simplified flow chart of the smoking dynamics computer program.

changes in humidity, barometric pressure, and temperature which, in turn, affect the accuracy of the system. Slight differences in calibration values before and after using the cigarette holder with a marijuana cigarette were noted. These differences were attributed to the build-up of residue on the glass holder during smoking. After the puff volume transducer was cleaned, the calibration values returned to those obtained before the cigarette was smoked.

The data acquisition and processing section computes puff volume, puff duration, inter-puff interval, cumulative volume, and cumulative smoking time on a puff-by-puff basis. Immediately following each puff, these parameters are displayed on the screen of a video terminal. An arbitary threshold of 20 A to D converter units was established for the flow signal in order to determine whether or not a puff was in progress. A puff was considered to be in progress if the flow value exceeded this threshold. Also, puff volumes less than 5 ml are considered artifactual and are discarded by the computer. The flow baseline is continuously sampled at 50 samples per second between puffs and averaged over 5 second intervals. Therefore, the flow baseline is automatically up-dated every 5 seconds during inter-puff intervals that exceed 5 seconds. After the last puff of the smoking sequence, which is signaled by the subject depressing a push-button switch connected to the computer's parallel I/O port, the program computes additional parameters regarding smoking dynamics. These include mean puff volume, mean puff duration, total smoking time, total smoke volume, percent of total volume for each puff, percent of total time for each puff, and a linear regression and correlation coefficient of puff volume versus puff duration.

The output and storage section of the program generates a hard-copy printout of smoking dynamic parameters and permits the user to store these data on disk in two different formats. One of the storage formats is compatible with a plotting program that drives the HP 225B X-Y plotter and permits quick and easy analysis of certain smoking parameters (e.g., puff volume versus cumulative time) in graphical form. The other format stores all smoking behavioral data in a large multidimentional array that allows easy editing and further processing (e.g., averaging data across subjects).

C. Evaluation of System Performance

Following development, the system performance was evaluated by drawiing different known volumes of both tobacco and marijuana through the puff volume transducer. A 200 ml glass syringe was used to draw these test volumes in progressively

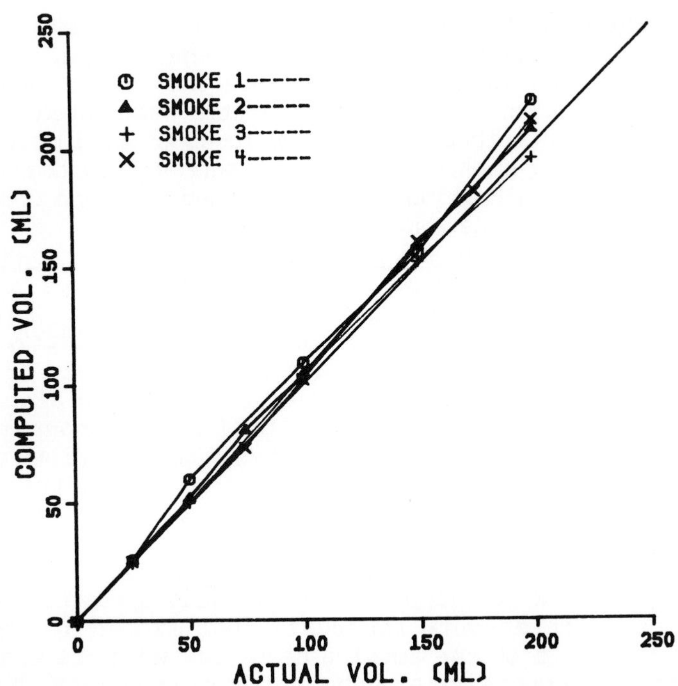

FIGURE 4. The relationship between computed volumes and actual volumes over a 0 to 200 ml range for 2 tobacco and 2 marijuana cigarettes. Known volumes within this range was drawn through the cigarettes using a 200 ml syringe.

increasing or decreasing 25 ml steps over a 200 ml range. The results of this procedure using four different cigarettes (2 unflitered tobacco and 2 marijuana) is shown in Figure 4. Computed volumes were plotted against actual volumes and compared with the line representing a correlation of one. Results indicate that the smoking dynamics system is linear over the range of 0 ml to 150 ml. This proved to be more than adequate siince we have observed most puff volumes fall within the 30 ml to 60 ml range.

A pilot study was conducted, using the smoking dynamics system, to evaluate the smoking characteristics of one marijuana smoker. He smoked on three different days, in a blind cross-over design, marijuana cigarettes of three different potencies (placebo, and 1.5% and 2.9% THC content marijuana). He was instructed to smoke in his customary way and to inhale all of each puff. System calibration using tobacco smoke was performed before testing the subject. A 'stop' button was depressed immediately following the subject's last puff. This caused the computer to store all smoking data on disk. Figure 5 is an example printout of the smoking dynamic parameters that were generated by the smoking of a 1.5% THC content marijuana cigarette.

Figure 6 shows the subject's puff volume smoking profile versus time. It can be seen that differences in THC content of the cigarettes did not significantly alter the puff volume smoking profile or total volume intake.

```
ENTER FILE NAME FOR DATA:*SUBJ31.DAT
DISK READING COMPLETE!
DO YOU WANT TO PRINT DATA ARRAY?Y
SMOKING DYNAMICS RESULTS:
NAME:
COMMENT:
VOL. CALIBRATION=  15.795    PUFFS=  17
BIRTHDAY . 4-10-54      WT=  185.000   HT=   187.960
TOTAL TIME= 460.600          TOTAL VOL.=    0.664
PUFFPUFF VOL   PUFF DUR   INT PUF I % VOLUME   % TIME
 1      48.914      1.400      0.000      7.365      0.000
 2      48.932      2.100     18.100      7.368      3.930
 3      60.684      1.900     18.400      9.137      3.995
 4      61.470      2.000     22.500      9.256      4.885
 5      59.998      1.900     29.600      9.034      6.426
 6      46.617      1.500     27.200      7.019      5.905
 7      50.882      1.500     27.200      7.661      5.905
 8      40.842      1.600     28.700      6.150      6.231
 9      40.461      1.300     21.500      6.092      4.668
10      35.509      1.300     25.200      5.347      5.471
11      34.350      1.700     25.400      5.172      5.515
12      26.087      1.200     27.500      3.928      5.970
13      28.072      1.100     34.500      4.227      7.490
14      17.323      1.000     25.700      2.608      5.580
15      18.365      0.800     30.100      2.765      6.535
16      26.268      0.800     30.600      3.955      6.644
17      19.355      0.800     32.900      2.914      7.143
AVG PUFF VOL=    39.066   AVG PUFF DUR=       1.406
SLOPE=    30.883   INTERCEPT=    -4.352   CORR COEF=       0.877
END OF DATA OUTPUT !
DO YOU WANT TO PRINT ANOTHER FILE? N

BYE!
STOP --
```

FIGURE 5. Example printout of smoking dynamics parameters for one marijuana (1.5% THC) cigarette smoker.

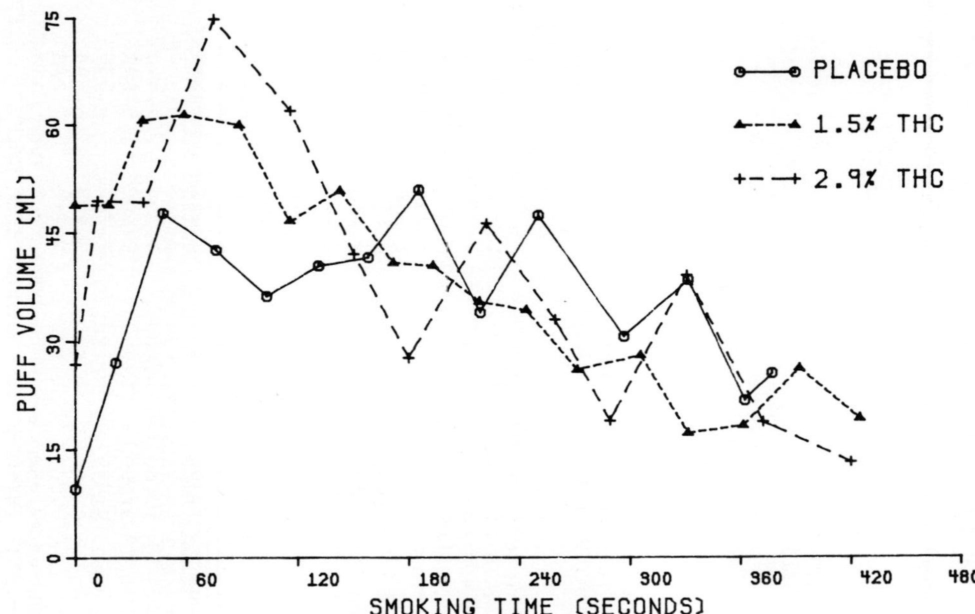

FIGURE 6. Graph showing one subject's puff volume smoking profile versus total smoking time for a placebo (circle), 1.5% THC (triangle), and 2.9% THC (+) dose levels.

III. CONCLUSIONS

A computer-based smoking dynamics system has been developed that allows us to evaluate the smoking behavior of marijuana cigarette smokers by measuring puff volume, puff duration, and inter-puff intervals. Performance evaluation indicates that puff volumes through an ignited marijuana cigarette can be measured accurately over a 0 to 150 ml range, and that system linearity is maintained over this range. Using this system to evaluate the smoking behavior of one subject smoking marijuana cigarettes of 0%, 1.5%, and 2.9% THC content, we found that there is little or no difference in this subject's puff volume profile between the three THC dose levels. Test results from this pilot experiment also indicates that the smoking dynamics system is easy to use, and that it performs well on a repeatable basis under actual smoking conditions.

REFERENCES

1. Chait, L. D., and Griffiths, R. R., Smoking behavior and tobacco smoke intake: Response of smokers to shortened cigarettes, Clin. Pharacol Therap. 32:90-97 (1982).
2. Creighton, D. E., Noble, J. J., and Whewell, R. T., Instruments to measure, record and duplicate human smoking patterns, in "Smoking Behavior", (R. E. Thornton, ed.), pp. 277-288. Churchill Livingstone, 1978.
3. Perez-Reyes, M., Di Guiseppi, S., Davis, K. H., Schindler, V. H., and Cook, C. E., Comparison of effects of marihuana cigarettes of three different potencies, Clin. Pharmacol. Therap. 31:617-624 (1982).
4. Rawbone, R. G., Murphy, K., Tate, M. E., and Kane S. J., The analysis of smoking parameters: inhalation and absorption of tobacco smoke in studies of human smoking behavior, in "Smoking Behavior", (R. E. Thornton, ed.), pp. 171-193. Churchill Livingstone, 1978.
5. Shortley, G., and Williams, D., Mechanics of fluids, in "Elements of Physics", Second edition, pp. 130-154. Prentice-Hall, 1955.
6. Warren, D. W., and DuBois, A. B., A pressure-flow technique for measuring velopharyngeal orifice area during continuous speech, The Cleft Palate J. 1:52-71 (1964).

DEVELOPMENTS IN CANNABINOID ANALYSES OF BODY FLUIDS: IMPLICATIONS FOR FORENSIC APPLICATIONS

Richard L. Hawks

Division of Research
National Institute on Drug Abuse
Rockville, Maryland

I. INTRODUCTION

While much of the pioneering research on the pharmacology and metabolism of cannabinoids carried out in the late sixties and early seventies was done with radiolabeled material, assays were also developed using a variety of analytical techniques, including gas chromatography (GC) with electron capture detection (EC), GC with flame-photometric detection, GC/mass spectrometry (MS), high-performance liquid chromatography (HPLC), HPLC/MS, radioimmunoassay (RIA), HPLC/RIA, thin layer chromatography (TLC), enzyme immunoassay (EMIT), and fluorometry (1-5). These techniques have supported significant research in the cannabis area but the techniques which have evolved as the most useful to the broadest experimental audience have been the RIA and the GC/MS.

Most of the analytical development in the past has concentrated on delta-9-tetrahydrocannabinol (THC), the primary pharmacologically-active component in marijuana. The development of highly sensitive analytical methods for THC in body fluids has been relatively slow for several reasons. Only very low doses of THC are necessary to produce pharmacological effects, so body fluid levels are generally in the low ng/ml range. There is an extensive and rapid metabolism and tissue distribution of THC which contributes to the rapid decrease in body fluid levels. Because THC is an essentially neutral molecule with high lipophilicity, it is difficult to separate from other substances in the biological matrix and has a strong tendency to bind non-specifically to tissue, protein and to the glass walls of vessels used in workup procedures (6,7).

ISBN 0-12-044620-0

In spite of these difficulties, considerable progress has been made over the past decade and assay methods in a number of labs have achieved sensitivity in the low nanogram range required for research studies. These methods, however, have required technical sophistication which was often beyond the reach of most forensic laboratories. Also, most of these methods have been directed at plasma or serum analyses where basic research emphasis in pharmacokinetics and pharmacology has been centered. Forensic applications often require methods suitable for tissue, urine and saliva or breath.

The basic reason for the shift in analytical researchin the direction of the forensic area has been due to the increasing concern about the use of marijuana by segments of our population where marijuana use might be particularly dangerous to the individual or to those around him. These groups include workers in industrial environments, where both their safety and that of their coworkers could depend on their sobriety, by military personnel, pilots, motor vehicle operators, etc. While research has attempted to define the extent of the risk to individuals and society, there has been a parallel effort to develop ways to identify users or those intoxicated to eliminate the risk.

Particular impetus to the new emphasis in cannabinoid assay development in the forensic area resulted from the commercial introduction of the EMIT system (1,4) by the Syva Company two and a half years ago. Up to this time there had been other methodologies available from commercial sources to perform cannabinoid immunoassays on urine, but these methods relied on RIA techniques employing tritium tracers, which require technical abilities beyond the reach of many forensic laboratories. The EMIT system provided a relatively simple method of cannabinoid screening and created a rapidly growing interest in such screening by organizations in which marijuana use is considered a cause for punitive measures.

Another reason for accelerated interest in this area has resulted from a massive testing and partial implementation of a urinalysis program for cannabinoids in the military. Approximately 2 years ago, the Department of Defense (DOD) reported a survey-by-questionaire of drug use in all branches of the armed forces. The results were very disturbing to both DOD and Congress. Chronic marijuana use exceeded 30% in some parts of the services.

In response, DOD has embarked on a program designed to deter the extensive use of marijuana in the services. Initial stages of massive screening programs have already been initiated using both the Syva EMIT urinalysis system and an RIA developed by Roche Diagnostics and marketed under its ABUSCREEN label. This is the first time that drug screening has been attempted on such a large volume of samples for a drug which presents such a difficult analytical problem. Many administrative difficulties are exacerbated as well in running a program where hundreds of thousands of samples must be tracked and the occurrence of a false positive analysis has such a great potential for consequences for the individual who contributed the urine sample. Therefore, much heavier responsibility is placed on the confirmation methodology of such a screening program.

The universally accepted method in the forensic community has been the GC/MS method, which unfortunately does not lend itself to high-volume confirmation work because of its cost and complexity. In response to this problem, the Armed Forces Institute of Pathology (AFIP) developed a gas-liquid chromatography method based on the extraction of 10 ml of urine. It employs a flame ionization detector and has a reported sensitivity of 20 ng/ml (8). This method has been chosen by the military as the primary confirmation method on which their program depends.

The reasons for the military's interest in urine screening is obviously due to their concern for combat readiness. However, in the case of the military, the issue of whether the individual is intoxicated or impaired at the time the sample is taken is not necessarily important. Punitive action can be based on the fact that an order to desist from marijuana or drug use has been disobeyed.

In the case of motor vehicle and industrial equipment operators, and others whose level of sobriety is a key safety factor, the primary forensic issue is the determination of intoxication or impairment rather than a "past history" of drug use.

II. ANALYTICAL FACTORS

There are many specific factors to be considered when cannabinoid assays are used in the forensic area, including the convenience of obtaining the sample to be analyzed and the usual concerns of sensitivity, specificity, and other technical aspects of the assay. If an individual's impairment is to be established, the interpretation of the analytical result becomes as important as the accuracy of the assay performed and requires a clear understanding of the pharmacokinetic parameters of THC and its metabolites.

In human studies it has been shown that 80% to 90% of the total dose of THC administered is excreted within 5 days, mostly (65%) in feces (9). The urinary fraction, which makes up the remaining 18% to 23% of the dose excreted, consists primarily of acidic metabolites, such as 11-nor-delta-9-THC-9-

carboxylic acid (9-carboxy-THC) and other related acids, which are excreted in detectable amounts for several days (10). Only about 5% of the total urinary fraction consists of neutral cannabinoids, with THC itself making up less than 1%. The endpoint of the renal pathway is therefore multi-oxygenated acidic metabolites. The feces fraction consists of approximately equal parts of neutral and acidic metabolites; 9-carboxy-THC making up about 29% of the extracted metabolites, THC about 8%, and 11-hydroxy-THC about 21% (11).

In plasma, after a smoked dose of marijuana, THC levels, which initially may rise to over 100 ng/ml, decrease rapidly to levels around 10 ng/ml within an hour and below one nanogram within 4-6 hours. 9-Carboxy-THC becomes detectable in blood within minutes and generally reaches a concentration which coincides with that of THC at about 20 minutes after the smoked dose. This gives credence to the hypothesis that a blood analysis that shows similar concentrations for both THC and 9-carboxy-THC could be an indication of very recent use of marijuana and perhaps of a high probability that the subject is in an intoxicated state.

Within 40 minutes after a smoked does, the plasma level may be below 10 ng/ml, which places considerable demand on a blood assay for THC. Analytical methodology less sensitive than 1 or 2 ng/ml is not likely to detect the presence of THC after four hours, except perhaps in a heavy chronic smoker. 9-Carboxy-THC, however, manifests a considerably longer time course and therefore provides a better indicator of previous smoking.

Because THC becomes rapidly undetectable by presently available blood analysis methods, some investigators have suggested that if any level of THC is detectable in blood at all, one can assume that the sample was taken at a time very close to the incident of smoking and that, therefore, the subject has a high probability of being intoxicated. This argument makes fairly broad assumptions concerning the presumptive concentrations of THC that can be related to specific types of impaired behavior. A recent study, which suggests that some heavy chronic smokers maintain "steady state" blood levels of THC in the low ng/ml range (12) due to accumulation in the body, will further complicate attempts to set specific and practical presumptive levels of impairment.

It appears from available data that only a blood level may correlate physiologically with an actual state of impairment. A urine sample which tests positive indicates prior use, but such an analysis cannot be directly related to impairment since cannabinoid metabolites can persist in the urine for several days after smoking a single cigarette (13).

When the result of an analysis on a single urine sample could potentially lead to punitive actions being taken against an individual, there are two key issues to be considered from a forensic analysis point of view. The first and most obvious is that the result must be accurate. A sample reported positive has significant and obvious consequences. When marijuana screening programs involve very large numbers of samples, in which high percentages of positives will result and require confirmation, the need for certainty puts particular demands on the confirmation technique itself, the quality assurance programs that the lab uses, and the care and documentation that is applied to the chain of custody associated with the transfer of the sample from the individual to the laboratory.

The second critical issue concerns what the positive assay tells us about the individual's marijuana-use habits. If the concern is merely to identify him or her as a smoker of marijuana, with little concern for whether the smoking occurred the previous hour or the previous week, then a urine analysis for metabolites of THC is sufficient information. An interpretation of impairment from a urine analysis is inappropriate in the absence of other corroborating evidence regardless of the level of metabolites found.

A quantitative measure of THC in blood has a higher probability of relating to the presumptive intoxication of the individual. In an attempt to determine whether it is feasible to establish a concentration of THC in blood that would be presumptive of impairment studies were initiated under a NIDA contract (14) at the Southern California Research Institute to study the effects of various doses of marijuana on behavioral tasks related to driving ability. Coincident with the behavioral study, a pharmacokinetic analysis of each subject based on plasma concentrations over time was performed. The sensitive behavioral tests were carried out periodically after the dose to provide a performance time-course curve which could be statistically compared to the pharmacokinetic blood-level curve. Analysis of this data is not yet complete, but what is obvious so far is that even though some consistency exists across individuals smoking a given dose of marijuana, in terms of expected blood levels, the associated performance effects of these doses do not show the same consistency. It is not yet clear whether a practical presumptive concentration of THC can be related to measurable impairment.

III. SOCIETAL FACTORS

Because of the recent availability of the Syva EMIT system and particularly the new portable version, the possibility of doing urinalyses for marijuana use has been extended into many new areas of our society. This interest has extended far beyond the forensic laboratory and screening programs are being considered by organizations which traditionally have not been involved with urinalysis (15). The relative ease of performing an assay with the EMIT system by non-technical personnel is a primary feature of the new portable version, but also one which sometimes encourages its use in an inappropriate manner. No method, regardless of how simple, can substitute for technical experience when an analysis carries significant consequences for the individual being tested.

There is little controversy concerning whether the armed forces have a right and obligation to determine who is a drug user and who is not. Also, there would probably be general agreement that certain individuals in positions of critical responsibility whose impairment could create a danger to others could be subjected to such a program. This could possibly include pilots, school-bus drivers, air-traffic controllers and so on.

Safety is an obvious reason for identifying drug users or drug-impaired individuals. More controversial rationales for screening programs in certain social or vocational settings are also subjects of current discussion. The issue of health and productivity are rationales for industrial interest in such programs and the basis for proposals to screen in public school systems. In private industry, the effect of drug use on health and job performance, which in turn affects productivity and the economics of doing business, is often as important a concern as the safety factor associated with an intoxicated individual. While industry recognizes alcohol as their primary drug problem, the use of marijuana among younger age groups is often equal to the use of alcohol, and, therefore, an issue of increasing concern.

Performance on the job becomes intertwined with potential susceptibility to blackmail when an illegal drug such as marijuana is concerned. This provides the rationale for the screening of law enforcement personnel and individuals who hold positions in our society of high public trust. Proposals have also been discussed for urine screening of professional athletes. These proposals are aimed more at combating the general use of marijuana in these population groups rather than identifying actual impairment of the individual at the time the sample is taken. Because drug-use habits rather than intoxication or impairment are being monitored by urinalysis programs, the issue of an individual's right to privacy will be an issue of continuing controversy and legal challenge.

Use of urinalysis in private industry and the resulting legal challenges will define where such programs can practically and legally be acceptable and under what circumstances. The resolution of these challenges will provide the basis for the acceptability in many of the other social settings for which cannabinoid urinalysis has been proposed.

If a program of urinalysis screening is considered for all employees in a nonspecific way, particular consideration must be given to the kind of employee behavior that is to be monitored. Since qualitative urinalysis for marijuana components cannot distinguish between the person using at the time the sample is taken from that person who may have used it a week prior, the issue arises as to how far a company can go in dictating the behavior of its employees when not on the job. The concern for the individual's right to privacy becomes an important issue. Also, the extent to which that right has to be acknowledged by his employer who may be concerned about whether the off-the-job drug use could lead to a situation where it becomes an on-the-job drug problem. Another factor is the degree of the punitive response to a positive urine analysis. Obviously, the concern for the ramifications of a positive sample would be different in the case where the company rule was to terminate on the basis of a positive analysis versus one where the rule was a requirement for drug counseling with a treatment and rehabilitation motive.

Programs of urinalysis in use now by private industry are generally used for preemployment screening or in the context of a referral for counseling or treatment of an employee who has been targeted because of an apparent drug problem. There have been challenges to preemployment screening programs that detect recent use of marijuana, but these challenges have largely been on the basis of questionable analyses rather than on the basis of the company's right to carry out such a program. The rights of the preemployment applicant are certainly less than that of the employee who has already been hired and has established a contractual arrangement with the company, but even applicants have recourse to legal precedent, which could form the basis of court challenges in the areas of privacy and discrimination. Whether such challenges are successful, and to what degree, will depend in part on the public perception of the sensitivity of the job for which application is being made. Clearly, the issue of cannabinoid urinalysis encompasses enough unprecedented issues that new legal and social ground will be broken during the next few years.

If screening is limited to the detection of impairment along the lines of alcohol screening, which is used regularly in industry, blood analysis is the body fluid with the greatest potential for a chemical marker of performance decrements. This will raise even more complicated legal analytical issues. Of primary importance will be the basis for associating particular impairment with blood levels of drug. It is in this very area where considerable efforts need to be made to better define the "time course" of impairment after smoking marijuana and the associated presumptive blood level for significant impairment. New findings of "steady state" blood levels in some regular users may significantly complicate this effort.

IV. DISCUSSION

Assuming that some of the programs under present consideration will be put in place, the economic impetus for developing better and less expensive confirmation methods for the presently available immunoassay methods will shape much of the research and development in the near future. Confirmation is very critical to forensic programs where the analysis ofa single sample with no corroborating evidence will provide the sole reason for punitive measures against the subject.

Confirmation by GC/MS, the presently accepted method of choice, is expensive because the sample must be hydrolyzed, extracted and then derivatized, a time consuming and therefore expensive process. Two techniques which appear promising in alleviating some of these problems in confirmation arehigh performance liquid chromatography (HPLC) with fluorescent or electrochemical detectors and high performance thin-layer chromatography (HPTLC). While systems such as the Syva EMIT and Roche ABUSCREEN are relatively inexpensive for carrying out large volume screening, the possibility of immunoassay systems being developed based on solid state techniques and designed for mass screening, at a lower cost per sample, may also become important.

As discussed previously, blood analyses do have the potential for providing information relevant to intoxication, but they are difficult to obtain for forensic purposes because of their invasive nature. Urine, which provides different information from a blood sample, also has problems associated with its acquisition and the information which it provides. Saliva and breath samples, on the other hand, are much easier to acquire for drug detection and both have been investigated for the presence of marijuana components after smoking. The use of TLC methods for detection of THC in saliva has been suggested by several investigators (16-20). This type of sample offers advantages in ease of collection, as well as by providing chemical information which may be as easy to obtain as a urine sample, but is more informative about an individual's time of drug use.

A study in humans using radiolabeled THC administered by intravenous injection failed to detect radioactivity in saliva samples (21). This suggests that neither THC nor its metabolites pass into the saliva or lung from the blood, and that cannabinoids detected in these matrices are sequestered in the mucous membranes during the smoking process and then slowly released into the saliva.

The use of breath as a screening medium has been investigated using solvent and cryogenic traps with subsequent analysis by HPLC/MS (22), and also using solid matrix traps followed by conventional RIA (23). The levels in breath appear to be lower than those found in saliva after smoking and use of such a medium for detection would consequently require relatively more sensitivity in the assay method as well as a more complex means of sample collection.

In a recent study, saliva samples from 5 subjects, who smoked standard marijuana cigarettes containing cannabis of approximately 2% potency, were collected over a 24 hour period (14). Analysis by RIA showed detectable levels of THC remaining in saliva several hours after smoking (24). These are illustrated in Fig.1. During the first hour somelevels exceeded 100 ng/ml, and levels above 5 ng/ml werestill detectable in many samples beyond 8 hours. The effect of food and drink on this time course remains to be determined.

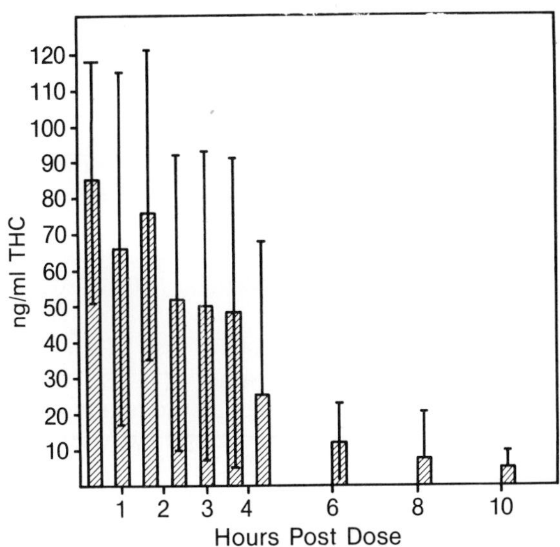

FIGURE 1. THC concentrations in mixed saliva samples from human subjects (N = 5) after smoking one marijuana cigarette (2% THC by weight). Concentrations expressed as means +/- S.D.

These results give further indication that saliva could be a useful fluid for presumptive detection of recent use. Even though no quantitative correlation can be made between saliva levels and intoxication, because only sequestered THC is being detected, the capacity to reduce the "past use" time-frame from weeks to hours could have useful research and forensic applications.

Underlying all the interest in drug screening for the purpose of identifying performance related problems is the concern that individuals who smoke marijuana will, in fact, be significantly impaired at the task in question. While the effects of marijuana on many types of performance have been demonstrated, the quantitative measures of such performance effects have not yet clearly defined their time course, nor have such studies established specific blood levels which can be presumptive of impairment. What is clear so far is that acute marijuana use affects cognitive and motor tasks in a negative manner, but the extent and duration of such effects varies with the task performed.

The need to characterize and quantitate these effects and their duration has obvious importance to the interpretation of a forensic analysis. The need is clear, therefore, to build on our present knowledge in the area of performance impairment related to marijuana and better define where and under what circumstances the rapidly evolving chemical techniques of marijuana-use detection can best and most legitimately be used.

Clearly the issues surrounding chemical analysis for the detection of marijuana use or impairment in our society will provide many new challenges and controversies in the near future.

REFERENCES

1. "Cannabinoid Assays in Humans" (R. E. Willette, ed.), National Institute on Drug Abuse Research Monograph, No. 7, DHEW Pub. (ADM) 78-339. Supt. of Docs., U.S. Govt. Print. Off., Washington, D. C., 1976.
2. "Cannabinoid Analysis in Physiological Fluids", (J. A. Vinson, ed.). ACS Symposium Series 98, Amer. Chem. Soc., Washington, D. C., 1979.
3. Foltz, R. L., Fentiman, Jr., A. F., and Foltz, R. B., "GC/MS Assays Abused Drugs in Body Fluids". National Institute on Drug Abuse Research Monograph, No. 32, DHEW Pub. (ADM) 80-1014. Supt. of Docs. U.S. Govt. Print. Off., Washington, D. C., 1980.

4. "Cannabinoid Assays in Body Fluids" (R. L. Hawks, ed.). National Institute on Drug Abuse Research Monograph, No. 42, DHHS Pub. (ADM) 82-1212. Supt. of Docs., U.S. Govt. Print. Off., Washington, D. C., 1982.
5. "Chromatography of Environmental Hazards, Volume 4: Drug of Abuse" (L. Fishbein, ed.). Elsevier Scientific Publishing Co., New York, 1982.
6. Garrett, E. R., Hunt, G. A., Physiochemical properties, solubility and proteins binding of delta-9-tetrahydrocannabinol, J. Pharm. Sci. 63:1056 (1974).
7. Fenimore, D. C., Davis, C. M., Whitford, J. H., and Harrington, C. A., Vapor phase silylation of laboratory glassware, Anal. Chem. 48:2289 (1976).
8. Whiting, J. D., and Manders, W. W., Confirmation of a tetrahydrocannabinol metabolite in urine by gas chromatography, J. Anal. Tox. 6:49-52 (1982).
9. Hunt, A. C., and Jones, R. T., Tolerance and disposition of THC in man, J. Pharm. Exp. Ther. 215:135-44 (1980).
10. Halldin, M.M., Carlsson, S., Kanter, S. L., Widman, M., and Agurell, S., Urinary metabolites of delta-1-tetrahydrocannabinol in man, Arzeim.-Forsch. 32:764-769 (1982).
11. Wall, M. E., Brine, D. R., Perez-Reyes, M., Metabolism of cannabinoids in man, in "The Pharmacology of Marijuana", Vol. 1 (M. C. Braude and S. Szara, eds.), pp. 93-116. Raven Press, New York, 1976.
12. Foltz, R., personal communication.
13. Clark, S., Turner, J., and Bastiani, R., "EMIT Cannabinoid Assay, Clinical Study No. 74, Summary Report". Syva Co., Palo Alto, CA, 1980.
14. Moskowitz, H., Southern California Research Institute, CA, samples collected under NIDA contract 271-76-3316.
15. "Urine Testing for Marijuana Use: Implications for a Variety of Settings", (M. Basinsky and G. K. Russell, eds.). The American Council on Marijuana and Other Psychoactive Drugs, Inc., Rockville, MD., 1981.
16. Forrest, I. S., Green, D. E., Rose, S. E., Skinner, G. C., and Torres, D. M., Fluorescent-labeled cannabinoids, Res. Commun. Chem. Pathol. Pharmacol. 2:787-792 (1971).
17. Melikian, A. P., and Forrest, I. S., Dansyl derivatives of delta-9- and delta-8-tetrahydrocannabinols, J. Pharm. Sci. 62:1025-1026 (1973).
18. Just, W. W., Werner, G., and Weichmann, M., Bestimmung von delta-1- and delta-1(6)-Tetrahydrocannabinol in Blut, Urin und Speichel von Haschisch-Rauchern, Naturwiss., 59:222-223 (1972).
19. Friedrich-Fiechtl, F., Spiteller, G., Just, W. W., Werner, G., and Weichmann, M., Au Nachweis und Identifizierung von Tetrahydrocannabinol in Biologischen Flussighkeiten, Naturwiss. 60:207-208 (1973).

20. Just, W. W., Filipovic, N., and Werner, G., Detection of delta-9-THC in saliva of men by means of thin-layer chromatography and mass-spectrometry, J. Chromatogr. 96:189-194 (1974).
21. Perez-Reyes, M., University of North Carolina, personal communication.
22. Valentine, J. L., Bryant, P. J., Gutshall, P. L., Gan, O. H. M., and Niu, H. C., Detection of delta-9-THC in human breath following marijuana smoking, Anal. Letters 12:867-880 (1979).
23. Soares, J. R., Grant, J. D., and Gross, S. J., Significant developments in radioimmunoassay methods applied to delta-9-THC and its 9-substituted metabolites, in "Cannabinoid Assays in Biological Fluids", (R.Hawks, ed.), pp. 44. NIDA Research Monograph, No. 42, DHHS Pub. (ADM) 82-1212. Supt. of Docs., U.S. Govt. Print. Off., Washington, D. C., 1982.
24. Cook, C. E., Research Triangle Institute, NC, performed under NIDA contract 271-80-3705.

RADIOIMMUNOASSAY FOR 11-HYDROXY-DELTA-9-TETRAHYDROCANNABINOL, MAJOR PSYCHOACTIVE METABOLITE OF DELTA-9-TETRAHYDROCANNABINOL

C. E. Cook, V. H. Schindler
C. R. Tallent, H. H. Seltzman
C. Warick, C. G. Pitt

Research Triangle Institute
Research Triangle Park, North Carolina

I. INTRODUCTION

The potential simplicity, speed and specificty of radioimmunoassys (RIA) led to consideration of this technique for the analysis of delta-9-tetrahydrocannabinol (THC) and/or its metabolites in biological materials. The production of antisera with high selectivity for specific cannabinoid molecules was required for this work, as was the preparation of appropriately labeled radioligands.

Since THC and its metabolites are small molecules, they must be linked to a large molecule (e.g., a protein) in order to evoke an immune response in animals. Landsteiner has shown that the position on a small molecule through which it is attached to a protein has a strong effect on the selectivity of the resulting antisera. Other molecules differing in substitution at that position can still have high affinity for the antibodies (1). Thus metabolically reactive sites should generally be avoided as the position of linkage to protein in design of an immunogenic conjugate.

II. RESULTS AND DISCUSSION

Early work on the metabolism of tetrahydrocannabinol indicated that reactions occurred in the 8 and 11 positions of the cannabinoid molecule. Although later work has shown that

ISBN 0-12-044620-0

other positions on the cannbinoid molecule are also subject to enzymatic modification, pathways involving the 8 and 11 positions still are responsible for the majority of human THC metabolites (2). When we began developing immunoassays for cannabinoid compounds, we therefore looked upon the amyl side chain as a logical point for attaching the molecule to protein in order to form an immunogenic conjugate. Other conjugates have been reported (see ref. 3 for a list), but we expected that this position of linkage should result in greatest exposure of the metabolicaly reactive 8 and 11 positions as well as of the phenolic group, aromatic ring and tricyclic ring structure. Thus the conjugate should stimulate the formation of relatively high affinity and selective antibodies.

As we have previously reported, conjugation of a 5'-carboxyl derivative of THC to bovine serum albumin by means of an amide bond proceeded well, and the resulting conjugate (Compound 1, Figure 1) was found to stimulate the formation of antibodies capable of binding THC with good selectivity, particularly versus the 11-nor-9-carboxylic acid metabolite. Because synthesis is easier in the delta-8-series, the initial conjugate was made from delta-8-THC derivatives (3,4). Later we prepared the corresponding delta-9-conjugates, but either antiserum could be used for the analysis of THC in plasma. Our procedure has been repeated in the delta-8-series by Owens et al. (5), who obtained similar results.

Initially tritium labeled delta-8-THC (6) was evaluated as the radioligand. Delta-8-THC was chosen for labeling because high specific activity tritium-labeled delta-9-THC has poor stability. Although this resulted in a heterologous system for the analysis of delta-9-THC, the high speecific activity attainable and the coonsiderable degree of cross-reactivity between delta-8- and -9-THC for the antibody permitted a useful assay. Because of the advantages often associated with iodine-125 as the radio-label, we then prepared [^{125}I]-5'-iodo-delta-9-THC (Compound 3, Figure 1)(7). We anticipated that because of the location of the iodine at the same position as that involved in formation of the immunogen, steric hindrance to antibody binding caused by this bulky atom would be minimized. Thus the iodinated molecule would be bound with sufficiently high affinity for it to be useful as a radioligand. This hope was justified by experience, and the combination of delta-9-antiserum and delta-8-radioligand has proved useful for the analysis of biological samples (3,8).

Somewhat similar strategy was used for the development of antisera to 11-nor-9-carboxy-delta-9-THC in plasma and urine. In this instance the chemistry had to be modified in order to distinguish the two ends of the molecule for coupling purposes. The resulting conjugate was thus an alkylamino substituted bovine serum albumin (Compound 2, Figure 1). The radio-

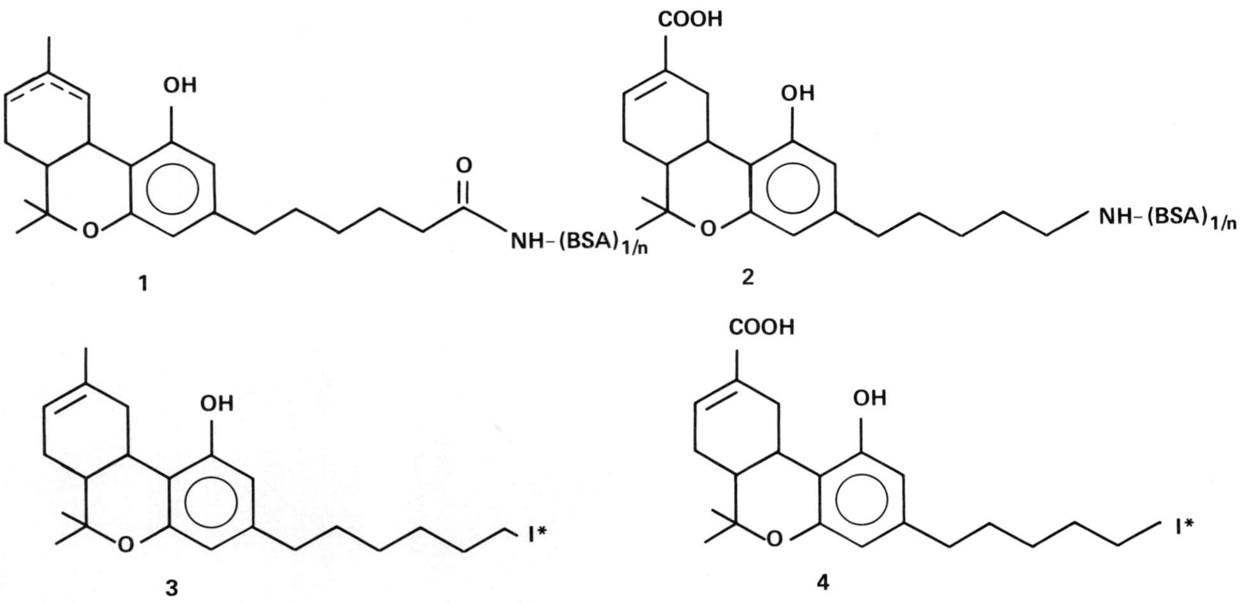

FIGURE 1. Conjugates and radioligands for cannabinoid analysis.

ligand employed was [^{125}I]-9-carboxy-5'-iodo-11-nor-delta-8-THC (Compound 3, Figure 1). Both the conjugate and the radioligand were prepared as the delta-8-isomers, but the antisera proved quite satisfactory for detection and analysis of the delta-9-carboxylic acid (4,9).

An analogous approach has now been applied to the analysis of 11-hydroxy-delta-9-THC. As Figure 2 shows, the 5'-bromo derivative of delta-8-THC was converted by acetate displacement, protection of the phenolic group as a silyl ether and reduction to the 5'-hydroxy compound. Oxidation of the hydroxyl group and protection of the aldehyde as the ethylene acetal was followed by standard conversion of the 11-position to an aldehyde with selenium dioxide and thence to an alcohol by sodium borohydride reduction. Use of tritium labeled sodium borohydride to reduce the aldehyde at position 11 yielded material labeled with tritium in the hydroxymethyl group. (A radiolabeled tracer is useful for determining incorporation into protein in the final conjugate.) Acid in acetone cleaved the ethylene acetal to the aldehyde (Compound 4, Figure 2).

In this route it is necessary to retain the protecting acetate group until after the aldehyde-protein coupling reaction has been carried out. In the case of delta-8-THC, the unprotected phenolic aldehyde was found to very readily undergo cyclization reactions to the benzocycloheptene derivatives shown in Figure 3. The aldehyde, still protected as the phenolic acetate, was then allowed to react with the amino groups of bovine serum albumin (Figure 4). As has been shown in the case of steroidal ketones (10), a Schiff base forms and is then reduced by sodium cyanoborohydride to the alkyl amine. Finally, mild hydrolysis under basic conditions removed the acetate group (4), leaving the dihydroxy conjugate containing 19 cannabinoid residues per molecule of BSA. This conjugate was used for the immunization of rabbits.

Figure 5 shows the synthesis of the required radioligand. 5'-Bromo-delta-8-THC was acetylated, oxidized to the 11-aldehyde and reduced to the 11-hydroxy compound. Displacement of the bromide with sodium iodide and then displacement with silver tosylate led to the 5'-tosylate which on treatment with ^{125}I-sodium iodide gave the required radioligand.

Rabbits were immunized by subcutaneous injection of the conjugate. A vigorous immunization schedule (illustrated in Figure 6) previously used by Owens et al. (5) for development of antisera to delta-8-THC was followed. Rabbits were bled 25 days after the initial immunization and then 10 or 11 days after each booster injection. After four months of immunizations, the rabbits were rested for three months and then booster injections were resumed. For the first four immunizations each rabbit received a subcutaneous injection of 200 ug of conjugate as an emulsion in equal volumes of saline and

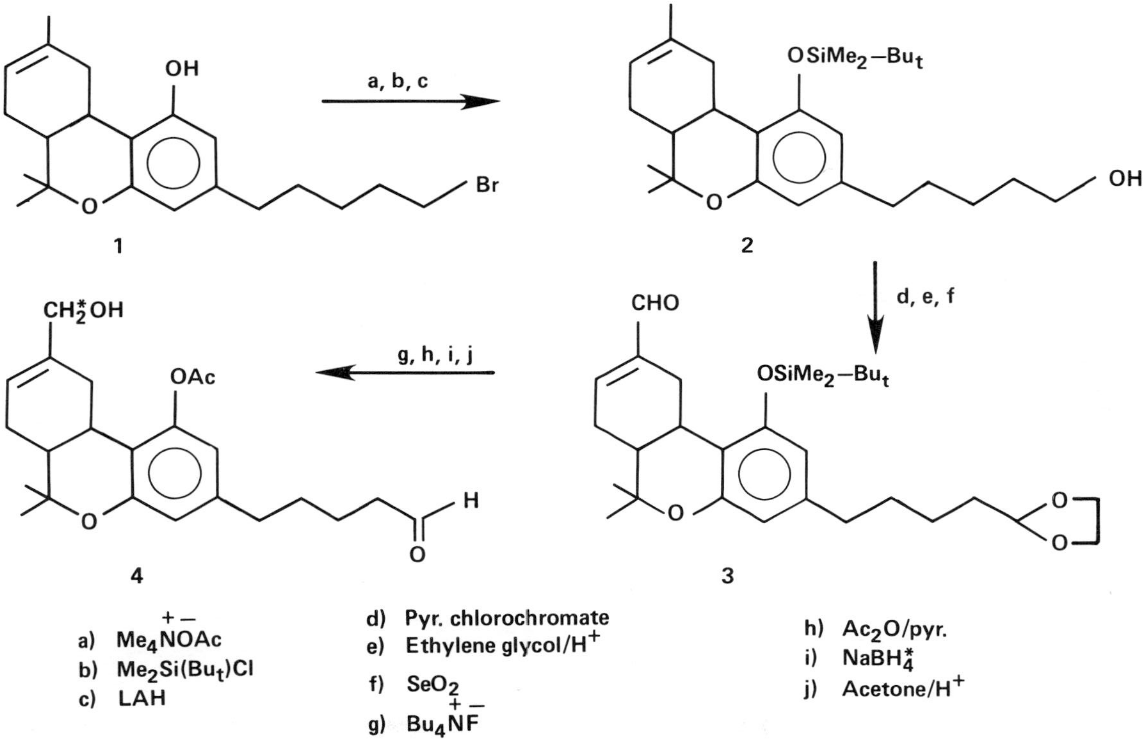

a) $Me_4\overset{+}{N}\overset{-}{O}Ac$
b) $Me_2Si(Bu_t)Cl$
c) LAH
d) Pyr. chlorochromate
e) Ethylene glycol/H^+
f) SeO_2
g) $Bu_4\overset{+}{N}\overset{-}{F}$
h) Ac_2O/pyr.
i) $NaBH_4^*$
j) Acetone/H^+

FIGURE 2. Synthesis of 11-hydroxy-delta-8-THC hapten. Reactants: a) $Me_4\overset{+}{N}OAc$; $Me_2Si(Bu_t)Cl$; c) LAH; d) Pyr. chlorochromate; e) Ethylene glycol/H^+; f) SeO_2; g) Bu_4NF; h) Ac_2O/pyr.; i) $NaBH_4$*; j) Acetone/H^+.

Freund's complete adjuvant. After that time 100 mcg of conjugate (in saline/Freund's incomplete adjuvant) per rabbit was used for the immunization. Antisera titers rose relatively rapidely, and by 80-100 days after initial immunization a 1:1000 initial dilution of antisera (which is equivalent to about 1:5000 final dilution) from all four rabbits bound over 50% of the radioligand. Antiserum 6 from rabbit 554 was chosen for more detailed study. This antiserum was used at an initial dilution of 1:15,000 which bound approximately 25-40% of the [^{125}I]-5'-iodo-delta-8-11-hydroxy-THC.

The ability of several cannbinoids to displace radioligand from this antiserum is illustrated in Figures 7-9. 11-Hydroxy-delta-9-THC exhibits quite reasonable affinity for the antiserum (Figure 7). With radioligand of the specific activity presently being used, a standard curve runs from 20-10,000 picograms with best results in the range from 50-5,000 picograms. THC itself has quite a low cross reactivity as measured by 50% displacement of radioligand (only 0.9%). (See ref. 11, footnote 4, for a discussion of this method of measuring cross-reactivity.) Cannabinol has even less (only 0.5%) and 9-carboxy-11-nor-delta-9-THC cross-reacts only minimally (0.15%).

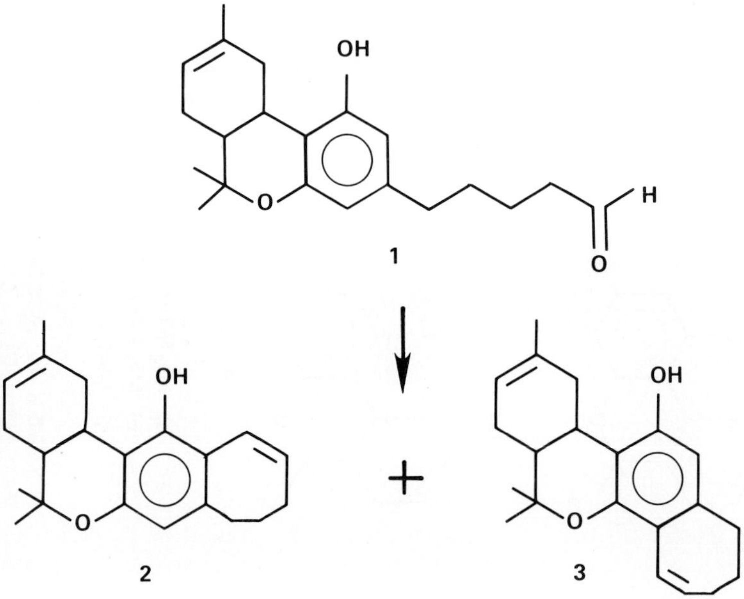

FIGURE 3. Cyclization of the aldehyde intermediate.

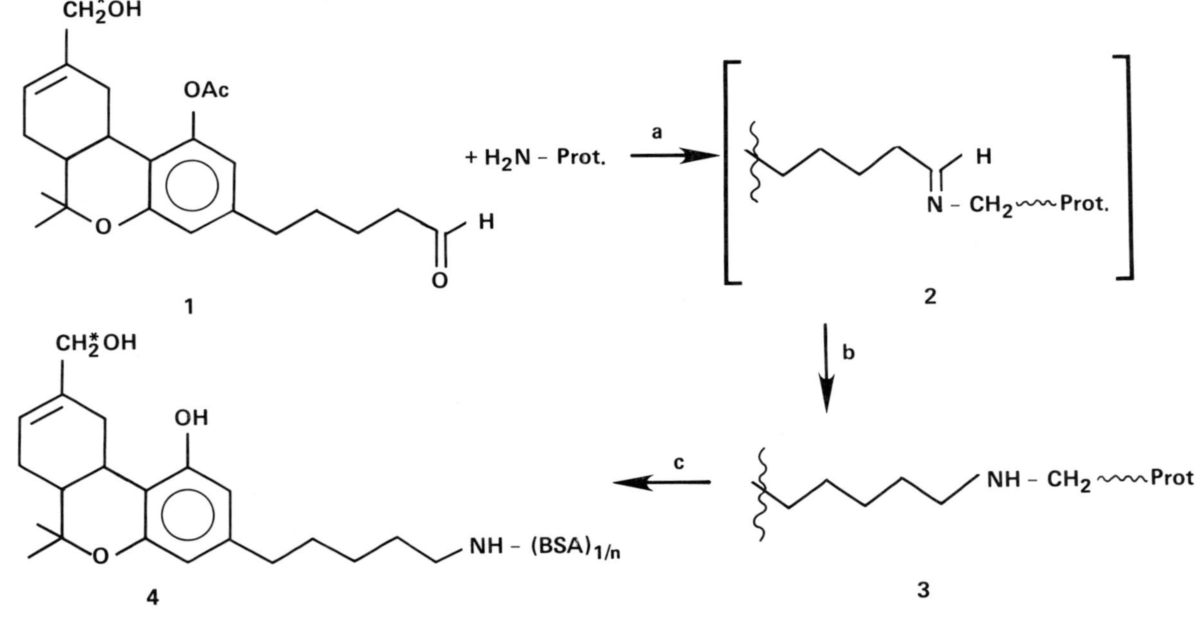

FIGURE 4. Synthesis of 11-hydroxy-delta-8-THC-BSA conjugate. Reactants: a) MeOH; b) $NaBH_3CN$; c) OH^-.

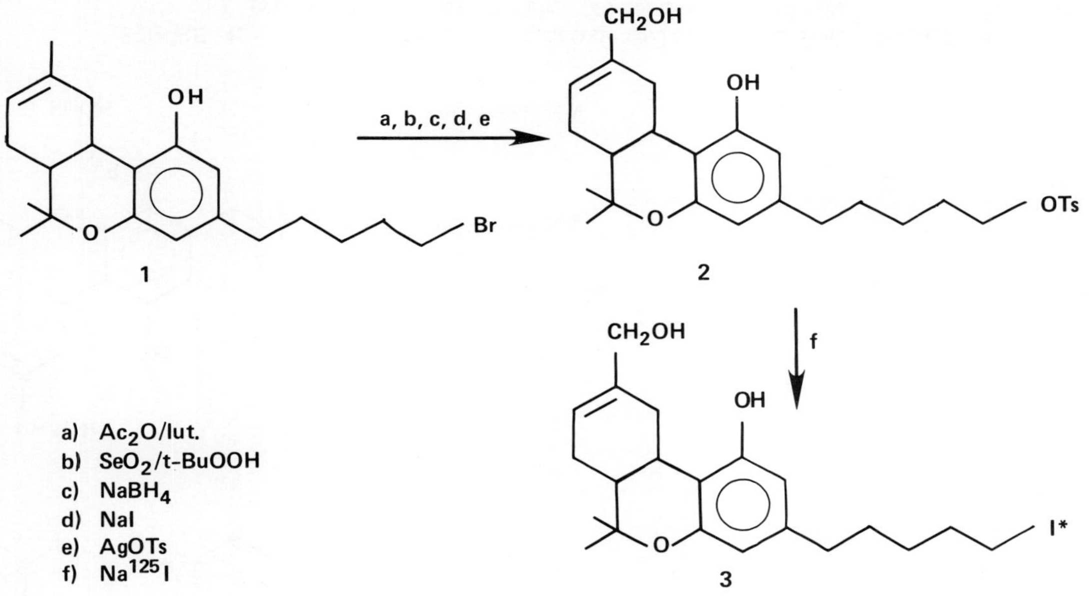

a) Ac_2O/lut.
b) SeO_2/t-BuOOH
c) $NaBH_4$
d) NaI
e) AgOTs
f) $Na^{125}I$

FIGURE 5. Synthesis of radioligand. Reactants: a) Ac_2O/lut.; b) SeO_2/t-BuOOH; c) $NaBH_4$; d) NaI; e) AgOTs; f) $Na^{125}I$.

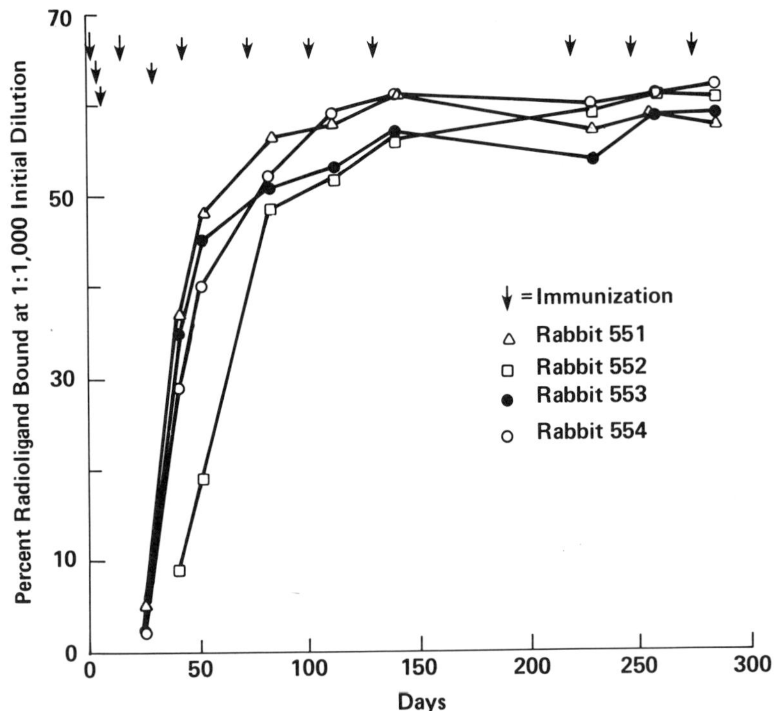

FIGURE 6. Development of antiserum to 11-hydroxy-delta-8-THC. Legend: arrows, immunization times; open triangle, rabbit 551; open square, rabbit 552; closed circle, rabbit 553; open circle, rabbit 554.

Fig. 8 illustrates the cross-reation of the antiserum with 8-hydroxy metabolites of THC. 8beta-Hydroxy-delta-9-THC gives minimal cross-reaction, and there is also less than 1% cross-reation with 8beta,11-dihydroxy-delta-9-THC. 8alpha- and 8alpha,11-dihydroxy-delta-9-THC present greater cross-reaction problems, on the order of 5-18%. Fortunately, 8alpha-hydroxylation represents a minor metabolic pathway for THC (2). 11-Hydroxycannabinol, however, cross-reacts strongly with the antiserum. Again in most instances this would not present problems in an analysis of plasma samples.

Figure 9 shows that the side chain hydroxylated metabolites of THC fall into a pattern which accords with expectations based on proximity of the hydroxyl to the point of conjugation. Thus, the two diastereoisomeric 1'-hydroxy-delta-9-THC compounds exhibit very little cross-reaction (less than 0.1%). Somewhat greater, but still minimal, cross-reaction is

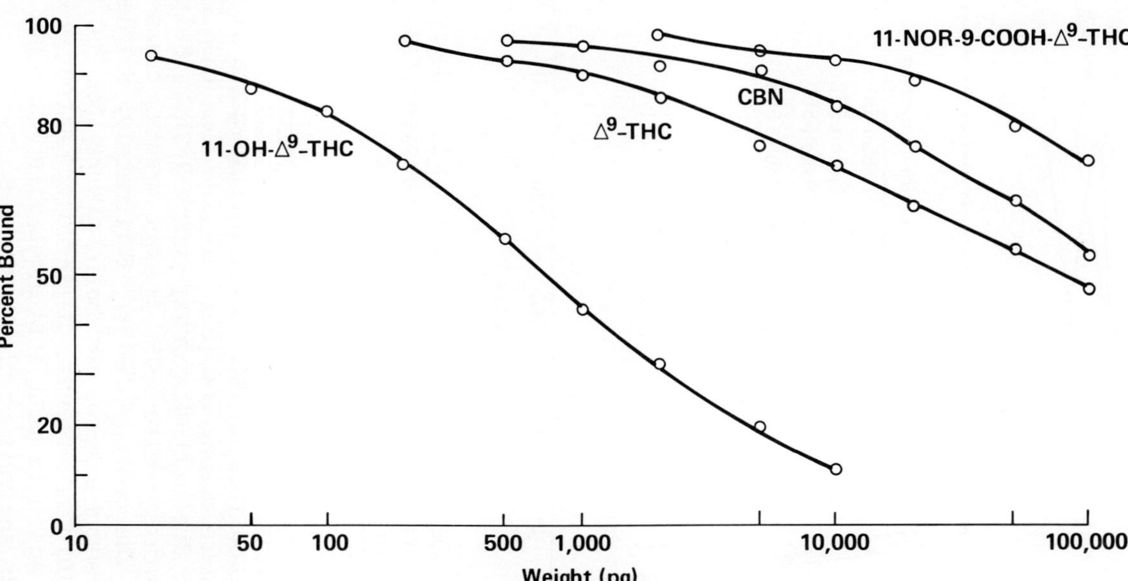

FIGURE 7. Cross-reactions of 11-hydroxy-delta-8-THC antiserum.

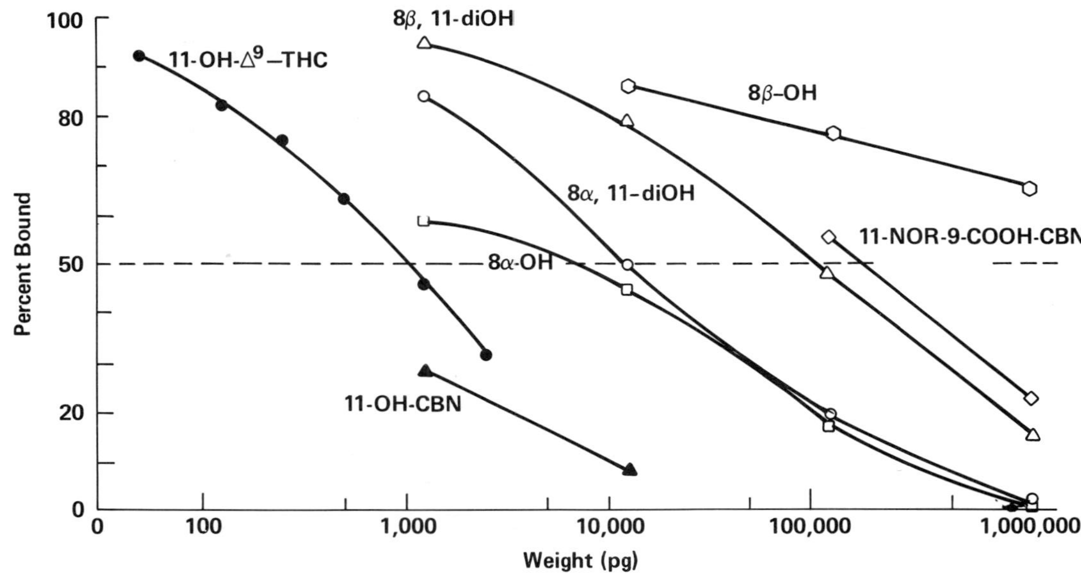

FIGURE 8. Cross-reaction of 11-hydroxy-delta-8-THC antiserum with some hydroxy metabolites.

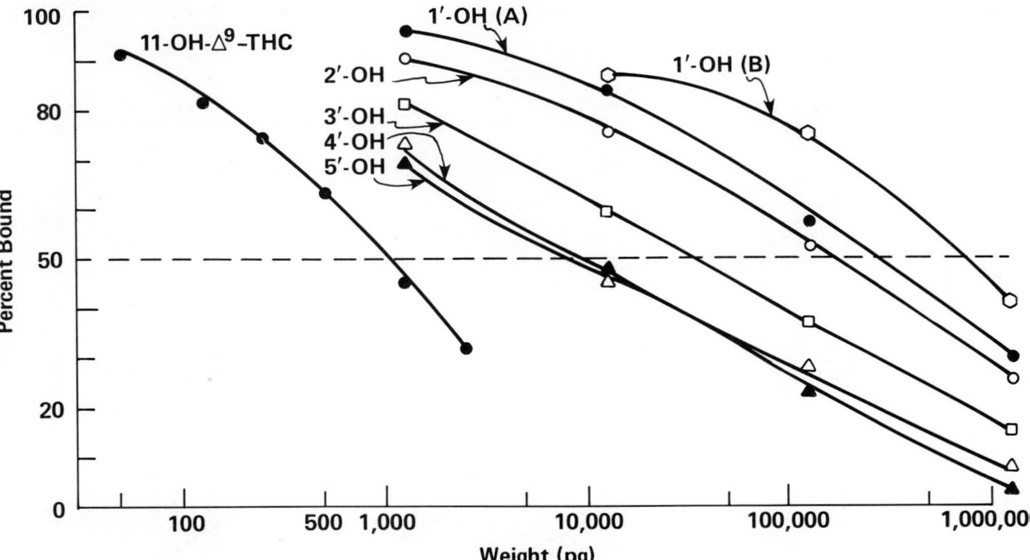

FIGURE 9. Cross-reaction of 11-hydroxy-delta-8-THC antiserum with side-chain hydroxy metabolites.

exhibited by the 2'-hydroxy-isomer. 3'-Hydroxy-delta-9-THC exhibits 3% cross-reaction and the 4'- and 5'-hydroxy metabolites have about 10% the relative affinity of 11-hydroxy-delta-9-THC. By comparison with the cross-reaction of THC, this suggest that a polar group close to the position of the amino function in the conjugate can enhance affinity for the antibody.

Figure 10 shows the procedure for analysis of plasma samples for 11-hydroxy-delta-9-THC. Plasma is diluted with methanol and the protein-free supernatant is then added to radiolabeled buffer, antiserum and solid plase second antibody (Immunobeads^R). Overnight incubation followed by centrifugation and washing results in a pellet containing the bound radioligand. Measurement of the radioactivity then allows the generation of the standard curve. Alternatively charcoal can be used to separate free and bound radioligand.

In summary, conjugation of 11-hydroxy-delta-8-THC to bovine serum albumin through a 5'-aminoalkyl linkage gives a material which stimulates the formation of antibodies capable of binding 11-hydroxy-delta-9-THC. Use of them in conjunction with [^{125}]-5'-iodo-11-hydroxy-delta-8-THC as a radioligand permits the analysis of 11-hydroxy-delta-9-THC is plasma sam-

100 μL Plasma

\+

400 μL Methanol

Aliquot 100 μL

Add radiolabel /buffer/antiserum/Immunobeads®

Incubate overnight (4° C)

Centrifuge and decant

Wash beads, centrifuge and decant

Measure ^{125}I

FIGURE 10. Analysis of plasma for 11-hydroxy-delta-9-THC.

ples. Standard curves range from 2-200 ng/mL. Cross-reactions with THC itself and with its 9-carboxy-11-nor metabolite are very low. Gratifyingly low affinities for other hydroxylated metabolites of THC are also observed, and plasma does not appear to interfere with the analysis at the levels measured. However, as is the case with any anlytical technique, care must be taken with regard to its use and to conclusions drawn from its application. After oral adminstration of THC to humans, for example, the 11-hydroxy metabolite constitutes a relatively large proportion of the psychoactive substances (2) and its analysis by the present radioimmuoassay would appear to be feasible. However, possible species differences, the presence of various other hydroxylated metabolites in plasma and their potential build-up on prolonged exposure, must be taken into consideration. In short, although this technique looks quite promising for the analysis of 11-hydroxy-THC in plasma, investigators should assure themselves that it is indeed applicable to their own situation.

REFERENCES

1. Landsteiner, K., "The Specificity of Serological Reactions", Dover Press, Inc., New York, 1962.
2. Wall, M. E., and Perez-Reyes, M. The Metabolish of delta-9-tetrahydrocannabinol and related cannabinoids in man, J. Clin Pharmacol. 21:1785-1895 (1981).
3. Cook, C. E., Radioimmunoassay of Cannabinoid Compounds, in "Cannabinoid Analysis in Physiological Fluids", J. A. Vinson ed., ACS Symposium Series 98, American Chemical Society, Washington, D.C., 137-154, 1979.
4. Cook, C. E., Seltzman, H. H., Schindler, V. H., Tallent, C. R., Chin, K. M., and Pitt, C. G. Radioimmunoassays for cannabinoids, in "Cannabinoid Assays in Biological Fluids", R. L. Hawks, ed., NIDA Monograph Series, In Press, 1982.
5. Owens, S. M., McBay, A. J., Reisner, H. M., and Perez-Reyes, M., ^{125}I Radioimmunoassay of delta-9-tetrahydrocannabinol in blood and plasma with a solid-phase-second-antibody separation method, Clin. Chem. 27:619-624, 1981.
6. Pitt, C. G., Seltzman, H. H., Setzer, S. R. and Williams, D. L. The synthesis of deuterium, carbon-14 and carrier-free tritium labeled cannabinoids, J. Label. Comp. 11:551-575 (1975).
7. Pitt, C. G., Seltzman, H. H. Setzer, S. R. and Williams, D. L. The preparation of 5'-iodo-iodine-125-delta-8-THC; a radioligand for the radioimmunoassay of cannabinoids, J. Label. Comp. Radiopharm. 17:681 (1979).

8. Cook, C. E., Hawer, M. L., Amerson, E. W., Pitt, C. G., Williams, D. L. and Willette, R. E., Tetrahydrocannabinol (THC) radioimmunoassay: Immunogen and novel iodine-125-radioligand based on 5'-substituted-delta-8-THC, Pharmacologist 18:291 (1976).

9. Cook, C. E., Schindler, V. H., Tallent, C. R., Seltzman, H. H., and Pitt, C. G., Radioimmunoassay for a major tetrahydrocannabinol (THC) metabolite, 11-nor-9-carboxy-delta-9-tetrahydrocannabinol (NCTHC), Federation Proceedings 40:278 (1981).

10. Muller, R., Scheuer, A., Gerdes, H., and Mosebach, K. O., Direkte Kupplung von Steroiden an Eiweiss durch reduktive Aminierung zur Gewinnung specifischer Antikorper, Fresenius Z. Anal. Chem. 290:164 (1978).

11. Cook, C. E., Tallent, C. R., Amerson, E. W., Myers, M. W., Kepler, J. A., Taylor, G. F. and Christense, H. D., Caffeine in plasma and saliva by a radioimmunoassay procedure, J. Pharmacol. Exp. Therap. 19:679-686 (1976).

NOVEL DERIVATIZATION METHODS IN THE ANALYSIS OF CANNABINOIDS

J. Rosenfeld

Department of Pathology
McMaster University
Hamilton, Ontario

I. INTRODUCTION

In the course of investigating the analytical chemistry of cannabinoids, we exploited phase transfer catalysis (PTC) as a general approach to the quantitative determination of these compounds and their metabolites (1). Predominantly this catalytic process was applied to the mass spectrometric determination of delta-9-tetrahydrocannabinol (THC) and 11-hydroxy-delta-9-THC (2,3). Recognizing that mass spectrometry was not a technique that could be widely used, we also began investigations into analysis of cannabinoids by gas chromatography with electron capture detection (GC/ECD) and used PTC in the analytical synthesis of electrophoric derivatives, such as the pentafluorobenzyl and the trifluoroethyl ethers of THC (1).

Derivatization of organic acids with phase transfer catalysis is based upon the transfer of an ion pair between ionized organic acid and a quaternary ammonium or phosphonium salt from aqueous into organic phase (4). If the organic phase contains an alkylating agent, such as methyl iodide (CH_3I) or pentafluorobenzyl bromide (PFBBr), the conjugate base of the organic acid is converted to the corresponding ester or ether. The schematics of the reaction mechanism appear in Figure 1.

While phase transfer catalysis offers several distinct advantages, such as simultaneous extraction and derivatization of analyte, speed of reaction and mild reactionconditions, there are some drawbacks. The first of these is that the phase transfer catalyst (in the case of cannabinoid analysis, the quaternary ammonium cation) co-extracts with the analyte. Thus the residue consists of a mixture of several nanograms of

ISBN 0-12-044620-0

analyte in approximately a milligram of co-extracted catalyst. Consequently methods have been developed to eliminate the co-extracted catalyst prior to analysis by GC or GC/MS (2,5-7). However, this extra step adds to the technical complexity of the procedures which utilized PTC as an approach to simplifying analytical methods. A second problem stems from the fact that this process is a liquid/liquid extraction and is thus relatively difficult to automate.

The latter point is particularly important. There is considerable interest in the medical applications of cannabinoids and cannabinoid-like drugs. These compounds will require investigation of their pharmacokinetics and pharmacodynamics. There are also legal requirements for determination of cannabinoids and cannabinoid metabolites. Thus, simplification and possible automation of cannabinoid analyses would be particularly useful.

Difficulties with co-extraction of the phase transfer catalyst have been encountered in organic synthesis. An elegant solution was proposed by Regen (8) and Tundo (9). These authors, working independently, demonstrated that the quaternary and phosphonium cations can be covalently linked to a solid insoluble support such as silica gel or polystyrene. The reaction is then carried out in a triphasic system of water, immiscible organic solvent (e.g. toluene), water and the solid catalyst. This approach has not been tested in analytical organic chemistry possibly because of the extended reaction times and elevated temperatures required. Nevertheless, the use of solid insoluble catalysts is generally recognized as a valid approach to automation and simplification of chemical processes (10-15).

This report describes two approaches to dealing with the problems encountered in the use of PTC. In the first approach, a reaction mechanism was developed that permits simultaneous extraction and derivatization of THC from aqueous medium in the absence of phase transfer catalyst. Secondly, a solid state synthesis of pentafluorobenzyl derivatives of THC was investigated. The latter reaction also eliminatesthe problem of co-extracted phase transfer catalyst but in addition provides an approach to automation of analytical derivatization reactions for the cannabinoids.

II. LIQUID/LIQUID BIPHASIC BENZYLATION REACTIONS

One approach to minimizing the problem of co-extraction of catalyst is simply to use less catalyst. The understanding of the mechanism of phase transfer catalysis suggest this is feasible if the leaving group of the alkylating agent is

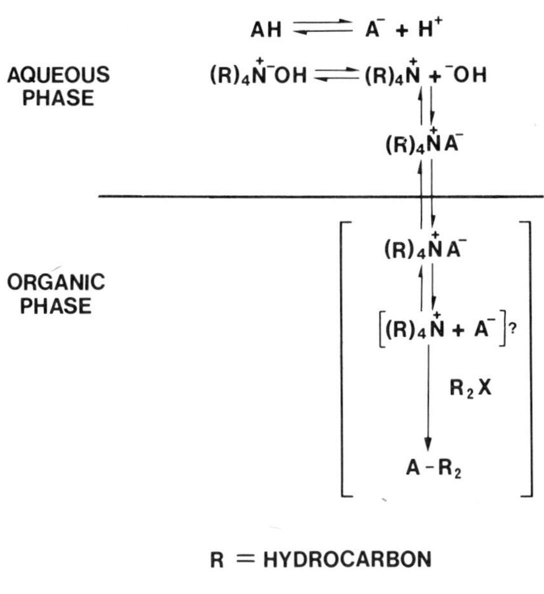

FIGURE 1. Schematic of phase transfer catalysis.

either chloride or bromide (16). In these instances after alkylation the resulting by-product is a tetra-alkyl ammonium bromide or chloride. These halogen/quaternary ammonium cation ion pairs are water-soluble and are transferred back into the aqueous phase to provide a further source of cationic phase transfer catalyst. Under these conditions it is conceivable that very small amounts of quaternary cation may be sufficient to catalyse the reaction (16).

We investigated the effect of decreasing the amount of catalyst in the PTC based derivatization of THC preparatory to GC-ECD analysis. Initial studies were carried out using BzBr (17) as a model for the electrophoric but expensive PFBBr. The latter reagent was used once the preliminary studies with the BzBr had been completed.

These investigations demonstrated that THC could be effectively converted to the benzyl (18) or pentafluorobenzyl ether (19) in a liquid/liquid biphasic system of methylene chloride/aqueous alkali but in the absence of phase transfer catalyst. This was a surprising finding. Phenols (and other organic acids) must be ionized in order to displace the bromide and such ionization can only take place in the aqueous phase. Conversely the ionized phenol must be transferred into the organic phase in order to react with alkylating agent

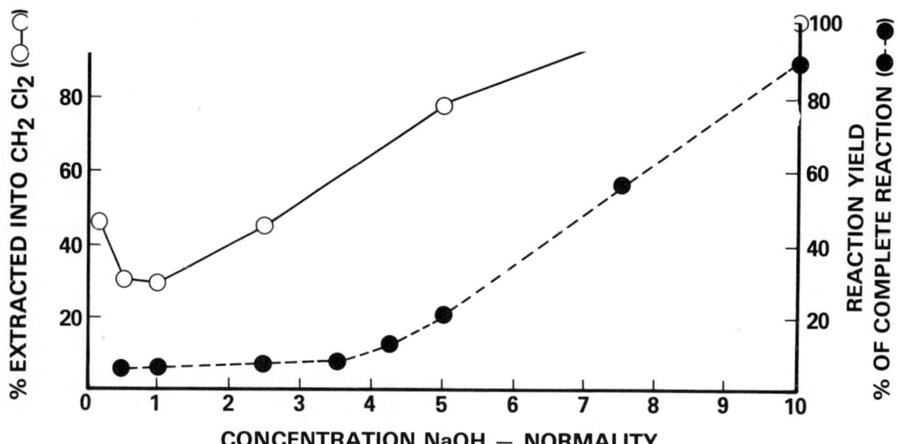

FIGURE 2. Benzylation of estradiol: The extraction efficiency (----) and reaction yield (- - -) as a function of NaOH concentration.

which is soluble only in organic solvents. It therefore appeared that some mechanism other than PTC was involved in the reaction between the phenolate anion and alkylating agent.

The high lipophilicity of THC suggested that the sodium salt of the phenol was sufficiently soluble in methylene chloride to permit the extraction of the sodium cation and the anion of THC as an ion pair. In fact studies on the partition of THC between alkaline phase and methylene chloride showed that sodium phenolate was partitioned to a great extent into the organic layer. However, studies with other phenols, as well as further investigations of the characteristics ofthe reaction, indicated that the lipophilicity of THC was not the critical factor in permitting the reaction to take place.

The question regarding the role of lipophilicity of the phenols was investigated by studying the reaction of more hydrophilic phenols such as beta-naphthol or estradiol. Just as in the case of THC, these phenols could also be benzylated or pentafluorobenzylated in a biphasic system of methylene chloride and aqueous alkali in the absence of phase transfer catalyst (18,19). The yield of the derivative was independent of the extraction efficiency of the sodium phenolate (Fig. 2).

The yield of benzyl or pentafluorobenzyl derivative was dependent upon the amount of derivatizing agent in the reaction mixture and the composition of the alkaline phase (Fig. 3). These data in Fig. 2 and 3 indicate that a salting-out process is not involved in the reaction, that the high lipo-

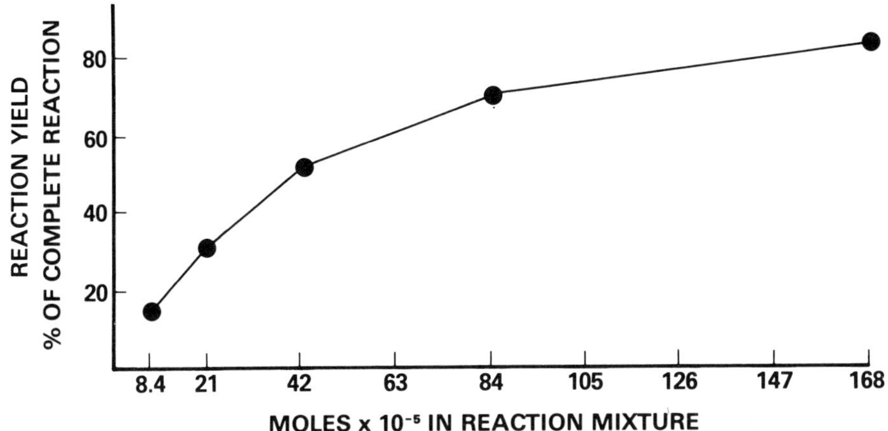

FIGURE 3. Benzylation of estradiol: Relationship between reaction yield and amount of benzyl bromide in the reaction mixture.

philicity of THC is not a prerequisite for derivatization, and that the derivatizing agent itself is involved in enhancing the reaction.

In the course of these investigations, several characteristics were discovered which may be particularly useful in analysis of cannabinoids. Firstly, the yield is independent of concentration of analyte. Secondly, the reaction is specific for phenols since no carboxylic acid of any molecular weight can be derivatized under these conditions (13,14). For instance hexadecanoic, octadecanoic, cosanoic and tetracosanoic acids could be extracted into the methylene chloride phase under these conditions but could not be derivatized. Significantly and in analogy with the data in Fig. 2, both phenols and carboxylic acids can be extracted into immiscible organic phase from aqueous phase (Table I).

Thirdly, the yield over a one hour reaction time and by inference the reaction rate, appears to be specific for the analyte, particularly THC. Whereas, THC can be quantitatively pentafluorobenzylated using 5 N NaOH, quantitative pentafluorobenzylation of estradiol requires 8 N NaOH and pentafluorobenzylation of beta-naphthol requires 10 N NaOH (Fig. 4) (18).

The mechanism of reaction that permits derivatizationof phenols in the biphasic system is unknown. Clearly, salting-out is insufficient to permit derivatization. The relationship between sodium hydroxide concentration and yield (Fig. 2) is reminiscent ofmicellular phenomena with the inflection

TABLE I. Extraction Results

Substrate	Composition of Aqueous Phase	Partition Ratios	% Reaction Yield
E_2	1 N NaOH	0.3	6
	1 N NaOH + 4 N NaCl	0.91	6
	5 N NaOH	8.84	20
	10 N NaOH	0.98	80
Palmitic acid	10 N NaOH	0.8	0

point being equal in volume to the critical micelle concentrations. In addition, the data in Fig. 3 shows that concentration of alkylating agent plays a significant role in promoting the reaction. It is possible that the bipolar molecules such as BzBr or PFBBr can act as micelle-forming species under certain critical conditions related to the concentration of hydroxide ion.

Liquid/liquid biphasic derivatizations have several potential advantages for the analysis of cannabinoids. These conditions dispense with the use of phase transfer catalyst; have an apparent specificity for phenols in the presence of carboxylic acids; and finally, exhibit a structural specificity for different analytes which permits quantitative derivatization of THC in the presence of other phenols that are less reactive. Nevertheless, there are some disadvantages to this reaction. Firstly, the reaction requires strong base, which couldresult in some problems with cannabinoid-like drugs that may be base-liable. In addition, pentafluorobenzyl bromide can be degraded or dimerized in the presence of strong base. Finally, the reaction conditions involve aliquid/liquid biphasic system. Such systems, as mentioned previously, are relatively difficult to automate.

III. AUTOMATION OF CHEMICAL PROCESSES

In considering automation of any chemical reaction, solid phase processes are frequently used (10-15). In addition to the earlier example of triphasic catalysis (8,9), there is also the classical work of Merrifield who used solid state synthesis to automate the construction of peptides and pro-

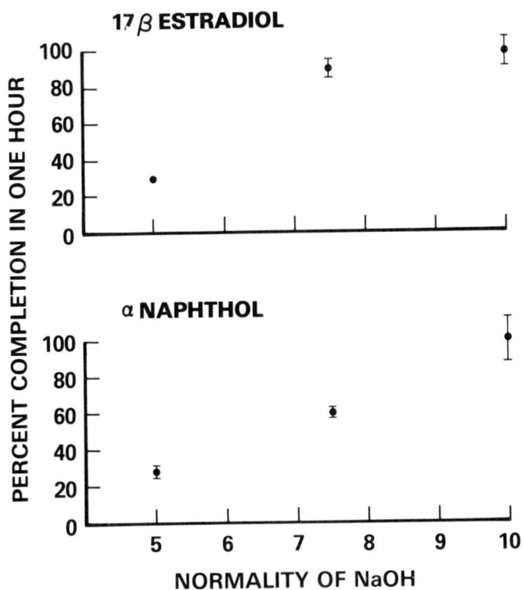

FIGURE 4. Pentafluorobenzylation of phenols. THC is quantitatively derivatized with 5 N NaOH.

teins. Analytical chemists have also used solid phase processes. Solid macroreticular resins, such as XAD2, have been extensively used either in semi-automated (13,14) or completely automated systems (15) for the isolation of organic analytes and aqueous matrices, including those of biological origin. In these systems the aqueous matrix is simply percolated through a column of the resin, which absorbs organic analytes. The inorganic salts, proteins and other highly hydrophilic material are removed by water wash while the absorbed lipophilic analytes or analytes with lipophilic moieties are retained on the surface of the resin. Following the aqueous wash, the adsorbed analytes are eluted with organic solvent. The technical simplicity and ease of manipulation of isolations that are based upon macroreticular resins is the basis for use of such resins in automation.

Our objective was to develop methods of equal technical simplicity that would affect simultaneous extraction and derivatization of cannabinoids from aqueous medium. Given the success of solid state processes in automation of synthetic and analytical procedures we focused our attention onsimilar techniques for combining the extraction and derivatization step for cannabinoids in aqueous matrix.

IV. SOLID PHASE SYNTHESIS

The basis for these investigations was the model of alumina catalyzed reactions reviewed by Posner in 1978 (20). The proposed mechanism is based upon both the electrophilic and nucleophilic reagents being adsorbed at proximal sites on the surface of the alumina. This concentration effect permits the reaction between the two reagents. We propose that if a system could be devised that would concentrate PFBBr and ionized analyte at proximal sites, we could also effect a derivatization of the analyte. However, the requirements of this system would have to be subject to certain constraints. The first of these would be compatibility with aqueous matrix at alkaline and neutral pH required to ionize either the cannabinoids or their _in vivo_ metabolites. Furthermore, the solid state would have to be compatible with organic solvent to permit elution in order to isolate the derivatized products.

This possibility that XAD2 could meet the stated requirements was strongly suggested by the recent report of the use of a column of XAD2 to preconcentrate analytes from as much as 5 ml of plasma percolated through a column of the resin (21). In this instance the organic analytes were absorbed in a sufficiently narrow band on the top of the column that backwashing from the resin onto an analytic HPLC column resulted in a small injection volume. This showed that analytes are highly concentrated on the resin. We reasoned that if the resin was impregnated with PFBBr or BzBr that this concentration effect on the analytes could affect the derivatization.

We now report that XAD2 impregnated with either PFBBr or BzBrcan effect a simultaneous isolation and derivatization of THC from aqueous medium (22). In this process the resin is impregnated with the reagent prior to the reaction. The impregnated resin is simply added to an aqueous solution containing THC and the mixture is shaken. During the reaction the ionized phenol is simultaneous absorbed and derivatization takes place on the surface of the resin with derivatized products being retained on the solid phase. At the end of the reaction the resin containing the absorbed and derivatized product is isolated by filtration and the derivatives are eluted with organic solvents.

We have applied this system to the pentafluorobenzylation of THC. The preliminary investigations showed that XAD2-mediated derivatization of THC from aqueous alkali is feasible. Significantly, we were able to obtain an 80% yield of the pentafluorobenzyl derivative using 0.1 N NaOH. Theseare considerably milder reaction conditions than those required for the reaction under conditions of biphasic liquid/liquid pentafluorobenzylation of THC in the absence of phase transfer catalyst.

The role of the resin in this reaction has yet to be deduced but it can fulfill at least two and possibly more functions. In the first instance it could act simply as a support or a dispersive phase for the PFBBr. In this case the function of the resin would be analagous to that of the methylene chloride in the biphasic benzylation reaction and the critical factors controlling the reaction would be the amount of pentafluorobenzyl bromide and the concentration of base (18,19). In the second instance it could act as a surface catalyst analagous to the action of alumina described by Posner (20).

The characteristics for the reaction of derivatization of THC are such that the function of the resin cannot be clearly deduced. For instance, in the biphasic pentafluorobenzylation of THC, 5N NaOH was required for quantitative derivatization. In contrast, the resin based process requires 0.1N NaOH thus suggesting a catalytic role for the resin. However, arguments can also be presented that the resin acts simply as a dispersive phase. The reaction conditions require impregnation of 50 mcl of pentafluorobenzyl bromide onto 100 mg of XAD2. The surface area for that weight of resin is 30 m^2. The derivatizing reagent is thus dispersed over a large surface area, increasing the interfacial contact between pentafluorobenzyl bromide and the alkaline solution. The importance of interfacial surface area was evidenced from the effect of shaking speed on the reaction yield (19). Successful derivatization with 0.1 NNaOH may simply reflect a very large interfacial contact area. However, using these reaction conditions we were able to derivatize carboxylic and barbituric acids (21). This was not feasible using biphasic alkylation conditions suggesting the resin has a catalytic role.

V. SUMMARY

We have investigated two alternatives to PTC-based derivatizations and extractions. In both instances the problem of co-extraction of catalyst was eliminated. Liquid/liquid biphasic derivatization was found to be phenol-specific relative to carboxylic and barbituric acids, which did not react under these conditions. Furthermore, in these reactions, THC reacted quantitatively under conditions which derivatized other phenols in low yield. The solid phase synthesis offers an approach to simplification of existing procedures as well as the potential for development of semi-automated or fully automated methods of sample preparation.

REFERENCES

1. "Cannabinoid Analysis in Physiological Fluids", p. 81. American Chemical Society Symposium Series #98, American Chemical Society, Washington, D. C., 1979.
2. Rosenfeld, J. M., and Taguchi, V. Y., Mass fragmentographic assay for 11-hydroxy-delta-9-tetrahydrocannabinol from plasma, Anal. Chem. 48:726 (1976).
3. Rosenfeld, J., The simultaneous determination of delta-9-tetrahydrocannabinol and 11-hydroxy-delta-9-tetrahydrocannabinol in plasma, Anal. Lett. 10:917 (1977).
4. "Handbook of Analytical Derivatization Reactions" (O. R. Knapp, ed.). Wiley Interscience, John Wiley and Sons, New York, 1979.
5. Hartvig, P., Gyllenhaal, O., and Hammarlund, M., Determination of saccharin in urine by electron-capture gas chromatography after extractive methylation, J. Chromat. 151:232 (1978).
6. Vessman, J., Johansson, M., Magnusson, P., and Stromberg, S., Determination of intact oxazepam by electron capture gas chromatography after an extractive alkylationreaction, Anal. Chem. 49:1545 (1977).
7. Ervik, M., and Gustavii, K., Application of the extractive alkylation technique to the gas chromatographic determination of chlorthalidone in plasma in nanograms quantities, Anal. Chem. 46:39 (1974).
8. Regen, S. L., Triphase Catalysis, Angew. Chem. Int. Ed. Engl. 18:421 (1979).
9. Tundo, P., Easy and economical synthesis of widely porous resins; very efficient supports for immobilized phase-transfer catalysts, J. Chem. Soc. Chem. Comm. (1978).
10. Gelbard, G., and Colonna, S., Anionic activation in polymer-supported reactions; nucleophilic substitutionwith anion-exchange resins; I. synthesis of alkyl phenyl ethers, nitrocarboxylic esters and x-alkyl-dicarbonyl compounds. J. Chem. Soc. Chem. Comm. 113 (1973).
11. Leznoff, C. C., The use of insoluble polymer supports in general organic synthesis. J. Amer. Chem. Soc. 100:327 (1978).
12. Manaeck, G., and Storck, W., Polymeric catalysts. Angew. Chem. Int. Ed. Engl. 17:657-670 (1978).
13. Weissman, N., Lowe, M. L., Beattie, J. M., and Demetrious, J. A., Screening methods for detection of drugs of

abuse in human urine, Clin. Chem. 17:875 (1971).
14. Pranitis, P. A. F., Milzoff, J. R., and Stolman, A., Extraction of drugs from biofluids and tissues with XAD2 resin, J. Forensic. Sci. 19:917 (1974).
15. St. Onge, L. M., Dolar, E., Anglim, M. A., and Least, C. J. Jr., Improved determination of phenobarbital, primidone and phenytoin by use of a preparative instrument for extraction, followed by gas chromatography, Clin. Chem. 25:1373 (1979).
16. Dockx, J., Quaternary ammonium compounds in organic synthesis, Synthesis 441 (1973).
17. Rosenfeld, J., unpublished data.
18. Rosenfeld, J. M., and Crocco, J. L., Specific pentafluorobenzylation of phenols in a biphasic system, Anal. Chem. 50:701 (1978).
19. Rosenfeld, J., Crocco, J., and Ling, T. L., Specific alkylation reactions--evidence for a novel reaction mechanism in biphasic mixtures, Anal. Lett. 13:283 (1980).
20. Posner, G. H., Organic reactions at alumina surfaces, Angew. Chem. Int. Eol. Eng. 17:487-496 (1978).
21. Hue, R. A., Mohammed, H. Y., and Cantwell, F. F., Precolumns of ambeolite XAD-2 for direct injection liquid chromatographic determination of methaqualone in blood plasma, Anal. Chem. 54:113-117 (|1982).
22. Rosenfeld, J., U.S. patent application No. 06/367,941, April 13, 1982.

Section III METABOLIC AND PHARMACOKINETIC ASPECTS

RECENT STUDIES ON THE PHARMACOKINETICS OF DELTA-1-TETRAHYDROCANNABINOL IN MAN*

Stig Agurell, Jan-Erik Lindgren, Agneta Ohlsson

Astra Lakemedel AB
Sodertalje, Sweden

and

Department of Pharmacology
Karolinska Institute
Stockholm, Sweden

Hampton K. Gillespie, Leo E. Hollister

Veterans Administration Medical Center
Palo Alto, California

I. INTRODUCTION

The purpose of the present paper is to summarize and integrate the results of five recent reports on the pharmacokinetics of delta-1-tetrahydrocannabinol (THC; delta-9-THC in the benzpyrene nomenclature) by our group (1-5). These studies have, from a pharmacokinetic point of view, followed very similar protocols and were designed to elucidate, e.g.:

- levels and interindividual variations in plasma levels of THC after different routes of administration.
- the systemic availability of THC after oral and smoke administration compared to the intravenous route.
- possible correlations between THC plasma levels and objective (heart rate) and subjective ("high") parameters.

---

*Supported by grants from the Swedish Medical Research Council and the Veterans Administration.

ISBN 0-12-044620-0

- any marked differences between one group of light and one group of heavy marijuana users with respect to pharmacokinetics and clinical response.

- investigate interactions between THC, cannabidiol (CBD) and cannabinol (CBN).

These studies will also be discussed in relation to other published findings in this area.

II. METHODS

The results discussed in the present paper are derived from five different studies (1-5), which were based on essentially similar protocols, but where, e.g., type of subjects (heavy and light users), timing and duration of sampling, and dose and mode of administration differed. Specific details are given in legends to figures or in the text.

A. Subjects

The subjects were between the ages of 18 and 36 and were almost all males who had previous experience with marijuana. All were in good mental and physical health, were on no current psychoactive medication, and none admitted to significant use of other social drugs than marijuana.

In two studies (4,5) groups of heavy and light users participated. The definition "heavy users" was used for subjects who smoked the drug at least once daily, whereas "light users" used the drug on a monthly basis. In addition to volunteered information, the classification of these subjects was reasonably confirmed by analysis of urine for THC metabolites and pre-experiment plasma THC levels.

For at least 24 hours prior to and for the duration of each trial subjects were asked to abstain from marijuana and alcohol.

B. Dose and Administration

Cannabinoids were administered to each subject in a random cross-over design according to the following general procedures.

1. Smoking. A marijuana cigarette containing a known amount of THC or a marijuana placebo cigarette spiked with a known amount of unlabelled or deuterium labelled THC was smoked in a fashion determined by the subject, such as to

obtain the maximum (except in ref. 5) desired high (usually within 5-7 min). The butt was extinguished in water and retained for analysis of residual THC. In this way the total amount of smoked THC could be determined.

2. Oral. A chocolate cookie was prepared containing 20 mg of THC added in ethanol solution.

3. Intravenous. Into the injection port of a rapidly flowing normal saline infusion, 5.0 mg of THC in 2.5 ml 95% ethanol was injected over a period of 2 min.

4. Blood Sampling. Three to 10 ml heparinized blood samples were drawn before administration of drug and at suitable time intervals for periods up to 4, 6, 10 or 48-72 hours -- as indicated by Figs. 1-10. Plasma was separated immedi-

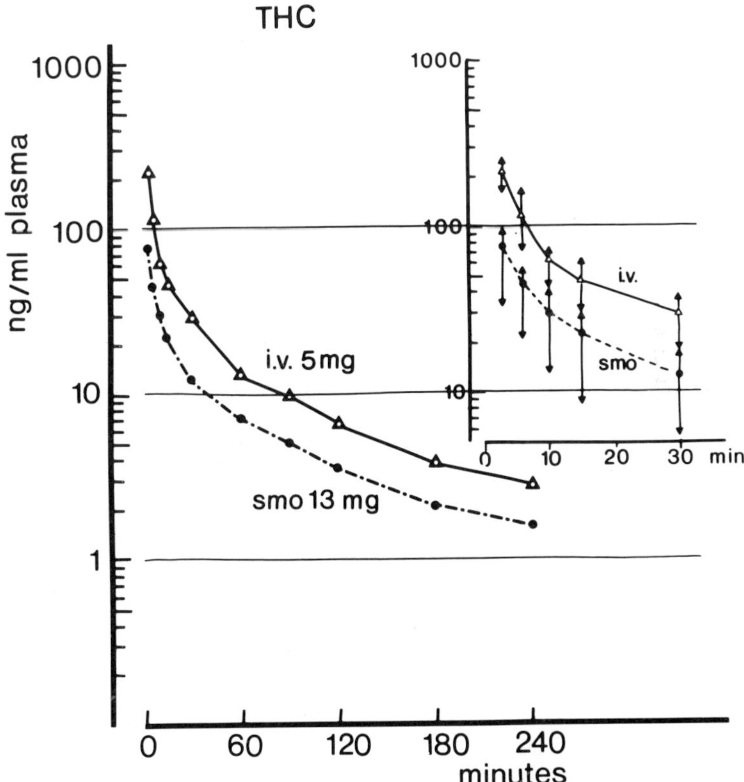

FIGURE 1. Mean plasma concentrations (n = 11) of THC after administration of 5.0 mg intravenously and 13.0 mg (mean value) by smoking (1). The insert shows in detail the average and range of plasma levels during the first 30 min.

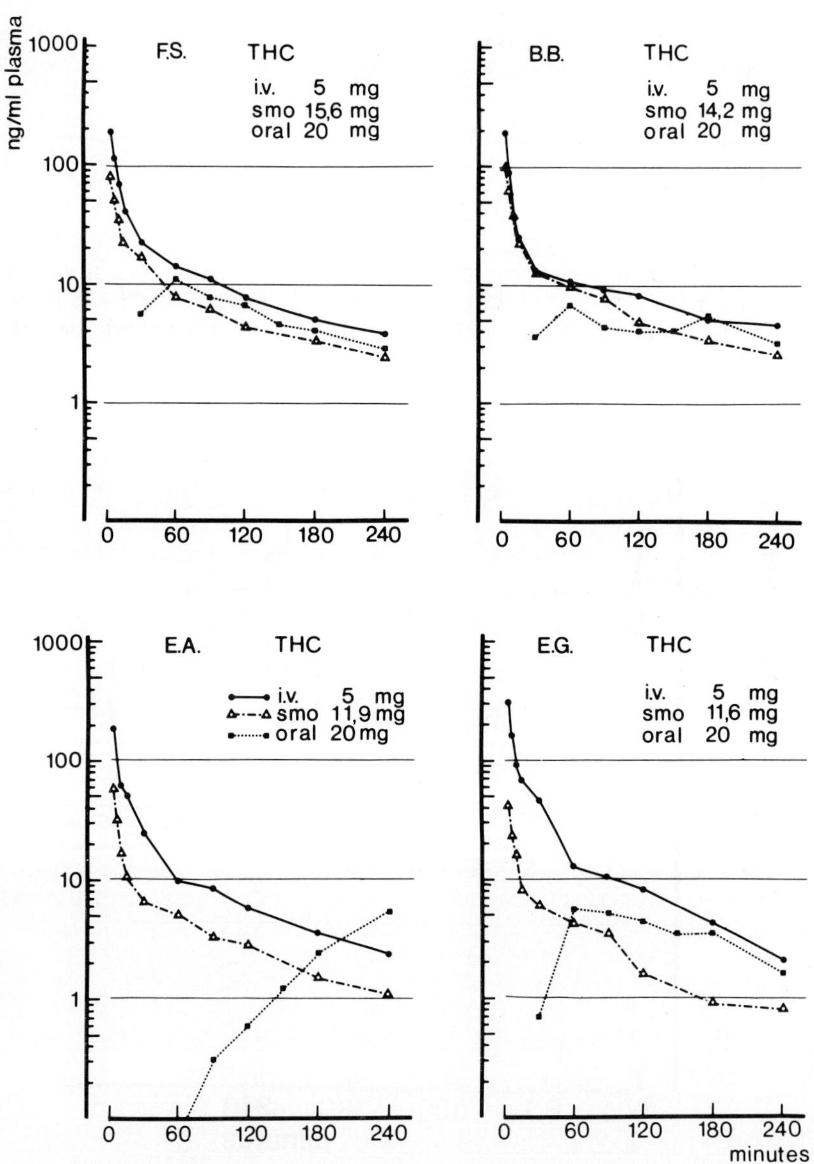

FIGURE 2. Individual plasma concentrations of THC in four subjects after administration of THC intravenously, orally and by smoking (1). The individual doses are stated in the figure.

ately and stored frozen in silanized glass tubes for subsequent assay.

5. Analysis of THC and Other Cannabinoids in Plasma. The present assay is described previously (4-6) and briefly, consists of an extraction of the cannabinoids from the plasma after addition of the appropriate deuterium-labelled internal standard. The extract is purified by liquid chromatography (6), concentrated, silylated and assayed by mass fragmentography (4,5). The assay is specific for THC, CBD, and CBN, as desired, and has a lower limit of sensitivity at 30-100 pg/ml (4,5).

6. Kinetic Analysis. The area under the plasma concentration curves (AUCs) for the investigated time periods were estimated using the trapezoidal rule. The systemic availability after smoking or oral administration was estimated by comparison of the AUC with that after intravenous administration.

7. Clinical Evaluation of Drug Effects. Pulse rates were recorded using earlobe monitors. Ratings of degree of subjective high on a global scale from 0-10 was made prior to and during the experiments. The raking 10 was equal to the highest "high" ever experienced by a subject.

III. RESULTS AND DISCUSSION

A. Plasma Levels of THC

Intravenous infusion of 5.0 mg THC over 2 min yielded average plasma levels around 200 ng/ml 3 min post infusion. Fig. 1 shows the rapid decline to about 3 ng/ml at 4 hours. The smoking of a THC cigarette over 5 to 7 min, until the desired high, yielded lower THC levels (Fig. 1), which were essentially parallel to the intravenous curve but at half the concentration. The group of users in this study (1) consisted of both heavy and light marijuana users who had smoked from 11.6 to 15.6 mg (average 13.0 mg) of the ca. 19 mg THC originally present in the cigarette.

The curves shown in Fig. 1 are average plasma curves but as indicated by the insert, an interindividual variation is noted, especially after smoking. Fig. 2 shows more clearly the interindividual variation among four of the eleven subjects participating in the study (1) after intravenous, oral and smoke administration. The variation in plasma THC levels is limited after intravenous but considerable after smoking.

The lower levels in subject E.G., e.g., result in a systemic availability of only 8% after smoking, compared, e.g., to 24% in subject B. B.

Oral administration of 20 mg THC in a chocolate cookie resulted in low (mean peak level 6 ng/ml) plasma concentrations of THC as shown in Fig. 3. Although this curve indicates a peak level at 60 min followed by a slow and steady decline, this mean plasma curve is actually representative for few subjects. As shown by the individual curves in Fig. 2, oral absorption of THC from a chocolate cookie is slow and erratic, e.g., subject B. B. shows two plasma peaks as does subject E. G., whereas subject E. A. did not peak until the 4 hour sample. This considerable interindividual variability in magnitude and rate of absorption of THC after oral administration was earlier observed by Perez-Reyes et al. (7) in a study with radio-labelled THC.

More plasma level data is subsequently discussed under other headings. Thus, THC levels during 48 hours after intravenous administration and smoking is illustrated in Figs. 6-7. As evident the mean levels are in the range 0.1-0.5 ng/ml, 10-48 hours after smoking 10 mg THC.

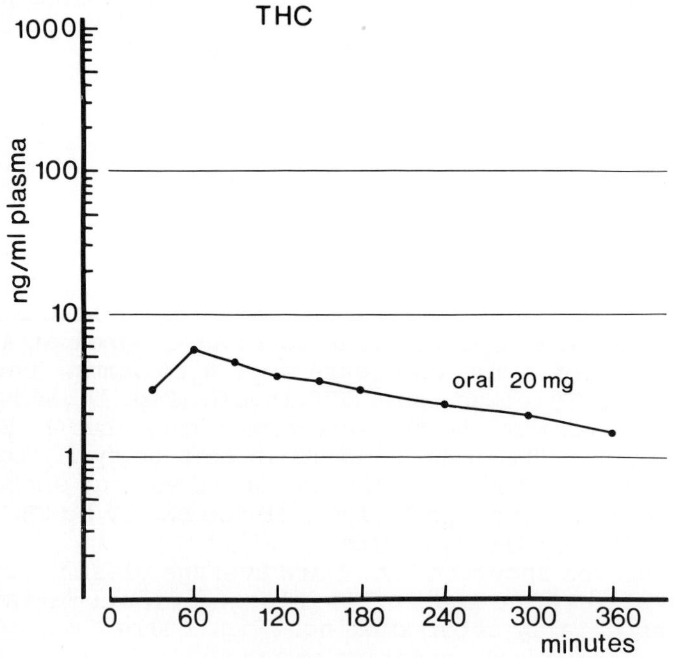

FIGURE 3. Mean plasma levels of THC (n = 11) after administration of 20 mg THC in a chocolate cookie (1).

B. Tolerance to THC. Induction of Metabolism or Tachyphylaxis?

Development of tolerance to the behavioural and pharmacological effects of THC is known after prolonged administration of high doses of THC to both man and animal (cf. 2,8-10). This tolerance could simply be a functional tolerance but could also be due to pharmacokinetic changes, e.g., induction of a faster THC metabolism. In fact, early observations by Lemberger et al. (10) indicated that the half-life of THC in chronic users of marijuana was shorter than that in naive users.

We have carried out two studies (2,5) to elucidate whether any pharmacokinetic differences exist between heavy and light users of marijuana (for definitions of "heavy" and "light" users see Methods).

In Fig. 4 is shown the average plasma levels of THC after intravenous administration to one group of heavy and one group of light users (2). The interindividual variations are

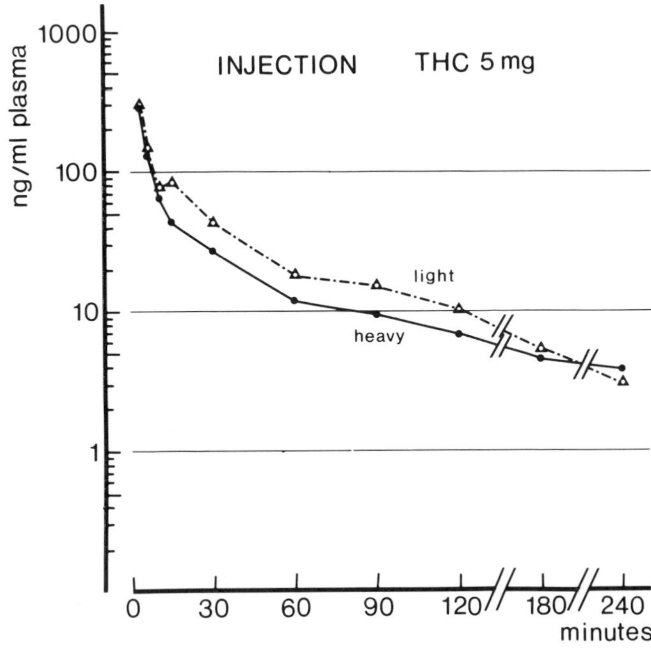

FIGURE 4. Average plasma concentrations of THC after intravenous administration of 5 mg of THC to heavy (n = 9) and light (n = 9) users (2).

greater in this study than in the previous (Fig. 1), but there is a trend (p = 0.08) that the heavy users may have lower plasma levels after injection than the light users. This possible difference in pharmacokinetics could perhaps partly be due to differences in weight (heavy users mean weight 74 kg, light users 68 kg).

In another experiment we studied plasma levels and some other pharmacokinetic parameters in light (n = 4) and heavy (n = 5) users who had been administered 5 mg of deuterium labelled THC intravenously (5). Using the labelled compound, we could study the plasma levels for 48-72 hours. As shown below in Fig. 6, this experiment also shows hints that heavy users might have lower plasma levels of THC than light users after the same intravenous dose. The difference is, however, not statistically significant and the magnitude of the difference is, conversely, certainly not great.

In a study where high doses of oral THC (180 mg/day) was administered for 10 to 12 days to a group of 6 subjects, Hunt and Jones (8) found a similar slight decrease in plasma levels of intravenously administered radio-labelled THC after the high THC administration. This decrease was due to an increase in the volume of distribution.

The conclusion from both of our studies (2,5) and that of Hunt and Jones (8) is that the development of tolerance to the cardiovascular and the psychological effects of THC cannot in a major way be due to changes in pharmacokinetic and metabolic parameters. Both Hunt and Jones and we do find pharmacokinetic differences -- more pronounced in Hunt and Jones' study -- but not differences that explain the development of tolerance as a pharmacokinetic difference. It should also be pointed out that the development of tolerance in Hunt and Jones' study was quite marked but marginal in our study (2). Our results also agree in general with those of Perez-Reyes et al. (11). The development of tolerance and the possible mechanisms for this has also been discussed by Cochetto et al. (12) and Domino et al. (13). The latter authors have also reanalyzed some of our studies from a pharmacokinetic point of view and drawn further conclusions. Although pharmacokinetic parameters in one group and clinical effects in another group are compared, their work (13) give interesting suggestions for future studies.

The importance of a faster metabolism of THC for the possible development of tolerance could also be assessed from total metabolic clearance data. Such data is, however, both scarce and ambiguous. In one study with delta-1-THC-d_3 (5), we found average plasma-clearance values may be somewhat overestimated since there were difficulties with the timing of the initial blood samples. Hunt and Jones (8) found that the metabolic clearance rose from a mean value of 605 ml/min to

977 ml/min in a group of 6 subjects after exposure to very high doses of THC orally. Since 80 per cent of THC in blood is in the plasma (8), these clearance values approach total hepatic blood flow. Hence an induction of drug-metabolizing liver enzymes would have little influence on the kinetics of smoked or intravenously administered THC. The clearance values found by Lemberger et al. (14) were, however, clearly lower.

The information on terminal half-life values for THC in man is controversial and usually based upon average plasma levels from groups of various sizes (cf. 13). Assessment of half-life values is indeed very dependent upon the precision with which the very low 24-72 hour THC levels can be assayed. We have limited our assessment to the statement that the terminal half-lives of THC in both light and heavy smokers appear to be more than 20 hours (5). Hunt and Jones (8) also found similar half-lives in both light and heavy users (average values 18-19 hours) whereas Lemberger et al. (14) and Domino et al. (13) -- using our data (2,5) -- suggest that the half-life in naive users may be longer (ca. 60-70 hours) than in heavy users (23-28 hours). Thus, the information is ambiguous but since the apparent terminal half-life of THC is probably controlled by the slow return of THC from the tissues, one would not expect a great influence on the half-life by metabolic changes (8).

Thus, a tentative conclusion might be that there seem to exist minor pharmacokinetic differences between light and heavy users of marijuana. These differences cannot, however, to any significant extent explain the development of tolerance in heavy users as a metabolic phenomena. Further, development of tolerance to various effects of marijuana in man seems to require very high daily doses of THC. Obviously tolerance can be due to a combination of various factors and tolerance to different effects of THC may vary.

C. Systemic Availability of THC

The conventional way to measure systemic availability (bioavailability) of a drug is to determine the ratio of the areas under the plasma levels vs. times curves (AUC) for equal oral and intravenous doses. One then has a rough measure of the oral absorption of the drug together with its presystemic elimination by, e.g., the gut and the liver. The systemic availability of THC is influenced by even more factors, e.g.:

- during smoking; by pyrolysis of THC in the cigarette, by loss of side stream smoke (smoke not inhaled), absorption by buccal membranes, possible metabolism in the lung (cf. 15) in addition to liver, etc.

- during oral administration; by chemical break-down in the acidic pH of the gastric juice as well as by the factors normally included in "first pass" metabolism.

We have studied the systemic availability of THC in a group of mixed users as well as in groups of light and heavy users. In Fig. 1 is shown the mean plasma levels of THC after smoking 13.0 mg vs. intravenous infusion of 5.0 mg THC (1). The estimated systemic availability ranged from 8 to 24 (mean 18 +/- 6 s.d.) per cent in this group of users with mixed experience. The same group of users were also administered 20 mg of THC in chocolate cookies (Fig. 3). As discussed earlier this plasma curve is indeed a composite of individual curves which differ greatly and often show slow and erratic absorption. The estimated systemic availability ranged from 4 to 12 (mean 6 +/- 3) per cent. Previous information in the literature is limited to an estimation by Hunt and Jones (8) of some early data collected by Lemberger et al. (16) which indicated an oral availability of some 2 per cent.

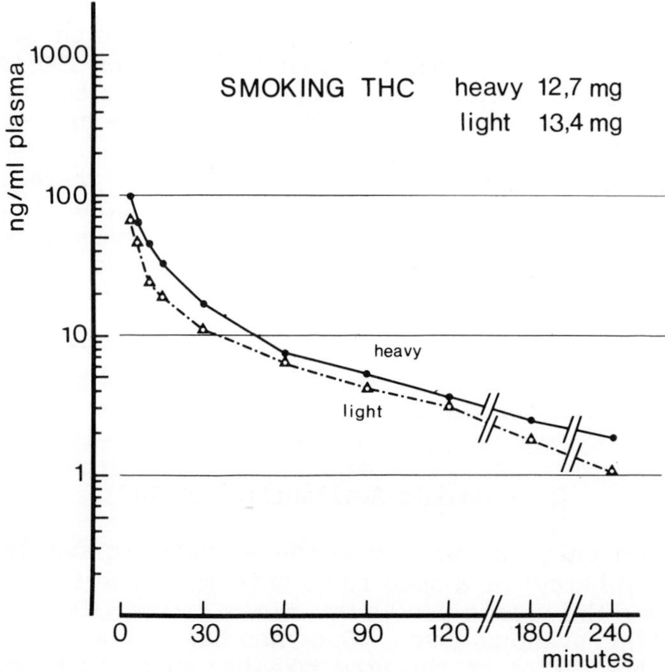

FIGURE 5. Mean plasma levels of THC in one group of heavy (n = 9) and one group of light (n = 9) users after smoking marijuana cigarettes. The average doses smoked were 12.7 and 13.4 mg, respectively. The groups are the same as in Fig. 4 (2).

The chocolate cookie oral administration of THC used by us (1) is one form of oral administration used by certain social groups in the San Francisco area and is not an optimal oral formulation. Indeed, previous work by Perez-Reyes et al. (7) has shown that certain adjuvants, such as sesame oil, are advantageous for absorption although interindividual variations are still considerable.

We also explored possible differences in the systemic availability of smoked THC in light vs. heavy users (2,5).

In one study (2) groups of light (n = 9) and heavy (n = 9) users were allowed to smoke marijuana cigarettes until their maximum desired high. Both groups smoked similar amounts (light users: 13.4 +/- 1.6 mg, heavy users: 12.7 +/- 1.3 mg) of THC. By comparing the $AUC_{0-4\ h}$ (Fig. 5) and assuming linear pharmacokinetics, the heavy users were found to have a statistically significant higher systemic availability than the light users (heavy users: 23 +/- 16%, range 6-56%, vs. light users: 10 +/- 7%, range 2-22%). The mean plasma levels

INJECTION THC-d_3 5 mg

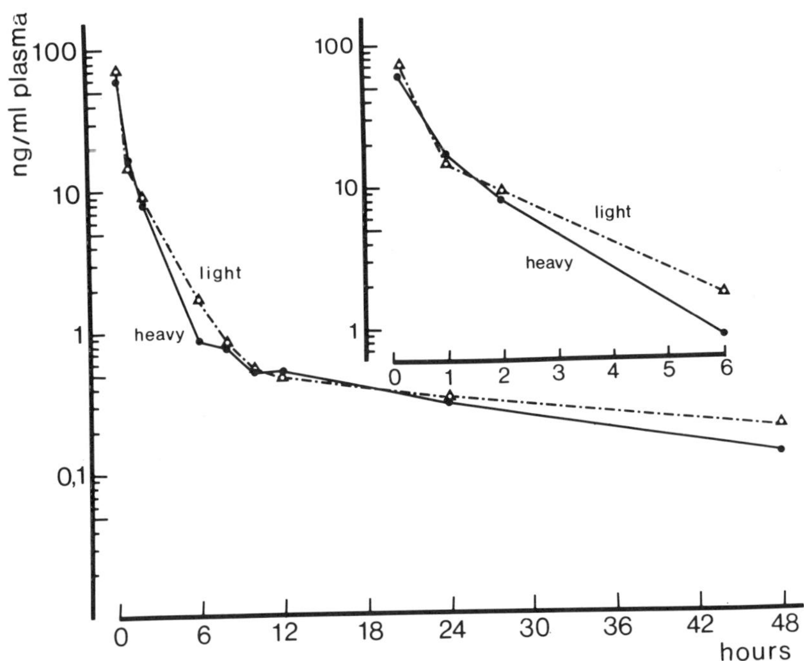

FIGURE 6. Average plasma levels of delta-1-THC-d_3 during 48 hours after intravenous administration to light (n = 4) and heavy (n = 5) users of 5.0 mg of delta-1-THC-d_3 during 2 min (5). Note that the first mean plasma level point is at 10 min. The insert shows average plasma concentrations during the first 6 hours.

after i.v. administration of 5 mg THC to the same groups are shown in Fig. 4. These results indicate that heavy marijuana users smoke more efficiently than light users and seem to prefer higher THC plasma levels.

In a similarly designed study (5) with heavy and light users, AUC for 48 or 72 hours were assessed after administration of 5.0 mg delta-1-THC-d_3 intravenously (Fig. 6) and 10 mg delta-1-THC-d_3 in a marijuana placebo cigarette (Fig. 7). Also here the systemic availability of THC after inhalation was higher in heavy (27 +/- 10%) than in light (14 +/- 1%) users.

From these studies comprising a limited number of subjects one might conclude that the amount of THC appearing in the systemic circulation after smoking varies greatly (10-fold) between individuals both in groups of heavy and light users. Heavy users, however, tend to smoke more efficiently (mean availability ca. 23-27%) than light users (mean availability ca. 10-14%).

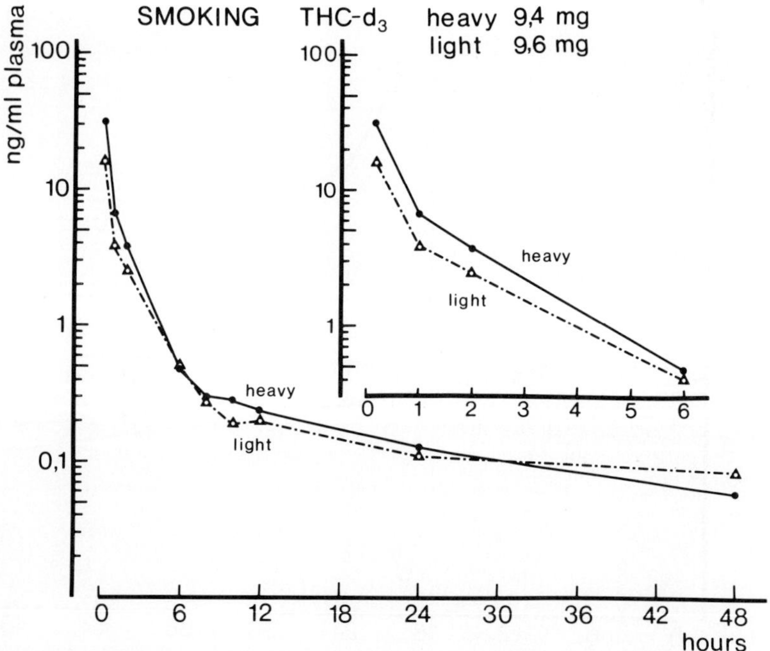

FIGURE 7. Mean plasma levels of delta-1-THC-d_3 after smoking a marijuana placebo cigarette spiked with 10 mg of delta-1-THC-d_3 (5). The average dose smoked by heavy users was 9.4 mg and by light users, 9.6 mg. Further details as in Figure 6.

The amount of THC appearing systemically after oral administration is low (ca. 6%) and also varies greatly. In addition to variations in AUC, the time to peak levels can vary between subjects, e.g., from 1 to 4 hours. This form of administration, however, tends to yield plasma levels of longer duration than by smoking.

D. Interactions of THC with Other Cannabinoids

There is reasonable evidence that the psychoactive effects of marijuana can roughly be equated with its content of THC per se or as carboxylic acids. Two other major cannabinoid constituents, cannabidiol (CBD) and cannabinol (CBN), however, occur together with THC. Studies in animals indicated that CBD could inhibit mixed function oxidases (cf. 4). Studies in man have yielded somewhat conflicting information on the pharmacological interaction between THC, CBD and CBN, but a pharmacokinetic interaction between THC and CBD was conceivable (cf. 4).

In one study we have now investigated the interaction in man of THC with CBD and CBN (4). Twenty mg of THC was administered orally together with placebo or 40 mg CBD or 40 mg CBN (4) in a randomized, cross-over fashion.

Fig. 8A shows the mean plasma level after oral administration of 20 mg THC. The plasma level is very similar to that found previously (Fig. 3). Co-administration of 40 mg of CBD — which would clearly be much higher than the CBD-dose one would normally expect -- gave no evidence of a pharmacokinetic interaction as judged from the plasma levels (Fig. 8B). Simultaneous oral administration of 20 mg THC with 40 mg CBN indicated a possible interaction, but the increase in THC levels is not statistically significant. Thus, these experiments, which were designed to find a maximal interaction if drug-metabolizing liver enzymes were involved, did not reveal any significant pharmacokinetic interactions between THC and the other two major cannabinoid components of marijuana.

E. Relations Between Plasma THC Levels and Pharmacological Effects

In some of our studies (1-3) clinical investigations of drug effects were carried out simultaneously with the pharmacokinetic assessment. Hence we have attempted to relate plasma concentrations of THC to one subjective measure, self-ratings of degree of intoxication ("high") and one objective measure, viz., pulse rate. Subsequently only relations to "high" are discussed.

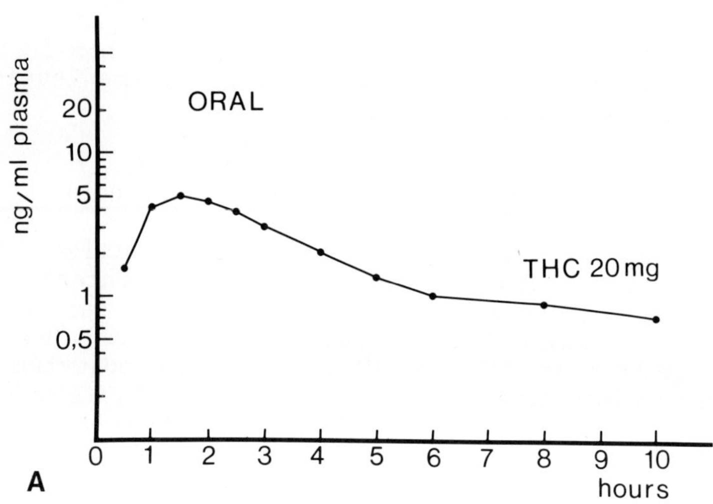

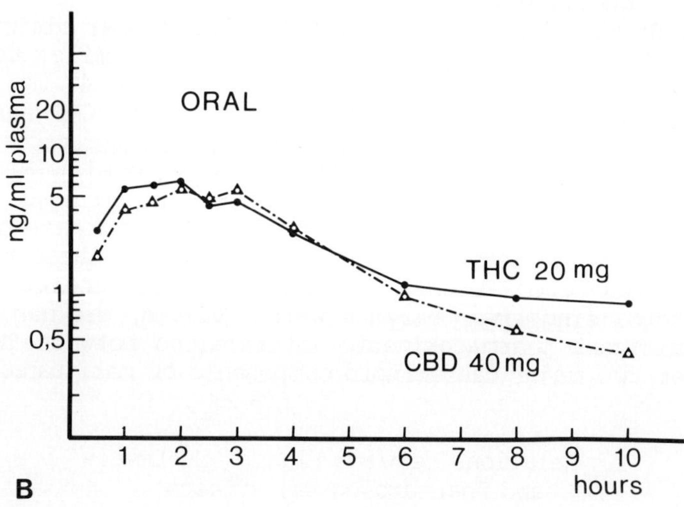

FIGURE 8A. Average plasma level of THC (n = 12) after oral administration of 20 mg THC in a chocolate cookie (4).

B. Average plasma levels of THC and CBD after oral administration of 20 mg THC together with 40 mg CBD.

C. Average plasma levels of THC and CBN after oral administration of 20 mg THC together with 40 mg CBN.

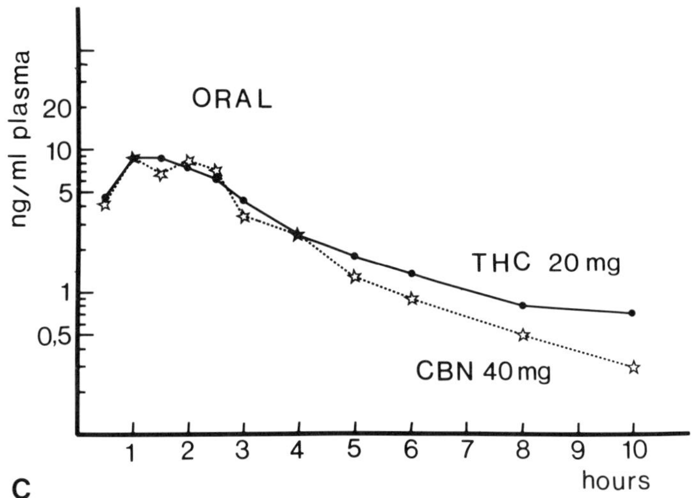

Fig. 9 shows the average plasma level after injection of 5.0 mg THC as does Fig. 1. In addition we have in Fig. 9 plotted the mean time course of "high" after this administration. Since these were an intravenous, 2-min injection, peak plasma concentrations were reached in the first sample, whereas the peak "high" was delayed to 15 min. Degrees of "high" were rated at 3, 6, 10, 15, 30, 60, etc. min, and it is not possible to define more precisely the average peak time for "high". By 3 hours the average THC level was ca. 4 ng/ml and the "high" was quite low and approached zero by 4 hours. Thus, looking at <u>mean curves</u> there seems to be a delay but also a reasonable correlation between levels and "high".

If we look at individual values as in Fig. 10, where plasma concentrations vs. perceived "high" have been plotted after intravenous injection of THC, a moderate correlation (r = 0.35) is evident. However, it is also evident that numerous single values show a poor correlation. This can also be seen from the total material (3) where a score of 10 in degree of "high" was recorded at THC plasma levels from 5 to 160 ng/ml and a score of 9 at 7 to 196 ng/ml after intravenous and smoke administration, respectively. Also, an attempt to find time periods when correlations between "high" and THC levels were better did not yield much more impressive correlations -- although the period from 10 to 120 min seems more reliable (3).

Thus, our conclusion is that although groups of values show a reasonable correlation between "high" and plasma THC levels, single values do not well reflect the degree of intoxication. One will not then be able to determine for a single individual the degree of intoxication from a single plasma value. Furthermore, it is not entirely clear to us that there is a clearcut correlation between a subjective "high" and psychomotor performance in, e.g., a driving test.

The relationship between plasma THC concentrations and pharmacolocigal effects (tachycardia and psychological "high") in man has recently also been investigated by Cocchetto et al. (12). Their analysis using hysteresis plots revealed that both heart rate and subjective psychological effects were elicited in a deep compartment relative to the plasma compartment. This is in agreement with our findings as is their finding that the time courses of tachycardia and "high" lagged behind the plasma THC time profiles. In fact Perez-Reyes et al. (17) find this delay so marked that they find the common notion

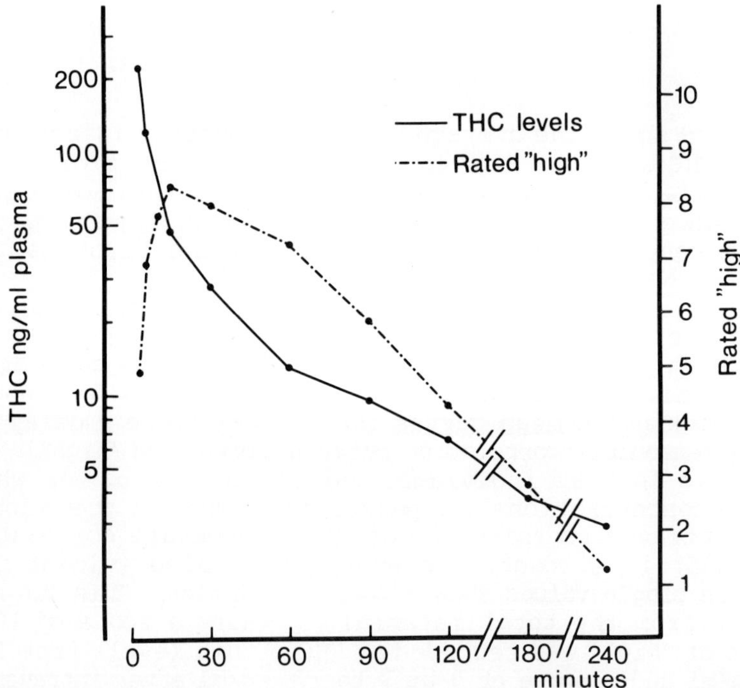

FIGURE 9. Time course of high (dashed line) in relation to plasma THC concentrations (solid line) after intravenous administration of 5 mg THC during 2 min (3). Average of 11 subjects.

that smokers titrate to the desired level of high is unrealistic! Cocchetto et al. (12) also conclude that plasma THC concentrations are poor predictors of physiological and psychological effects. Such a view is, however, not held by Domino et al. (13).

One possible explanation -- apart from a deep compartment -- for the out of phase relation between plasma THC concentrations and pharmacological effects, could be the formation of an active metabolite responsible for the main activity, e.g., the psychological high. Fig. 11 shows the time course of high after intravenous administration of 5 mg THC during 2 min, smoking a marijuana cigarette containing 19 mg THC (average smoked amount 13 mg), and administration of 20 mg THC by the oral route (3). As evident from Fig. 11, the pattern of high is similar both after intravenous administration of THC and smoking. The plasma THC profiles are also similar (Fig. 1). The time course for high after oral administration is lagging

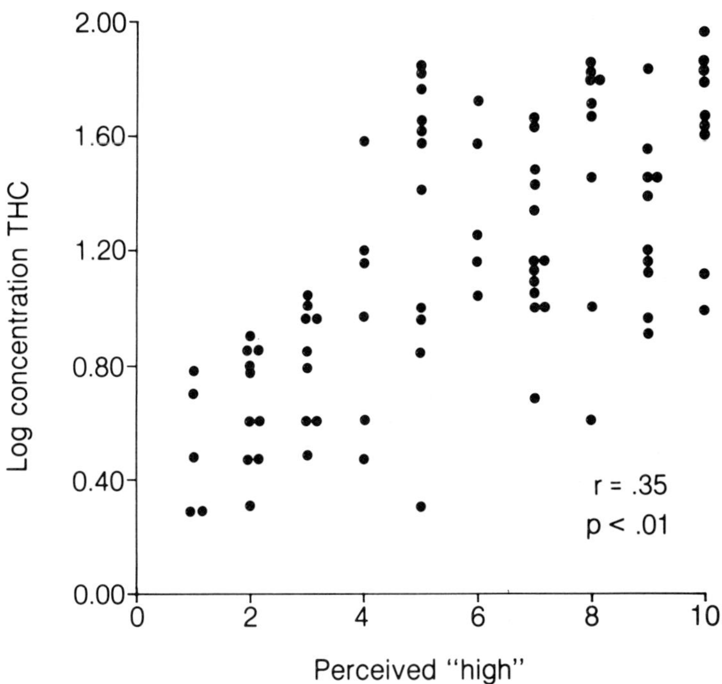

FIGURE 10. Correlations between log concentrations of plasma THC and perceived high following intravenous injection of 5 mg THC. (3).

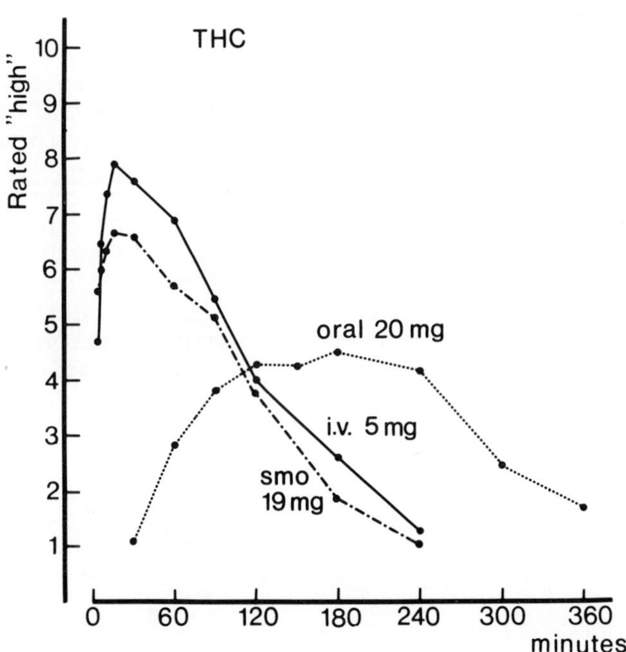

FIGURE 11. Time course of high ratings following three modes of administration: 5 mg of THC intravenously, 20 mg orally, and smoking a cigarette containing 19 mg of THC (average of 13 mg smoked by 11 subjects).

behind the plasma level even more, from 1 to 3 hours (Figs. 3,11) The contribution of metabolites to the activity of THC has been discussed by us (1,3) and others (18). To summarize, it is, however, not very likely that 7-hydroxy-delta-1-THC -- the potential candidate -- could contribute in a major way after smoke or intravenous administration. After oral administration it does, however, probably contribute to the effects of THC itself and could explain the further delay.

ACKNOWLEDGMENTS

S. Anderson kindly made the illustrations and B. Anderson typed the manuscript.

REFERENCES

1. Ohlsson, A., Lindgren, J.-E., Wahlen, A., Agurell, S., Hollister, L. E., and Gillespie, H. K., Clin. Pharmacol. Therap. 28:409 (1980).
2. Lindgren, J. E., Ohlsson, A., Agurell, S., Hollister, L. E., and Gillespie, H., Psychopharmacol. 74:208 (1981).
3. Hollister, L. E., Gillespie, H. K., Ohlsson, A., Lindgren, J.-E., Wahlen, A., and Agurell, S., J. Clin. Pharmacol. 21:171S (1981).
4. Agurell, S., Carlsson, S., Lindgren, J.-E., Ohlsson, A., Gillespie, H., and Hollister, L., Experientia37:1090 (1981).
5. Ohlsson, A., Lindgren, J.-E., Wahlen, A., Agurell, S., Hollister, L. E., and Gillespie, H. K., Biomed. Mass. Spectr. 9:6 (1982).
6. Ohlsson, A., Lindgren, J.-E., Leander, K., and Agurell, S., in "Cannabinoid Assays in Humans" (R. E. Willette, ed.), p. 48. NIDA Research Monograph 7, NIDA, Rockville, 1976.
7. Perez-Reyes, M., Lipton, M. A., Timmons, M. C., and Wall, M. E., Clin. Pharmacol. Therap. 14:48 (1973).
8. Hunt, C. A., and Jones, R. T., J. Pharmacol. Therap. 215:35 (1980).
9. Nowlan, R., and Cohen, S., Clin. Pharmacol. Therap. 22:550 (1977).
10. Lemberger, L., Silberstein, S. D., Axelrod, J., and Kopin, I. J., Science 170:1320 (1970).
11. Perez-Reyes, M., Timmons, M. C., and Wall, M. E., Arch. Gen. Psychiatry 31:89 (1974).
12. Cocchetto, D. M., Owens, S. M., Perez-Reyes, M., DiGuiseppi, S., and Miller, L. L. Psychopharmacol. 75:158 (1981).
13. Domino, L. E., Domino, S. E., Domino E. F., Presented at "Cannabinoids 82," Louisville, KY, 1982. 14. Lemberger, L., Tamarkin, N. R., Axelrod, J., and Kopin, I. J., Science 173:72 (1971).
15. Halldin, M. M., Widman, M., Isaac, H., Ryrfeldt, A., and Nilsson, E. J., Pharm. Pharmacol. Submitted for publication.
16. Lemberger, L., Weiss, J. L., Watanabe, A. M., Galanter, I. M., Wyatt, R. J., and Cardon, P. V., N. Engl. J. Med. 286:685 (1972).
17. Perez-Reyes, M., DiGuiseppi, S., Davis, K. H., Schindler, V. H., and Cook, C. E., Clin. Pharmacol. Therap. 31:617 (1982).
18. Wall, M. E., and Perez-Reyes, M., J. Clin. Pharmacol. 21:178C (1981).

METABOLISM, DISPOSITION AND PHARMACOKINETICS OF DELTA-9-TETRAHYDROCANNABINOL IN MALE AND FEMALE SUBJECTS*

Monroe E. Wall, Brian M. Sadler
Dolores Brine, Harold Taylor

Research Triangle Institute
Research Triangle Park, North Carolina

Mario Perez-Reyes

University of North Carolina
Chapel Hill, North Carolina

I. INTRODUCTION

It is well established that delta-9-tetrahydrocannabinol (THC) (I, Fig. 1) is the active psychoactive constituent found in *Cannabis sativa* (commonly referred to as "marijuana") (15). In recent years, a number of reports have appeared dealing with the potential therapeutic activity of THC. Its activity as an anticonvulsive agent and its potential for reducing intraocular pressure have been reviewed (4,5). Of highest interest and now well established is the antiemetic activity exhibited by THC (18,24). Knowledge of the metabolism, disposition and pharmacokinetics of any drug scheduled for therapeutic use is of great value to rational planning of dose schedules.

Although there have been a number of reports on the metabolism and disposition of THC (11,12,14,19) (cf.13,28,33 for reviews), the studies have been conducted predominantly with male volunteers. Sex differences have been observed in respect to metabolism of drugs (25) and steroids (9) by microsomal enzymes. It has been reported that microsomes from male

*Supported by NIDA grant DA-02424.

ISBN 0-12-044620-0

rats metabolize THC faster than those from females (2), and that a THC distillate was more potent in female rats than males in terms of behavioral response (6). Therefore, it was important to determine whether the sex differences observed with rodents would be noted in the metabolism and disposition of THC in humans.

This report presents a detailed comparison of the metabolism, disposition, and pharmacokinetics of THC in women and men.

II. MATERIALS AND METHODS

A. Subjects

Subjects who participated in the study were all healthy, female and male, paid volunteers, with normal weight in relation to their height and eating normal diets. All were familiar with the recreational use of marijuana. The female subjects had been taking oral contraceptives for at least six months prior to the study. Six male and six female volunteers were used for both the intravenous (iv) and oral (po) studies. The protocol required that different individuals be utilized in each study to minimize exposure to radiolabeled THC used in these studies.

The characteristics for the female and male subjects who volunteered for the iv studies expressed as X +/- S.D. were, respectively: age (years) 23 +/- 3 and 23+/- 2; weight, (kg) 54 +/- 7 and 72 +/- 9; height (cm), 163 +/- 7 and 175 +/- 6. Corresponding characteristics for female and male subjects in the oral group were, respectively: age 21.5 +/- 4.4 and 25.8 +/- 5.1; weight, 56.4 +/- 1.7 and 66.2 +/- 8.7; height, 165 +/- 5.5 and 175 +/- 6.9.

B. Chemicals and Materials

Tritium labeled THC-1',2'-$^3H_2$ or THC-4',5'-$^3H_2$, specific activity 150-165 mcC/mg; unlabeled THC (I); 11-hydroxy-delta-9-THC (II); and 11-nor-delta-9-THC-9-carboxylic acid (III) were obtained from the National Institute on Drug Abuse. Precoated thin-layer chromatography (TLC) plates, 20 x 20 cm, Silica Gel 60F-254 (E. Merck, Darmstadt, West Germany) were used for all chromatographic analyses. For scintillation counting, a fluor was utilized consisting of a mixture of Triton X-100/toluene/ Omnifluor (1 liter:2 liter:18 g).

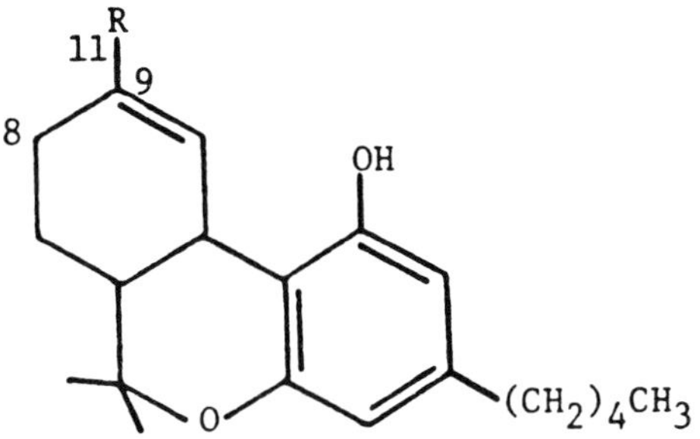

I.	Δ^9-Tetrahydrocannabinol	R = CH_3
II.	11-Hydroxy-Δ^9-Tetrahydrocannabinol	R = CH_2OH
III.	11-nor-Δ^9-Tetrahydrocannabinol-9-Carboxylic Acid	R = COOH

FIGURE 1. Chemical formula for THC and its major metabolites.

C. Drug Administration

Tritium labeled THC was mixed with unlabeled drug for all dosage forms. For the iv study an ethanolic solution of THC containing approximately 150 mcC of tritium was mixed with human serum albumin (Abbott) to form a microsuspension according to the method of Perez-Reyes et al. (22). By means of an infusion pump, the preparation was administered over a 20-30 min period to six female and six male volunteers; the mean THC doses were approximately 2.2 and 4.0 mg, respectively.

In the case of the oral studies, 15 or 20 mg of THC (females and males, respectively) containing 150 mcC of radiolabeled were dissolved in 0.5 ml of sesame oil and administered in two gelatin capsules.

D. Pharmacological Measurements

To measure the magnitude of the psychological effects produced by the administration of THC, the subjects were asked to rate their degree of "high" at frequent intervals during the 90-180 min of the studies by a standard technique (20,23). Since the most consistent physiological effect of THC is cardiac acceleration, the heart rate was continuously recorded from 10 min before drug administration and for 90-180 min thereafter.

E. Sample Collections

Blood samples were drawn at frequent intervals during the first hours of the experiments through an indwelling needle in one of the arm veins and by independent venipunctures thereafter. The blood samples were heparinized and centrifuged. The plasma obtained was immediately placed in frozen storage prior to analyses. The total urine excreted was collected at timed intervals for 72 hr, and total feces collected for the same interval of time.

F. Analytical Procedure

The basic procedure utilizes TLC to separate cannabinoid fractions, followed by scintillation counting of the radioactivity found in the separated zones.

Plasma, urine, and feces samples were analyzed for total drug, total non-conjugated and conjugated cannabinoids, THC, 11-hydroxy-delta-9-THC, and 11-nor-delta-9-THC-9-carboxylic acid by a slight modification of the procedure described by Wall et al. (31).

The major modifications were: (1) TLC developing system, for neutral cannabinoids: chloroform, ethanol, acetone, t-butanol, 92:1:3:5; for acid cannabinoids: plates pretreated in acetone, acetic acid 100:3, and dried at 110°; developing solvent was chloroform,acetone,acetic acid 60:45:0.5; and (2) extraction of urine. It had been found that preliminary chromatography on Amberlite XAD-2 resin can be omitted. The acidified urine could be extracted directly with diethyl ether.

The above procedure has been shown to give results comparable to those obtained by GC/MS procedures (30).

G. Pharmacokinetic and Statistical Analysis

The concentrations of drug in the plasma of each subject (Cp) were weighted at $1/Cp^2$, $1/Cp$, and 1 and fitted to the biexponential curve ($Cp = Ae^{-alpha \cdot t} + Be^{-beta \cdot t}$) (7), using the computer program NONLIN (17). Only data points after the peak concentration of drug in the plasma were fitted. From the three weighted analyses, the estimate of the smaller exponent which had the smallest standard deviation was used as the estimate of beta for each individual. In a few isolated cases in which the number of observed concentrations in the plasma was seven or less or when the coefficient of variation of beta was large, the data were weighted as before and fit with a monoexponential curve ($Cp = Be^{-beta \cdot t}$). An F-test was performed in order to justify the use of the lower order model ($P > 0.1$). The estimate of the absorption rate constant for THC was found by adding an absorption term ($Ce^{-gamma \cdot t}$) to the equation which represented the concentration of THC in the plasma after its oral administration and fitting all observed data points using NONLIN (17).

Cumulative urine data (U_C) were fitted with the equation $U_C = U_{inf.} (1-e^{-kt})$ (7). The first deviation of this equation was evaluated at four or five times for which there were corresponding plasma samples. The renal clearance (Cl_R) for each subject was estimated by taking the mean of $(dUc/dt)/Cp$ at those points.

The areas under the plasma concentration curves (AUC) were calculated from 0 to 48 hr or from 0 to 72 hr by the trapezoidal rule. The area under the curve from the last data point (48 to 72 hr) to infinity represented less than 2% of AUC in all cases and was considered to be negligible. The total clearance of drug from the plasma (Cl_T) was calculated as V_d = Dose/beta x AUC). Half-lives (t/2) were calculated from the fitted exponents ($lambda_i$ = alpha, beta, or gamma) as $t/2 = 0.693/lambda_i$.

Weighted means were used whenever the variance of an individual parameter was estimated (viz. beta and Cl_R). In these cases the formulas of Meiers were used (16).

Correlation analysis was done for the subjective "high" and heart rate data vs the concentrations of THC, total cannabinoids, 11-hydroxy-delta-9-THC, and 11-nor-delta-9-THC-9-carboxylic acid in the plasma. The subjective "high" was expressed as a percent of the maximum "high" for each subject. The heart rate was expressed as the percent increase over the basal heart rate for each subject. The coefficients of correlation (r) were determined for pooled groups of subjects using the CORR procedure in Statistical Analysis Systems (SAS). Correlation coefficients were compared using Fisher's Z-transformation of r (26).

Unless otherwise stated, statistical significance was determined at the 0.05 level.

III. RESULTS

A. Correlation of Plasma Cannabinoid Levels and Pharmacodynamic Measurements

Figure 2 (a-d) compares over a 2-3 hr period the mean

INTRAVENOUS

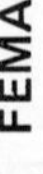

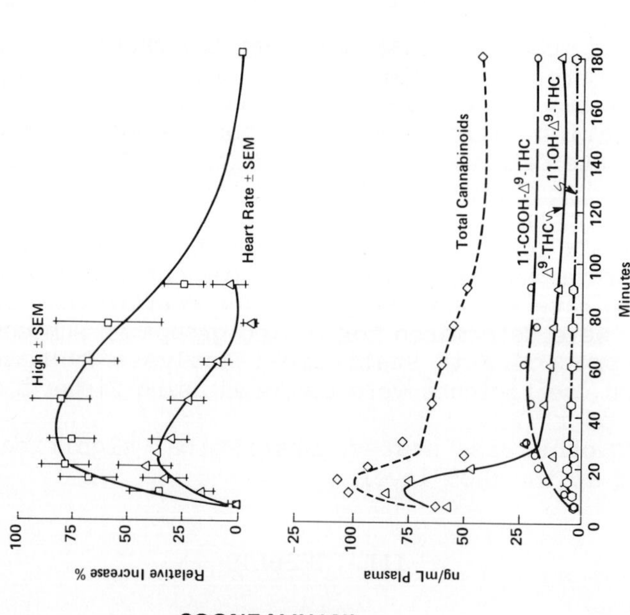

(a)

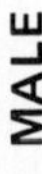

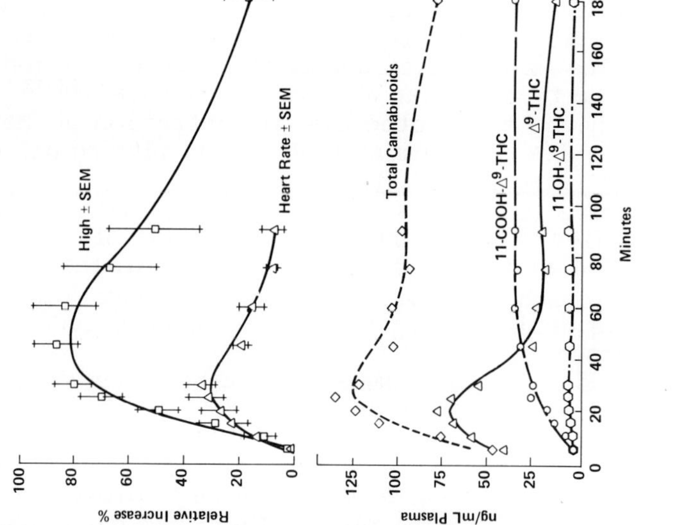

(b)

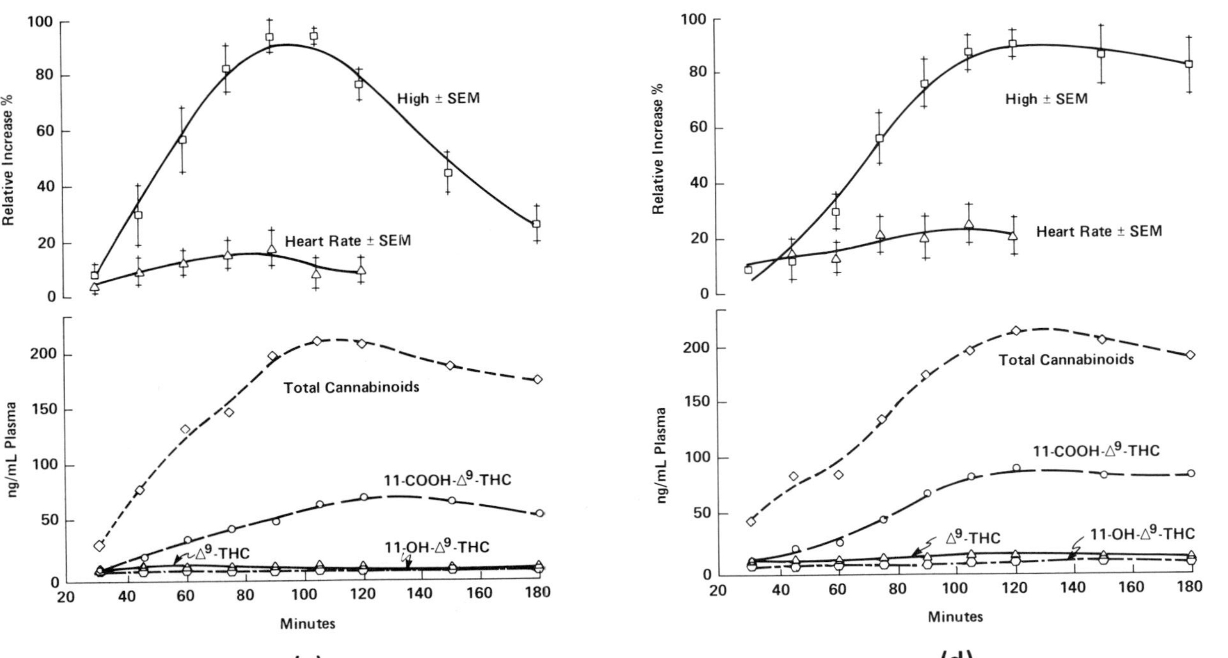

FIGURE 2. Concentration of THC and its major metabolites in plasma and their effect on subjective high and heart rate. Panels a and b represent the data from female and male subjects, resp., after intravenous administration of THC. Panels c and d represent the data from female and male subjects, resp., after oral administration of THC. Subjective high is presented as a percentage of the maximum response for each subject. Heart rates are presented as the percent increase above the heart rate prior to dosing. All curves represent the means of six subjects.

plasma concentration of THC and metabolites with the mean subjective "high" and mean heart rate of male and female subjects. Table I presents the correlation analysis of the data. In general for both sexes and both administration routes, total cannabinoid plasma levels provided better correlation with heart rate and psychological effects than corresponding THC plasma concentrations. After both iv and po administration to male subjects, correlation of THC plasma levels with heart rate was observed; $p < 0.05$. In general, no correlation of THC plasma levels with mean subjective "high" could be found.

B. Metabolism and Excretion

The plasma concentrations of THC and major metabolites at various time periods are presented in Tables II (iv administration) and III (po administration). A similar pattern was observed for both sexes. THC plasma levels decreased rapidly after iv infusion of drug was terminated (usually 15-25 min). After 1-1.5 hr, a much slower decrease in plasma THC levels was noted (cf. Fig. 3,4).

The active metabolite, 11-hydroxy-delta-9-THC (II), was present in the plasma in low concentrations, varying from 5-10% of THC levels at most time periods. The inactive metabolite 11-nor-delta-9-THC-9-carboxylic acid (III) was the major metabolic product found in plasma. Conjugated cannabinoids (defined as the radiolabeled plasma fraction insoluble in diethyl ether) were absent.

After oral administration, the composition of plasma cannabinoids was again similar for both sexes, exhibiting, however, characteristic differences from the data obtained after iv dosing. The major differences noted were (1) that after po administration, THC plasma levels increased to rather constant concentrations up to 4-6 hr after dosing, and (2) that the ratio of the plasma levels of active metabolite II relative to those of parent drug I showed a considerable increase (cf., Tables II and III). After oral administration, the concentrations of acid metabolites also increased considerably over the levels noted after iv dosing, and small quantities of conjugated cannabinoids were noted.

C. Urinary Excretion.

THC was excreted in urine as non-conjugated or conjugated acid metabolites (Tables IV, V). The mean cumulative cannabinoid excretion found in 72 hr after iv administration was 16.7 +/- 2.6% and 15.2 +/- 4.2% of the total dose for females and

TABLE I. Correlation of "High" and Heart Rate with Plasma Levels of THC and Metabolites

Correlation Coefficient (r)[a] for 6 Subjects

Cannabinoid	Male (iv)		Female (iv)		Male (po)		Female (po)	
	High	Heart	High	Heart	High	Heart	High	Heart
Δ^9-THC	-0.0998	0.5460*	0.0879 (0.0399)	-0.0187 (0.0785)	0.0729	0.4840*	0.3862*	0.2348
Total Drug	0.4674*+	0.7393*	0.1072 (0.2873)	0.1433 (0.4752)*+	0.5438*+	0.6093*	0.6409*+	0.1352

[a]R values receiving an asterisk showed significance at $P < 0.05$. R values in parentheses under the heading "Female (iv)" were obtained by dropping the data of one subject.

[+]Total drug significantly better correlated with parameter than Δ^9-THC ($P < 0.05$).

TABLE II. THC and Metabolites Found in Human Plasma after Intravenous Administration

ng/ml (Mean ± SD)

Time (hr)	Total Cannabinoids	Nonconjugated Cannabinoids	Polar Acids	11-nor-Δ^9-THC-9-COOH	11-OH Δ^9-THC	Δ^9-THC
			Six Female Subjects - Average Dose 2.2 mg			
* 0.08	62 ± 18	62 ± 18	Trace	0.6 ± 0.3	0.7 ± 0.4	58 ± 17
0.17	102 ± 31	102 ± 31	4.1 ± 1.5	4.8 ± 1.0	2.3 ± 1.5	85 ± 26
0.25	107 ± 40	106 ± 40	11 ± 2.2	13 ± 4.2	3.6 ± 2.4	75 ± 40
0.33	93 ± 39	92 ± 39	16 ± 3.1	16 ± 6.5	3.8 ± 2.8	47 ± 30
0.5	77 ± 22	76 ± 21	15 ± 6.4	22 ± 7.4	3.2 ± 2.3	23 ± 12
* 1.0	60 ± 13	60 ± 14	15 ± 8.6	24 ± 10	2.5 ± 1.14	12 ± 6.1
* 1.5	49 ± 6.3	48 ± 6.2	11 ± 4.6	21 ± 7.3	1.6 ± 0.7	8.7 ± 2.7
* 3.0	43 ± 3.8	48 ± 4.9	11 ± 4.7	18 ± 6.4	1.1 ± 0.6	7.9 ± 3.0
6.0	30 ± 3.4	30 ± 3.0	5.3 ± 1.9	14 ± 4.2	0.5 ± 0.3	5.6 ± 2.4
* 12.0	24 ± 7.5	23 ± 7.9	3.2 ± 1.0	12 ± 7.8	Trace	4.4 ± 3.7
* 24.0	16 ± 2.3	16 ± 2.1	2.4 ± 1.2	8.0 ± 3.1	Trace	2.7 ± 1.3
48.0	11 ± 3.2	11 ± 3.3	1.8 ± 1.4	4.8 ± 1.5	Trace	2.3 ± 1.1
			Six Male Subjects - Average Dose 4.0 mg			
0.08	46 ± 20	46 ± 20	1.1 ± 1.0	1.3 ± 0.8	0.5 ± 0.4	41 ± 20
* 0.17	75 ± 19	75 ± 22	5.0 ± 3.4	5.5 ± 2.6	1.4 ± 0.8	59 ± 21
0.25	110 ± 34	109 ± 35	8.8 ± 5.9	11 ± 7.5	2.7 ± 1.6	70 ± 30
0.33	123 ± 33	122 ± 33	17 ± 6.7	15 ± 3.2	3.0 ± 1.4	63 ± 34
0.42	135 ± 46	133 ± 46	20 ± 7.8	21 ± 15	3.6 ± 1.2	71 ± 34
0.5	122 ± 41	120 ± 40	25 ± 7.4	24 ± 9.0	3.7 ± 2.3	55 ± 31
* 0.75	102 ± 28	100 ± 28	29 ± 10	31 ± 11	3.1 ± 1.8	25 ± 5.2
1.0	103 ± 35	100 ± 34	29 ± 12	34 ± 13	2.8 ± 1.2	23 ± 8.3
* 1.25	93 ± 28	91 ± 29	24 ± 9.7	33 ± 18	2.7 ± 0.6	18 ± 2.9
1.5	97 ± 33	94 ± 31	25 ± 8.9	34 ± 15	3.0 ± 0.7	20 ± 6.2
* 2.0	93 ± 31	91 ± 30	27 ± 9.8	38 ± 16	2.2 ± 0.6	19 ± 6.2
2.5	90 ± 31	87 ± 30	23 ± 11	35 ± 15	2.1 ± 1.0	16 ± 6.3
3.0	78 ± 29	76 ± 29	18 ± 7.8	34 ± 14	1.4 ± 0.6	13 ± 5.9
6.0	57 ± 19	55 ± 20	12 ± 3.6	28 ± 12	0.7 ± 0.3	6.8 ± 2.8
* 8.0	52 ± 26	50 ± 26	10 ± 3.5	27 ± 15	0.6 ± 0.3	6.2 ± 3.5
12.0	34 ± 12	33 ± 13	6.5 ± 3.0	15 ± 6.5	Trace	5.0 ± 1.0
24.0	31 ± 14	29 ± 13	5.5 ± 2.6	15 ± 7.6	Trace	3.7 ± 1.2
* 30.0	32 ± 12	29 ± 13	6.7 ± 2.3	16 ± 7.0	Trace	3.8 ± 1.8
48.0	24 ± 11	21 ± 10	4.4 ± 2.0	11 ± 5.2	Trace	3.2 ± 1.8

*Five subjects

TABLE III. THC and Metabolites Found in Human Plasma after Oral Administration

ng/ml (Mean ± SD)

Time (hr)	Total Cannabinoids	Nonconjugated Cannabinoids	Polar Acids	11-nor-Δ^9-THC-9-COOH	11-OH Δ^9-THC	Δ^9-THC
Six Female Subjects - Average Dose 15 mg						
0.50	28 ± 26	26 ± 26	11 ± 14	4.1 ± 3.9	1.4 ± 1.3	4.8 ± 4.6
0.75	76 ± 58	69 ± 53	27 ± 23	15 ± 10	3.8 ± 4.2	9.0 ± 8.4
1.0	112 ± 67	104 ± 63	49 ± 27	27 ± 18	3.7 ± 2.8	7.7 ± 5.9
1.25	146 ± 61	135 ± 56	56 ± 23	41 ± 21	4.2 ± 2.6	8.4 ± 5.3
1.5	196 ± 66	184 ± 65	91 ± 31	48 ± 28	5.5 ± 2.6	9.1 ± 4.7
1.75	210 ± 53	194 ± 54	79 ± 28	62 ± 28	5.9 ± 2.8	9.4 ± 4.5
2.0	207 ± 40	192 ± 40	80 ± 21	68 ± 20	5.3 ± 1.6	7.4 ± 2.2
2.5	185 ± 32	173 ± 33	70 ± 26	64 ± 10	4.5 ± 2.5	7.2 ± 3.8
3.0	172 ± 34	160 ± 39	70 ± 26	51 ± 14	4.4 ± 2.9	6.8 ± 3.1
4.0	140 ± 30	130 ± 31	50 ± 22	48 ± 8.0	2.5 ± 1.7	6.2 ± 3.2
6.0	119 ± 30	109 ± 30	45 ± 17	38 ± 8.6	1.6 ± 0.9	5.4 ± 4.2
8.0	96 ± 39	95 ± 37	29 ± 19	39 ± 13	1.2 ± 0.5	3.8 ± 2.3
12.0	76 ± 23	68 ± 24	25 ± 15	28 ± 6.4	0.9 ± 0.5	3.2 ± 1.9
24.0	56 ± 11	48 ± 11	16 ± 3.7	21 ± 6.4	0.7 ± 0.5	1.9 ± 0.6
30.0	46 ± 12	39 ± 10	19 ± 8.2	15 ± 2.6	Trace	1.5 ± 1.0
48.0	35 ± 11	27 ± 10	8.4 ± 3.0	12 ± 7.4	Trace	0.9 ± 0.5
72.0	28 ± 10	23 ± 11	7.7 ± 3.9	8.4 ± 5.3	Trace	0.8 ± 0.9
Six Male Subjects - Average Dose 20 mg						
0.75	84 ± 14	62 ± 18	39 ± 8	18 ± 6	2.7 ± 0.8	9.1 ± 4.0
1.0	85 ± 42	81 ± 40	29 ± 19	23 ± 12	3.4 ± 3.1	8.0 ± 7.3
1.25	134 ± 41	127 ± 39	52 ± 26	47 ± 22	3.8 ± 1.9	11 ± 9.3
1.5	173 ± 41	164 ± 42	60 ± 27	66 ± 32	5.2 ± 1.7	11 ± 6.6
1.75	194 ± 51	185 ± 51	58 ± 20	82 ± 39	5.1 ± 2.1	13 ± 7.5
2.0	213 ± 68	201 ± 69	66 ± 17	89 ± 40	6.6 ± 3.4	13 ± 9.1
2.5	204 ± 61	191 ± 62	56 ± 26	80 ± 39	5.9 ± 3.0	14 ± 9.7
3.0	190 ± 67	180 ± 68	57 ± 13	82 ± 37	5.6 ± 3.2	11 ± 8.2
4.0	176 ± 68	167 ± 67	45 ± 19	82 ± 36	5.6 ± 3.6	11 ± 6.6
6.0	142 ± 47	134 ± 46	42 ± 11	62 ± 31	4.0 ± 1.8	10 ± 6.0
8.0	122 ± 37	115 ± 37	36 ± 10	51 ± 21	3.4 ± 2.3	8.4 ± 4.8
11.0 - 12.0	94 ± 31	87 ± 31	25 ± 9	37 ± 18	1.9 ± 1.3	6.4 ± 3.9
24.0	63 ± 22	56 ± 23	15 ± 4	29 ± 14	1.3 ± 1.2	3.3 ± 2.4
30.0	51 ± 15	44 ± 13	14 ± 4	23 ± 8	0.8 ± 0.6	3.2 ± 2.1
48.0	38 ± 12	30 ± 11	10 ± 3	14 ± 6	0.6 ± 0.5	2.2 ± 1.7
72.0	25 ± 7	17 ± 7	6 ± 3	8 ± 5	Trace	1.0 ± 0.6

TABLE IV. THC and Metabolites Found in Human Urine after Intravenous Administration Cumulative % Dose* (Mean ± SD)

		Nonconjugated Cannabinoid			Conjugated Cannabinoids		
Time (hr)	Total Cannab.	Total	Polar Acids	11-nor-Δ^9-THC-9-COOH	Total	Polar Acids	11-nor-Δ^9-THC 9-COOH
Six Female Subjects - Average Dose 2.2 mg							
1-1.5	1.8 ± 1.3	1.2 ± 0.9	0.8 ± 0.5	0.08 ± 0.04	0.6 ± 0.5	0.1 ± 0.1	0.05 ± 0.02
3	4.1 ± 0.2	2.6 ± 0.3	1.8 ± 0.5	0.4 ± 0.1	1.4 ± 0.4	0.3 ± 0.1	0.1 ± 0.06
6	5.4 ± 1.9	3.6 ± 1.1	1.9 ± 0.8	0.6 ± 0.3	1.8 ± 0.9	0.4 ± 0.2	0.2 ± 0.08
11-12	7.5 ± 1.2	4.9 ± 0.6	2.6 ± 0.9	0.9 ± 0.4	2.4 ± 0.9	0.5 ± 0.2	0.2 ± 0.03
24	11 ± 2	7.1 ± 1.6	3.3 ± 1.1	1.8 ± 1.0	3.7 ± 0.9	0.8 ± 0.3	0.4 ± 0.07
48	14 ± 2	14 ± 2	4.1 ± 1.3	2.6 ± 1.3	5.1 ± 1.4	1.0 ± 0.3	0.5 ± 0.05
72	16 ± 3	10 ± 3	4.4 ± 1.6	3.2 ± 1.7	5.5 ± 1.5	1.2 ± 0.3	0.6 ± 0.08
Six Male Subjects Average Dose 4.0 mg							
1.5-2	3.2 ± 1.1	2.1 ± 0.6	1.6 ± 0.7	0.3 ± 0.3	1.2 ± 0.6	0.3 ± 0.2	0.1 ± 0.1
2.5-3	4.9 ± 4.1	3.9 ± 3.2	1.5 ± 1.2	0.8 ± 0.8	1.9 ± 1.7	0.4 ± 0.4	0.3 ± 0.2
6	4.4 ± 0.1	2.8 ± 0.1	1.4 ± 0.1	0.6 ± 0.3	1.6 ± 0.3	0.3 ± 0.1	0.2 ± 0.2
11-12	5.9 ± 2.4	3.8 ± 1.5	1.5 ± 0.7	1.0 ± 0.7	2.1 ± 0.9	0.4 ± 0.1	0.3 ± 0.2
24	10 ± 5	6.4 ± 2.3	2.5 ± 0.9	2.0 ± 1.4	3.9 ± 1.5	0.7 ± 0.3	0.6 ± 0.5
48	14 ± 4	8.4 ± 2.3	5.8 ± 3.2	2.8 ± 1.6	5.2 ± 1.3	1.0 ± 0.3	0.8 ± 0.5
72	15 ± 4	9.5 ± 2.8	3.4 ± 1.1	3.2 ± 1.7	6.0 ± 1.7	1.1 ± 0.3	0.9 ± 0.5

*Data may not be consecutive due to missing values.

TABLE V. THC and Metabolites Found in Human Urine after Oral Administration Cumulative % Dose* (Mean ± SD)

Time (hr)	Total Cannab.	Nonconjugated Cannabinoid: Total	Nonconjugated Cannabinoid: Polar Acids	Nonconjugated Cannabinoid: 11-nor-Δ^9-THC-9-COOH	Conjugated Cannabinoids: Total	Conjugated Cannabinoids: Polar Acids	Conjugated Cannabinoids: 11-nor-Δ^9-THC-9-COOH
Six Female Subjects - Average Dose 15 mg							
1.25-1.5	0.9 ± 0.8	0.6 ± 0.5	0.4 ± 0.3	0.1 ± 0.1	0.4 ± 0.3	0.1 ± 0.1	0.1 ± 0.1
4	6.2 ± 2.0	3.6 ± 0.7	1.9 ± 0.3	0.8 ± 0.1	2.6 ± 1.3	1.0 ± 0.6	0.6 ± 0.6
5-6	5.5 ± 0.6	2.6 ± 0.6	1.7 ± 0.1	0.5 ± 0.4	2.9 ± 1.3	0.9 ± 0.5	0.8 ± 0.5
8	8.8 ± 1.9	4.7 ± 0.7	2.5 ± 0.4	1.0 ± 0.2	4.1 ± 1.3	1.8 ± 0.7	0.9 ± 0.6
11	9.4 [illegible].4	4.6 ± 1.2	2.7 ± 0.5	1.0 ± 0.5	4.8 ± 1.9	2.0 ± 0.8	1.1 ± 0.7
24	12.5 ± 3.0	6.3 ± 0.7	3.4 ± 0.7	1.4 ± 0.4	6.2 ± 2.6	2.4 ± 1.2	1.4 ± 0.8
30	14.1 ± 3.5	6.8 ± 0.7	3.9 ± 0.9	1.5 ± 0.5	7.3 ± 3.4	2.9 ± 1.5	1.6 ± 1.1
48	15.4 ± 3.0	7.7 ± 0.8	4.0 ± 0.7	1.9 ± 0.5	7.7 ± 2.9	2.9 ± 1.4	1.8 ± 1.0
72	15.9 ± 3.6	8.1 ± 1.0	4.3 ± 1.0	1.9 ± 0.5	7.8 ± 3.4	2.9 ± 1.5	1.8 ± 1.1
Six Male Subjects - Average Dose 20 mg							
1.5-2	1.3 ± 0.3	0.7 ± 0.1	0.47 ± 0.01	0.118 ± 0.004	0.5 ± 0.2	0.3 ± 0.1	0.12 ± 0.01
2.5-3	2.4 ± 0.3	1.4 ± 0.1	0.8 ± 0.1	0.3 ± 0.2	1.0 ± 0.2	0.5 ± 0.1	0.2 ± 0.1
4	3.7 ± 0.2	1.9 ± 0.3	1.1 ± 0.2	0.5 ± 0.2	1.8 ± 0.5	0.6 ± 0.2	0.5 ± 0.1
6	5.7 ± 1.0	3.1 ± 0.6	1.6 ± 0.1	0.8 ± 0.3	2.6 ± 0.3	1.1 ± 0.2	0.7 ± 0.1
8	5.9 ± 0.6	3.3 ± 0.6	1.8 ± 0.1	0.9 ± 0.4	2.6 ± 0.2	1.0 ± 0.2	0.7 ± 0.3
11	8.1 ± 0.8	4.4 ± 0.8	2.2 ± 0.1	1.2 ± 0.5	3.7 ± 0.5	1.5 ± 0.1	0.9 ± 0.4
24	10.3 ± 2.1	5.5 ± 1.4	2.7 ± 0.4	1.7 ± 0.8	4.8 ± 1.0	1.9 ± 0.5	1.2 ± 0.3
30	11.2 ± 2.0	5.9 ± 1.4	2.8 ± 0.4	1.8 ± 0.9	5.3 ± 1.0	2.1 ± 0.5	1.3 ± 0.3
48	12.7 ± 1.8	6.5 ± 1.5	3.0 ± 0.4	2.0 ± 0.9	6.1 ± 1.0	2.4 ± 0.5	1.5 ± 0.4
72	13.4 ± 2.0	6.9 ± 1.6	3.2 ± 0.4	2.2 ± 1.0	6.5 ± 1.1	2.5 ± 0.5	1.6 ± 0.4

*Data may not be consecutive due to missing values.

males, respectively; after po administration corresponding values were 15.9 +/- 3.6% and 13.4 +/- 2.0%. Analyses were conducted for neutral non-conjugated and conjugated cannabinoids but only traces were found. The composition of the cannabinoid urinary metabolites was similar for both sexes. After iv administration the ratio of non-conjugated to conjugated fraction increased, the non-conjugated-conjugated ratio approximating 1:1 at many time periods. The 11-nor-acid metabolite (III) and the less well defined "polar acid" fraction were the major constituents in urine. Other acid metabolites intermediate in polarity were present but were not quantitated.

D. Fecal Excretion

After iv administration, mean cumulative cannabinoid excretion in feces after 72 hr was 25 +/- 19% and 20 +/- 16% for female and male, respectively; after po administration corresponding values were 48 +/- 6% and 53 +/- 19%. The composition of cannabinoids found in the feces was similar for both sexes but was affected by the route of administration (cf. Tables VI and VII). In general, the cannabinoids in feces were non-conjugated -- the conjugate fraction amounting to only 5-10% of the total. After iv administration, both the 11-hydroxy and 11-nor-acid metabolites comprised the major components of the cannabinoid fractions which were analyzed; whereas after po administration, the 11-nor-acid was the major metabolite.

E. Pharmacokinetic Parameters

Figures 3 and 4 present graphical plots of the observed and calculated THC plasma concentrations vs time. The observed and calculated data were in agreement and consistent with a two compartment model with a biexponential decline in plasma levels as a function of time. The mean values of certain pharmacokinetic parameters are shown in Table VIII. After iv administration, the t/2 values for the rapid disposition alpha-phase calculated for THC were 0.4 and 0.6 hr, female, and male, respectively. Corresponding terminal phase (beta) half-lives were 29 and 36 hr, respectively. After oral administration, the t/2 values fo the absorption phase (gamma-phase) were 0.7 and 0.9 hr, female and male, respectively; t/2 of alpha-phase 3.8 and 3.9 hr; and t/2 beta-phase 25 hr for both sexes. Biological half-lives were also calculated from the beta-exponentials of metabolites (Table VIII). The terminal phase half-lives of the total drug and 11-nor-acid approx-

TABLE VI. THC and Metabolites Found in Human Feces after Intravenous Administration Cumulative % Dose* (Mean ± SD)

Time (hr)	Total Feces**	MeOH Soluble** Non-conjugated	MeOH Soluble** Conjugated	MeOH Insoluble**	Nonconjugated Polar Acids	Nonconjugated 11-nor-Δ^9-THC 9-COOH	Nonconjugated 11-OH Δ^9-THC	Nonconjugated Δ^9-THC
Four Female Subjects - Average Dose 2.2 mg								
21-24	9 ± 11	7 ± 9	0.4 ± 0.4	1.4 ± 2.0	1.2 ± 1.3	2.3 ± 2.8	4.4 ± 6.5	0.4 ± 0.5
44.5-48	19 ± 17	15 ± 13	1.0 ± 0.4	0.9 ± 0.5	2.2 ± 1.7	4.4 ± 4.5	2.3 ± 1.4	0.9 ± 0.8
72	26 ± 19	19 ± 14	1.2 ± 0.4	5.0 ± 4.7	2.9 ± 1.9	5.9 ± 5.5	3.1 ± 1.6	1.3 ± 0.8
Five Male Subjects - Average Dose 4.0 mg								
24	14 ± 11	11 ± 9	0.6 ± 0.5	1.9 ± 1.8	1.0 ± 1.0	2.2 ± 1.8	4.1 ± 4.5	0.8 ± 1.2
48	40 ± 6	32 ± 6	2.2 ± 0.1	5.7 ± 0.6	3.3 ± 2.7	5.9 ± 4.7	10 ± 3	2.0 ± 0.6
72	35 ± 11	27 ± 10	1.9 ± 0.7	5.9 ± 2.2	2.9 ± 1.7	6.3 ± 2.6	9.9 ± 5.7	2.7 ± 1.4

*Data may not be consecutive due to missing values.

**Total feces, MeOH soluble, and MeOH insoluble were measured independently.

TABLE VII. THC and Metabolites Found in Human Feces after Oral Administration Cumulative % Dose* (Mean ± SD)

		MeOH Soluble**			Nonconjugated			
Time (hr)	Total Feces**	Non-conjugated	Conjugated	MeOH Insoluble**	Polar Acids	11-nor-Δ^9-THC-9-COOH	11-OH Δ^9-THC	Δ^9-THC
			Five Female Subjects - Average Dose 15 mg					
22-24	9 ± 11	7 ± 8	2.1 ± 2.4	2 ± 2	1.1 ± 1.8	1.4 ± 1.8	0.8 ± 1.0	1.3 ± 1.3
48	37 ± 6	24 ± 2	4.2 ± 1.4	8 ± 1	4.4 ± 1.8	6.1 ± 0.5	3.0 ± 0.6	2.8 ± 0.6
72	48 ± 6	33 ± 3	4.4 ± 2.0	11 ± 2	6.0 ± 2.2	8.1 ± 1.7	4.0 ± 0.3	4.1 ± 1.9
			Six Male Subjects - Average Dose 20 mg					
24	24 ± 24	18 ± 19	1.8 ± 1.9	4 ± 5	2.3 ± 2.3	4.3 ± 4.5	1.9 ± 2.1	2.8 ± 2.9
40-48	55 ± 13	39 ± 11	5.1 ± 0.8	12 ± 4	5.8 ± 0.9	11 ± 2	4.0 ± 1.1	5.6 ± 3.5
72	53 ± 18	39 ± 12	4.0 ± 2.3	11 ± 6	6.1 ± 2.2	11 ± 5	3.7 ± 1.2	5.7 ± 1.7

*Data may not be consecutive due to missing values.

**Total feces, MeOH soluble, and MeOH insoluble were measured independently.

TABLE VIII. Mean Values of Pharmacokinetic Parameters[a]

DRUG FORM	AUC/DOSE i.v.	AUC/DOSE p.o.	β[c] i.v.	β[c] p.o.	$t_{\frac{1}{2}\beta}$[b] i.v.	$t_{\frac{1}{2}\beta}$[b] p.o.	V_d[d] i.v.	Cl_T i.v.	Cl_R[c] i.v.	Cl_R[c] p.o.
	(min/ml) x 10^3		(hr^{-1}) x 10^2		(hr)		(liters)	(ml/min)	(ml/min)	
MALES										
Total Drug	28 (10)	13 (4)	1.6 (1.0)	1.8 (0.6)	43	39	226 (129)	40 (16)	4.5 (0.7)	14.3 (1.1)
Δ^9-THC	4.2 (1.0)	0.8 (0.5)	2.0 (1.7)	2.7 (0.7)	36	25	734 (444)	248 (62)	-	-
11-OH-Δ^9-THC	-	-	4.6 (1.8)	3.8 (2.3)	15	18	-	-	-	-
11-nor-Δ^9-THC-9-COOH	-	-	1.3 (1.2)	2.8 (0.8)	55	25	-	-	1.6 (0.1)	4.4 (0.6)
FEMALES										
Total Drug	26 (8)	16 (2)	2.3 (1.4)	1.4 (0.7)	31	48	130 (87)	44 (24)	8.0 (0.9)	14.2 (2.5)
Δ^9-THC	5.5 (2.1)	0.6 (0.3)	2.4 (2.8)	2.8 (1.4)	29	25	523 (217)	197 (50)	-	-
11-OH-Δ^9-THC	-	-	2.1 (3.0)	5.8 (2.2)	33	12	-	-	-	-
11-nor-Δ^9-THC-9-COOH	-	-	2.8 (1.1)	1.9 (1.3)	25	37	-	-	1.8 (0.4)	4.2 (0.7)

(a) Figures in parentheses are standard deviations.
(b) Calculated from mean β.
(c) Weighted mean and standard deviation.
(d) Apparent volume of distribution corrected for β.

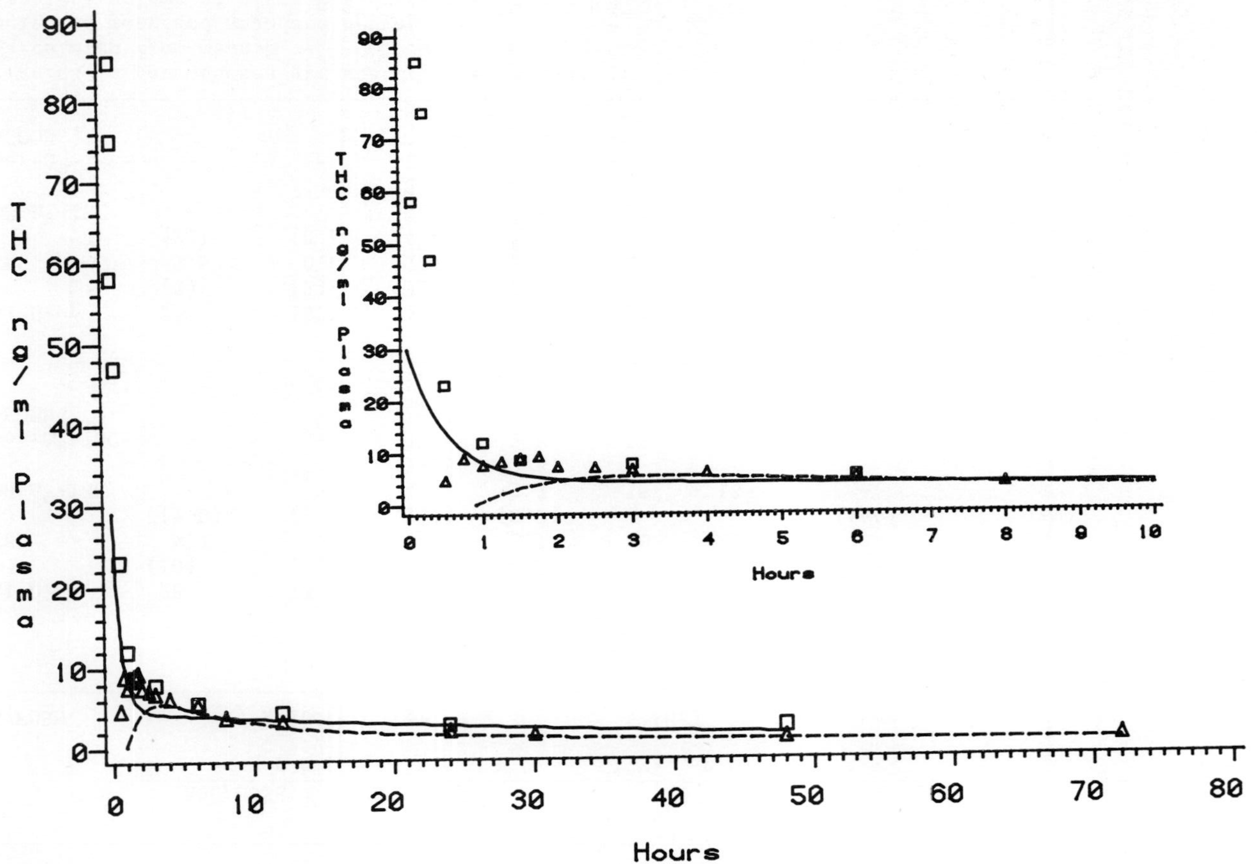
THC ng/ml Plasma
Hours
90
80
70
60
50
40
30
20
10
0
0
10
20
30
40
50
60
70
80
THC ng/ml Plasma
Hours
0
1
2
3
4
5
6
7
8
9
10

imated those noted for THC. AUC/Dose calculated for total drug and THC were similar for both sexes. The magnitude of the area uder the curve corrected for dose, calculated for total cannabinoids and THC, was unaffected by the sex of the subjects, but was markedly influenced by the route of administration, cf., Table VIII. The values obtained after po dosing were much lower than the corresponding values noted after iv administration. The volume of distribution corrected for beta was of the same order for both sexes, approximately 10 l./kg. Total clearance values were also of the same order for both sexes, 197 and 248 mL/min for females and males, respectively. Renal clearance values for 11-nor-delta-9-THC-9-carboxylic acid were of the same order for both sexes (1.5-2.0 mL/min). There seemed to be some increase in these values after oral administration, although the difference may not be significant.

IV. DISCUSSION

Although the metabolism of THC in man has received extensive study (cf.10,28,32,33 for reviews), previous studies have been conducted largely with male volunteers (31). Moreover, in most of the earlier studies, analyses of plasma for THC or metabolites were not conducted for sufficiently long periods to obtain reasonable estimates for beta-parameters and corresponding half-lives. The studies reported in this paper present a comprehensive study of the metabolism, excretion and pharmacokinetics of THC administered to female and male volunteers by iv and oral dosing. In agreement with other workers (3,8), we could not demonstrate a consistent relationship between plasma THC concentrations and subjective "high" or heart rate. With male volunteers correlation was observed (iv and po, Table I) between THC levels and heart rate. However, better correlation was observed for both sexes between the total cannabinoid plasma concentrations found after iv or po administration and both heart rate and psychological "high". This relationship is probably coincidental. However, we have noted that the shape of the plots for total cannabinoids, "high", and heart rate shown in Figs. 2a-d, which depict these

FIGURE 3. Observed and calculated concentrations of THC in plasma of female subjects. The observed data represent the means of six subjects for oral (triangles) and intravenous (squares) administration of THC. The corresponding calculated curves (oral ---; intravenous ——) were constructed from the weighed parameter means from individual fitted plasma data.

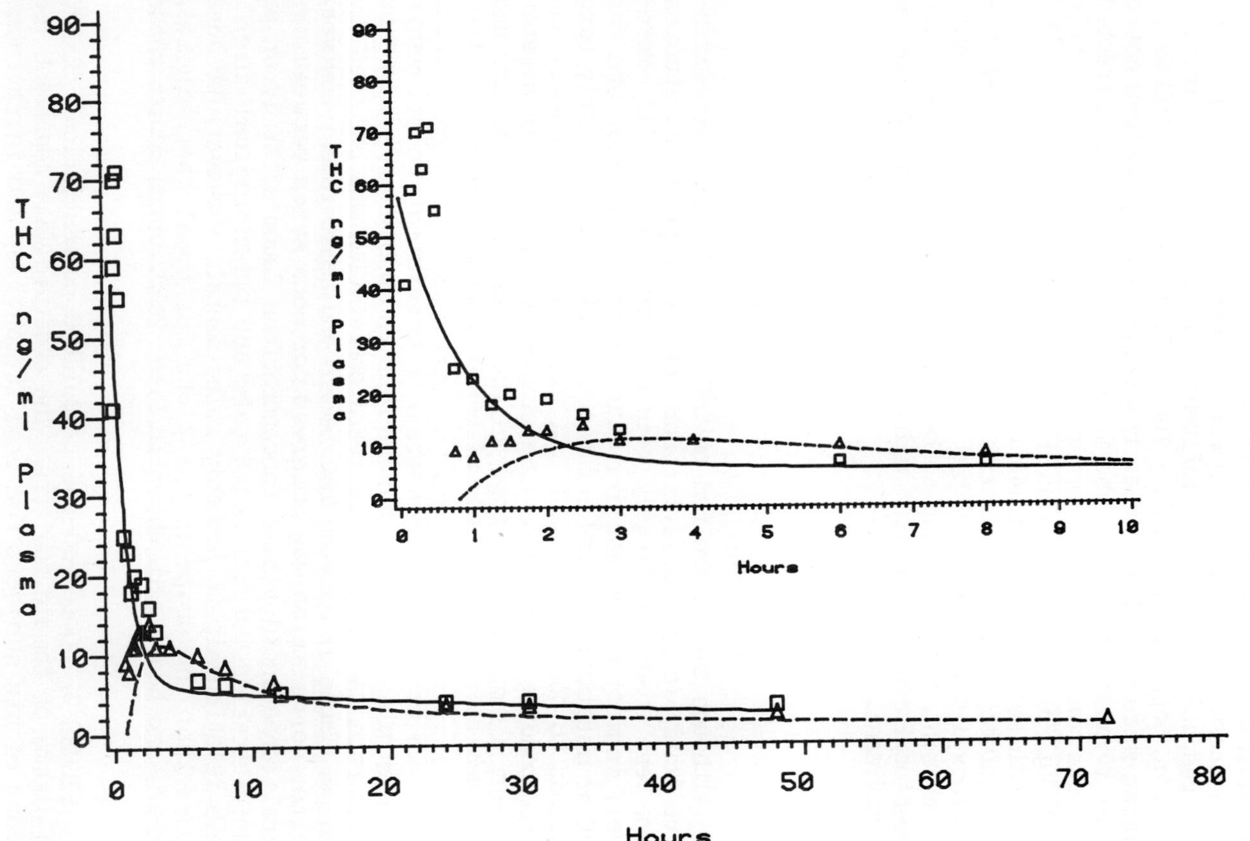
THC ng/ml Plasma
Hours
THC ng/ml Plasma
Hours

correlations, and the plots of THC concentration in mouse brain vs time after iv administration, are similar (21,29). In the mouse model it has been shown (21,29) that after iv administration of cannbinoids, brain concentrations of parent drug reach a maximum within 0.5 min after administration, and a steady state is maintained for at least 30 min before brain levels decrease; whereas, mouse plasma cannabinoid levels decreased rapidly. If similar effects occur in man, this would account for psychological effects persisting for long time periods after plasma cannabinoid levels have decreased.

It is now well established from _in vitro_ and _in vivo_ animal studies and _in vivo_ in man that THC is extensively metabolized by liver enzymes (27,28). In man allylic hydroxylation at the C-8 or C-11 positions by microsomal enzymes convert the parent drug to metabolites hydroxylated at C-8 (8-alpha or 8-beta), C-11, or both positions. Hydroxylation in the side chain frequently occurs in animals but many not be an important process in man. The primary alcohol at C-11 is metabolized to the corresponding 11-nor-acid or more polar acids by liver alcohol-dehydrogenase enzymes.

Our studies indicate that after administration of THC, no significant differences in metabolic pattern or excretion were observed between women and men. As noted in our earlier studies (31), certain major differences can be noted due to the route of administration. Of particular interest are the differences noted in the ratio of plasma THC (I) concentration to that of its 11-hydroxy metabolite (II). After iv administration, the ratio of II:I varies from 1:10-20; whereas after oral administration, the ratio increases to 1:2. The increase in the plasma levels of II after oral administration has been noted in our earlier studies (28,31). We attribute this to first-pass effects which both increase the concentration of II and decrease that of I. The increased proportion of the active 11-hydroxy metabolite may account for the fact that the subjective "high" noted with subjects receiving oral THC dosing is of the _same order_ as noted with subjects receiving iv dosing, even though in the latter case THC plasma concentrations are initially _much higher_. Previous studies with mice have shown that THC metabolites with one additional hydroxyl moiety (8-beta, 11, or 3') penetrate the blood-brain barrier more rapidly and achieve much higher concentrations in

FIGURE 4. Observed and calculated concentrations of THC in plasma of male subjects. The observed data represent the means of six subjects for oral (triangles) and intravenous (squares) administration of THC. The corresponding calculated curves (oral ---; intravenous ——) were constructed from the weighed parameter means from individually fitted plasma data.

the brain than parent drug (21,29).

The cannabinoid acids, which include the 11-nor acid (III), as well as other less defined and more polar compounds, constitute the end products of cannabinoid metabolism. These acids comprised the major metabolite fraction found in plasma, urine and feces. No differences were found in the metabolism of these compounds that could be attributed to differences in sex. However, the route of administration did play a role, particularly in the degree of conjugation. We define urinary cannabinoid conjugates as the radiolabeled fraction that cannot be extracted from urine with diethyl ether. After oral administration, concentration of the conjugated fraction in urine was larger than the comparable fraction found after iv dosing. Similarly, in the feces, after iv administration, little conjugation was noted, whereas the concentration of total conjugates increased after oral administration. Little is known about the composition of the cannabinod conjugate fraction except that some of it can be hydrolyzed by glucuronidase. This represents at times only a small fraction of the total conjugates. The nature of the remaining forms of conjugation is still largely unknown.

Acidic cannabinoids comprise almost the entire cannabinoid fraction found in the urine. Neutral cannabinoids, both free and conjugated, are found only in trace quantity. Urinary excretion is the minor route of elimination of cannabinoids. Approximately 13-16% of the total dose is found in urine after 72 hr with both administration routes and for both sexes.

As noted previously (31), biliary excretion via the feces is the major route of cannabinoid excretion. Approximately 30% of the total dose was recovered in feces after iv administration, and about 50% after oral administration. The composition of the cannabinoids found in the feces is noteably different from the pattern of urinary metabolites. Fecal cannabinoids were found only in the non-conjugated form. In addition to acid metabolites, neutral cannabinoids, particularly 11-hydroxy-delta-9-THC, were important constituents. Whether the cannabinoids are excreted partially or totally as conjugates in bile and then enzymatically cleaved by endogenous intestinal enzymes or enzymes from microbial flora is uncertain. In the rat, an animal in which THC is also excreted in metabolized form primarily in feces (1), biliary cannulation studies of animals dosed with THC demonstrated that 60% of the metabolites were eliminated as water-soluble conjugates (34).

Pharmacokinetic parameters were similar for both sexes but differed in some cases due to the administration route. After termination of iv infusion of THC, the plasma decay curves for THC, when plotted as concentration vs time, yielded a biexponential curve which could be fitted by a digital computer program to provide a non-linear regression analysis of the curve (17), from which could be calculated the constants of the equation: $C = Ae^{-alpha.t} + Be^{-beta.t}$. The actual and calculated plots of THC concentrations vs time (Figs. 3,4) are in reasonable agreement. The half-lives calculated for THC from the terminal phase constant beta were in excellent agreement for both sexes and both routes of administration, the range being 25-36 hr (Table VIII). Similar values were noted for total drug and the 11-nor-acid metabolite. Our results were in excellent agreement with an earlier study by Lemberger et al. (14), which covered approximately the same time period (72 hr) as our study. These workers report terminal phase half-lives of 28 hr for subjects who were experienced marijuana users. They noted similar half-lives for total radioactivity (total drug) and "ether extractable" radioactivity (which may have included the 11-nor-acid metabolite).

Similar apparent volumes of distribution were found for THC after iv administration of the drug to female and male volunteers. The high values observed, 523 and 734 liters (9.9 and 10.2 l./kg), are in accord with the results reported by Lemberger et al. (14) and can be ascribed to sequestration of the lipid soluble drug in fatty tissues.

After oral administration of THC, the values for AUC/dose were of the same order for both sexes but were markedly lower than corresponding values noted after iv dosing. The bioavailability of THC ranged from 10.9% (female) to 19.0% (male). Ohlsson et al. (19) report a systemic availability of 6% for THC utilizing a protocol with a shorter time period and a different vehicle for the drug.

From Table VII, it can be noted that the maximal quantity of THC found in feces ranges from 3-6% of the total dose, some of which may be due to biliary excretion. It follows therefore that absorption of THC through the gastrointestinal wall was high. Consequently, the low bioavailability of THC observed in our studies after oral administration must be due to extensive biotransformation of the drug by liver enzymes as a result of the "first pass" effect.

Renal clearance values Cl_R were determined for non-conjugated 11-nor-delta-9-THC-9-carboxylic acid, which is the major acidic metabolite found in urine. It should be noted that a number of other acids are present, some of which are probably included in what we term the polar acid fraction. In accord with the previously discussed pharmacokinetic data, no differences in Cl_R values were found due to the sex of the subjects. The data does indicate increased renal clearance after oral administration. The reason for this is not clear-cut. Possibly there may be greater saturation of the binding protein in plasma by the higher levels of the 11-nor-acid metabolite formed after oral administration. The renal clearance values were not corrected for plasma binding as this constant has never been determined for the 11-nor-acid. In all likelihood, it would be of the order of at least 80-90% based on other cannabinoids binding values. Even correcting for an assumed 90% plasma binding of the 11-nor-acid (III), it is evident that the clearance ratio would be much lower than unity compared to inulin. This suggests that the metabolite may be subject to reabsorption (7).

REFERENCES

1. Agurell, S., Nilsson, I. M., Ohlsson, A., and Sanberg, F., Elimination of tritium-labelled cannabinoids in the rat, Biochem. Pharmacol. 18:1195-1201 (1969).
2. Burstein, S., and Kupfer, D., Hydroxylation of trans-delta-1-tetrahydrocannabinol by hepatic microsomal oxygenase, Ann. N. Y. Acad. Sci. 191:61-66 (1971).
3. Cocchetto, D. M., Owens, S. M., Perez-Reyes, M., Guiseppi, S. D., and Miller, L. L., Relationship between plasma delta-9-tetrahydrocannabinol concentration and pharmacologic effects in man, Psychopharmacol. 75:158-164 (1981).
4. Cohen, S., Therapeutic aspects, in "Marijuana research findings" (R.C. Peterson, ed.), pp. 199-215. NIDA Research Monograph, No. 31, U.S. Government Printing Office, Washington, D. C. 1980.
5. Cohen, S., and Stillman, R. C., (eds.), "The Therapeutic potential of marihuana". Plenum Medical Book Co., New York, 1976.
6. Cohn, R., Barnes, P., Barratt, E., and Pinch, J., Sex differences in response to marijuana extract in rats, Pharmacologist 13:297 (1971).
7. Gibaldi, M., and Perrier, D., "Pharmacokinetics". M. Dekker, Inc., New York, 1975.
8. Hollister, L. E., Gillespie, H. K., Ohlsson, A., Lindgren, J. E., Wahlen, A., and Agurell, S., Do plasma concentrations of delta-9-tetrahydrocannabinol reflect the degree of intoxication? J. Clin. Pharmacol. 21:171S-177S (1981).
9. Kuntzman, R., Schneidman, K., Jacobson, M., and Conney, A. H., Similarities between oxidative drug-metabolizing enzymes and steroid hydroxylases in liver microsomes, J. Pharmacol. Exp. Ther. 146:280-285 (1964).
10. Lemberger, L., Metabolism of the tetrahydrocannabinols, in "Advances in Pharmacology and Chemotherapy" (S. Garattini, A. Goldin, and F. Hawking, eds.), pp. 222-225. Academic Press, New York, 1972.

11. Lemberger, L., in "Marihuana, Chemistry, Biochemistry and Cellular Effects" (G. G. Nahas, ed.), pp. 169-178, Springer-Verlag, New York, 1976.
12. Lemberger, L., Axelrod, J., and Kopin J. J., Metabolism and disposition of tetrahydrocannabinols in naive subjects and chronic marihuana users, Ann. N. Y. Acad. Sci. 191:142-154 (1971).
13. Lemberger, L., and Rubin, A., The physiological disposition of marijuana in man, Life Sci., 17:1637-1642 (1975).
14. Lemberger, L., Tamarkin, N. R., Axelrod, J., and Kopin, J. J., Delta-9-tetrahydrocannabinol: Metabolism and disposition in long-term marijuana users, Science 173:72-74 (1971).
15. Mechoulam, R., (ed.), "Marijuana: Chemistry, pharmacology, metabolism and clinical effects". Academic Press, New York, 1973.
16. Meier, P., Variance of a weighted mean, Biometrics 9:59-73 (1953).
17. Mettler, C. M., Elfring, G. L., and McEwen, A. J., "A users manual for NONLIN and associated programs". Revised edition, The Upjohn Company, Kalamazoo, MI, 1976.
18. Milne, G. M., Johnson, R. M., Wiseman, E. H., and Hutcheson, D. E., Therapeutic progress in cannabinoid research, J. Clin. Pharmacol. 21:Suppl. Aug.-Sept. (1981).
19. Ohlsson, A., Lindgren, J. E., Wahlen, A., Agurell, S., Hollister, L. E., and Gillespie, B. A., Plasma delta-9-tetrahydrocannabinol concentrations and clinical effects after oral and intravenous administration and smoking, Clin. Pharmacol. Ther. 28:409-416 (1980).
20. Perez-Reyes, M., Lipton, M. A., Timmons, M. C., Wall, M. E., Brine, D. R., and Davis, K. H., Pharmacology of orally administered delta-9-tetrahydrocannabinol, Clin. Pharmacol. Ther. 14:48-55 (1973).
21. Perez-Reyes, M., Simmons, J., Brine, D., Kimmel, G. D., Davis, K. H., and Wall, M. E., Rate of penetration of delta-9-tetrahydrocannabinol and 11-hydroxy-delta-9-tetrahydrocannabinol to the brain of mice, in "Marihuana; Chemistry, biochemistry and cellular effects" (G. G. Nahas, ed.), pp. 179-185. Springer-Verlag, New York, 1976.
22. Perez-Reyes, M., Timmons, M. C., Lipton, M. A., Davis, K. H., Wall, M. E., Intravenous injection in man of delta-9-tetrahydrocannabinol and 11-OH-delta-9-tetrahydrocannabinol, Science 177:633-634 (1972).
23. Perez-Reyes, M., and Wall, M. E., Pharmacology of delta-9-tetrahydrocannabinol and other cannabinoids, in "Treatment of cancer chemotherapy induced nausea and vomiting" (D. S. Poster, J. S. Penta, and S. Bruno, eds.), Masson Publishing, New York, 1981.

24. Poster, D. S., Penta, J. S., and Bruno, S., in "Treatment of cancer chemotherapy induced nausea and vomiting". Masson Publishing, New York, 1981.
25. Quinn, J. P., Axelrod, J., and Brodie, B. B., Species, strain and sex differences in metabolism of hexobarbitone, amidopyrine, antipyrine and aniline, Biochem. Pharmacol. 1:152-159 (1958).
26. Snedecor, G. W., and Cochran, W. C., "Statistical methods", Sixth Edition, pp. 185-188. The Iowa State University Press, Iowa City, 1967.
27. Wall, M. E., The _in vitro_ and _in vivo_ metabolism of tetrahydrocannabinol, Ann. N. Y. Acad. Sci. 191:23-29 (1971).
28. Wall, M. E., The chemistry and metabolism of cannabinoids, in "The inter-agency committee on new therapies for pain and discomfort", pp. 1-74. Report to the White House, USDHEW, PHS, NIH, Bethesda, MD, 1979.
29. Wall, M. E., and Brine, D. R., Applications of mass spectrometry in cannabinoid research, in "Marihuana: Biological effects" (G. G. Nahas and W. D. M. Paton, eds.), pp. 15-43. Pergamon Press, New York, 1979.
30. Wall, M. E., Brine, D. R., Bursey, J. T., and Rosenthal, D., Analytical methods for the determination of cannabinoids in biological meterials, in "Cannabinoid Assays in Humans" (R. E. Willette, ed.), pp. 107-117. NIDA Research Monograph, No. 7, U.S. Government Printing Office, Washington, D. C., 1976.
31. Wall, M. E., Brine, D. R.,and Perez-Reyes, M., The metabolism of cannabinoids in man, in "Pharmacology of marihuana" (M. C. Braude and S. Szara, eds.), pp.93-113. Raven Press, New York, 1976.
32. Wall, M. E., Perez-Reyes, M.: Metabolism of delta-9-THC, in "Treatment of cancer chemotherapy-induced nausea and vomiting" (D. Poster, J. S. Penta, and S. Bruno, eds.), pp. 93-110. Masson Publishing USA, Inc., New York, 1981.
33. Wall, M. E., and Perez-Reyes, M., The metabolism of delta-9-tetrahydrocannabinol and related cannabinoids in man, J. Clin, Pharmacol. 21:178S-189S (1981).
34. Widman, M., Nordqvist, M., Agurell, S., Lindgren, J. E., Sandberg, F., Biliary excretion of delta-1-tetrahydrocannabinol and its metabolites in the rat, Biochem. Pharmacol. 23:1163-1172 (1974).

ACIDIC METABOLITES OF DELTA-1-TETRAHYDROCANNABINOL EXCRETED IN THE URINE OF MAN*

M. M. Halldin, M. Widman

Department of Pharmacognosy
Faculty of Pharmacy, BMC
Uppsala, Sweden

S. Agurell

Astra Lakemedel AB
Sodertalje, Sweden

L. E. Hollister, S. L. Kanter

Veterans Administration Medical Center
Palo Alto, California

I. INTRODUCTION

Early in 1970 the major primary route of cannabinoid metabolism hydroxylation at the allylic C-7 position was identified (1-3). Since then extensive research has led to the elucidation of a number of the major pathways involved in the metabolism of the cannabinoids and especially delta-1-tetrahydrocannabinol (THC). The metabolism has been studied in several species including rat, mouse, rabbit, dog, guinea-pig and rhesus monkey. However, much less is known about the metabolism of THC in man. In Fig. 1, known metabolic pathways of THC are shown. Hydroxylation (or oxygenation) occurs at the allylic positions as well as on the side chain. Epoxidation of the double bond has also been observed. The monohydroxy-

*Supported by grants from the Swedish Medical Research Council, NIDA and the Veterans Administration.

ISBN 0-12-044620-0

lated products may undergo further hydroxylations as well as oxidation to the corresponding acids. The side chain canbe cleaved and oxidized to acids. Most monooxygenated THC metabolites are pharmacologically active (4). The most abundant type of secondary metabolites of THC are the glucuronides (5-7). In addition to the glucuronides, esters of fatty acids with cannabinoids or primary metabolites of cannabinoids have been observed (8,9).

When our study in man was initiated there was limited knowledge about the fate of THC in man. Wall and colleagues had identified 7-hydroxy-, 6-alpha-hydroxy-, and 6-beta-hydroxy- together with 6,7-dihydroxy-delta-1-THC in human plasma and feces after oral administration, i.v. injection or smoking (10,11). However, in the urine of man, Wall et al. have shown that the concentration of neutral cannabinoids is negligible and that delta-1-THC-7-oic acid and acids of increasing polarity are the major urinary metabolites. Thus far delta-1-THC-7-oic acid and its glucuronide were the only urinary metabolites identified (7,11,12). The purpose of our study was to elucidate the structures of the hither-to unidentified acidic metabolites of THC excreted in the urine of man.

II. EXPERIMENTAL

Three healthy male volunteers participated in this study. They received 20-30 mg of THC in a chocolate cookie on three to four different occasions separated by 48 h. One person received radiolabelled THC (29.1 MEq/mg). Urine was collected daily up to 72 h after the last administered dose. Drug administration and collections of urine samples have been described in detail (13). The urine samples were extracted and metabolites separated and isolated as previously reported (13,14).

The isolated metabolites were identified by matching their mass spectra and chromatographic data (LC, TLC and GC) to reference compounds and to published data (15-17).

III. RESULTS AND DISCUSSION

About 90% of the radioactivity in the urine was recovered by extraction. No unchanged THC could be detected. Eighteen acidic metabolites (Table I) were isolated and identified as described (13,14). Structures of the four most abundant metabolites are shown in Fig. 2. The most prominent metabolite of all was delta-1-THC-7-oic acid (1) which accounted for

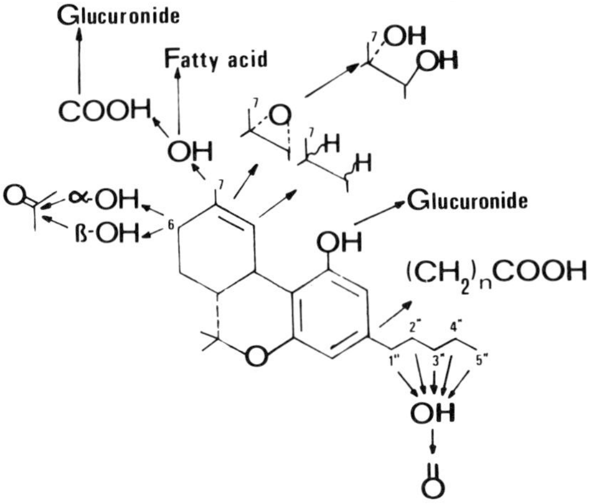

FIGURE 1. Major metabolic pathways for THC.

27% of total radioactivity in the urine. The second and third most abundant metabolites were 4",5"-bisnor-delta-1-THC-7,3"-dioic acid (16) and 4"-hydroxy-delta-1-THC-oic acid (6), which accounted for 8% and 5% of the radioactivity, respectively. The side-chain unsaturated 1",2"-dehydro-4",5"-bisnor-delta-1-THC-7,3"-dioic acid (18) was found in smaller amounts (3%). The remaining fourteen metabolites were present in less than 1% or in trace amounts.

In addition to the 7-oic acid (1) only one more monocarboxylic acid identified as the 4",5"-bisnor-delta-1-THC-3"-oic acid (2) was found in minor amounts. There were 7-oic acids (3-7) hydroxylated at C-1" to C-4" positions of the side chain accounting in all for about 8% of the radioactivity. Side-chain acids (8-13) oxidized at C-2" to C-4" positions coupled with hydroxylations at either C-7, C-6-alpha or C-6-beta positions accounted for about 5%. The dicarboxylic acids (14-18), which accounted for about 15% of the radioactivity in the urine, were oxidized at C-7 position coupled with oxidations at C-1", C-2", C-3" or C-4" positions of the side chain. Of all metabolites isolated in the urine of man, metabolite 1was the only metabolite with an intact side chain. The remaining seventeen metabolites (~30%) have the side chain hydroxylated, further oxidized or shortened.

Allylic oxidation occurred at either C-6 or C-7 position. Metabolites with a 7-hydroxy or a 7-carboxy function predominated. Allylic attack at the C-6 position yielded mainly 6-beta-hydroxy derivatives of monocarboxylic acids. No metabo-

TABLE I. Structure and Relative Abundance of Acidic Metabolites of Delta-9-THC Isolated from Human Urine

Metabolite	R_1	R_2	R_3	Rel.Ab.*
1 Delta-1-THC-7-oic acid	COOH	H	C_5H_{11}	4+
2 4",5"-bisnor-delta-1-THC-3"-oic acid	CH_3	H	C_2H_4COOH	+
3 1"-OH-delta-1-THC-7-oic acid	COOH	H	$C_5H_{10}OH$	t
4 2"-OH-delta-1-THC-7-oic acid	COOH	H	$C_5H_{10}OH$	+
5 3"-OH-delta-1-THC-7-oic acid	COOH	H	$C_5H_{10}OH$	+
6 4"-OH-delta-1-THC-7-oic acid	COOH	H	$C_5H_{10}OH$	2+
7 3",4",5"-trisnor-delta-1-THC-2"-oic acid	COOH	H	C_2H_4OH	+

8	7-OH-3",4",5"-trisnor-delta-1-THC-2"-oic acid	CH_2OH	H	CH_2COOH	+
9	7-OH-4",5"-bisnor-delta-1-THC-3"-oic acid	CH_2OH	H	C_2H_4COOH	+
10	6-beta-OH-3",4",5"-trisnor-delta-1-THC-2"-oic acid	CH_3	beta-OH	CH_2COOH	+
11	6-beta-OH-3",4",5"-bisnor-delta-1-THC-3"-oic acid	CH_3	beta-OH	C_2H_4COOH	+
12	6-alpha-OH-5"-bisnor-delta-1-THC-3"-oic acid	CH_3	alpha-OH	C_3H_6COOH	t
13	2",3"dehydro-6-alpha-OH-5"-nor-delta-1-THC-4"oic acid	CH_3	alpha-OH	C_3H_4COOH	t
14	2",3",4",5"-tetranor-delta-1-THC-7,1"-dioic acid	COOH	H	COOH	t
15	3",4",5"-trisnor-delta-1-THC-7,2"-dioic acid	COOH	H	CH_2COOH	t
16	4",5"-bisnor-delta-1-THC-7,3"-dioic acid	COOH	H	C_2H_4COOH	3+
17	5"-nor-delta-1-THC-7,4"-dioic acid	COOH	H	C_3H_6COOH	t
18	1",2"-dehydro-4",5"-bisnor-delta-1-THC-7,3"-dioic acid	COOH	H	C_3H_4COOH	+

*Rel.Ab. = Relative Abundance: +, 2+, 3+, 4+ indicate minor to major metabolite, quantification by radioactivity and GC. t = trace amount.

lite was found with a 6-hydroxy coupled with a 7-carboxy function nor were 6,7-dihyroxylated acidic metabolites detected, although these compounds have earlier been identified in animals (18). However, these latter metabolites may stillbe found in the more polar fractions, which were eluted from Sephadex LH-20 and have not been investigated so far. Neither ketones nor aldehydes from oxidized allylic hydroxyl groups were detected nor was any aromatization of the terpene ring noted as reported in the rhesus monkey (19).

Oxidation of the pentyl side chain is known to be a common metabolic pathway for THC in different animals (4,20). Our study shows that the side chain is easily oxidized also in man. All urinary metabolites but one showed a pentyl side chain hydroxylated or further oxidized to an acid or shortened. Oxidation occurred at all positions of the side chain from C-1" to C-4" with the C-3" position being mainly attacked. The side chain acids might be formed by initial hydroxylation followed by oxidation via a keto derivative to the acid. However, no such intermediate was detected in the urine of man but side-chain keto derivatives of cannabinoids have been reported (21,22). Another route of formation of side-chain acids could involve beta-oxidation. Metabolite 7 with a shortened hydroxylated side chain might be an intermediate of metabolite 15 derived from beta-oxidation of metabolite 17. The unsaturated metabolites 13 (tentative structure) and 18 could be formed by the activity of dehydrogenase enzymes on metabolites 12 and 16, respectively. Delta-1-THC-7-oic acids coupled with a carboxy function in the side chain have so far also been found in rabbit urine (15,16).

The remaining radioactivity in the urine was due to compounds more polar than the metabolites already identified. Whether these metabolites are conjugated metabolites and/or more oxygenated acidic metabolites remains to be clarified. Conjugates have earlier been identified in the urine of man (7). We were unable to identify the glucuronic acid conjugate of delta-1-THC-7-oic acid, which has been proposed to be a major urinary metabolite of THC in man (7). An explanation could be that the ester conjugate was hydrolysed from extraction at pH 12 and/or from being stored frozen before analysis (cf. 23).

In vitro metabolic studies on THC using the 10000 g supernatant of human livers indicated that side-chain oxidation of THC was of minor importance in man (24). Yet there are side-chain oxidized metabolites excreted in the urine of man. The discrepancy between *in vitro* and *in vivo* studies could be due to the fact that side-chain oxidation predominantly occurs by enzymes from tissues other than the liver. The complex *in vivo* metabolite pattern could also be due to enterohepatic circulation. Furthermore, one has to remember that the uri-

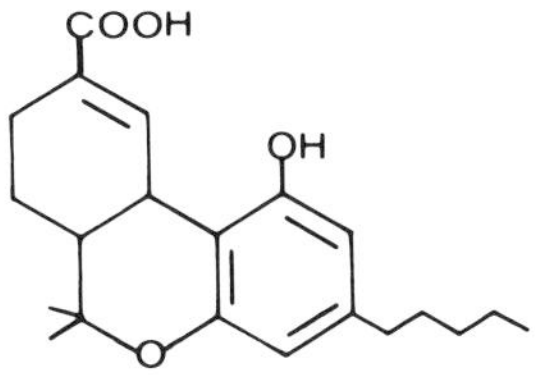

Δ^1-THC-7-oic acid

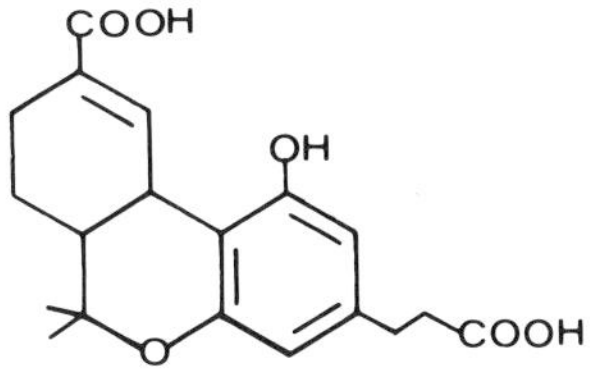

4'',5''-bisnor-Δ^1-7,3''-dioic acid

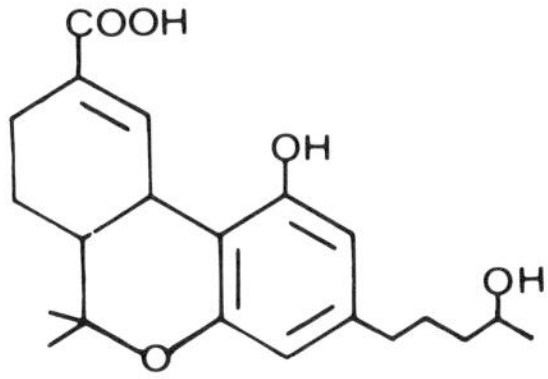

4''-hydroxy-Δ^1-THC-7-oic acid

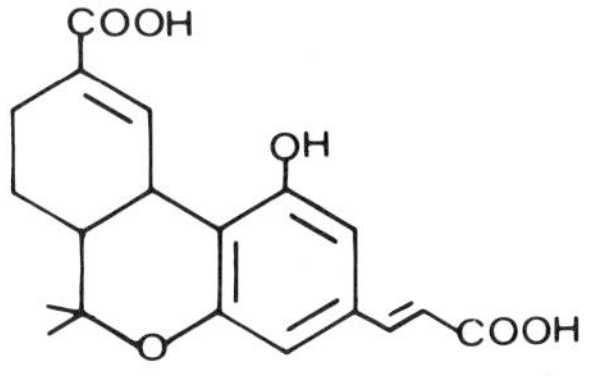

1'',2''-dehydro-4'',5''-bisnor-Δ^1-THC-7,3''-dioic acid

FIGURE 2. Structures of the four most abundant urinary metabolites of THC in man following oral administration.

nary metabolites hitherto identified account for less than 10% of the given dose. The main excretory route for THC in man is via the bile and the metabolic pattern of THC there might be quite different to that in the urine.

REFERENCES

1. Foltz, R. L., Fentiman, A. F., Leighty, E. G., Walter, J. L., Drewes, H. R., Schwartz, W. E., Page, T. F., and Truitt, E. B., Science 168:844 (1970).
2. Nilsson, I. M., Agurell, S., Nilsson, J. L. G., Ohlsson, A., and Sanberg, F., Science 168:1228 (1970).
3. Wall, M. E., Brine, D. R., Brine, G. A., Pitt, C. G., Freudentahl, R. I., and Christensen, H. D., J. Amer. Chem. Soc. 92:3466 (1970).
4. Mechoulam, R., and Edery, H., in "Marihuana: Chemistry Pharmacology, Metabolism and Clinical Effects" (R. Mechoulam, ed.), pp. 101-103. Academic Press, New York, 1973.
5. Levy, S., Yagen, B., and Mechoulam, R., Science 200:1391 (1978).
6. Pallante, S., Lyle, M. A., and Fenselau, C., Drug. Metab. Dispos. 6:389 (1978).

7. Williams, P. I., and Moffat, A. C., J. Pharm. Pharmacol. 32:445 (1980).
8. Leighty, E. G., Fentiman, A. F., and Foltz, R. L., Res. Commun. Chem. Pathol. Pharmacol. 14:13 (1976).
9. Yisak, W., Agurell, S., Lindgren, J.-E., and Widman, M., J. Pharm. Pharmacol. 30:462 (1978).
10. Wall, M. E., Brine, D. R., Pitt, C. G., and Perez-Reyes, M., J. Amer. Chem. Soc. 94:8579 (1972).
11. Wall, M. E., Brine, D. R., and Perez-Reyes, M., in "Pharmacology of Marihuana" (M. C. Braude and S. Szara, eds.), pp. 93-113. Raven Press, New York, 1976.
12. Kanter, S. L., and Hollister, L. E.
13. Halldin, M. M., Carlsson, S., Kanter, S. L., Widman, M., and Agurell, S., Arzeim.-Forsch./Drug. Res. 32:764 (1982).
14. Halldin, M. M., Andersson, L. K. R., Widman, M. and Hollister, L. E., Arzneim.-Forsch./Drug Res. 32:1135 (1982).
15. Nordqvist, M., Lindren, J.-E., and Agurell, S., J. Pharm. Pharmacol. 31:231 (1979).
16. Nordqvist, M., Agurell, S., Rydberg, M., Falk, L., and Ryman, T., J. Pharm. Pharmacol. 31:238 (1979).
17. Harvey, D. J., Biomed. Mass Spectrom. 8:579 (1981).
18. Harvey, D. J., Martin, B. R., and Paton, W. D. M., in "Mass Spectrometry in Drug Metabolism" (A. Frigero and E. Ghisalberti, eds.), pp. 403-428. Plenum Press, New York, 1977.
19. Ben-Zvi, Z., Berger, J. R., Burstein, S., Sehgal, P. K., and Varanelli, C., in "Pharmacology of Marihuana" (M. C. Braude and S. Szara, eds.), pp. 63-75. Raven Press, New York, 1976.
20. Mechoulam, R., in "Handbook of Experimental Pharmacology" (F. Hoffmeister and G. Stille, eds.), pp. 119-134. Springer Verlag, Berlin, 1981.
21. Yisak, W., Widman, M., and Agurell, S., J. Pharm. Pharmacol. 30:554 ((1978).
22. Harvey, D.J., and Paton, W. D. M., Res. Commun. Subst. Abuse 2:193 (1981).
23. Upton, R. A., Bushin, J. N., Williams, R. L., Holford, N. H. G., and Riegelman, S., J. Pharm. Sci. 69:1254 (1980).
24. Halldin, M. M., Widman, M., v. Bahr, C., Lindgren, J.-E., and Martin, B., Drug Metab. Dispos. 10:297 (1982).
25. Mechoulam, R., McCallum, N. K., and Burstein, S., Chem. Reviews 76:75 (1976).

SINGLE DOSE KINETICS OF CANNABIDIOL IN MAN[1]

A. Ohlsson,[2] J. E. Lindgren
S. Andersson, S. Agurell

Department of Pharmacology
Karolinska Institute
Stockholm, Sweden
and
Astra Lakemedel AB
Sodertalje, Sweden

H. Gillespie, L. E. Hollister[3]

Veterans Administration Medical Center
Palo Alto, California

I. INTRODUCTION

Cannabidiol (CBD) is one of the main constituents in most Cannabis preparations. CBD possesses no psychotomimetic activity in humans in contrast to the highly active delta-1-tetrahydrocannabinol (THC) the major compound in the plant (1-3). However, CBD has anticonvulsant properties in animals and possibly also in man (4,5), and, consequently, the potential of CBD as an antiepileptic drug is under investigation. Despite CBD being a main constituent of Cannabis preparations and an interest in the medical use of CBD, very few reports have been published concerning the kinetics of this cannabinoid (3,8). This report presents data on the single dose kinetics of CBD after smoking and intravenous administration.

---

[1]Supported by the Medical Research Council.
[2]Provided with a travel grant from the Swedish Academy of Pharmaceutical Sciences.
[3]Supported by the Veterans Administration Medical Center.

ISBN 0-12-044620-0

II. METHODS

A. Subjects

Five healthy young men volunteered to participate in this study. All had previous experience with marijuana ranging from infrequent to frequent use. All were in good physical and mental health and none were taking other psychoactive drugs. Prior to the trial, subjects were asked to abstain from cannabis for at least 72 hours and from alcohol for at least 24 hours.

B. Compounds

Deuterium-labeled CBD (CBD-d_2; Fig. 1) was administered to follow the plasma levels without disturbances from non-allowed smoking of cannabis during the experiment. The synthesis of CBD-d_2 as well as CBD-d_7 (see Fig. 1 for labeling), the latter was used as internal standard, have been described earlier (9). The unlabeled CBD in CBD-d_2 was 1.4% and in CBD-d_7 0.3%. The d_2-content in the internal standard was 0.4%. The chemical purity checked by gas chromatography was over 92%.

C. Doses and Routes of Administration

Deuterated CBD, <u>viz</u> CBD-d_2, was administered by an intravenous injection during 2 minutes of 20 mg.--a technique used

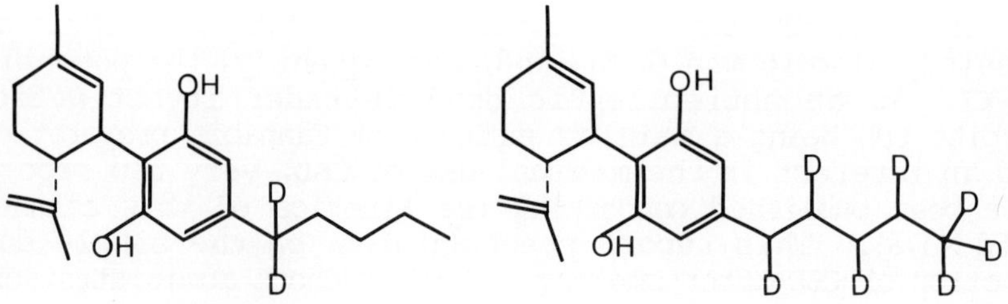

FIGURE 1. Structural formulas of deuterium labeled CBD, CBD-d_2, and CBD-d_7, the internal standard.

earlier for THC (10)--and by smoking marijuana placebo cigarettes (furnished by NIDA, Rockville, MD) spiked with 20 mg of the compound. The smoked dose was estimated by subtracting the remaining amount of CBD in the butt from the original amount in the cigarette (11). No exchange of deuterium atoms was observed after the smoking process. The two trials were performed in a randomized order with at least one week between the treatments.

D. Blood Sampling

Blood samples were drawn prior to the sessions and at 3, 6, 10, 15, 30, 60, 90, 120, 180 and 240 minutes after termination of smoking or intravenous injection. The samples were collected in heparinized glass tubes and immediately centrifuged. The plasma, usually 3 ml, was transferred to silanized glass vials and stored at $-20^{o}C$ until analysis.

E. Analytical Procedure

After addition of internal standard, the plasma samples were extracted with organic solvents and purified by liquid chromatography according to a method described earlier (8,9). The trimethylsilylated CBD extracts were submitted to the mass spectrometric quantification. The gas chromatographic-mass spectrometric procedure, using a LKB 2091-051 instrument, has been described previously (8). The base peaks $[M-68]^{+\cdot}$ in the mass spectra of the disilylated CBD analogues were selected for monitoring: m/z 392 for CBD-d_2 and 397 for CBD-d_7. The standard curves with a range of 0.04-10 ng/ml and 10-2000 ng/ml (Fig. 2) were prepared by mixing different dilutions from stock solutions.

F. Pharmacokinetic Analysis

The area under the plasma concentration versus time curve (AUC), for the time 0-240 minutes, were estimated using the trapezoidal rule. The systemic availability of CBD-d_2 after smoking was calculated by comparisons of the AUC with that obtained after intravenous injection.

III. RESULTS AND DISCUSSION

The single dose kinetics of deuterium labeled cannabidiol

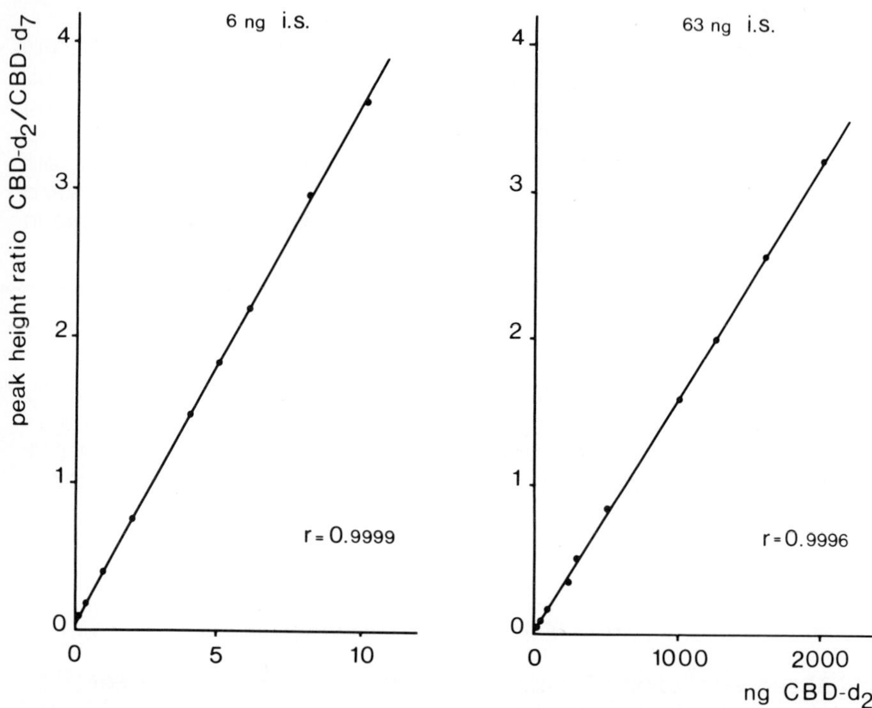

FIGURE 2. Standard curves for CBD-d_2, 0-10 ng/ml and 10-2000 ng/ml.

(CBD-d_2, Fig. 1) has been studied in man after intravenous injection of 20 mg and by smoking a placebo marijuana cigarette spiked with 20 mg CBD-d_2. The average dose smoked was estimated to 19.2 +/- 0.3 mg by subtracting the compound remaining in the butt from the original amount in the cigarette. The plasma levels were followed for four hours and the mean plasma levels for the five subjects are shown in Fig. 3. After both routes of administration a marked fall in the plasma levels occurred during the first fifteen minutes whereafter the levels declined smoothly. At three minutes the plasma levels were 684 +/- 240 (mean +/- S.D.) (range 356-972) ng/ml at fifteen minutes and had declined to 10.3 +/- 4.5 (range 3.4-15.5) ng/ml at four hours. These values, except for the earliest time points, are in good agreement with those determined in an earlier report (3), where plasma levels of 20 mg tritium labeled CBD was followed in man after intravenous infusion. Since a more rapid infusion time was used in the present study, higher initial plasma levels were obtained.

After smoking, a plasma curve with a very similar slope as the curve after intravenous administration was achieved. However, the plasma levels after smoking were lower 114 +/- 62

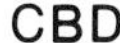

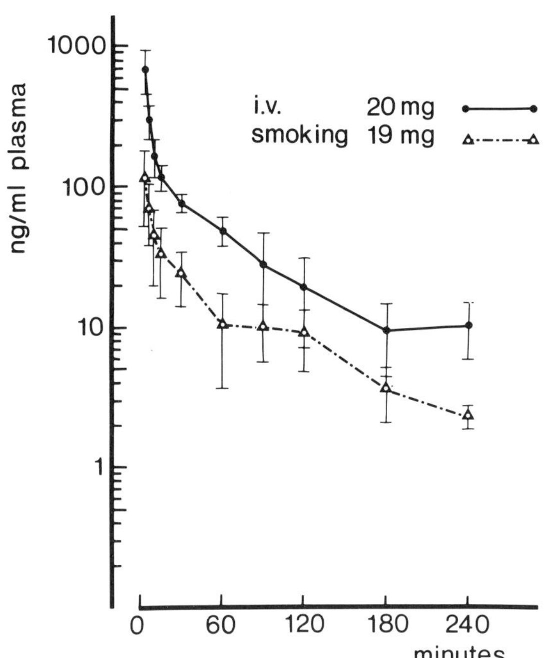

FIGURE 3. Mean plasma curves (mean +/- SD) of CBD-d_2 after intravenous administration and smoking in five healthy users.

(range 42-191) at three minutes, 33 +/- 17 (range 12-51) at fifteen minutes and 2.3 +/- 0.05 (range 1.9-2.8) ng/ml at four hours.

Both after smoking and infusion the shape of the mean plasma curves of CBD-d_2 very much resemble those obtained after THC administration in a previous study with a similar experimental design (10). However, doses given were lower for THC and therefore the actual plasma levels were lower.

The interindividual variations in plasma levels were relatively small, both after smoking and infusion. A greater difference in the individual plasma levels after smoking could perhaps have been expected since the subjects smoked in their usual fashion. Rather small interindividual differences after smoking THC have also been noted (10).

The AUC and estimated availability in the five subjects are listed in Table I. The subjects smoked very similar amounts, range 18.8-19.4 mg of CBD-d_2, a dose that was very close to the injected dose of 20 mg. The estimated systemic availability was 31 +/- 13 (range 10-42) % of CBD-d_2 after

TABLE I. Kinetic Parameters of CBD-d_2 Disposition in Man after Intravenous Administration (20 mg) and Smoking

Subject	Intravenous AUC[a]	Smoking: Estimated Amount Smoked (mg)	Smoking: AUC[a]	Smoking: Estimated Systemic Availability (%)
PF	9.13	19.4	3.69	42
BM	10.54	19.3	3.17	31
IP	14.78	19.3	1.45	10
RP	11.44	18.8	3.14	29
IW	12.93	19.0	4.99	41
Mean[b]	11.76 (2.18)	19.2 (0.3)	3.29 (1.27)	31 (13)

[a]AUC = $\frac{AUC_{1-240}}{(ng/ml) \times min} \times 10^{-3}$

[b]Mean (+/- S.D.).

smoking. The main loss of CBD is probably due to pyrolysis and disappearance of CBD through the side-stream smoke during the smoking process.

The estimated systemic availability after smoking an average of 13.0 mg THC was 18 +/- 6 (range 7-25) % in a group of subjects with a comparable use of cannabis as the presently investigated group. If that possible difference in availability of the cannabinoids is due to differences in the transfer of the cannabinoids during the smoking process, or due to metabolic or kinetic factors is not yet known.

REFERENCES

1. Hollister, L. E., Experientia, 29:825-826 (1973).
2. Perez-Reyes, M., Timmons, M. C., David, K. H., and Wall, M. E., Experentia, 29:1368-1369 (1973).
3. Wall, M. E., Brine, D. R., and Perez-Reyes, M., in "The Pharmacology of Marihuana" (M. C. Braude and S. Szara, eds.), pp. 93-113. Raven Press, New York, 1976.
4. Karler, R., and Turkanis, S. A., in "The Therapeutic Potential of Marihuana" (S. Cohen and R. C. Stillman, eds.), pp. 383-397. Plenum Press, New York, 1976.

5. Karler, R., and Turkanis, S. A., in "Marihuana: Biological Effects" (G. G. Nahas and W. D. M. Paton, eds.), pp. 619-641. Pergamon Press, New York, 1979.
6. Cunha, J. M., Carlini, E. A., Pereira, A. E., Ramos, O. L., Pimentel, C., Gagliardi, R., Sanvito, W. L., Zander, N., and Mechoulam, R., Pharmacology 21:175-185 (1980).
7. Carlini, E. A., and Cunha, J. M., J. Clin. Pharmacol. 21:417S-427S (1981).
8. Agurell, S., Carlsson, S., Lindgren, J. E., Ohlsson, A., Gillespie, H., and Hollister, L. E., Experentia 37:1090-1091 (1981).
9. Ohlsson, A., Lindgren, J. E., Leander, K., and Agurell, S., in "Cannabinoid Assay in Humans" (R. E. Willette, ed.), pp. 48-63. NIDA Research Monographs Series 7, U. S. Government Printing Office, Washington, D.C., 1976.
10. Ohlsson, A., Lindgren, J. E., Wahlen, A., Agurell, S., Hollister, L. E., and Gillespie, H. K., Clin. Pharmacol Ther. 28:409-416 (1980).
11. Agurell, S., and Leander, K., Acta. Pharm. Suec. 8:391-402 (1971).

THE PHARMACOKINETICS OF DELTA-9-TETRAHYDROCANNABINOL IN MAN AFTER SIMULTANEOUS INTRAVENOUS AND ORAL ADMINISTRATION*

Brian M. Sadler
Monroe E. Wall

Research Triangle Institute
Research Triangle Park, North Carolina

Mario Perez-Reyes

University of North Carolina
Chapel Hill, North Carolina

I. INTRODUCTION

Cannabinoid research recently has been branched into a number of clinically important areas. Mechoulam cited several potential clinical applications for delta-9-tetrahydrocannabinol (THC) and related cannabinoids, including the treatment of glaucoma, nausea, ulcers, and hypertension (1). As a result the metabolism and disposition of THC have been studied to a great degree (2,3).

One piece of important information which has been lacking has been an accurate measure of the bioavailability of orally administered THC. Ohlsson et al. reported bioavailability of THC at 0.06, but their study terminated in six hours and used a chocolate cookie as a vehicle (4). Wall et al. reported values of 0.11 and 0.19 for female and male subjects, respectively, using sesame oil capsules, but their protocol prohibited the simultaneous administration of oral and intravenous doses of the same subjects.

---

*Supported by NIDA grant DA-02424.

ISBN 0-12-044620-0

This study is an effort to assess the bioavailability of THC in male subjects after simultaneous administration of a tracer intravenous (i.v.) dose and a 20 mg oral dose.

II. MATERIALS AND METHODS

A. Subjects

Six, healthy, male paid volunteers of average height and weight and eating normal diets were used in this study. All had used marijuana in a recreational manner.

B. Chemicals and Materials

[^{3}H]-delta-9-THC, THC, and various standard cannabinoids were obtained from the National Institute on Drug Abuse (NIDA). Precoated thin layer chromatography (TLC) plates, 20 x 20 cm, silica gel 60F-245 (E. Merck, Dramstadt, West Germany) were used for all TLC. Scintillation counting was performed using Triton X-100:toluene:Omniflor (1 l.:2 l.:18 g). Radioimmunoassay (RIA) kits for THC and 9-COOH-11-nor-delta-9-THC were obtained through NIDA from Dr. C. E. Cook (Research Triangle Institute, Research Triangle Park, NC).

C. Drug Administration

Each subject was given a single-bolus intravenous injection of [^{3}H]-delta-9-THC (0.141 mg/123 mcCi) dispersed in human serum albumin (5) and a simultaneous oral dose of 19.98 mg THC dissolved in sesame oil (0.5 ml) and administered in a gelatin capsule.

D. Sample Collection

Blood samples were drawn by means of an indwelling venous catheter for the first 4 hours and by independent venipuncture for all other periods. Samples were taken from all subjects for 24 hours. Samples from three subjects were collected for 96 hours. Samples from three subjects were collected for 96 hours. Urine samples were obtained for all subjects for 24 hrs while feces was collected only for the three subjects studied for 96 hours.

E. Analytical Procedure

The procedure described by Wall et al. (3), as modified in Wall et al. (6), was used for quantitation of tritiated cannabinoids. Briefly, the system involves solvent extraction followed by TLC and scintillation spectrophotometry. Non-radiolabeled THC and 9-COOH-11-nor-delta-9-THC were assayed by RIA according to published procedures (7,8). Gas chromatography/mass spectrometry (GC/MS) was used to quantitate the 11-OH-metabolite of THC in plasma (9).

F. Pharmacokinetics

All nonlinear curve fitting was done using NONLIN (10). Plasma concentrations of $[^3H]$-delta-9-THC were weighted as $1/C^2$ and fitted with a biexponential function. The cumulative urinary excretion curves (A_e vs. time) for total $[^3H]$-cannabinoids and $[^3H]$-9-COOH-11-nor-delta-9-THC were fitted with a monoexponential accumulation function. The first derivative of the fitted curve was evaluated at at least six time points for which there were corresponding plasma values (C_i) for the species, respectively, and the renal clearances calculated as the mean of $(dA_e/dt)_i/C_i$. AUC (0-t) for $[^3H]$-delta-9-THC and THC were calculated by use of the log-trapezoidal rule. AUC (t-infinity) was calculated by use of the weighted mean estimate of lambda_z (or beta) and the last observed plasma concentration. AUC (0-infinity) was adjusted to account for the area contributed by any THC present at t = 0. Standard formula were used for all pharmacokinetic calculations (11).

III. RESULTS

The concentrations of $[^3H]$-delta-9-THC and its major metabolites in plasma are present in Table I. The concentration of $[^3H]$-delta-9-THC in plasma is plotted in Figure 1 along with the fitted biexponental curve. A mean elimination phase half-life of 50 hours was observed. The mean terminal phase volume of distribution (V_z) was 578 +/- 76 (mean +/- S.E.M.) liters. The total body clearance of $[^3H]$-delta-9-THC from plasma (CL) was 135 +/- 13 ml/min.

The concentrations of THC, 9-COOH-11-nor-delta-9-THC, and 11-OH-delta-9-THC in plasma as determined by RIA and GC/MS are presented in Table II. The observed and fitted concentration of THC in plasma is plotted in Figure 2. The systemic bioavailability (f) of orally administered THC was 0.13 +/- 0.02.

TABLE I. [^{3}H]-Delta-9-THC and Metabolites Found in Human Plasma after Intravenous Administration of 0.141 mg [^{3}H]-delta-9-THC and Oral Administration of 19.98 mg THC

	ng/ml								
				Acids			Neutrals		
Time	Total Cannabinoids	Total Free	Total Conjunction	Total Acid	Polar	11-COOH	Total Neutrals	11-OH	Δ^9-THC
5 min	6.4 ± 2.1	6.1 ± 2.0	0.24 ± 0.1	0.84 ± 0.3	0.35 ± 0.2	0.39 ± 0.2	5.3 ± 2.1	0.36 ± 0.2	4.6 ± 1.9
10	5.1 ± 1.4	4.8 ± 1.3	0.35 ± 0.2	2.3 ± 0.5	1.0 ± 0.5	0.96 ± 0.6	2.5 ± 1.1	0.41 ± 0.3	1.8 ± 0.8
20	4.6 ± 1.0	4.2 ± 1.0	0.36 ± 0.1	2.6 ± 0.5	1.4 ± 0.5	0.83 ± 0.4	1.6 ± 0.5	0.21 ± 0.1	1.3 ± 0.5
30	4.3 ± 0.8	4.0 ± 0.9	0.30 ± 0.2	2.8 ± 0.5	1.0 ± 0.5	1.31 ± 0.7	1.3 ± 0.5	0.17 ± 0.05	0.97 ± 0.4
60	3.8 ± 0.5	3.3 ± 0.5	0.36 ± 0.2	2.4 ± 0.2	0.83 ± 0.4	1.26 ± 0.7	0.96 ± 0.4	0.11 ± 0.05	0.76 ± 0.3
90	3.5 ± 0.5	3.1 ± 0.6	0.37 ± 0.3	2.4 ± 0.4	1.1 ± 0.2	0.91 ± 0.5	0.75 ± 0.4	0.10 ± 0.06	0.58 ± 0.3
120	3.3 ± 0.5	2.9 ± 0.5	0.41 ± 0.2	2.2 ± 0.3	1.2 ± 0.1	0.61 ± 0.2	0.67 ± 0.4	0.07 ± 0.02	0.52 ± 0.3
150 a	3.0 ± 0.3	2.7 ± 0.2	0.35 ± 0.1	2.2 ± 0.3	1.0 ± 0.08	0.72 ± 0.2	0.45 ± 0.09	0.06 ± 0.02	0.34 ± 0.1
180	3.1 ± 0.5	2.8 ± 0.6	0.27 ± 0.1	2.3 ± 0.4	0.97 ± 0.3	0.87 ± 0.3	0.52 ± 0.3	0.06 ± 0.02	0.40 ± 0.3
4 hr	2.7 ± 0.5	2.5 ± 0.5	0.18 ± 0.1	2.1 ± 0.4	0.62 ± 0.5	1.1 ± 0.6	0.41 ± 0.2	0.05 ± 0.02	0.31 ± 0.1
6	2.3 ± 0.4	2.1 ± 0.3	0.23 ± 0.2	1.7 ± 0.3	0.55 ± 0.3	0.91 ± 0.5	0.36 ± 0.1	0.04 ± 0.01	0.28 ± 0.1
8	2.0 ± 0.4	1.8 ± 0.3	0.23 ± 0.2	1.5 ± 0.3	0.58 ± 0.3	0.57 ± 0.4	0.30 ± 0.09	0.03 ± 0.01	0.24 ± 0.1
11	1.7 ± 0.2	1.5 ± 0.2	0.16 ± 0.1	1.2 ± 0.2	0.48 ± 0.3	0.55 ± 0.3	0.33 ± 0.2	0.03 ± 0.01	0.27 ± 0.2
24	1.1 ± 0.2	1.0 ± 0.2	0.12 ± 0.05	0.84 ± 0.1	0.34 ± 0.2	0.30 ± 0.1	0.19 ± 0.07	0.02 ± 0.01	0.14 ± 0.1
30 b	0.81 ± 0.04	0.67 ± 0.04	0.14 ± 0.03	0.49 ± 0.03	[c]0.21 ± 0.1	[c]0.17 ± 0.1	0.18 ± 0.06	0.02 ± 0.01	0.15 ± 0.04
48 b	0.61 ± 0.05	0.49 ± 0.06	0.12 ± 0.06	0.38 ± 0.06	0.11 ± 0.04	0.20 ± 0.1	0.11 ± 0.00	0.01 ± 0.01	0.10 ± 0.00
72 b	0.41 ± 0.06	0.30 ± 0.05	0.11 ± 0.02	0.18 ± 0.05	0.06 ± 0.01	0.070 ± 0.01	0.12 ± 0.02	0.01 ± 0.01	0.11 ± 0.01
96 b	0.31 ± 0.06	0.22 ± 0.08	0.08 ± 0.03	0.15 ± 0.08	0.04 ± 0.01	0.073 ± 0.07	0.07 ± 0.00	trace	0.062 ± 0.00

[a]Mean of 5 subjects
[b]Mean of 3 subjects
[c]Mean of 2 subjects

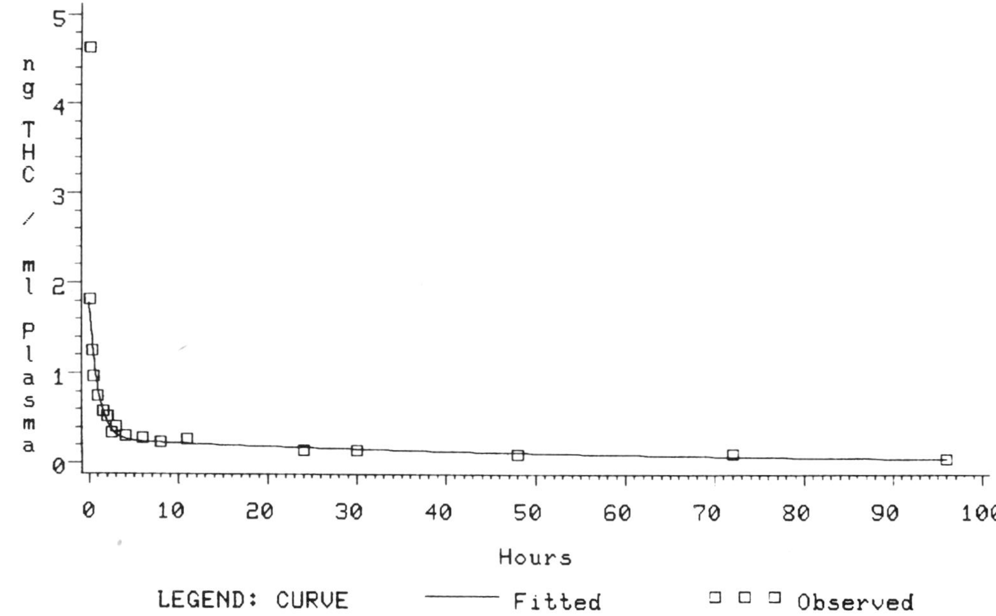

FIGURE 1. $[^3H]$-delta-9-THC (0.141 mg) was administered i.v. simultaneously with an oral dose of non-radiolabeled THC (19.98 mg) to six male subjects. The observed concentrations of tritiated THC in the plasma were weighed as $1/C^2$ and fitted with a biexponential function using NONLIN. The fitted (solid line) and observed (open squares) curves are presented above.

The cumulative excretion of radiolabeled cannabinoids in urine and feces is presented in Tables III and IV, respectively. After 72 hours 21 +/- 1% and 40 +/- 2% of the administered radiolabel was accounted for in urine and feces, respectively. Cumulative urinary excretion of total tritiated cannabinoids and tritiated 9-COOH-11-nor-delta-9-THC were fitted with an exponential accumulation function using NONLIN.

TABLE II. THC, 11-Nor-9-carboxy- and 11-Hydroxy-delta-9-THC in Human Plasma (see text for doses)

IV Dose 0.141 mg $[^3H]$-Δ^9-THC

Oral Dose 19.98 mg Δ^9-THC

	ng/ml					
	Δ^9-THC		11-Nor-9-COOH-Δ^9-THC		11-OH-Δ^9-THC	
Time	(n)		(n)		(n)	
0'	(6)	2.8 ± 1.5	(6)	13.7 ± 12.3		
5'	(6)	7.3 ± 2.3	(6)	17.4 ± 12.4		
10'	(6)	4.0 ± 1.5	(6)	17.6 ± 13.7		
20'	(6)	3.4 ± 1.8	(6)	17.3 ± 13.5		
30'	(6)	5.1 ± 3.1	(6)	20.9 ± 18.4	(5)	1.5 ± 1.1
60'	(6)	19.4 ± 13.2	(6)	101.8 ± 74.5	(5)	7.8 ± 1.3
90'	(6)	20.7 ± 4.3	(6)	206.9 ± 79.1	(6)	9.5 ± 2.1
120'	(6)	21.2 _ 5.3	(6)	223.8 ± 23.6	(5)	8.4 ± 2.1
150'	(5)	17.6 ± 6.1	(5)	231.0 ± 58.1	(5)	6.9 ± 2.4
180'	(6)	14.4 ± 2.9	(6)	214.7 ± 71.4	(6)	5.2 ± 1.5
4h	(6)	9.7 ± 1.5	(6)	136.1 ± 30.8	(5)	3.2 ± 0.9
6h	(6)	8.5 ± 3.6	(6)	103.9 ± 27.3	(6)	2.3 ± 0.8
8h	(6)	10.0 ± 6.7	(6)	97.6 ± 32.8	(5)	2.0 ± 1.1
11h	(6)	6.0 ± 1.2	(6)	82.0 ± 23.8	(5)	1.4 ± 0.5
24h	(6)	4.4 ± 1.5	(6)	50.6 ± 25.8		
30h	(3)	3.6 ± 0.4	(3)	25.1 ± 9.7		
48h	(3)	2.6 + 0.4	(3)	17.6 ± 4.2		
72h	(3)	2.3 ± 0.5	(3)	9.2 ± 3.4		
96h	(3)	2.3 ± 0.7	(3)	7.1 ± 4.0		

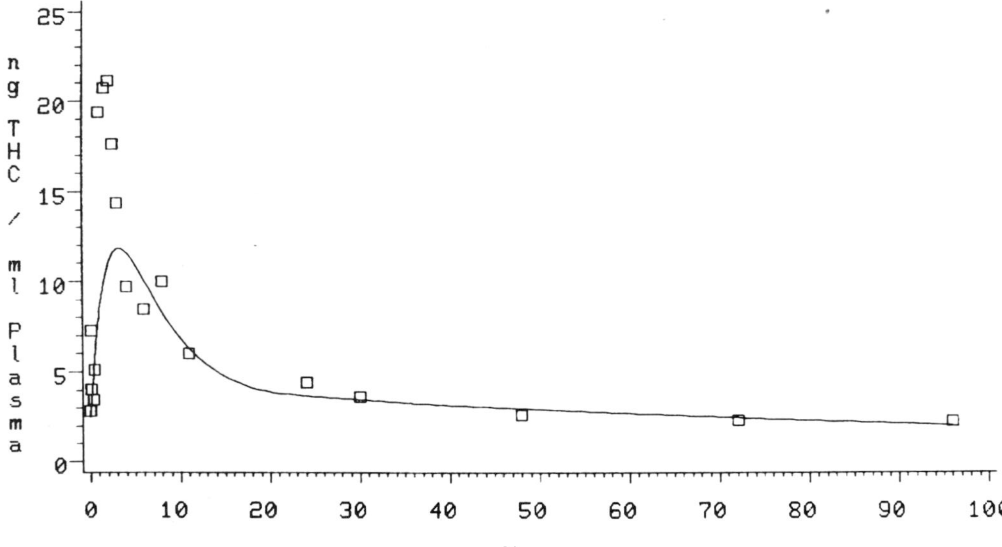

FIGURE 2. THC (19.98 mg) was administered orally with a simultaneous dose of tritiated THC (0.141 mg, i.v.) to six male subjects. RIA was used to determine the plasma concentrations of THC, which were weighted as $1/C^2$ and fitted with a triexponential function using NONLIN. The fitted (solid line) and observed (open squares) curves are presented above.

TABLE III. [^{3}H]-Delta-9-THC and Metabolites Found in Human Urine after Intravenous Administration of 0.141 mg [^{3}H]-delta-9-THC and Oral Administration of 19.98 mg THC Expressed in Cummulative % Dose

			Free Acids			Free Neutrals		
Sample (n)	Total Cannabinoids	Total Free	Total Acids	Polar Acids	11-COOH-Δ^9-THC	Total Neutrals	11-OH-Δ^9-THC	Δ^9-THC
0-4h (5)	4.5 ± 2.2	3.3 ± 1.9	3.3 ± 1.8	1.8 ± 0.8	0.9 ± 0.8	0.05 ± .03	0.02 ± .01	.006 ± .001
6-11h (3)	5.7 ± 0.8	3.9 ± 0.4	3.8 ± 0.3	1.8 ± 0.4	1.2 ± 0.4	0.07 ± .02	0.02 ± .01	.005 ± .003
24h (4)	12.4 ± 2.6	8.7 ± 1.6	8.6 ± 1.6	3.4 ± 0.8	3.4 ± 0.8	0.12 ± .02	0.05 ± .02	.01 ± .008
30h (2)	16.6 ± 0.8	11.4 ± 0.3	11.2 ± 0.2	4.3 ± 0.2	5.1 ± 0.6	0.14 ± .01	0.06 ± .01	.02 ± .008
48h (2)	19.2 ± 1.0	13.0 ± 0.5	12.9 ± 0.5	4.8 ± 0.4	5.6 ± 0.6	0.16 ± .02	0.07 ± .01	.02 ± .009
72h (2)	21.3 ± 1.6	14.5 ± 1.0	14.4 ± 1.0	5.2 ± 0.6	6.4 ± 0.4	0.17 ± .03	0.07 ± .02	.03 ± .01
96h (2)	22.3 ± 2.2	15.2 ± 1.4	15.1 ± 1.3	5.4 ± 0.7	6.7 ± 0.3	0.18 ± .04	0.08 ± .02	.03 ± .01

			Cleaved Acids			Cleaved Neutrals		
Sample (n)	Total Conjugated	Total Cleaved	Total Acids	Polar Acids	11-COOH-Δ^9-THC	Total Neutrals	11-OH-Δ^9-THC	Δ^9-THC
0-4h (5)	1.2 ± 0.7	0.7 ± 0.4	0.7 ± 0.4	0.3 ± 0.2	0.11 ± .06	0.05 ± .03	.01 ± .01	.007 ± .000
6-11h (3)	1.8 ± 0.5	1.1 ± 0.4	1.0 ± 0.4	0.4 ± 0.2	0.24 ± .08	0.07 ± .03	.02 ± .01	.01 ± .008
24h (4)	3.7 ± 1.0	2.2 ± 0.7	2.1 ± 0.7	0.8 ± 0.3	0.41 ± .04	0.12 ± .03	.04 ± .01	.03 ± .004
30h (2)	5.2 ± 0.5	3.0 ± 0.7	3.0 ± 0.5	1.1 ± 0.5	0.46 ± .03	0.17 ± .01	.05 ± .01	.02 ± .007
48h (2)	6.2 ± 0.4	3.5 ± 0.7	3.4 ± 0.4	1.3 ± 0.5	0.54 ± .08	0.19 ± .01	.06 ± .01	.02 ± .01
72h (2)	6.8 ± 0.6	3.9 ± 0.8	3.8 ± 0.5	1.4 ± 0.5	0.62 ± .09	0.21 ± .02	.06 ± .01	.03 ± .01
96h (2)	7.1 ± 0.7	4.0 ± 0.9	4.0 ± 0.5	1.4 ± 0.6	0.64 ± .08	0.22 ± .02	.07 ± .01	.03 ± .01

TABLE IV. [^{3}H]-Delta-9-THC and Metabolites Found in Human Feces after Intravenous Administration of 0.141 mg [^{3}H]-delta-9-THC and Oral Administration of 19.98 mg THC Expressed as Cummulative % Dose

(n)		Total Cannabinoids	Fecal Residue	Methanol Extract		
				Total Methanol Extract Cannab.	Total Free	Total Conjugates
(1)	8h	0.06	0.006	0.05	0.05	0.004
(1)	24h	11.6	1.2	10.4	10.0	0.4 ± 0.3
(2)	48h	21.3 ± 15.4	2.8 ± 1.6	18.5 ± 13.9	17.7 ± 13.2	0.9 ± 0.7
(2)	72h	39.6 ± 2.7	6.5 ± 1.4	33.1 ± 4.1	31.0 ± 4.5	2.1
(1)	96h	45.8	6.3	39.5	37.6	2.0

(n)		Methanol Extract					
		Acids			Neutrals		
		Total Acids	Polar Acids	11-COOH-Δ^9-THC	Total Neutrals	11-OH-Δ^9-THC	Δ^9-THC
(1)	8h	0.03	0.004	0.02	0.01	0.006	0.005
(1)	24h	5.5	1.5	2.5	4.5	3.1	0.9
(2)	48h	10.3 ± 7.8	2.9 ± 2.1	5.0 ± 3.5	7.3 ± 5.4	4.9 ± 3.9	1.8 ± 0.8
(2)	72h	19.5 ± 2.2	5.2 ± 1.0	10.1 ± 0.6	11.5 ± 2.3	7.3 ± 2.3	3.1 ± 0.3
(1)	96h	23.7	6.5	12.2	13.9	9.4	3.0

The observed and fitted curves are presented in Figure 3. The renal clearances of total tritiated cannabinoid and [^{3}H]-9-COOH-11-nor-delta-9-THC were calculated by dividing the first derivative of the fitted accumulation curves by corresponding concentrations in the plasma. The renal clearances were 7.9 +/- 0.3 ml/min and 11.1 +/- 0.8 ml/min for total cannabinoids and 9-COOH-11-nor-delta-9-THC, respectively.

IV. DISCUSSION

The observed concentrations of cannabinoids in various biological samples in this experiment are in general consistent with the previous work of Wall et al (6). The elimination half-life reported here (50 hours) is longer than that reported by Wall et al (6). This may be accounted for by the fact that THC with a higher specific activity was used in the present study and more accurate estimates of the concentrations of THC at 72 and 96 hours were obtained.

Plasma samples taken before dosing revealed the presence of small amounts of THC in the plasma. Subjects were asked to refrain from the recreational use of marijuana for at least two days prior to the start of the experiment. The AUC (0-infinity) was corrected for the levels of THC at zero time by subtracting C_0/beta from the AUC for each subject.

The contribution of the present work is that for the first time the systemic bioavailability of orally administered THC was assessed after simultaneous oral and IV administration of the drug. Simultaneous use of two routes of administration appeared to have no significant effect on the pharmacokinetic parameters of either when used alone. The relatively low bioavailability (f = 0.13) is likely due to a significant first pass effect in the liver since previously reported values for oral absorption of THC are over 90% (6,12). This value for the bioavailability of THC is higher than that reported by Ohlsson et al. (4) and is probably due to the difference in the choice of oral vehicles. Sesame oil appears to be the more effective vehicle.

ACKNOWLEDGMENTS

The authors express their thanks to Carolyn Foust and Elizabeth Strawn for their technical assistance.

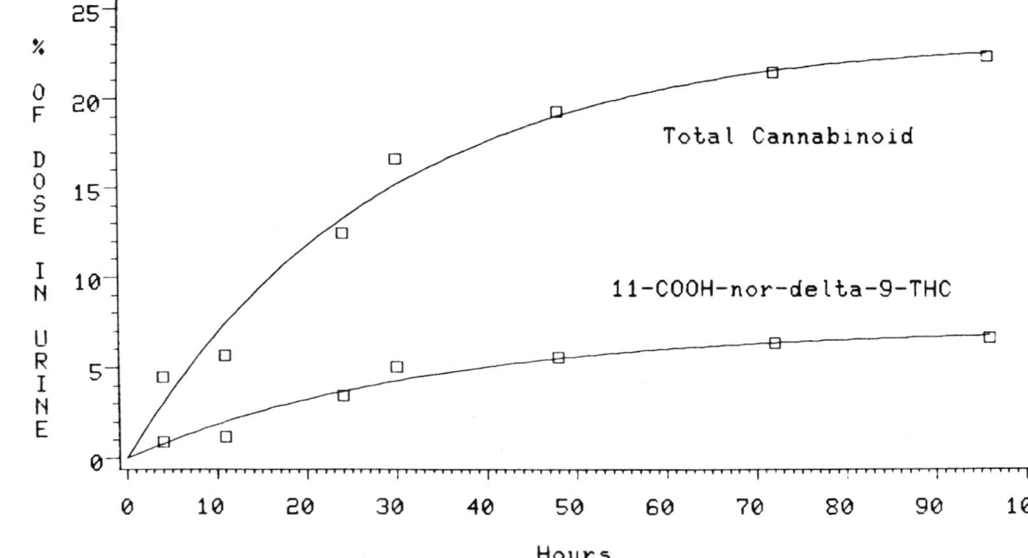

FIGURE 3. Drug was administered as in Fig. 2. The cummulative excretion of radiolabel and of [^{3}H]-11-COOH-delta-9-THC was fitted with a monoexponentail accumulation function using NONLIN. The fitted (solid line) and observed (open squares) curves are presented above.

REFERENCES

1. Mechoulam, R., J. Clin. Pharmacol. 21:23 (1981).
2. Lemberger, L., and Rubin, A., Life Sci. 17:1637 (1975).
3. Wall, M. E., Brine, D. R., and Perez-Reyes, M., The metabolism of cannabinoids in man, in "Pharmacology of Marihuana" (M. C. Braude and S. Szara, eds.), p. 93. Raven Press, New York, 1976.
4. Ohlsson, A., Lindgren, J. E., Wahlen, A., Agurell, S., Hollister, L. E., and Gillespie, B. A., Clin. Pharmacol. Ther. 28:409 (1980).
5. Perez-Reyes, M., Timmons, M. C., Lipton, M. A., Davis, K. H., and Wall, M. E., Science 177:633 (1972).
6. Wall, M. E., Sadler, B. M., Brine, D. R., Taylor, H., and Perez-Reyes, M., Metabolism, disposition and pharmacokinetics of delta-9-tetrahydrocannabinol in male and female subjects, submitted to Clin. Pharmacol. Therap. 1982.
7. Cook, C. E., Schindler, V. H., Tallent, C. R., Chin, K. M., and Pitt, C. G., Radioimmunoassay for cannabinoids, in "Cannabinoid Assays in Biological Fluids" (R. L. Hawks, ed.), NIDA Research Monograph No. 42, U.S. Government Printing Office, Washington, D. C., 1982.
8. Cook, C. E., Schindler, V. H., Tallent, C. R., Seltzman, H. H., and Pitt, C. G., Fed. Proc. 40:278, Abstr. 245 (1981).
9. Wall, M. E., Brine, D. R.,Bursey, J. T., and Rosenthal, D., Detection and quantitation of tetrahydrocannabinol and its metabolites, in "Cannabinoid Assays in Humans" (R. E. Willette, ed.), p. 197. NIDA Research Monograph No. 7, U.S. Government Printing Office, Washington, D. C., 1976.
10. Metzler, C. M., Elfring, G. L., and McEwen, A. J., "A Users Manual for NONLIN and Associated Programs". The Upjohn Company, Kalamazoo, MI, revised edition, 1976.
11. Allen, L., Kimura, K., MacKichan, J., and Ritschel, W. A., (eds.), "Manual of Symbols, Equations & Definitions in Pharmacokinetics". Committee for Pharmacokinetic Nomenclature of the American College of Clinical Pharmacology, Philadelphia, PA 1982.
12. Lemberger, L., Axelrod, J., Kopin, J. J., Ann. N. Y. Acad. Sci. 191:142 (1971).

MARIJUANA: ABSORPTION OF DELTA-1-TETRAHYDROCANNABINOL BY SMOKING. A PRELIMINARY STUDY

S. Agurell

Department of Pharmacology
Karolinska Institute
Stockholm, Sweden

and

Astra Lakemedel AB
Sodertalje, Sweden

K. Leander

Department of Organic Chemistry
University of Stockholm
Stockholm, Sweden

M. Asberg

Department of Psychiatry
Karolinska Hospital
Stockholm, Sweden

I. INTRODUCTION

In another paper (1) we have reviewed the systemic availability of delta-1-tetrahydrocannabinol (THC) by smoking. It was found -- although interindividual variations were large, in fact 10-fold -- that heavy users of marijuana had significantly higher systemic availability (bioavailability) of THC than light users (mean values: 23-27% vs. 10-14%). We now wish to report some previously unpublished material, which albeit limited in size, may suggest a possible reason why

ISBN 0-12-044620-0

heavy users smoke more efficiently than light users as judged from the THC plasma concentrations after smoking equal amounts of THC (1).

II. METHODS

A marijuana preparation containing mainly leaf material (4.0% THC) was strained through a sieve (3 mm mesh size). Known amounts (450-500 mg) of the material were rolled into "joint"- type cigarettes using cigarette papers.

Two groups of volunteers were used: 1. Experienced cannabis smokers, 2. Regular tobacco cigarette smokers

TABLE I. Amount of THC Absorbed by Marijuana Cigarette Smokers From Smoking 1.00 g of Marijuana

	Amount of THC (mg)		
Subject	Transferred	Exhaled During Smoking	Absorbed - by Difference
Smoked as marijuana cigarette:			
I Q	10.9	1.7	9.2 (84%)
AA	9.3	1.5	7.8 (84%)
T C	6.2	0.6	5.6 (90%)
T L	9.5	0.3	9.2 (97%)
I Q	10.9	1.3	9.6 (88%)
T L	9.1	2.7	7.4 (81%)
Average:	9.3	1.4	8.1 (87 +/- 6% s.d.)
Smoked as tobacco cigarette:			
I Q	10.9	5.1	5.8 (53%)
A A	9.4	6.6	3.2 (34%)
T L	9.5	5.6	4.9 (52%)
I Q	10.9	6.9	4.0 (37%)
Average:	10.2	6.1	4.5 (44 +/- 10% s.d.)

A. Transfer Experiment

Seven male, experienced cannabis smokers and three male, regular tobacco smokers participated in this experiment. Each subject smoked the full cigarette up to a mark, which left a half inch butt, in 10-15 puffs using a Cambridge glass fibre filter (2). The Cambridge filter is commonly used to determine the amount of tar in tobacco cigarettes. THC and other cannabinoids were collected on the glass fibre dish. Cannabinoids were eluted from the filter with methanol and the amount of THC quantitated by gas chromatography (2).

B. Absorption Experiment

Only experienced cannabis smokers (n = 4) participated in this experiment. Each subject was first allowed to smoke a marijuana cigarette connected to a Cambridge filter to determine the transfer of THC as described above. Then, he smoked another cigarette of the same weight without the filter during the inhalation phase but exhaling through a Cambridge filter. This allowed a rough estimate of the THC not absorbed in the respiratory tract. Thus, the THC absorbed (Table I) was calculated as the difference between the amount of THC trapped in the filter connected to the first cigarette and the THC being exhaled from the second cigarette.

The study was approved by the Ethics Committee of the Karolinska Institute and the National Board of Health.

III. RESULTS AND DISCUSSION

The transfer experiment was designed to reveal if there were any marked differences in the amount of THC carried by the main stream smoke if the marijuana cigarette was smoked as a marijuana cigarette (with deep inhalations and retention of "smoke" for a few seconds) or as a tobacco cigarette (with superficial inhalations).

As shown in Table II, the experienced marijuana smokers using deep inhalations did not achieve significantly higher transfer of THC with the main stream smoke than the regular tobacco smokers.

The absorption of THC during the smoking process was estimated as described under Methods. These subjects were all experienced marijuana smokers as well as tobacco smokers. They were asked to smoke the marijuana cigarette either as a marijuana cigarette or as a regular tobacco cigarette. The material is quite limited (Table I) but suggests that over 80%

TABLE I. Amount of THC in Smoke Condensate Obtained by Smoking 1.00 g of Marijuana Cigarette Containing 4.0% THC

	Subject*	THC (mg)
Smoked as marijuana cigarette	L A	8.6
	T C	6.2
	B T	7.1
	I Q	10.9
	A A	9.3
	I Q	11.0
	A A	9.6
	T L	9.5
	C K	11.3
	I Q	10.2
Average (+/- S.D.):		9.4 (1.7)
Smoked as tobacco cigarette	I Q	10.3
	A A	9.6
	I L	6.8
	M I	8.1
	L A	9.1
Average (+/- S.D.):		8.8 (1.4)

*Note that some subjects participated in more than one experiment.

of the THC in the main-stream smoke is retained and absorbed by marijuana smokers using their typical inhalation technique.

If the marijuana cigarette was smoked as a tobacco cigarette less than 50% of the THC was absorbed.

Thus, the present results indicate that experienced marijuana smokers use a technique with deep inhalations that may be of less importance for the transfer of THC by the main-stream smoke but of considerable importance for the amount of THC absorbed in the lungs during the smoking process. Conversely, our recent finding (1) that heavy marijuana users smoke more efficiently than light users might be explained by a more effective retention and absorption of THC in the lungs, than by a more efficient transfer of THC with the main-stream smoke.

REFERENCES

1. Agurell, S., Lindgren, J. E., Ohlsson, A., Gillespie, H., and Hollister, L., Recent studies on the pharmacokinetics of delta-1-tetrahydrocannabinol in man, This volume.
2. Agurell, S., and Leander, K., Acta. Pharm. Suec. 8:391 (1971).

RELATION OF PLASMA DELTA-9-THC CONCENTRATIONS TO SUBJECTIVE "HIGH" IN MARIJUANA USERS: A REVIEW AND REANALYSIS[1]

Laurence E. Domino[2]
Steven E. Domino[3]
Edward F. Domino

Department of Pharmacology
University of Michigan
Ann Arbor, Michigan

I. INTRODUCTION

Since Gaoni and Mechoulam (1) and Mechoulam and Gaoni (2, 3) first described the isolation and synthesis of delta-9-tetrahydrocannabinol or THC (which is also called delta-1-tetrahydrocannabinol, delta-1-THC) as the major active ingredient of hashish, a great deal of research has been directed toward its measurement in blood and tissues and its pharmacokinetics. Lemberger et al. (4-6) were the first to study the blood levels of ^{14}C-THC in man. Their research stimulated a great deal of research and controversy regarding possible metabolic and dispositional differences in normal volunteers compared to long-term marijuana smokers. Lemberger et al. showed that labeled THC given i.v. disappeared from the plasma of chronic marijuana smokers with a half-life of 28 hr as compared to 57 hr in nonusers. The apparent volumes of distribution did not differ between the two groups. Within 10 min after i.v. administration, these investigators found the 11-hydroxy metabolite in the blood of both groups. It was also present in the urine and feces of both groups for more than

[1]Supported in part by the Psychopharmacology Research Fund
[2]Present Address: Department of Psychiatry, University of Michigan, Ann Arbor, Michigan.
[3]Present address: Vanderbilt University Medical School, Nashville, Tennessee.

ISBN 0-12-044620-0

one week. Hence, it was readily apparent that following a single dose of THC, accumulation and persistence of active and inactive metabolites readily occurred.

Subsequently, Lemberger et al. (7) studied the temporal correlation between the psychological effects of labeled THC and blood levels after different routes of administration. They reported that the psychologic effects of oral or inhaled ^{14}C-THC were temporally correlated with plasma levels of THC and its metabolites in human volunteers who professed to be chronic marijuana users. In addition, these investigators observed that, of various routes of administration, the greatest and most prolonged radioactivity was obtained following inhalation of smoked spiked marijuana, and least after oral administration. These studies as well as those of other investigators were reviewed by Lemberger et al. (5). Lemberger (8) stressed the importance of methodology in detecting the small amounts of THC as well as active metabolites. Specificity as well as sensitivity also determine how long after dosing the cannabinoids are measured in blood and, hence, the complexity of the pharmacokinetic models proposed.

Agurell and his colleagues (11) used various methods, including radiolabeled and later gas chromatographic-mass spectrometric (GC/MS) methods, to study the metabolic fate of various tetrahydrocannabinols. Agurell et al. (12) reported on the pharmacokinetics of delta-8-tetrahydrocannabinol (delta-8-THC) in man after smoking and the relationship of blood levels to physiological and psychological effects. They chose to study delta-8-THC because of the relative ease of synthesis of deuterated derivatives for GC-MS analysis. Their data in general are in agreement with the human data based upon radiolabeled THC. They were able to show that the increase in heart rate was well correlated with the plasma levels of delta-8-THC, whereas the alterations in mental performance were more delayed and prolonged than the peak delta-8-THC plasma level. They suggested that, from a pharmacokinetic model point of view, the receptors for altering heart rate were in a "shallow compartment," whereas those for a psychological "high" were in a "deep compartment." The possible role of active metabolites was also stressed. In any event, these investigators pointed out that if, by analogy, the effects of delta-8 and delta-9-THC are similar, plasma levels of THC were not an entirely relevant parameter for determining performance decrement.

The role of active THC metabolites further complicates the picture. Wall et al. (13) also pointed out the extensive biotransformation of various cannabinoids in animals and man. The fact that some metabolites of THC are active further suggests that no simple relationship between plasma levels and marijuana induced "high" would be expected. However, in the case of 11-OH-delta-9-THC, one of the active metabolites of THC, its pharmacokinetics are similar to those of THC itself (14).

Lindgren et al. (15) determined the plasma concentrations of THC given by smoking and i.v. administration to groups of light and heavy users of marijuana. The marijuana cigarettes contained about 19 mg of THC. A dose of 5.0 mg of THC was given i.v. The investigators used a mass fragmentographic assay for THC as described by Ohlsson et al. (16-18). After i.v. injection of THC, the area under the curve for 0 to 240 min for the plasma levels of THC tended to be lower in the heavy users compared to the light users, but this was not statistically significant ($p = 0.08$). Inasmuch as a marijuana "high" is almost gone by 4 hr after either i.v. administration or via inhalation (18), these investigators only determined THC plasma levels up to 4 hr and were not able to confirm or deny the finding of Lemberger et al. (4-6) that the "apparent" terminal or beta-phase half-life of THC was shorter in chronic marijuana users. Likewise, in the smoking experiments, Lindgren et al. (15) were unable to determine any significant difference in plasma levels of THC between light and heavy users. They did note a tendency ($p = 0.06$) that heavy users showed higher THC levels, probably due to more efficient smoking than light users. The area under the curve for 0 to 240 min of the THC plasma levels was also greater in the heavy users ($p < 0.05$), again suggesting more efficient smoking by heavy users. The psychological effects on both groups from i.v. administration and inhalation were comparable. Their findings were similar to those of Perez-Reyes et al. (19) who found no differences in total plasma radioactivity or the amount of ^{14}C-THC needed i.v. to produce a maximal "high" in infrequent and frequent marijuana users. Hence, the findings of Lindgren et al. (15) and Perez-Reyes et al. (19) are in agreement with each other, but do not confirm or deny the findings of Lemberger and associates regarding a very marked reduction in the late half-life of THC in heavy marijuana users. Furthermore, insofar as maximal high is concerned, both studies find no difference in light vs. heavy users. Neither sensitivity nor tolerance to THC was observed.

Ohlsson et al. (20) studied the single dose kinetics of deuterium labeled THC in light and heavy cannabis users by both i.v. administration and smoking. Plasma levels of $^{2}H_3$-delta-9-THC were measured for 48 to 72 hr. After 5.0 mg i.v. or 8.6 to 9.9 mg by smoking, there was little difference between both groups with regard to the amounts smoked or plasma levels and areas under the curve. Heavy cannabis users tended to have statistically significantly higher THC levels by preference. A plasma clearance of 760 to 1190 ml/min and an elimination half-life of THC of more than 20 hr were calculated. This study, like their previous one, showed no evidence for either sensitivity or tolerance to THC in heavy users.

Hollister et al. (21) addressed the question of whether THC levels reflected the state of cannabis intoxication in 11 volunteers. They gave about 19 mg of THC in a marijuana cigarette for smoking, 20 mg of THC orally in a chocolate cookie, and 5 mg i.v. These investigators then measured THC in the plasma up to 4 hr after administration by the GC/MS method of Ohlsson et al. (16). In addition, both heart rate and subjective "high" were measured. The increases in pulse rate often returned to baseline or below even while the patient felt "high" and still had plasma concentrations of THC above 5 ng/ml. They concluded that the relationship between pulse rate and plasma concentrations of THC was similar to that previously observed by Agurell et al. (12) for delta-8-THC. Hollister et al. also pointed out that they saw no clear cut relationship between plasma concentrations of THC and the degree of intoxication in contrast to the case for ethyl alcohol.

Hunt and Jones (22) administered 30 mg of THC orally every 4 hr for 10 to 12 days to six subjects in an attempt to induce tolerance. They tested the hypothesis that development of tolerance may be due to alterations in THC biotransformation and disposition. Labeled ^{14}C-THC was given i.v. before and after the chronic oral doses of THC. The plasma and urine levels of labeled THC and metabolites were measured by HPLC separation and scintillation counting. Development of tolerance was accompanied by a statistically significant increase in the apparent volume of distribution from 2.6 to 6.4 liter/70 kg man and the plasma clearance increase from 605 to 977 ml/min. The steady state volume of distribution was not altered. The half-life for THC was unchanged (19.6 vs 18.7 hr) while the terminal half-life for the metabolites increased from 48.7 to 52.9 hr. The steady state volume of distribution was not changed (626 vs 742 liter/70 kg). Hunt and Jones (22) proposed a four compartment mammalary model with elimination from the central compartment to explain their data. The mean terminal half-lives of THC of 18.7 to 19.6 hr were shorter than those reported by Lemberger et al. (6) of 28 hr for chronic users. Since the Hunt and Jones subjects were experienced marijuana users, they could not provide data on the observation of Lemberger et al. of a 57 hr terminal half-life of THC in non-users.

Valentine (23) studied the plasma levels of THC in four male volunteers following smoking marijuana cigarettes with three different doses of THC. Plasma samples were analyzed for THC using a HPLC-MS assay for up to 12 hr post-smoking. The mean data for each dose could be fitted to a two compartment model with no absorption phase. No dose dependent pharmacokinetics were noted. A compartmental model was described that was consistent with the earlier reports of Lemberger et al. (5, 6).

Although the use of compartmental models in pharmacokinetics is currently a hotly debated issue, we have used a compartmental model approach in which subjective "high" was fit to a compartment (presumably brain) other than the plasma compartment. The results obtained indicate that, after about 1 hr, plasma levels of THC predict subjective "high" when these two compartments are in equilibrium. The results of this reanalysis are presented herein to act as a stimulus for further research on the relationship of plasma THC levels to degree of mental impairment.

II. METHODS

We have assumed that the effects of THC are related to its concentration at active sites and is dose related. Although no specific THC receptors have been found to date, it is reasonable to assume that there is a specific site of action for THC in the brain, with a dose response curve which may be modeled by the Hill equation (24).

We reanalyzed the reported data of Ohlsson et al. (20) and Lindgren et al. (15) according to a three compartment model with amounts in the second compartment related to the pharmacologic action, i.e., subjective "high." Ohlsson et al. administered five mg i.v. of deuterium-labeled THC ($^2H_3$-THC) to four light and five heavy marijuana users who ranged in age from 18-35 yr. Plasma levels of $^2H_3$-THC in plasma was extracted and purified by liquid chromatography, silylated and assayed via mass fragmentography. The assay is reported to be sensitive to approximately 0.1 ng/ml THC. Mean subjective "high" for light and heavy users were obtained from Lindgren et al. (15) under similar conditions. Subjects in this group consisted of 16 men and 2 women between the ages of 19 and 35, with 8 men and one women in each group. The three compartment model which we used in a reanalysis of this data may be illustrated as follows:

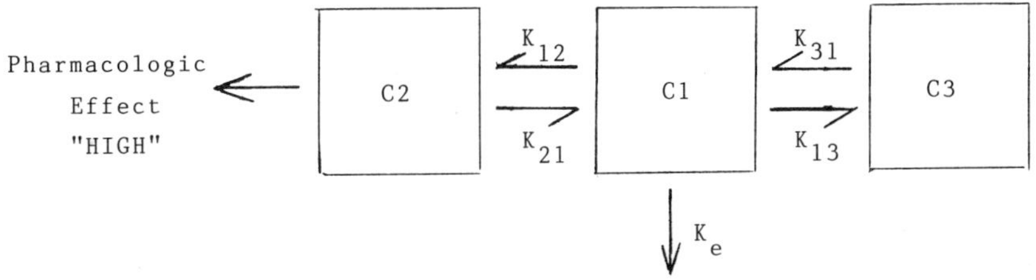

Standard abbreviations are used for the first order rate parameters, and are similar to those proposed by Hull (25). C1, C2, and C3 are "compartments", of which amounts in C2 were related to the time course of subjective "high" by means of the Hill equation (24):

$$E = E_{max} A^S / (1/Q + A^S)$$

E = pharmacologic effect, which in this case is subjective "high". E_{max} is the maximal effect, which is assumed to be 10. "A" is the amount of drug at an active site, which is related to concentration by the relationship: concentration = amount/volume of distribution. The Hill equation has been shown to be valid in classical pharmacological receptor assays (26,27). It predicts zero and maximal response, is sigmoidal in shape, and is continuous over the entire dose range. The use of a three compartment model was justified when F-test (28) was used on the NONLIN plasma curve fit to individual subjects.

NONLIN (29) was used with weights of reciprocal concentration to fit a three exponential equation to mean plasma concentrations in light and heavy users. First order rate parameters were calculated according to the method of Wagner (30). Amounts in the second compartment were calculated utilizing standard techniques (31). Mean subjective "high" in light and heavy users were fit according to the Hill equation by means of NONLIN regression with weights of reciprocal "high".

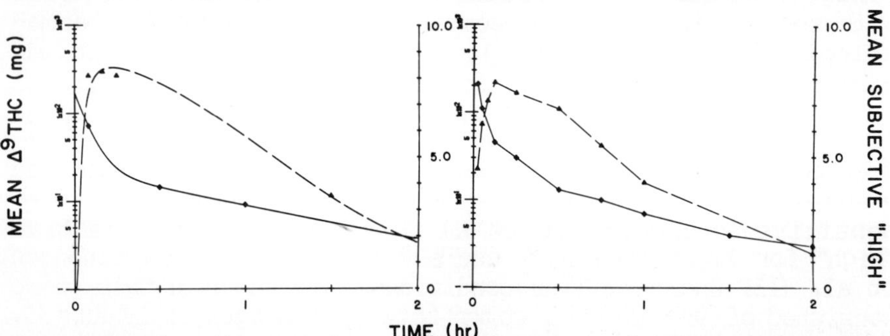

FIGURE 1. Comparison of plasma THC levels and subjective "high" after 5 mg i.v. THC. The solid line in the left graph is the triexponential fit of mean plasma THC levels from Ohlsson et al. (20), and the dashed line is the predicted time course of subjective "high" in light marijuana users based on "second" compartment amounts. The right graph shows actual mean data without curve fitting of THC plasma concentrations and subjective "high" from Hollister et al. (21) in a mixed group of light and heavy marijuana users. THC concentrations on the y-axis range from 1 to 1000 ng//ml.

CSTRIP (32) was used for initial estimates for the NONLIN fit of the plasma curve. The initial estimates for the Hill equation were obtained by linear regression of Log [Amount of THC in compartment 2] vs. Log ["high" / Max "high" - "high")]. A pharmacokinetic model for light and heavy users was also determined for smoke administration on the same subjects for mean plasma concentrations by nonlinear regression utilizing NONLIN. Calculation of first order rate parameters was performed utilizing the same method.

III. RESULTS

The time course of subjective "high" after an i.v. dose of THC appeared to show a course with initial elevation, peak effect at 15 min, followed by a decline. The calculated results for light marijuana users are shown in the left panel of Fig. 1, while the second panel shows the reported mean data of Hollister et al. (21) for a group of mixed light and heavy users. Note the general similarity, as subjective "high" rises while plasma levels of THC fall at early time points.

Mean plasma levels of THC are shown in Fig. 2 for light and heavy marijuana users following i.v. administration of 5 mg THC. A model for each group of the distribution of THC into the compartment which contains the presumed active site is shown in Fig. 3. Compartment 2 was assumed to contain the active site. It can be seen that the model predicts an equilibration and subsequent parallel decline of THC in plasma at approximately 40-60 min.

Table I shows the parameters of the pharmacodynamic model. These results are preliminary and are meant only for generation of further testable hypotheses.

IV. DISCUSSION

The use of models in scientific endeavors provides methods of obtaining new hypotheses and must be judged according to parsimony and predictive value. Clearly, distribution into brain cannot be studied directly in humans, and even imaging methods such as PET (Position Emission Tomography) require use of compartmental models for analysis (33). Despite such analysis, total brain levels may not correlate with a pharmacologic effect, as specific as well as nonspecific binding is measured. For example, no significant decreases in total brain concentrations of THC were found in groups of tolerant and nontolerant dogs and pigeons (34,35). When synaptic vesicles were isolated from brain, Martin et al. (34,35) reported a significant decrease in THC concentrations in this fraction of the brains of tolerant dogs.

There is a complex relationship between the ingestion of marijuana and the time course of its subjective effects. The peak subjective "high" occurs about 15-30 min following smoking of marijuana, and about 15 min following i.v. injection of THC. Plasma levels of THC are elevated initially, and appear to be falling as subjective high increases. Although it was suggested that regional distribution at the site of action in the brain might account for the dissociation between plasma levels and subjective high (4), the discovery of active metab-

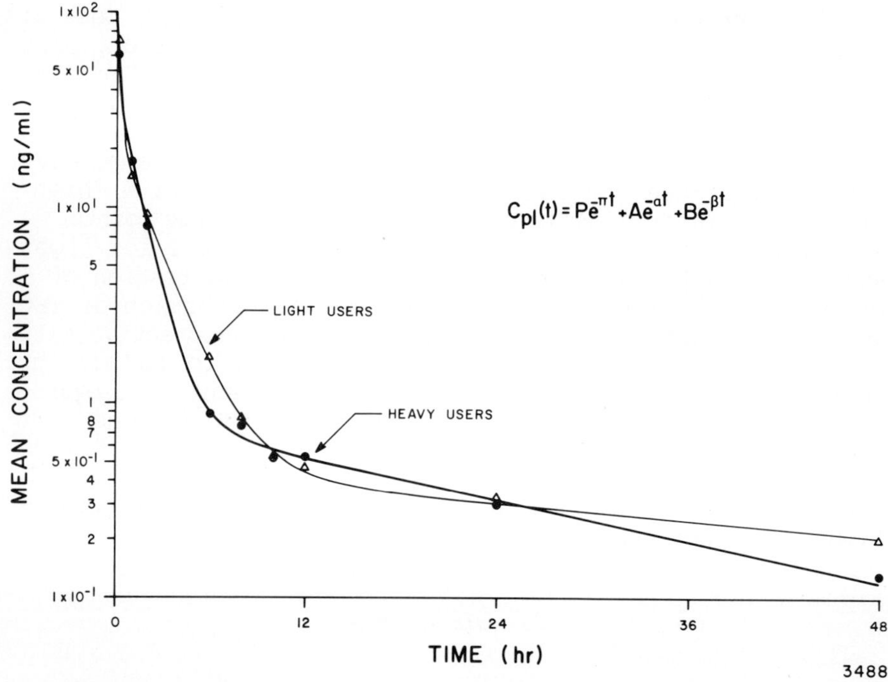

FIGURE 2. Mean plasma concentrations of deuterated THC in light and heavy marijuana users after a 5 mg i.v. dose. Mean plasma concentrations of $^2H_3$-THC in four light (open triangles) and five heavy (solid circles) marijuana users were determined by Ohlsson et al. (20). The solid lines are the fit according to the model described in the text. Parameters for light users are: P = 151 ng/ml, pi = 6.53 h^{-1}, A = 22.4 ng/ml, alpha = 0.483 h^{-1}, B = 0.460 ng/ml, beta = 0.0168. For heavy users: P = 85.9 ng/ml, pi = 7.13 h^{-1}, A = 38.4 ng/ml, alpha = 0.839 h^{-1}, B = 0.844 ng/ml, beta = 0.0405.

olites of THC focused efforts upon the possible correlation between the appearance of these substances in plasma and the time course of subjective "high". Thus subjective "high" was seen to parallel the plasma time course of 11-OH-delta-9-THC (14), and polar metabolites of THC (13). Temporal correlation alone of subjective high and plasma levels of possible active metabolites is not sufficient to determine the relative importance of distribution vs. metabolism in the onset of subjective "high;" metabolites must also distribute into brain. We describe a model which assumes only distribution and a dose-

TABLE I. Pharmacodynamic Model of Deuterated THC in Light and Heavy Marijuana Users*

First Order Rate Parameters		Use Level: Light i.v. (N = 4)	Heavy i.v. (N = 5)	Light Smoking (N = 4)	Heavy Smoking (N = 5)
K_{12}	h^{-1}	3.34	3.00	4.13	3.27
K_{21}	h^{-1}	1.35	2.95	1.65	1.91
K_{13}	h^{-1}	0.643	0.499	0.776	0.598
K_{31}	h^{-1}	0.0234	0.0548	0.0302	0.0523
K_e	h^{-1}	1.68	1.50	1.40	1.93
V_d (central)	1	31.7	43.6		
Hill Parameters					
S		2.03	1.28		
Q		1.17	0.95		

*This table lists the parameters calculated from mean plasma data reported by Ohlsson et al. (20) and Lindgren et al. (15) according to the model outlined in the text. The kinetic parameters for smoking were fit to mean plasma THC only. Standard abbreviations are used for the parameters and are similar to those proposed by Hull (25).

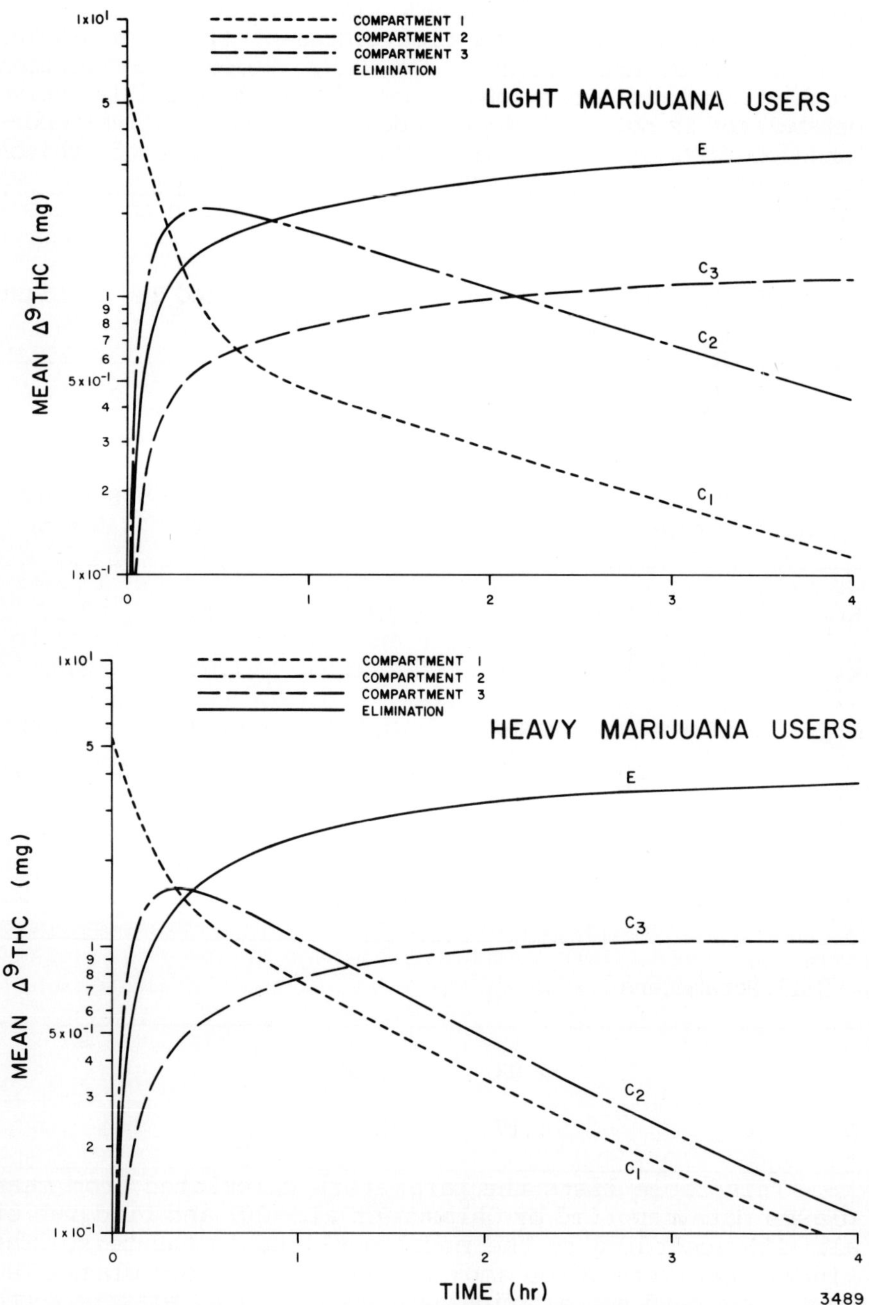

COMPARTMENT 1
COMPARTMENT 2
COMPARTMENT 3
ELIMINATION
LIGHT MARIJUANA USERS
E
C_3
C_2
C_1
MEAN Δ^9THC (mg)
1x10^1
5
1
9
8
7
6
5x10^{-1}
4
3
2
1x10^{-1}
0
1
2
3
4
COMPARTMENT 1
COMPARTMENT 2
COMPARTMENT 3
ELIMINATION
HEAVY MARIJUANA USERS
E
C_3
C_2
C_1
MEAN Δ^9THC (mg)
TIME (hr)
3489

relationship ofTHC to subjective "high". Following these assumptions, a time course of subjective "high" is predicted to occur which is similar to that observed.

The model suggests several hypotheses, two of which follow. Hypothesis 1: The time course of marijuana subjective "high" is determined by the delivery of THC and its active metabolites to brain. Prediction: Following pseudoequilibrium between blood and active sites in brain, plasma levels of THC and its active metabolites will correlate with subjective "high."

The model predicts a parallel decline between the active site and blood approximately 40 min following an i.v. dose in heavy users, and 60 min in light users of marijuana. A plasma concentration-response curve may, therefore, be predicted to apply at any time following the attainment of this equilibration. We have converted amounts in the "second" compartment to equivalent plasma concentrations after pseudoequilibrium, and present the resultant relationship between plasma levels and mean subjective "high" in Fig 4. There appears to be a relative right shift predicted in the concentration response curve for heavy users, suggesting tolerance. The estimates at plasma concentrations greater than 20 ng/ml are extrapolations, and hence, are not predicted to be as reliable as estimates at lower plasma concentrations.

The predictions of Fig 4 are testable under further empirical conditions. Preliminary evidence may support such a concept, as can be seen when completely separate data from Perez-Reyes et al. (36) is plotted. Three men and three women who smoked from 4 to 12 marijuana cigarettes a month were administered three different potencies of marijuana: 1.32%, 1.97% and 2.54% THC. The subjective "high" was determined. Contrary to the authors' opinion of a lack of correlation, after sixty min following smoking, mean plasma concentrations of THC significantly correlated with mean subjective "high". Addition of the 45 min points lowered the correlation. These data are shown in Fig. 5. Half maximal effect was seen at 15 ng/ml, which is between the bounds predicted from the model shown in Fig. 4. This group of marijuana users would, in fact, corre-

FIGURE 3. Amounts of deuterated THC in each compartment of a three compartment open model in light and heavy marijuana users. The "second" compartment, which is presumed to contain the site of action of THC, shows a peak at about 15-20 min with a parallel decline with plasma starting 60 min following an i.v. dose of 5 mg of THC in light users, and 40 min in heavy users. Compartmental amounts were based on the model described in the text.

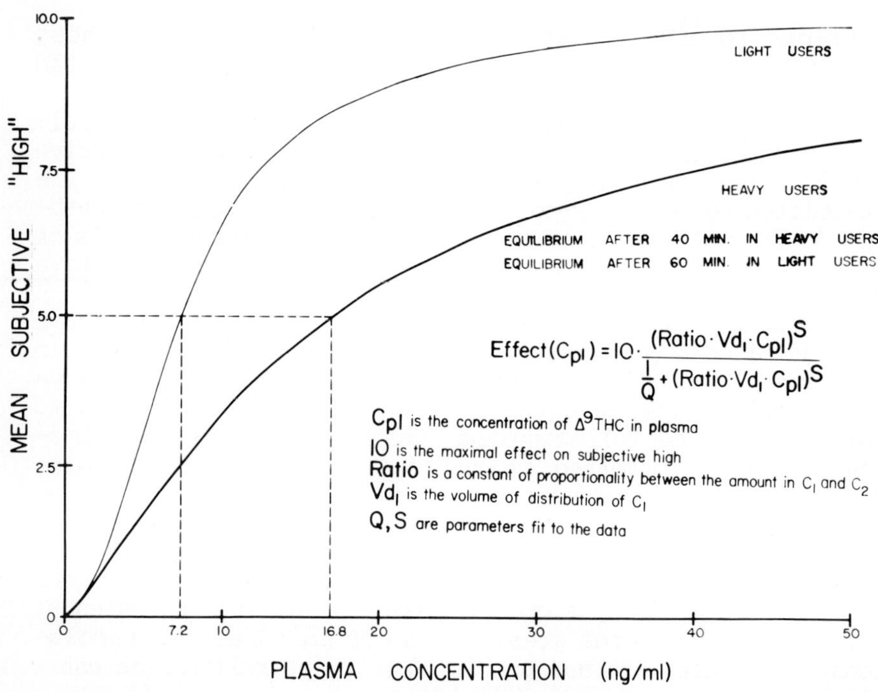

FIGURE 4. Relation of plasma THC concentration vs. subjective "high" estimates in light and heavy marijuana users at pseudoequilibrium. Following equilibration of THC between blood and active sites in brain, plasma concentrations of THC are predicted to show a dose-response relationship with subjective "high." The presence of large amounts of active metabolites would invalidate this specific relationship, and correlation would be better predicted to arise from concentrations of THC and active metabolites.

spond to slightly less frequent smokers than the heavy smokers of Ohlsson et al. (20).

Hypothesis 2: The elimination of THC from the body is determined by slow (net) release of THC from tissues (perhaps fat). Prediction: Calculations of half-life in man from blood data measured with current analytic techniques may underestimate terminal half-life when compared to that determined from fat (or other tissue).

Wagner (24,30) has discussed artifacts in calculated terminal half-lives when plasma levels fall to limits of detectability before all tissues equilibrate with blood. Thereis, in addition, much evidence which supports the possibility of a prolonged half-life of THC. Kreuz and Axelrod (37) have noted a terminal half-life of 5 days of THC in the rat when calcu-

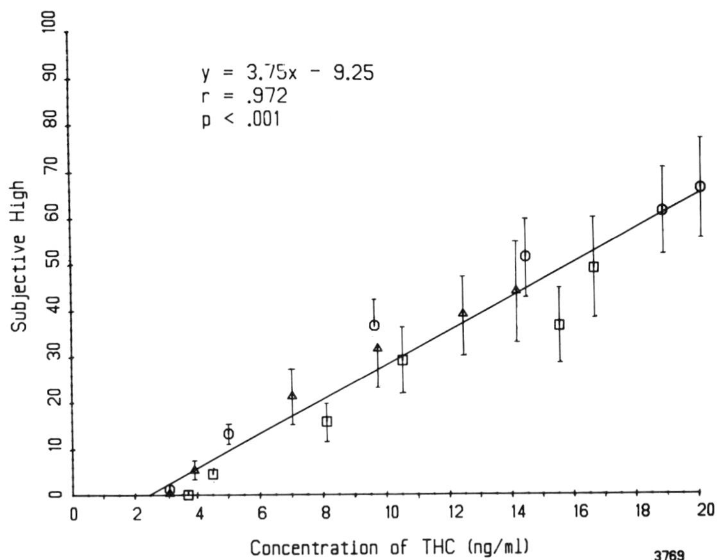

FIGURE 5. Correlation of plasma THC concentration and subjective "high" after pseudoequilibrium. The data of Perez-Reyes et al. (36) are shown for time points 60 min following smoking of 1.32% (triangles), 1.97% (squares), and 2.54% (circles) THC cigarettes. Error bars correspond to +/- S.E.M.

lated from fat and Garrett and Hunt (38) predicted a terminal half-life of 8 days in the dog.

The prediction of this model is consistent with findings of Hunt and Jones (22) that enhanced metabolism of THC will have a minimal effect on its terminal phase half-life. Our model suggests that the rate of metabolism (and excretion) is at least 50-100 times faster than release from tissue stores.

The prediction of a prolonged half-life of THC is of potential importance in the clinical treatment of patients with substance abuse, and is consistent with clinical reports of a relatively prolonged detoxification phase associated with treatment of marijuana dependence (39,40). Simultaneous measurement of plasma and some representative measurements of THC fat concentrations may provide clarification of this point.

The above two hypotheses are readily testable with additional research and will allow one to further understand the complex pharmacology of THC. Furthermore, additional new data will help validate or reject the present compartmental model which predicts that plasma THC levels correlate with subjective "high".

ACKNOWLEDGMENTS

We wish to thank Drs. Agurell, Ohlsson and colleagues for preprints and reprints of their extensive papers referred to in this manuscript and Kenneth E. Domino for programming assistance.

REFERENCES

1. Gaoni Y. and Mechoulam, R.: Isolation, structure and partial synthesis of an active constituent of hashish, J. Amer. Chem. Soc. 86:1646-1647 (1964).
2. Mechoulam, R., and Gaoni, Y.: A total synthesis of dl-delta-1-tetrahydrocannabinol, the active constituent of hashish, J. Amer. Chem. Soc. 87:3273-3275 (1965).
3. Mechoulam, R., and Gaoni, Y.: The absolute configuration of Delta-9-tetrahydrocannabinol, the major active constituent of hashish, Tetrahedron Lett. 12:1109-1111 (1967).
4. Lemberger, L., Silberstein, S. D., Axelrod, J., and Kopin, I. J.: Marihuana: Studies on the disposition and metabolism of Delta-9-tetrahydrocannabinol in man, Science 170: 1320-1322 (1970).
5. Lemberger, L., Axelrod, J., and Kopin, I. J.: Metabolism and disposition of tetrahydrocannabinols in naive subjects and chronic marijuana users, Ann. N. Y. Acad. Sci. 191:142-154 (1971).
6. Lemberger, L., Tamarkin, N. R., Axelrod, J., and Kopin, I. J.: Delta-9-tetrahydrocannabinol: Metabolism and disposition in long-term marihuana smokers, Science 173:72-74 (1971).
7. Lemberger, L., Weiss, J. L., Watanabe, A. M., Galanter, I. M., Wyatt, R. J., and Cardon, P. V., Delta-9-tetrahydrocannabinol. Temporal correlation of the psychologic effects and blood levels after various routes of administration, N. Engl. J. Med. 286:685-688 (1972).
8. Lemberger, L., Pharmacokinetics of delta-9-tetrahydrocannabinol and its metabolites: Importance and relationship in developing methods of detecting cannabis in biologic fluids, in "Marihuana-Chemistry, Biochemistry and Cellular Effects" (G. G. Nahas, W. D. M. Paton and J. E. Idanpaan-Heikkila, eds), pp. 169-178. Springer-Verlag, New

York, 1976.

9. Lemberger, L., and Rubin, A.: Minireview--The physiologic disposition of marihuana in man, Life Sci. 17:1637-1642 (1975).

10. Lemberger, L., and Rubin A., The Cannabinoids, in "Physiologic Disposition of Drugs of Abuse," p. 269-310. Spectrum Publications, Inc., New York, 1976.

11. Agurell, S., Dahmen, J., Gustafsson, B., Johasson, U. B., Leander, K., Nilsson, I., Nilsson, J. L. G., Nordqvist, M., Ransay, C. H., Ryrfeldt, A., Sanberg, F., and Widman M, Metabolic Fate of Tetrahydrocannabinol, in "Cannabis Derivatives--Pharmacology and Experimental Psychology" (W. D. M. Paton and J. Crown, eds), p. 16-38. Oxford Univ. Press, London, 1972.

12. Agurell, S., Levander, S., Binder, M., Bader-Bartfai, A., Gustafsson, B., Leander, K., Lindgren, J. E., Ohlsson, A., and Tobisson, B., Pharmacokinetics of Delta-8-tetrahydrocannabinol (delta-6-tetrahydrocannabinol) in man after smoking -- Relations to physiological and psychological effects, in "Pharmacology of Marihuana," Vol. 1 (M. C. Braude and S. Szara, eds), p. 49-61. Raven Press, New York, 1976.

13. Wall, M. E., Brine, D. R., and Perez-Reyes, M., Metabolism of cannabinoids in man, in "Pharmacology of Marihuana," Vol. 1 (M. C. Braude and S. Szara, eds), p. 93-113. Raven Press, New York, 1976.

14. Lemberger, L., Crabtree, R. E. and Rowe, H. M., 11-Hydroxy-delta-9-tetrahydrocannabinol: Pharmacology, disposition, and metabolism of a major metabolite of marihuana in man, Science 177: 62-64 (1972).

15. Lindgren, J. E., Ohlsson, A., Agurell, S., Hollister, L., and Gillespie, H., Clinical effects and plasma levels of delta-9-tetrahydrocannabinol (delta-9-THC) in heavy and light users of cannabis, Psychopharmacol. 74:208-212 (1981).

16. Ohlsson, A., Lindgren, J. E., Leander, K., and Agurell, S., Detection and quantification of tetrahydrocannabinol in blood plasma, in "Cannabinoid Assays in Humans," NIDA Research Monograph No. 7 (R. E. Willette, ed) p. 48-63. National Institute on Drug Abuse, Rockville, MD., 1976.

17. Ohlsson, A., Studies on the Synthesis, Metabolism and Kinetics of Cannabinoids. Doctoral Dissertation, Faculty of Pharmacy, Uppsala University. Almqvist and Wiksell International, Stockholm, Sweden, 1980.

18. Ohlsson, A., Lindgren, J.E., Wahlen, A., Agurell, S., Hollister, L. E., and Gillespie, H. K., Plasma delta-9-tetrahydrocannabinol concentrations and clinical effects after oral and intravenous administration and smoking, Clin. Pharmacol. Ther. 28:409-416 (1980).

19. Perez-Reyes, M., Timmons, M. C., and Wall, M. E., Long-term use of marihuana and the development of tolerance or sensitivity to delta-9-tetrahydrocannabinol, Arch. Gen. Psychiat. 31:89-91 (1974).
20. Ohlsson, A., Lindgren, J. E., Wahlen, A., Agurell, S., Hollister, L. E., and Gillespie, H. K., Single dose kinetics of deuterium labeled delta-9-tetrahydrocannabinol in heavy and light cannabis users, Biomed. Mass Spec. 9:6-10 (1982).
21. Hollister, L. E., Gillespie, H. K., Ohlsson, A., Lindgren, J. E, Wahlen, A., and Agurell, S., Do plasma concentrations of delta-9-tetrahydrocannabinol reflectthe degree of intoxication? J. Clin. Pharmacol. 21:171S-177S (1981).
22. Hunt, C. A., and Jones, R. T., Tolerance and disposition of tetrahydrocannabinol in man, J. Pharmacol. Exp. Ther. 215:35-44 (1980).
23. Valentine, J. L., Pharmacokinetics of delta-9-tetrahydrocannabinol in humans following marijuana smoking, The Pharmacologist 23: 203 (1981).
24. Wagner, J. G., Relations between drug concentration and response, J. Mond. Pharm. 14:279-310 (1971).
25. Hull, C. J., Symbols for compartmental models, Editorial, Br. J. Anesth. 51: 815-817 (1979).
26. Wagner, J. G., "Fundamentals of Clinical Pharmacokinetics," pp. 317-318. Drug Intelligence Publications, Hamilton, Ill., 1975.
27. Paalzow, L. K. and Edlund, P. O., Multiple receptor responses: A new concept to describe the relationship betweenpharmacological effects and pharmacokinetics of a drug: Studies on clonidine in the rat and cat, J. Pharmacokinet. Biopharmaceut. 7:495-510 (1979).
28. Boxenbaum, H. G., Riegelman, S., and Elashoff, R. M., Statistical estimations in pharmacokinetics, J. Pharmacol. Biopharm. 2:123-148 (1974).
29. Metzler, C. M., Elfring, G. L., and McEwen, A. J., A package of computer programs for pharmacokinetic modeling, Biometrics 38:562-563 (1974).
30. Wagner, J. G., Linear pharmacokinetic equations allowing direct calculation of many needed pharmacokinetic parameters from the coefficients and exponents of polyexponential equations which have been fitted to the data, J. Pharmacokin. Biopharm. 4:443-467 (1976).
31. Benet, L. Z., General treatment of linear mammalary models with elimination from any compartment as used in pharmacokinetics, J. Pharm. Sci. 61:536-541 (1972).
32. Sedman, A. J. and Wagner, J. G., CSTRIP, a Fortran IV Computer program for obtaining initial polyexponential parameter estimates, J. Pharm. Sci. 65:1006-1010 (1976).

33. Phelps, M. E., Maziotta, J. C., ad Huang, S. C., Review-Study of cerebral function with positron computed tomography, J. Cereb. Blood Flow Metab. 2:113-162 (1982).
34. Martin, B. R., Dewey, W. L., Harris, L. S., and Beckner, J. S., ^{3}H-delta-9-tetrahydrocannabinol tissue and subcellular distribution in the central nervous system and tissue distribution in the central peripheral organs of tolerant and nontolerant dogs, J. Pharmacol. Exp. Ther. 196:12-144 (1976).
35. Dewey, W. L., McMillan, D. E., Harris, L. S., and Turk, R. F., Distribution of radioactivity in brain of tolerant and nontolerant pigeons treated with ^{3}H-delta-9-tetrahydrocannabinol, Biochem. Pharmacol. 22:399-405 (1973).
36. Perez-Reyes, M., DiGuiseppi, S., Davis, K. H., Schindler, V. H. and Cook, C. E., Comparison of effects of marihuana cigarettes of three different potencies, Clin. Pharmacol. Ther. 31:617-624 (1982).
37. Kreuz, D. S., and Axelrod, J., Delta-9-tetrahydrocannabinol: Localization in body fat, Science 179:391-392 (1973).
38. Garrett, E. R., and Hunt, C. A., Pharmacokinetics of delta-9-tetrahydrocannabinol in dogs, J. Pharm. Sci. 66:395-407 (1977).
39. Dackis, C. A., Pottash, A. I. C., Annitto, W., and Gold, M. S., Persistence of urinary marijuana levels after supervised abstinence, Amer. J. Psychiat. 139:1196-1198 (1982).
40. Dackis, C. A., Pottash, A. I. C., and Gold, M. S., Letter to the Editor, Amer. J. Psychiat. 140:656 (1983).

URINARY CANNABINOID EXCRETION PATTERNS

Richard J. Bastiani

Syva Company
Palo Alto, California

I. INTRODUCTION

Investigators have shown that the rate of excretion of the many urinary metabolites and cannabinoid constituents following active smoking of marijuana is variable from individual to individual as well as for a single individual over time. Although the peak psychoactive and physiologic effects appear within 2-3 minutes and can last from 90 to 120 minutes after smoking a single cigarette, elevated excretion of urinary metabolites occurs within hours after exposure and levels have been shown to remain detectable for many days (1-11).

Since the variability in excretion of metabolites coupled with variabilities in fluid intake, frequency of urination and differences in kidney function exist, correlation of urine values with intoxication or time since use may not be feasible. It has been reported, however, that delta-9-tetrahydrocannabinol (THC) is more rapidly metabolized in chronic users than naive users and that frequent users often exhibit basal urinary values that exceed peak values attained by infrequent users (12-14).

The present study, therefore, was designed to monitor daily urine samples from several subjects following an alternating smoking/abstension protocol over a 25 day period. Comparison of the sample results to the dosing schedule was done in order to determine: the duration of positive results, the presence of observable trends in metabolite excretion and the existence of differences in excretion patterns for frequent vs. less frequent users.

The Cannabinoids: Chemical,
Pharmacologic, and Therapeutic Aspects

ISBN 0-12-044620-0

II. MATERIALS AND METHODS

The clinical aspects of this study were conducted at the University of North Carolina, Department of Psychiatry, by Dr. Mario Perez-Reyes. The subjects involved were selected volunteers from a group well known to Dr. Perez-Reyes and his staff and who had been found reliable in previous marijuana clinical research.

Three male and three female subjects, all experienced marijuana users, were asked to refrain from smoking for seven days prior to the beginning of the investigation. Subjects DF_2 and DM_3 stated that they were frequent users (~ daily). Subjects DF_1, DF_3, DM_1 and DM_2 were less frequent users (1-4 times/week). All subjects in this study also provided blood samples for a concurrent study conducted by Dr. Mario Perez-Reyes (15). After 7 days of abstinence from marijuana use, each subject provided a baseline urine sample. Using a randomized, double-blind sequence, subjects were required to smoke one marijuana cigarette each week for three weeks. Standardized cigarettes were obtained from the National Institute on Drug Abuse (NIDA) and contained 1.32%, 1.97% or 2.54% of THC. The subjects were required to refrain from further marijuana use for the duration of the study and for 10 days following the last cigarette. Urine samples were collected daily for the duration of the smoking study and for 10 days after smoking the third cigarette.

Subjects were instructed to provide the samples from the first urination each morning. On the days that a cigarette was smoked, the urine sample was collected prior to smoking in

TABLE I. Multiple Dose Study: Dosing Sequence

Subject	Stated frequency of prior use	Dosing Sequence (%THC/cigarette)		
		Day 1	Day 8	Day 15
Males:				
DM1	1-4x/week	2.54	1.97	1.32
DM2	1-4x/week	1.32	2.54	1.97
DM3	~ daily	1.97	1.32	2.54
Females:				
DF1	1-4x/week	2.54	1.32	1.97
DF2	~ daily	1.32	1.97	2.54
DF3	1-4x/week	1.97	2.54	1.32

TABLE II. Performance Characteristics: EMIT-d.a.u. and EMIT-st Urine Cannabinoid Assays

Parameter	EMIT-d.a.u. Semiquantitative Assay	EMIT-st Qualitative Assay
Cutoff Calibrator Concentration	20 ng/ml 8-THC Acid*	100 ng/ml 8-THC-Acid*
Sensitivity	ca. 20 ng/ml Cannabinoids	ca. 100 ng/ml Cannabinoids
Minimal concentration detected as Positive with 95% confidence	50 ng/ml Cannabinoids	200 ng/ml Cannabinoids
Confidence limit at 0 ng/ml for Negative response	at least 95% confidence	at least 95% confidence
Specificity:	Class Specific for Cannabinoids: delta-9-THC 11-Nor-delta-9-THC-9-carboxylic Acid 11-Hydroxy-delta-9-THC 8-beta-Hydroxy-delta-9-THC 8-beta,11-Dihydroxy-delta-9-THC	

*Performance of the 11-nor-delta-8-THC-9-carboxylic acid (8-THC Acid) employed in the calibrators has been shown to produce a response essentially equivalent to that of the 11-nor-delta-9-THC-9-carboxylic acid metabolite.

the morning; the samples collected on days 2, 9 and 16 were the first samples collected following smoking.

The individual dose sequence for each subject is given in Table I.

A. Analytical Method

Analytical determinations on the urine samples were conducted by the Clinical Studies Laboratory, Syva Company. All clinical samples were sent blind and included control specimens. The sample code was supplied following analysis.

The EMIT-st and EMIT-d.a.u. Cannabinoid Assays employ a homogeneous enzyme immunoassay technique for the microanalysis of specific compounds in biological fluids (16-18). A drug is labeled with an enzyme, and when the enzyme-labeled drug becomes bound to an antibody against the drug, the enzyme's activity is reduced. Drug in a sample competes with the enzyme-labeled drug for the antibody binding sites, thereby decreasing the antibody-induced inactivation of the enzyme. Active enzyme converts NAD^+ to NADH, resulting in an absorbance change that is measured photometrically (EMIT-st) or spectrophotometrically (EMIT-d.a.u.). The enzyme activity in the sample mixture is compared against the activity of the Cutoff calibrator in order to interpret the result. Samples producing a response greater than the Cutoff calibrator response are interpreted as Positive; those producing a response less than the Cutoff calibrator response are interpreted as Negative.

The EMIT-d.a.u. Cannabinoid assay is a semiquantitative technique employing a Negative (0 ng/ml), a Cutoff (20 ng/ml) and a Medium (75 ng/ml) calibrator. The Emit-st Cannabinoid assay is a qualitative technique employing one Cutoff calibrator (100 ng/ml). The performance characteristics of the assays are given in Table II.

The methods detect the presence of THC by assay of urinary cannabinoid constituents and metabolites. Both assays are most sensitive to 11-nor-delta-9-THC-9-carboxylic acid and to 11-hydroxy-delta-9-THC (12,14). Since it has been shown that 12 hours following the administration of THC, less than half of the total 11-nor-delta-9-THC-9-carboxylic acid is present in unconjugated form, the assays are also designed to be sensitive to both conjugated (glucuronide) and unconjugated forms of urinary metabolites (19).

III. RESULTS

A. EMIT-d.a.u. Analysis

All samples were frozen on the day of collection and thawed on the day of analysis. All the samples from each subject were assayed as a batch and were, thus, compared to the same Low Calibrator response for interpretation. Samples and calibrators were analyzed in duplicate; the results are expressed as the average of two determinations.

The daily sample responses for each subject are plotted in Figure 1. In order to compare intersubject variability, the results are presented as the differences obtained between the Low Calibrator response and the sample response.

As can be seen in Figure 1, the excretion pattern for each individual is different; however, general trends can be observed. All subjects produced a Positive response the day following smoking. And, in most cases, each of the three peaks occurred the day following smoking and each peak response was followed by responses that exhibited a declining trend over time. In several cases, it was noted that as the daily responses approached that of the Cutoff calibrator, the results vascillated between Positive and Negative interpretations. This effect is expected when excretion of cannabinoids decreases to the sensitivity level of the assay (20 ng/ml) and can be due primarily to normal variations in the urine.

Of the subjects who admitted to less frequent prior use (DF_1, DF_3, DM_1 and DM_2), all produced a pre-dosing Negative specimen on Day 1. Following smoking episodes, each subject generally produced 2-5 consecutive Positive samples followed by declining values until the last dose. As can be seen from the Figure, although some variability is apparent, peaks corresponding to the doses smoked which are followed by declining trends during the abstension periods are observable.

For the frequent prior-users (DF_2 and DM_3), after six days of abstinence from marijuana use, the pre-smoking (Day 1) samples produced Positive results; the sample from subject DF_2 exceeded the response of the 75 ng/ml Calibrator. With the exception of three samples obtained during the third week of the study, these subjects also remained consistently Positive for the duration of this investigation. In fact, positive samples were still being obtained at the end of the study, which was 10 days following the final smoking episode. These results illustrate the results of previous studies showing that chronic and/or high doses of marijuana can produce an accumulation of cannabinoid constituents in the body that are detectable in the urine for 10 days or longer with this analytical method (20,21).

Samples from subjects DF_2 and DM_3 are representative of chronic and/or high dose marijuana use. These subjects consistently produced higher responses than samples from other subjects and also produced the greatest number of consecutive Positive responses of the subjects studied. These analytical findings are consistent with the known marijuana smoking habits of the subjects.

For all subjects, following the peak occurring after the third dose, the responses obtained gradually declined; by Day 25, all subjects had produced at least one sample which was designated as negative.

No correlation between the % THC in the dose administered and the responses obtained was calculated.

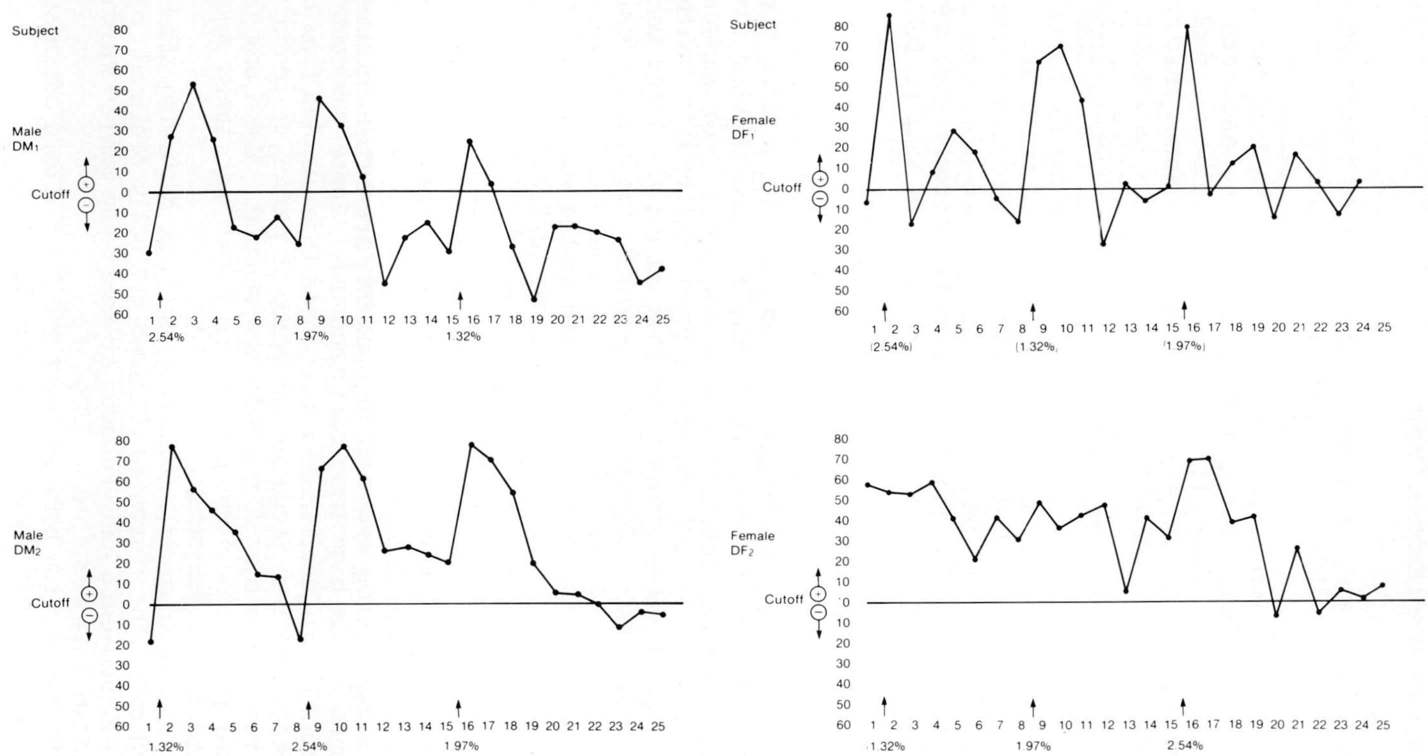

Subject
Male
DM1
Cutoff
2.54%
1.97%
1.32%
Male
DM2
Cutoff
1.32%
2.54%
1.97%
Subject
Female
DF1
Cutoff
(2.54%)
(1.32%)
(1.97%)
Female
DF2
Cutoff
1.32%
1.97%
2.54%

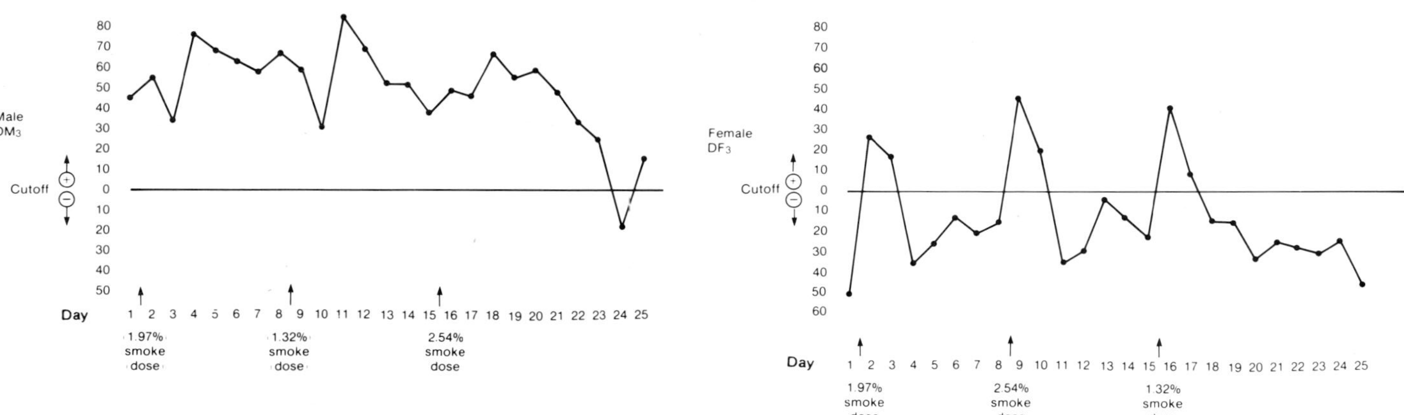

FIGURE 1. Males and Females: Individual Values vs. Time (Days). Samples response is expressed as the of the low Calibrator - of the sample; Cutoff response is expressed as "O".

B. Comparison of Daily Total Positive Values (EMIT-d.a.u.)

The data in Figure 1 was combined (Figure 2) and the percent of Positive samples was calculated for each day. From the figure it can be seen that 100% of the subjects produced positive samples one day after smoking which declined to approximately 50% 6 days after smoking and to 30% after 9 to 10 days.

C. Analysis of Samples by EMIT-st and Comparison Results with EMIT-d.a.u. Results

In order to illustrate the detectability of cannabinoids as a function of assay sensitivity, all samples were subsequently analyzed using the EMIT-st qualitative assay. As can be seen in Figure 3, since the EMIT-st assay has a 100 ng/ml sensitivity vs. 20 ng/ml for the EMIT-d.a.u. assay, interpretation of sample responses using the ST cutoff resulted in significantly fewer total Positive results. In general, however, following each smoking episode, excretion of cannabinoids was sufficient to produce at least one sample that was analyzed as positive.

From the Figure 1, it can be seen that the less frequent users produced no more than a total of 3 positive EMIT-st responses following each dose. These subjects also produced consecutively negative results for the final 9 days of the study. Of note was subject DM_1 who, although he smoked the three weekly doses, produced responses less than that of the 100 ng/ml calibrator for the duration of the study.

In contrast, the frequent smokers (DF_2 and D_3)excreted cannabinoids at levels consistently detectable by the 20 ng/ml D.A.U. cutoff as well as the 100 ng/ml ST cutoff for the first two weeks of the study. Following the final dose, subject DM_3 excreted sufficient cannabinoids to produce 7 consecutive responses by both assays. And, on the 10th day following the final dose, this subject also produced positive responses by both assays. Although samples from subject DF_2 produced responses greater than D.A.U. 20 ng/ml calibrator for 8 of the final 10 days of the study, only the first 4 samples collected after smoking contained sufficient cannabinoids to also produce responses greater than the 100 ng/ml ST cutoff. Again, the variability seen from subject to subject can be attributed to differences in excretion rates as well as to normal variabilities in urine; the excretion patterns observed, however, appeared to be related to the subject's prior frequency of use as well as to the doses smoked.

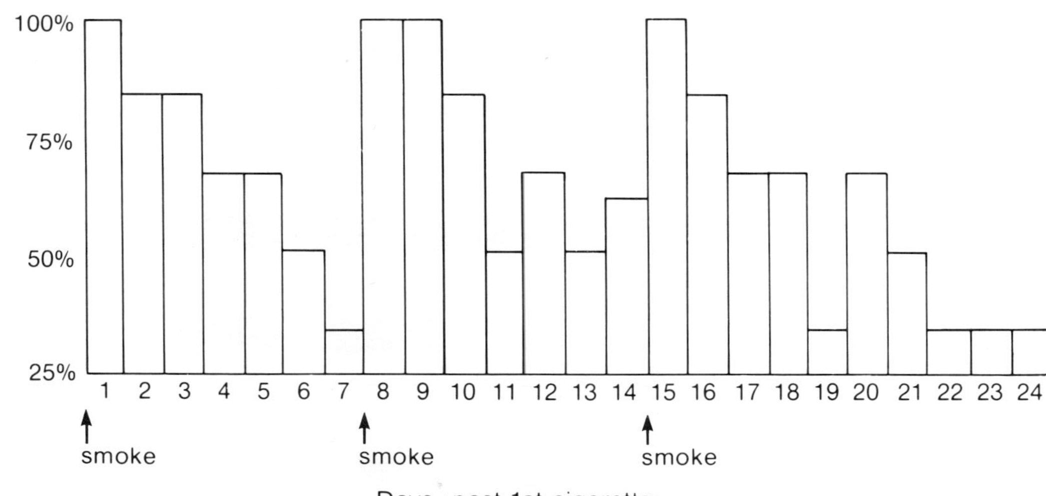

FIGURE 2. Percent of Samples Producing Positive Responses (First Urine Post-Smoking - 10 Days Following Final Cigarette)

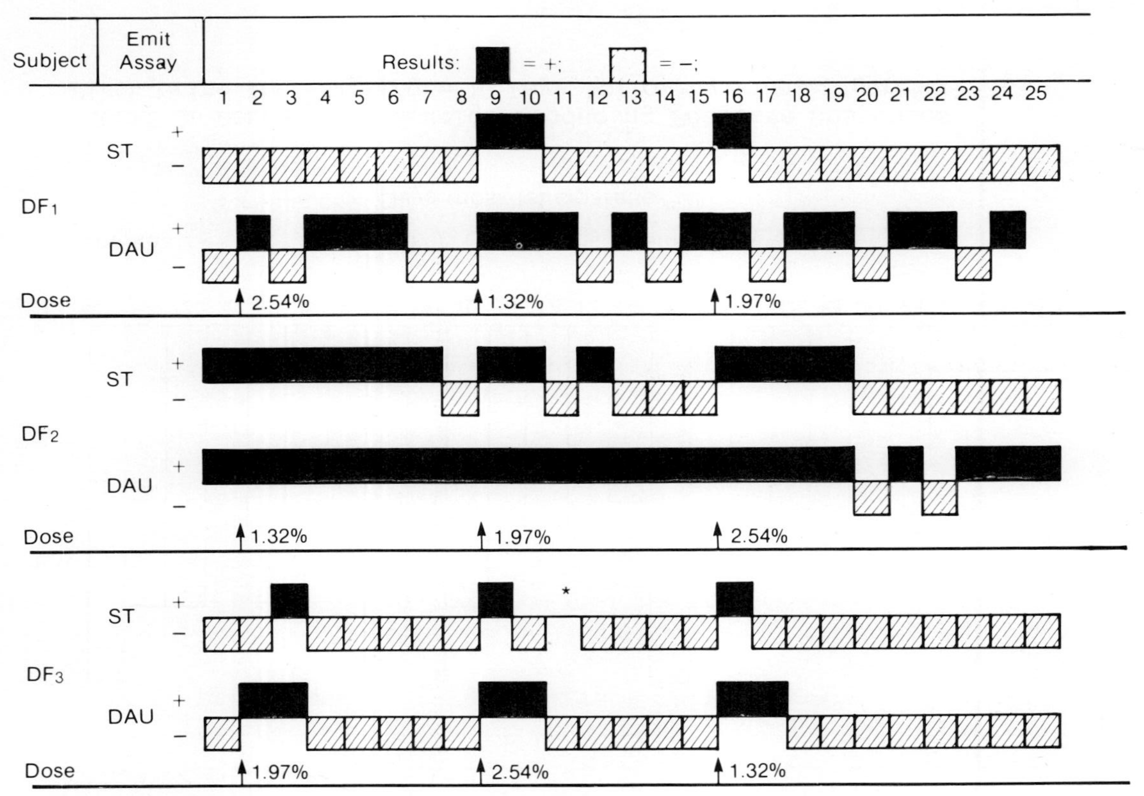
Subject
Emit Assay
Results: = +; = −;
1 2 3 4 5 6 7 8 9 10 11 12 13 14 15 16 17 18 19 20 21 22 23 24 25
DF1
ST
DAU
Dose
2.54%
1.32%
1.97%
DF2
ST
DAU
Dose
1.32%
1.97%
2.54%
DF3
ST
DAU
Dose
1.97%
2.54%
1.32%
*

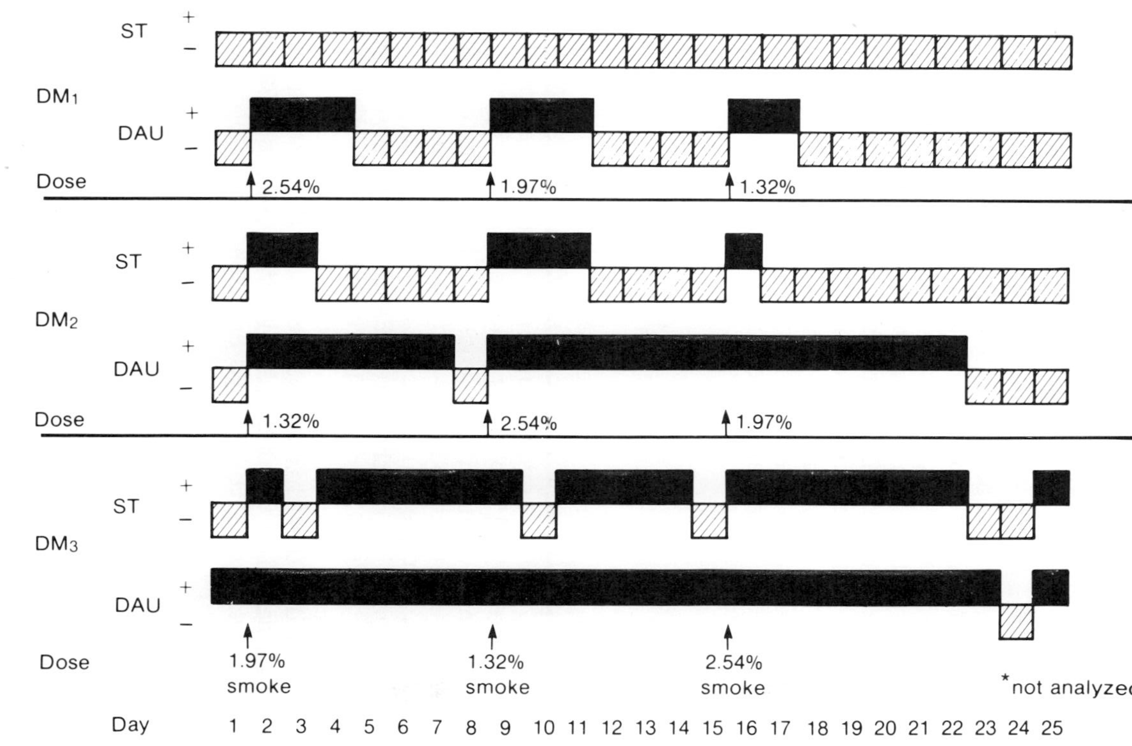

FIGURE 3. EMIT-st and EMIT-d.a.u. Comparison of Results for the Same Samples

D. Creatinine Study

Since the volume of urine produced can have an effect on the apparent concentration of a given substance, ng THC metabolite per mg creatinine was calculated for each sample. The results were then compared day to day and to each smoking episode in order to normalize the trends observed by analysis of the EMIT-d.a.u. data for possible dilution effects.

As can be seen from Figure 4, the ng THC metabolite per mg creatinine excretion patterns exhibit three distinct peaks that occur following smoking. Over time, the responses obtained declined between cigarettes and after the last cigarette until the end of the study. Although variability was apparent, the results exhibited patterns that appeared to be similar to those observed from the EMIT results. And, consistent with the EMIT data, the more frequent users (DF_2 and DM_3) were found to excrete cannabinoids at higher levels for greater numbers of consecutive days than the less frequent users.

E. Results Comparison

The results of these studies are consistent with the results of two previously reported smoking studies (20) also conducted by Dr. Perez-Reyes. In those studies, a total of 3 males and 4 females (all experienced users of marijuana) were asked to abstain from use for 6 days, to then smoke two 9 mg THC cigarettes within two hours and to abstain from further use for 10 days. Urine collected daily for 10 days and was stored and analyzed using the EMIT-d.a.u. assay. By comparing the total number of Positive results obtained each day following dosing (Figure 5), the trend was very similar to that observed following the third cigarette in the present study. Initially all samples produced Positive results; 45% of the samples were positive after 5 days and 25% after 10 days.

IV. DISCUSSION

A. EMIT-d.a.u.

Significant individual and subject to subject variability was observed; however, three peak responses corresponding to the smoking episodes were observed. In all cases, samples collected the day following smoking contained sufficient metabolites to produce Positive results. For the seventh through the tenth day of abstention, no more than 30% of the samples collected produced Positive results.

In general, the highest responses observed were those on the day following smoking; the responses then showed a general tendency to decline until the next dose. By the fourth day following the final cigarette, the responses obtained from all subjects showed a tendency to decline; no responses equal to or greater than the peak following the third cigarette were observed for the remainder of the study.

Of the less frequent users, all produced pre-smoking, Day 1 samples that were interpreted as Negative. Generally these subjects were found positive 2-5 days after each dose. In contrast, frequent users produced pre-smoking Positive responses and remained Positive for almost the duration of the 25 day study. Thus, the excretion patterns for both groups were dissimilar and the duration of detectable cannabinoid excretion was greater for the frequent users.

B. EMIT-st

Of the subjects who began the study with pre-smoking Negative results, all produced Positive responses for 1-3 days. These subjects also produced Negative results for the final nine days of abstinence following the third cigarette.

The two frequent users (DM_3 and DF_2) produced a greater number of consecutive daily Positive responses following each dose; both subjects produced as many as seven consecutive daily responses following one cigarette. By the tenth day following the final dose, subject DM_3 excreted sufficient metabolites to produce a Positive response; all other subjects had produced at least 6 consecutive daily Negative responses.

The trends observed were consistent with previous studies, and were confirmed when the data from both EMIT-st and EMIT-d.a.u. determinations were analyzed relative to creatinine excretion.

V. SUMMARY

Although general patterns were observed in the results obtained, the results are not indicative of intoxication or the time elapsed since using marijuana. In general, however, the difference in the duration of consecutive Positive responses for less frequent users versus frequent users appeared to be the result of cannabinoid metabolite excretion due not only to the doses administered but to the subject's previous habit of frequent use.

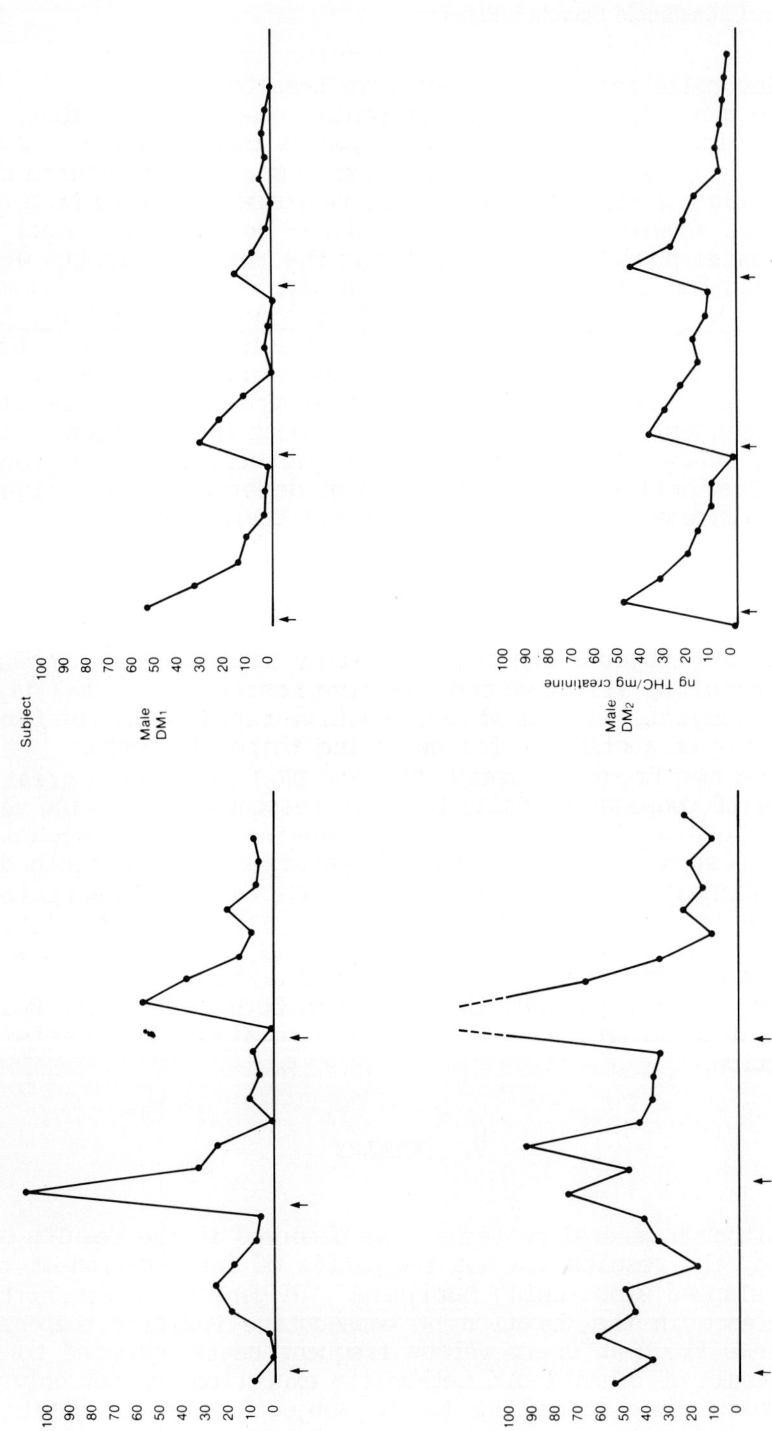
Subject
Male
DM_1
Male
DM_2
ng THC/mg creatinine
100
90
80
70
60
50
40
30
20
10
0

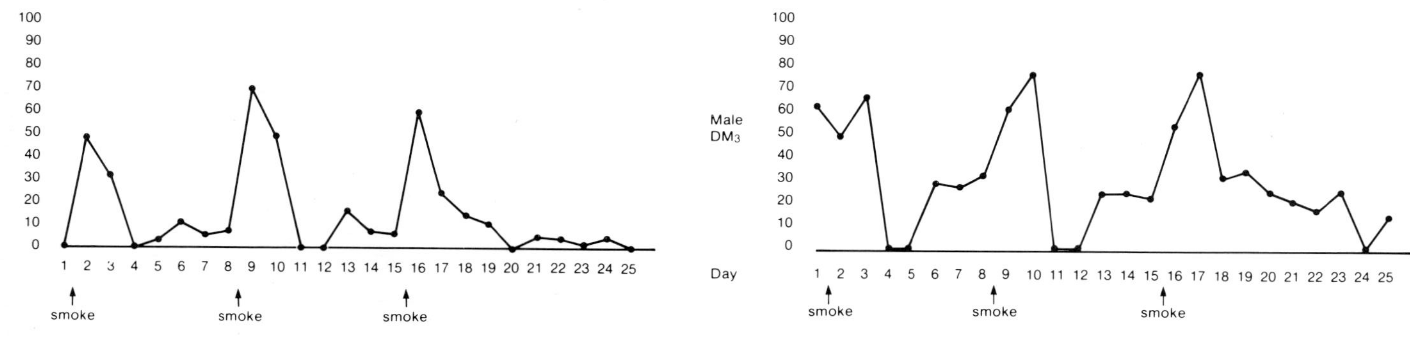

FIGURE 4. Males and Females - ng THC metabolite per mg creatinine per day.

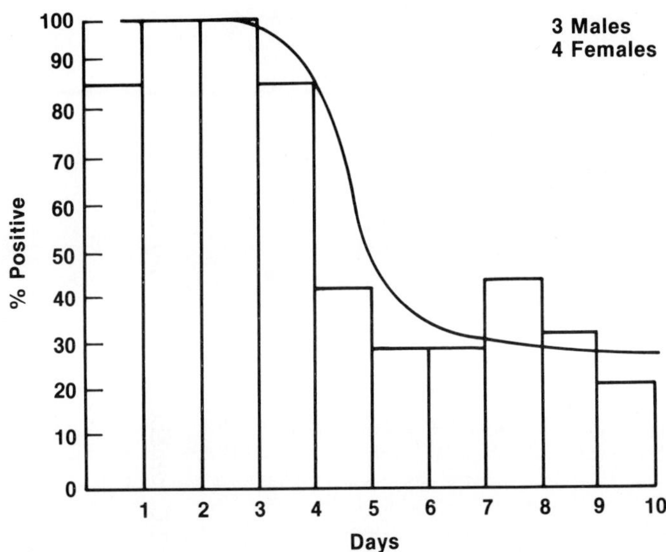

FIGURE 5. Percent of EMIT-d.a.u. Positive responses obtained per day following smoking of two marijuana cigarettes (n = 7).

EMIT-d.a.u. urinary excretion patterns, following weekly smoking episodes in a three week period, exhibited cyclic peak and decline profiles which allowed differentiation of each smoking episode. Peak response occurred 1-2 days after smoking and less frequent users remained Positive for 2-5 days while frequent users remained Positive for up to 10 days. A general declining trend followed the peak level, for all subjects.

Excretion patterns were highly individual, however cannabinoids were also detectable by the EMIT-st 100 ng/ml calibrator for up to 10 days following smoking for frequent users while less frequent users produced no more than 3 EMIT-st Positives following any dose.

Data on blood levels of THC, psychological rating and heart rate acceleration of these subjects were also collected according to a double blind protocol. All three parameters could be correlated with dose of marijuana (15).

REFERENCES

1. American Academy of Pediatrics, Committee on Drugs: Effects of marijuana on man, Pediatr. 56:134-143 (1975).
2. Hollister, L. E., Kanter, S. L., Moore, F., et al., Marijuana metabolites in urine of man, Clin. Pharmacol. Ther. 13:849-855 (1972).
3. Seventh Annual Report to the U.S Congress from the Secretary of Health, Education, and Welfare, NIDA: Marijuana and health, 1977.
4. Martin, W. R., General problems of drug abuse and drug dependence, in "Drug addiction I", (W. R. Martin, ed.) pp. 3-40. Springer-Verlag, New York, 1977.
5. Karler, R., Chemistry and metabolism, in "Marijuana research findings: 1976" (R. C. Petersen, ed.) pp. 55-66. NIDA Research Monograph 14, 1977.
6. Alli, B. A., Marijuana and the adolescent, J. Natl. Med. Assoc. 70:677-680 (1978).
7. Report of AMA Council on Scientific Affairs: Health aspects of marihuana use, Conn. Med. 42:377-380 (1980).
8. Perez-Reyes, M., Lipton, M. A., Timmons, M. C. et al.; Pharmacology of orally administered delta-9-tetrahydrocannabinol, Clin. Pharmacol. Ther. 14:48-55 (1973).
9. Wall, M. E., Brine, D. R., and Perez-Reyes, M., Metabolism of cannabinoids in man, in "The pharmacology of marijuana". (M. C. Braude and S. Szara, eds.), pp. 93-116. Raven Press, New York, 1976.
10. Lemberger, L, Axelrod, J., and Kopin, I. J.; Metabolism and disposition of tetrahydrocannabinols in naive subjects and chronic marijuana users, Ann. N. Y. Acad. Sci. 191:142-154 (1971).
11. Ohlsson, A., Lindgren, J., Wahlen, A., Agurell, S., Hollister, L. E., and Gillespie, H. K., Plasma concentrations of delta-9-tetrahydrocannabinol and clinical effects following three routes of administration, Clin. Pharmacol. Ther. (in press).
12. Rodgers, R., Crowl, D. P., Eimstaad, W. M., et al.; Homogeneous enzyme immunoassay for cannabinoids in urine, Clin. Chem. 24:95-100 (1978).
13. Harris, L. S., Dewey, W. L. and Razdan, R. K., Cannabis: Its chemistry, pharmacology and toxicology, in "Drug Addiction II", (W. R. Martin, ed.) pp. 371-431. Springer-Verlag, New York, 1977.
14. Rowley, G. L., Armstrong, T. A., Crowl, C. P. et al., Determination of THC ad its metabolites by EMIT homogeneous enzyme immunoassay -- a summary report, in "Cannabinoid assay in humans". (R. E. Willette, ed.), pp. 28-32. NIDA Research Monograph 7, 1976.

15. Perez-Reyes, M., et al., J. Clin. Pharmacol. Ther. 31:617-624 (1982).
16. Rubenstein, K. E., Schneider, R. S., and Ullman, E. F., "Homogeneous" enzyme immunoassay: A new immunochemical technique, Biochem. Biophys. Res. Commun. 47:846-851 (1972).
17. Bastiani, R. J., Phillips, R. C., Schneider, R. S., et al., Homogeneous immunochemical drug assays, Amer. J. Med. Tech. 39:211-216 (1973).
18. Rubenstein, K. E., Homogeneous enzyme immunoassay today, Scand. J. Immunol. Suppl 7:57-62 (1978).
19. Green, D. E., Chao, E. C., Loeffler, K. O. et al., Quantitation of delta-9-tetrahydrocannabinol and its metabolites in human urine by probability based matching GC/MS, in "Cannabinoid Analysis in Physiological Fluids", (J. A. Vinson, ed.), pp. 93-113. ACS Symposium Series, 1979.
20. Clark, S., Turner, J., and Bastiani, R., EMIT Cannabinoid Assay: Clinical Study No. 74: Summary Report, Syva Company, Palo Alto, CA., 1980.
21. Marijuana and the EMIT Cannabinoid Assay, Syva Company, June 1981.

URINE EXCRETION PATTERNS OF CANNABINOIDS AND THE CLINICAL APPLICATION OF THE EMIT-d.a.u. CANNABINOID URINE ASSAY FOR SUBSTANCE ABUSE TREATMENT

Joseph E. Manno
Kenneth E. Ferslew*
Barbara R. Manno

Department of Pharmacology and Therapeutics
Section on Toxicology
Louisiana State University School of Medicine
Shreveport, Louisiana

I. INTRODUCTION

Although the use of urine drug screens has provided a valuable adjunct to treatment of individuals who abuse drugs, the commonly used analytical methodology of thin layer and gas liquid chromatography has not been used to screen for the presence of cannabinoids. In addition, the long duration of excretion of cannabinoids (1,2) requires that a quantitative or semi-quantitative determination be made to differentiate between various patterns of marijuana use and long term excretion of cannabinoids in the absence of recent marijuana use.

The clinical availability of the EMIT-d.a.u. Cannabinoid Urine Assay has provided an analytical technique that will semi-quantitatively determine the concentration of "total cannabinoids" in urine. The antibody used in the enzyme immunoassay technique will react not only with delta-9-tetrahydrocannabinol (THC) but also with its principal urinary metabolite, 11-nor-delta-9-THC-9-carboxylic acid and other metabolites, including 11-hydroxy-, 8-alpha-hydroxy-, and 8-beta-11-hydroxy-delta-9-THC in both their conjugated and non-

*Present address: East Tennesee State University, School of Medicine, Department of Pharmacology, Johnson City, TN.

ISBN 0-12-044620-0

conjugated forms. The minimum detectable concentration for the assay is 20 ng of cannabinoids per milliliter of urine and the 95% confidence limit is at 50 ng/ml (3), which makes the test extremely sensitive and capable of detecting both recent marijuana use and chronic excretion of cannabinoids. The assay is available in kit form. One kit is designed for use with a semi-automated assay system (described above) and another is designed for use with a single test instrument and has a cut-off of 100 ng/ml (4).

The purpose of this investigation was to determine if excretion patterns of cannabinoids, as measured by the EMIT-d.a.u. cannabinoids assay, were similar to those reported by previous investigators (1,2). We also wanted to determine if excretion patterns in clinical situations are the same as those in more controlled experimental conditions.

II. MATERIALS AND METHODS

All urine assays were performed using the EMIT-d.a.u. Cannabinoid Urine Assay (Syva Company, Palo Alto,CA). Results were reported as nanograms of cannabinoids per milliliter of urine by comparing reaction rates of patient specimens to a standard concentration curve constructed using the negative, low (20 ng/ml) and medium (75 ng/ml) calibrators supplied with the assay kit. All urine specimens were kept frozen for storage and thawed just prior to analysis.

Urine creatinine concentrations were also determined on all urines using the Centrifichem System 400 centrifugal analyzer and the Centrifichem Creatinine Assay kit and standards (Baker Instruments Corporation, Pleasantville, NY).

A thin-layer chromatography drug screen (5) was also performed on each urine to determine if non-cannabinoid drugs known to cross-react with the Emit reagents were present.

Urine cannabinoid concentrations (UCC) were expressed as nanograms/milliliter of urine and nanograms/milligram of creatinine. In order to determine the urinary excretion patterns of the cannabinoids, marijuana cigarettes (6) calibrated (7) to deliver 37.5 mcg/kg or 75 mcg/kg THC were administered to 12 normal male volunteers who had reported casual marijuana use. Each subject received both cigarettes at different times with at least one week separating the smoking periods. Urine specimens were collected at two hours after smoking and each successive morning for seven consecutive days following the smoking period.

In another phase of this investigation, the UCC from clients in treatment at substance abuse clinics who had their urines assayed weekly was correlated with their reported patterns of marijuana use.

In addition, 250 random urines obtained from marijuana smokers under treatment in substance abuse clinics were assayed for UCC.

UCC expressed as ng cannabinoids/ml urine was determined by comparing the patient's assay reaction rate to that of the standard curve. Concentrations expressed as ng cannabinoid/mg creatinine were determined by dividing the ng cannabinoid/ml urine concentration by the urine creatinine concentration.

III. RESULTS

The UCC's resulting from smoking either the 37.5 mcg/kg THC or 75 mcg/kg THC marijuana cigarettes are represented in Figures 1 and 2. The data is plotted as the mean value from 12 subjects. UCC may be read from the cannabinoid concentration scale on the y-axis. Urine creatinine concentrations for the same time periods are shown above the UCC and values can

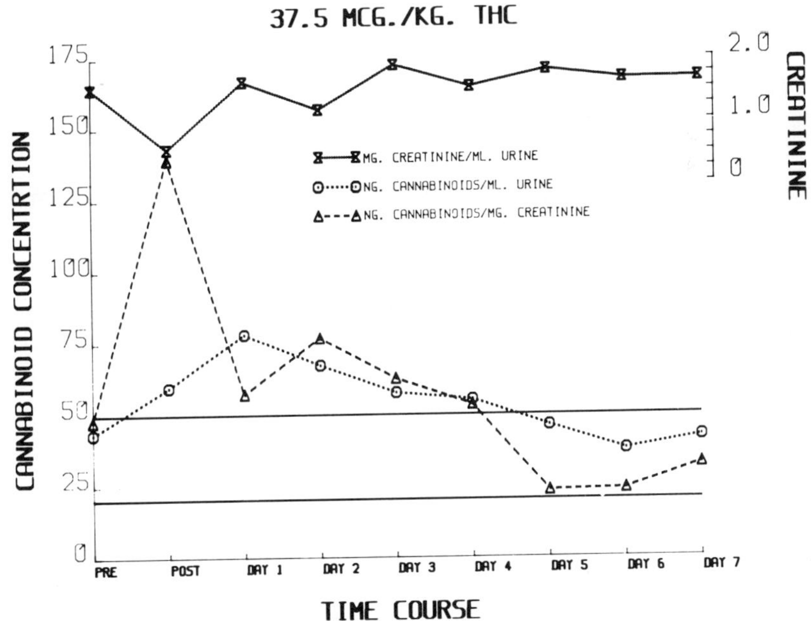

FIGURE 1. Urine cannabinoid concentrations resulting from smoking cigarettes delivering 37.5 mcg/kg THC.

be read from the creatinine scale in the upper right corner of the figure. Actual values with their standard deviations are shown in Table I. It should be noted that the urines collected prior to smoking contained a UCC of approximately 50 ng cannabinoids/ml urine.

There was no statistically significant ($p < .01$) difference between the UCC when reported in terms of cannabinoids/ml urine or as cannabinoids/mg creatinine except at the 2 hr. post-smoking time period.

Figure 3 shows representative data from individuals who had Emit-d.a.u. Cannabinoid assays performed on a weekly basis as part of their regular monitoring in a substance abuse clinic. It can be seen that the rise and fall in UCC correlated more closely to reported marijuana smoking when the assay results were reported as ng cannabinoid/mg creatinine. There were three instances where UCC correlated to reported marijuana smoking only if the results were expressed as ng cannabinoids/mg creatinine. These were: patient A, week 1; Patient C, week 9 and Patient D, week 10. The UCC data from patient B expressed as ng/ml urine suggested that the client smoked at weeks 4 and 5. UCC data from this same patient

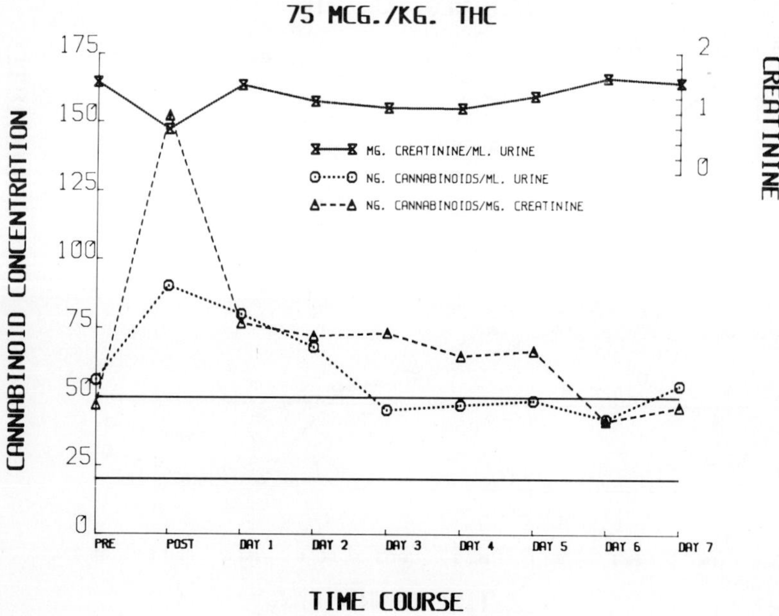

FIGURE 2. Urine cannabinoid concentrations resulting from smoking cigarettes delivering 75 mcg/kg THC.

expressed as ng/mg creatinine indicated that smoking did not occur, a conclusion that correlated with the history.

Data obtained from 250 random urines as shown in Table I. There was no statistically significant difference between UCC when reported by either unit of measure.

No drugs known to cross-react with the Emit-d.a.u. Cannabinoid assay were detected by the thin-layer chromatography urine drug screens.

IV. DISCUSSION

The Emit-d.a.u. Urine Cannabinoid Assay can be used for detecting marijuana use. Because the antibody can cross-react with several of the known metabolites of THC as well as with conjugated and non-conjugated metabolites, the assay is extremely sensitive (3). The metabolites of THC are excreted slowly (1,2) over a period of days to a week(s) and their

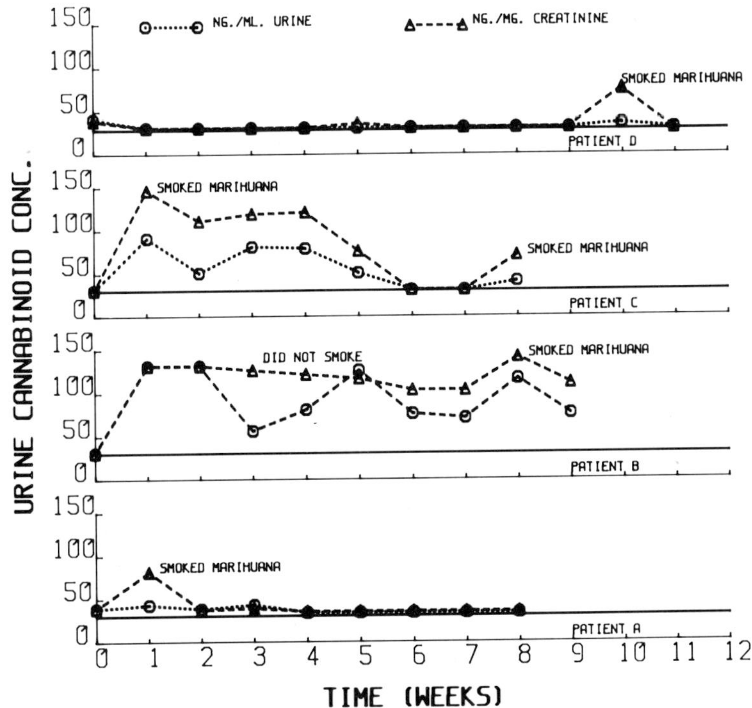

FIGURE 3. Weekly urine cannabinoid concentrations from patients being monitored in a substance abuse clinic.

TABLE I

THC Dose	Period		Concentration Urine (mL.)	Concentration Creatinine (mg.)
Random	Pre-Smoking	Mean	72.22	74.93
		S.D.	26.32	70.54
		Min.	12.00	6.90
		Max.	175.00	385.30
37.5 mcg/kg	Pre-Smoking	Mean	43.25	47.65
		S.D.	36.58	52.80
		Min.	0.00	0.00
		Max.	127.00	182.54
	Post-Smoking	Mean	59.35	139.29
		S.D.	33.40	73.27
		Min.	9.00	47.09
		Max.	127.00	280.41
	Day 1	Mean	78.02	56.94
		S.D.	24.99	28.71
		Min.	47.50	16.26
		Max.	124.00	128.63
	Day 2	Mean	67.06	76.51
		S.D.	29.13	83.38
		Min.	24.50	24.69
		Max.	132.00	346.10
	Day 3	Mean	57.42	62.36
		S.D.	34.26	100.64
		Min.	0.00	0.00
		Max.	124.75	382.94
	Day 4	Mean	55.02	53.22
		S.D.	39.93	75.15
		Min.	10.50	8.88
		Max.	121.50	293.07
	Day 5	Mean	45.94	23.00
		S.D.	42.77	20.35
		Min.	0.00	0.00
		Max	133.50	61.41
	Day 6	Mean	37.48	23.57
		S.D.	39.41	24.83
		Min.	0.00	0.00
		Max	131.00	83.06
	Day 7	Mean	42.04	32.40
		S.D.	38.00	35.56
		Min.	0.00	0.00
		Max.	121.50	127.75

THC Dose	Period		Concentration Urine (mL.)	Concentration Creatinine (mg.)
75 mcg/kg	Pre-Smoking	Mean	55.90	46.82
		S.D.	47.83	44.52
		Min.	0.00	0.00
		Max.	146.50	148.73
	Post-Smoking	Mean	90.10	152.11
		S.D.	27.74	71.26
		Min.	36.50	28.79
		Max.	124.25	294.96
	Day 1	Mean	79.79	76.52
		S.D.	25.90	44.80
		Min.	45.00	19.21
		Max.	131.00	155.46
	Day 2	Mean	67.81	71.91
		S.D.	28.53	48.75
		Min.	24.50	13.84
		Max.	112.00	187.50
	Day 3	Mean	45.08	72.99
		S.D.	26.13	101.49
		Min.	0.00	0.00
		Max.	102.00	400.00
	Day 4	Mean	46.83	64.49
		S.D.	35.17	104.91
		Min.	0.00	0.00
		Max.	103.50	414.00
	Day 5	Mean	48.37	66.37
		S.D.	39.09	99.37
		Min.	5.00	3.14
		Max.	117.50	386.72
	Day 6	Mean	41.65	41.01
		S.D.	32.00	53.37
		Min.	0.00	0.00
		Max.	120.25	207.55
	Day 7	Mean	53.75	46.04
		S.D.	39.09	43.05
		Min.	14.25	8.05
		Max.	117.50	151.12

concentrations in urine are in the range detectable by the assay, therefore it is possible to detect marijuana use for several days to weeks after smoking. Since the psychologic or pharmacologic effects of smoking marijuana dissipate within a period of up to several hours (7), the results of the urine test cannot be reliably related to drug effects.

Our initial data from random urines suggested that there was no difference in cannabinoid concentrations (see Table I) when reported in concentration per ml urine or mg creatinine. Mean data from 12 subjects also indicated that there was no significant difference in urine cannabinoid concentrations, when expressed by the two units, except at the 2 hour post-smoking time. Examination of clinical data from individuals using marijuana, however, indicates that differences in excretion patterns occur when expressed by the two differentunits. Data from individual patients (Figure 3) demonstrates that UCC, when expressed as ng/ml urine, does not correspond to admitted marijuana smoking activity in all cases.

Our clinical implementation of the assay is to detect both casual and chronic marijuana use. In order to differentiate between recent marijuana use, it is necessary to adjust for changes in UCC caused by urine dilution or concentration and to determine if the UCC increases or decreases with time. A urine drug screen is also performed on each urine to rule out false positives due to drugs known to cross-react with the antibody.

We developed the following procedure (8) to facilitate use of the assay. After intake, each client's urine is assayed for cannabinoids. The UCC expressed in both units is recorded on graph paper correlated to collection time. Client urines are then tested at weekly intervals until the urine concentration falls below our cut-off (set at 30 ng/ml urine). It is expected that the urine concentration of cannabinoids will decrease and become undetectable within several days to weeks depending on the previous marijuana use patterns.

During this "return to baseline" period, any increases in UCC that are 50% higher than the previous UCC are attributed to marijuana use. To reduce the likelihood of random changes in UCC due to dilution or concentration of urine being improperly interpreted as marijuana use, we adjust the UCC by means of urine creatinine concentrations. The use of this procedure gives clients the maximum benefit for interpretation of test results. Once the client's UCC has decreased to that concentration below our assay cut-off, testing is performed on a less frequent and random basis. Subsequent UCC above our cut-off are considered to be caused by marijuana use.

V. CONCLUSION

We have found the EMIT-d.a.u. Cannabinoid Assay to be useful for detecting and monitoring marijuana use in a urine surveillance program. With the limited data that we have gathered, we feel that it is necessary to express UCC concentrations both in terms of ng/ml urine and ng/mg creatinine when attempting to monitor marijuana use patterns.

ACKNOWLEDGMENTS

Our sincere appreciation is given to Dr. Richard L. Hawks, Research Technology Branch, National Institute on Drug Abuse, for supplying us with the marijuana cigarettes along with his continued support of this project. Also, we are very grateful to Dr. Richard Bastiani, Vice President for Clinical Studies, Syva Company, for the supply of Urine Cannabinoid Assay kits needed for the controlled clinical investigation. We also wish to thank Mrs. Susie Jobe for her editorial assistance in the preparation of this manuscript.

REFERENCES

1. Lemberger, L., The pharmacokinetics of delta-9-tetrahydrocannabinol and its metabolites: Importance and relationship in developing methods for detecting cannabis in biologic fluids, in "Marihuana: Chemistry, Biochemistry, and Cellular Effects", (G. G. Nahas, W. D. M. Paton and J. E. Idänpään-Heikkilä, eds.), pp. 169-178. Springer-Verlag, New York, 1976.
2. Wall, M. E., Brine, D. R., and Perez-Reyes, M., Metabolism of cannabinoids in man, in "The Pharmacology of Marijuana" (M. C. Braude and S. Szara, eds.), pp. 93-116, Raven Press, New York, 1976.
3. Emit-d.a.u. Urine Cannabinoid Assay, product brochure. Syva Co., Palo Alto, CA 94303.
4. EMIT-st Urine Cannabinoid Assay, product brochure, Syva Company, Palo Alto, CA 94303.
5. Urine Drug Screening procedure. Clinical Toxicology Laboratory - Manual of Procedure. L.S.U. Medical Center, Shreveport, Louisiana 71130.
6. Marijuana cigarettes were obtained through Dr. Richard Hawks, National Institute on Drug Abuse, Rockville, MD. Doses were individualized based on the subject's weight

by removing sufficient marijuana from cigarettes containing 0.86%, 1.54% or 1.83% THC to deliver the desired dose.

7. Manno, J. E., Kiplinger, G. F., Haine, S. E., Bennett, I. F., and Forney, R. B., Comparative effects of smoking marijuana or placebo on human motor and mental performance, Clin. Pharmacol. Ther. 11:808-815 (1970).
8. Manno, J. E., and Manno, B. R., Urine cannabinoid assay. A manual prepared for professionals using the Cannabinoid Assay supplied by the Clinical Toxicology Laboratory (Copyrighted, 1982).

PHARMACOKINETICS OF DELTA-9-TETRAHYDROCANNABINOL IN RABBITS AND MICE WITH MEASUREMENTS TO THE LOW PICOGRAM RANGE BY COMBINED GAS CHROMATOGRAPHY/MASS SPECTROMETRY USING METASTABLE ION DETECTION*

D. J. Harvey, J. T. A. Leuschner
D. R. Wing, W. D. M. Paton

Department of Pharmacology
Oxford University
Oxford, United Kingdom

I. INTRODUCTION

Although a large number of assays have now been reported for delta-9-tetrahydrocannabinol (THC) (4,28,30), none is sufficiently sensitive to measure the drug in plasma to levels below about 100 pg/ml. Consequently pharmacokinetic studies of the drug are scarce as the levels reached during the elimination phase are well below this figure. Nevertheless, Lemberger et al. (19) have obtained a value of 56 hours for the elimination half life in non-users of the drug based on measurements with [^{14}C]THC and a somewhat lower value of 28 hours (20) in experienced users. Wall and Perez-Reyes (29) in studies using GC/MS have reported values of 33.2 +/- 4.7 and 22.7 +/- 4 hours for male and female subjects, respectively, following intravenous administration and values of 32.4 +/- 4.7 and 24.5 +/- 10.0 for the same subjects after an oral dose. However, measurements were only made to 48 hours. Ohlsson et al. have concluded that the final phase is not reached until at least 72 hours and was probably not achieved in their study which indicated a value of 20 hours (25). Experiments with dogs by Garrett and Hunt using electron-capture GLC and radiolabelling have indicated a half life of

*Supported by a Medical Research Council Programme Research Grant and the Wellcome Trust.

ISBN 0-12-044620-0

around 8 days with the plasma curve exhibiting up to 5 exponential phases (7).

It is evident from these studies that for meaningful results to be obtained, the assay must be capable of measurement to the low picogram/ml or even the high femtogram/ml range, that is, some two or three orders of magnitude better than existing assays. This range is in fact within the capability of existing techniques, such as GC/MS, providing that pure compounds are examined. However, these levels are not usually achieved when drugs such as THC are measured in extracts of biological media, because co-extracted lipids invariably generate ions of the same nominal mass as those required for measurement of the drug and contribute significantly to the background noise level. Extensive purification stages are thus a feature of most available assays. Reducing the polarity of the extracting solvent gives improved signal: noise ratios as demonstrated by Rosenthal et al. (27) and further improvement can be achieved by increasing the selectivity of the mass spectrometer either by reducing the number of ions produced by means of chemical ionization (5) or by using high resolution to select ions of a given composition rather than of a specific nominal mass.

In this paper we report the use of a highly sensitive assay for THC in plasma and tissues based on GC/MS with metastable ion monitoring. This technique, first introduced by Gaskell and Millington for steroid analysis (6), increases the selectivity of a double focussing mass spectrometer by monitoring a metastable transition from the first field free region. Ions of the same nominal mass as that monitored but formed from a different precursor ion will not be transmitted by the electrostatic analyser. As most of these ions arise from the residual lipids, the final signal:noise ratio is greatly improved and hence high sensitivity can be achieved. The present assay is capable of measuring THC in plasma to 5 pg/ml and in tissue to 200 pg/g (wet weight) using a tetradeuterated analogue of cannabinol (CBN) as the internal standard; details of the plasma assay have been published (9). This paper describes the assays and their application to the study of THC pharmacokinetics in rabbits and mice together with corresponding measurements in tissues. Finally application to the measurement of THC levels in ocular fluids and tissues and in erythrocyte membranes will be described.

II. METHODS

A. Materials

THC (98% pure by GLC) was obtained from NIDA. [1',1',2',2'-$^2H_4$]CBN was synthesized from [1',1',2',2'-$^2H_4$]THC (13) by dehydrogenation with chloranil (22-24). N,O-Bis-(trimethylsilyl)trifluoroacetamide (BSTFA) and "Diazald" were obtained from Aldrich Chemical Co. All solvents were distilled twice before use and all glassware was silanized with a 5% solution of dichlorodimethylsilane in toluene followed by treatment with methanol.

B. Quantitation of THC in Plasma

Full details of recovery and estimates of precision have been published (9). [$^2H_4$]CBN in ethanol was added to the plasma sample at a concentration such that the final THC and [$^2H_4$]CBN GLC peak heights were comparable, and allowed to equilibrate with plasma proteins for at least 30 min. The cannabinoids were extracted 3 times with 2 ml of redistilled hexane each sample being agitated for 2 min on a vortex mixer. Samples were centrifugated at 1,500 g for 10 min to break the resulting emulsion and the combined extracts were evaporated to dryness with a nitrogen stream in a 0.3 ml conical vial. The residue was taken up in methanol (ca 20 mcl) and an excess of ethereal diazomethane, prepared from "Diazald" was added. After 2 min the solution was again blown to dryness and dissolved in BSTFA (20 mcl). The mixture was heated for 10 min at 60° and aliquots (0.1-5 mcl) were examined by GC/MS. Standard curves were constructed by adding known amounts of THC and [$^2H_4$]CBN to the plasma and extracting them by the above procedure.

C. Quantitation of THC in Tissues

Samples of the tissue (ca. 2 g) were chopped and homogenized in isotonic saline. [$^2H_4$]CBN was added and the cannabinoids were extracted as described above. Before the methylation stage, the extract was chromatographed in chloroform on a 5 g column (1 cm diameter) of Sephadex LH-20 and the fraction eluting between 18 and 37 ml was collected. This was evaporated to dryness in a 0.3 ml conical vial, methylated and trimethylsilylated as described above. For fat samples, two passes through the column were necessary in order to reduce the triglyceride levels sufficiently.

D. GC/MS

Metastable GC/MS analysis was performed with a V.G. Analytical 70/70 F mass spectrometer interfaced via a glass jet separator to a Varian 2440 gas chromatograph. It was fitted with a 2 m x 2 mm (ID) glass column packed with 3% SE-30 on 100-120 mesh Gas Chrom Q (Applied Science Laboratories Inc., State College). The injector, column, separator and ion source temperatures were 300°, 220°, 300° and 280°C, respectively, and helium at 30 ml/min was used as the carrier gas. The mass spectrometer slits were opened to give flat-topped peaks at a resolution of about 700 and the magnet was tuned to $\underline{m}/\underline{z}$ 371, the $[M-CH_3]^+$ ion from the trimethylsilyl (TMS) derivative of THC, with the accelerating voltage at 4 kV. The accelerating voltage was then raised to 4.16 kV to bring the metastable ion into focus and the source controls were optimized for maximum sensitivity. The trap current was 1 mA and the electron energy 70 eV.

E. Pharmacokinetics of THC in Rabbits

THC in Tween 80 and isotonic saline was injected over 30 sec into the marginal ear vein of 4 female New Zealand white rabbits (ca. 2 kg) at doses of 1 mg/kg, n = 4 (rabbits 2-4 and 9) and 0.1 mg/kg, n = 1 (rabbit 7). Blood samples, 0.5-1 ml for early time periods and 3-5 ml for later fractions, were collected into heparinized tubes at intervals from the marginal ear vein of the ear not used for the injection, starting immediately after the injection and continuing until the drug could no longer be detected. The plasma was separated by centrifugation and stored at -2°C until required for analysis. Some 6-7 weeks later the animals were treated with the same dose of the drug daily for either 8 (n = 2, rabbits 2 and 3) or 22 days (n = 1, rabbit 4) and blood sampling was commenced immediately after the last dose. In a further set of experiments, 4 rabbits (Nos. 8-11) were treated as above with 1 mg/kg of THC, plasma samples were collected and the animals were killed at 28 h 40 min, 54 h 35 min, 191 h 50 min and 240 h after treatment. Samples of brain, spleen, lung, heart, peritoneal fat and renal fat were collected for THC analysis as described above. A further 4 rabbits (Nos. 13-16) were treated daily for 8 days and killed at 96 h 20 min, 192 hr 5 min, 264 h and at 406 h 45 min after the last dose. Tissues were sampled as above.

F. Pharmacokinetics of THC in Mice

Groups of 4 mice (male, Charles River, CD-1, 23-25 g) were treated with THC in Tween 80 and isotonic saline into the tail vein at a dose of 10 mg/kg. The animals were killed by cervical dislocation at various times after drug treatment and blood (pooled from all animals at each time point) and brain samples were collected. These were treated as above.

G. Measurement of THC in Ocular Fluids and Tissues

Female New Zealand white rabbits (2 kg) were anaesthetized with chloralose and urethane, and aqueous humour was collected by insertion of a fine needle through the centre of the cornea into the anterior chamber, the fluid being allowed to flow continuously into a silanized glass vial at or slightly above the level of the eye. THC (1 mg/kg) in Tween 80 and isotonic saline was administered into the marginal ear vein and the accumulated aqueous humour was collected at intervals together with a plasma sample. The animals were killed from 3-5 hours after drug administration, the eyes were removed and vitreous humour, lens and uvea were collected. Levels of THC in these fluids and tissues were measured as described above for plasma. Full experimental details will be published later.

H. Measurement of THC in Mouse Erythrocyte Membranes

Groups of 4 mice were treated with THC in Tween 80 and isotonic saline by injection into the tail vein at a dose of 10 mg/kg and killed at various times after drug administration. The pooled blood samples from mice killed at each time point were centrifuged to collect the erythrocytes and the membranes were prepared by the method of Hanahan and Ekholm (8). THC was extracted and measured as described above for plasma and protein was measured by the method of Lowry et al. (21).

III. RESULTS AND DISCUSSION

The assay relies mainly for its high sensitivity achieved by monitoring a metastable ion rather than a fragment ion. By increasing the accelerating voltage of the spectrometer to a value that gives the parent ion an amount of energy equal to that lost during the metastable transition in the first field-free region, it is possible to transmit the fragment ions from

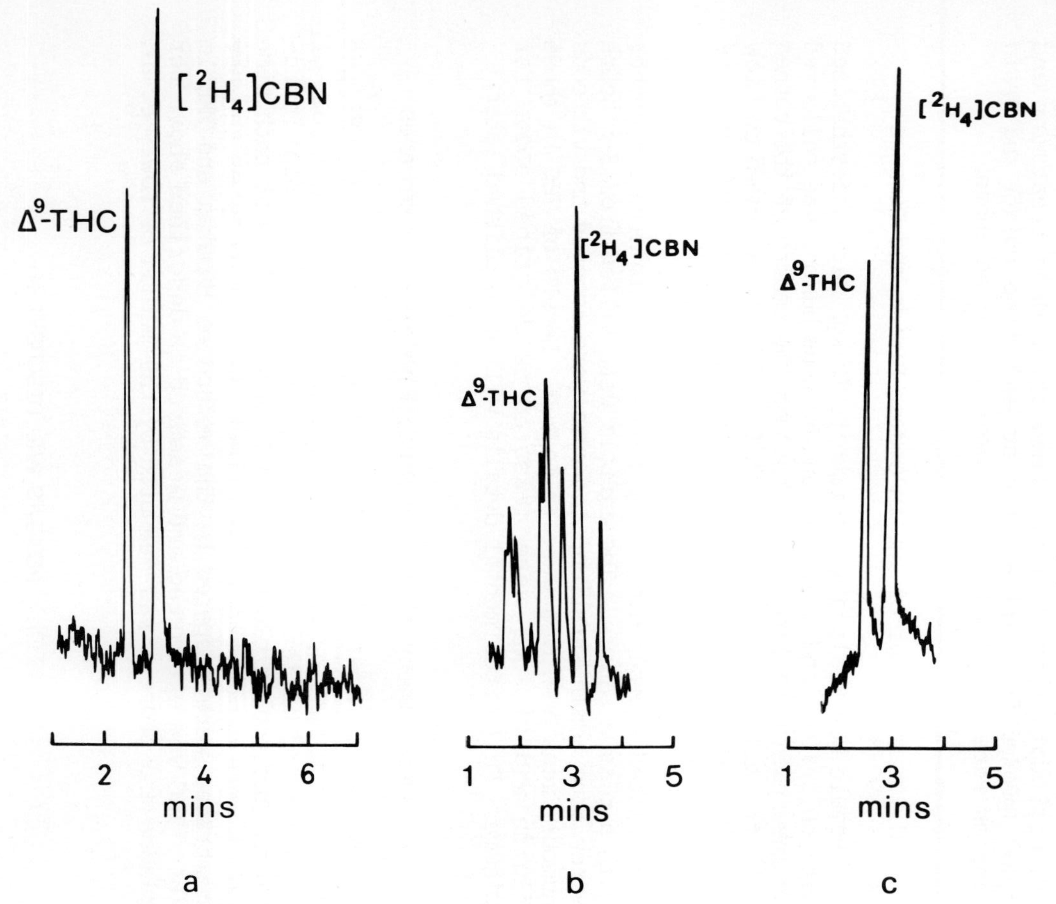

Δ9-THC
[2H4]CBN
2
4
6
mins
a
Δ9-THC
[2H4]CBN
1
3
5
mins
b
Δ9-THC
[2H4]CBN
1
3
5
mins
c

THC formed by metastable transition and, at the same time, filter out most of the lipid-derived ions which are formed by different mechanisms. For this assay, the TMS derivatives of THC were chosen; previous work with conventional single ion monitoring of free THC and of several derivatives has shown that derivatization considerably improves the sensitivity although little difference is seen if the derivative is changed (12). This latter effect arises as the result of charge localization remote from the derivatized function, at the pyran oxygen. The most prominant metastable ion in the mass spectrum of the TMS derivative of THC corresponds to the loss of a methyl group from the molecular ion ($M^+ > [M-CH_3]^+$, *m/z* 386 > *m/z* 371). Although greater selectivity could possibly be achieved by choosing a more specific transition, the other metastable ions in the spectra gave a weaker response and thus lower overall sensitivity. Using the $M^+ > [M-CH_3]^+$ metastable transition, a detection limit for THC TMS ether of about 500 fg was established.

It has been reported that greater precision can be obtained with mass spectrometric quantitation if single rather than multiple ion recording is adopted (18). This is because changes in the electric and magnetic fields are not involved and thus instrumental variables are minimized. As monitoring two metastable transitions with ions of different mass would require simultaneous alteration of two fields, single ion detection would appear to offer the most accurate method of ion monitoring. This internal standard must therefore separate from THC on the GLC column and have the same metastable transition. For this assay, CBN, labelled with four deuterium atoms in the side-chain to provide the same molecular weight and metastable ion, fulfilled these requirements and was adopted. The labels appeared stable; no exchange of the benzylic deuteriums has been observed in two years of use. Retention times and response factors were appropriate as can be seen from Fig. 1a.

When these compounds were added to and then extracted from plasma and derivatized with BSTFA alone, some residual lipid

FIGURE 1. Metastable ion chromatogram (*m/z* 386-371) of:

a) THC (10 pg) and 1',1',2',2'-$^2H_4$ CBN (20 pg) as their TMS derivatives;

b) the same concentrations of those compounds added to plasma, extracted with hexane and converted to TMS derivatives;

c) the effect of methylation with diazomethane prior to TMS formation. The THC peak corresponds to about 7 pg extracted from plasma. Reprinted from ref. 9 with permission.

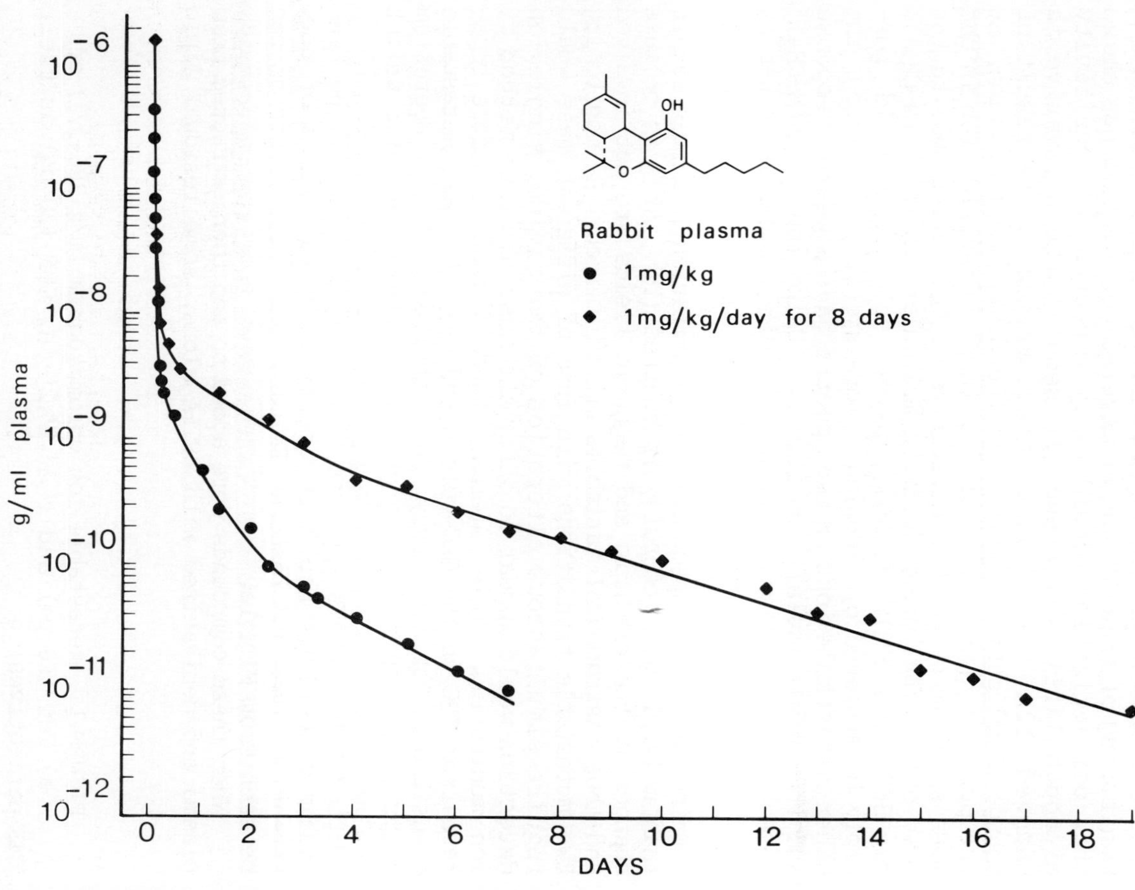
OH
O
Rabbit plasma
1mg/kg
1mg/kg/day for 8 days
g/ml plasma
10^{-6}
10^{-7}
10^{-8}
10^{-9}
10^{-10}
10^{-11}
10^{-12}
0
2
4
6
8
10
12
14
16
18
DAYS

was still detected as shown in Fig. 1b. From its comparative GLC behaviour on SE-30 and OV-17 columns, it appeared to consist of fatty acids and, therefore, the extract was methylated with diazomethane prior to TMS ether formation. This selectivity methylated the acids and removed them from the chromatogram while leaving the THC free to be converted into its TMS ether. No reaction of THC or CBN with diazomethane was observed even after 2 hours. This chromatogram resulting from this double derivation technique is shown in Fig 1c and contains essentially no residual peaks from endogenous lipids. The recovery of the cannabinoids was around 70-80% (9), enabling THC to be measured in plasma to 5 pg/ml.

A. Pharmacokinetics of THC in Rabbits

Pharmacokinetic studies of THC in the rabbit showed that the plasma levels fell rapidly after dosing and then declined much more slowly, a pattern already observed for THC in several species. The drug could be detected for up to 8 days following a single 1 mg/kg dosed and for at least 19 days after an 8 day treatment with the same dose (Fig.2). After a 22 day treatment (10) with 1 mg/kg of the drug, THC could be measured to 26 days (Fig. 3).

Pharmacokinetic parameters were calculated by computer using the least squares non-linear regression program, NONLIN (23), with a weighting of $1/y^2$. The best fits were obtained using triexponential curves, but variable estimates of the rate constants and thus half-lives were obtained for the early phases as shown in Table I. This suggested that more phases were probably resolvable with the inclusion of additional measurements taken at early times and the computer was resolving different phases in the various rabbits. The data from rabbit 2 could in fact be fitted to a four exponential plot. Thus from these results, it would appear that the plasma curve can be fitted by at least four exponentials. Garrett and Hunt (7) in their experiments with dogs resolved 5 phases with half-lives in phases 2-5 showing close similarity to the four phases resolved in these rabbit studies. Insufficient samples were taken from the rabbits immediately after drug administration to observe the first phase reported by Garrett and Hunt (7); this had a half-life less than 1 min. The half-life of the terminal phase ranged from 2049.6 to 3558.7 min (34.16 to 59.3 hours) with a mean of 2642.1 min (44.03 hours).

FIGURE 2. THC levels in rabbit plasma after single (circles) and 8 daily (diamonds) intravenous doses of 1 mg/kg of the drug.

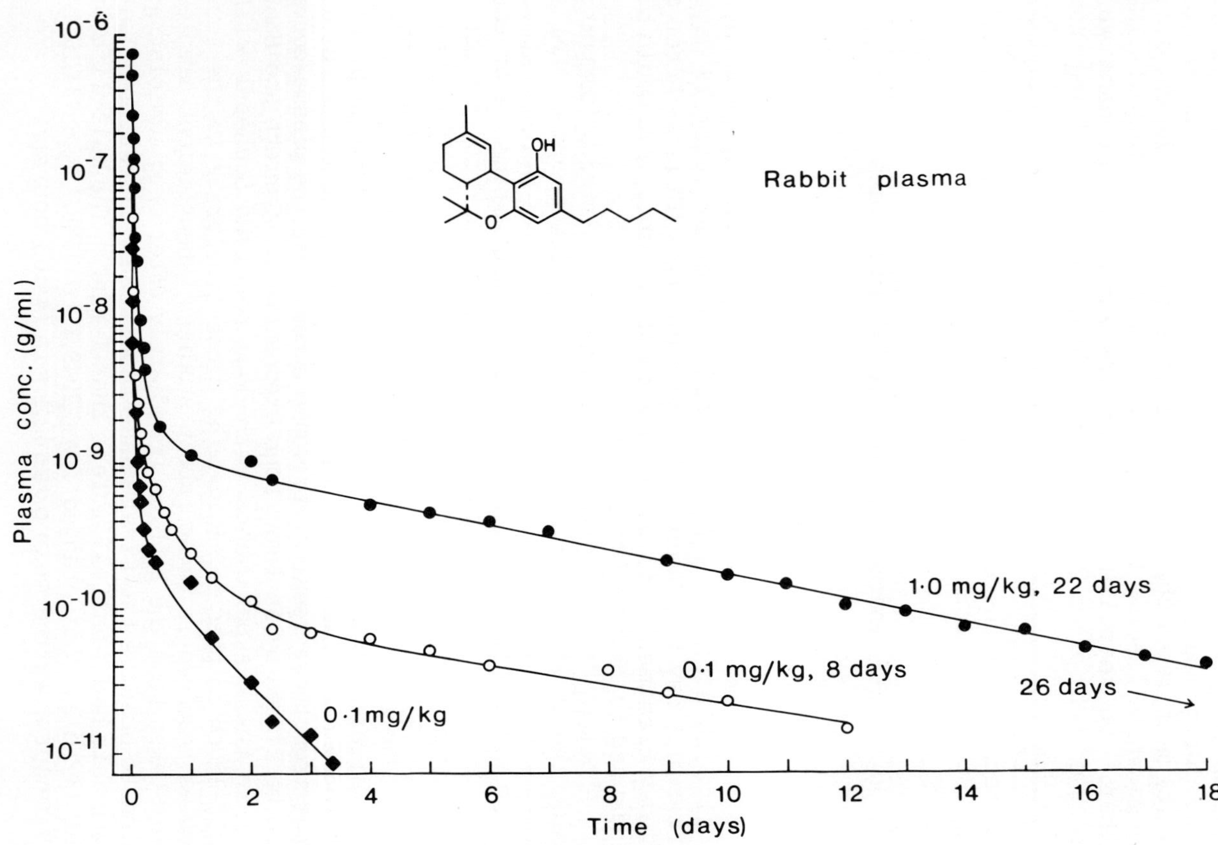
Rabbit plasma
OH
O
Plasma conc. (g/ml)
10^{-6}
10^{-7}
10^{-8}
10^{-9}
10^{-10}
10^{-11}
1·0 mg/kg, 22 days
0·1 mg/kg, 8 days
26 days
0·1mg/kg
0
2
4
6
8
10
12
14
16
18
Time (days)

Three phases were also resolved in the plasma curves of rabbits 2 and 3 when these were treated with 1 mg/kg of the drug for 8 days. Rabbits 13 and 15, which also received multiple doses, were treated for studies of tissue levels of the drug and fewer blood samples were taken. Consequently only two phases were resolved. Plasma levels in all rabbits were considerably higher than after the single dose and the half-lives of the terminal phase were most consistent (mean 74.6 +/- 1.7 hours, S.E.M.) reflecting better equilibration with the tissue forming the final compartment. The volume of distribution was calculated as 301.6 +/- 70.0 l. (n = 4), whereas under the conditions of acute administration a value of 57.3 +/- 10.1 l. (n = 4) was found. The single rabbit treated with this dose of THC for 22 days gave a value for the terminal half life of 83.0 h and a volume of distribution of 393.3 l.

Although THC could only be measured in plasma for 80 hours after a single dose of 0.1 mg/kg THC, the plasma concentration curve matched that from the 1 mg/kg-treated rabbits when multiplied by a factor of 10 to compensate for the difference in dose. Insufficient data points were collected for the final phase to be resolved. However, after the 8 day treatment with this dose, the plasma levels were considerably elevated and when compensation was made for the dose difference, the curve again matched that obtained from rabbits treated with 1 mg/kg of the drug for 8 days, although the terminal phase showed a longer half-life at 120.0 h. The elimination of THC thus appears to be independent of dose and thus of saturable metabolic processes and to be governed by slow release of the sequestered drug from tissues.

This conclusion was also reached by calculation of the plasma clearance values from the area under the curve (AUC). The mean value for the four rabbits treated singly with 1 mg/kg of THC was 59.1 +/- 5.9 (S.E.M.) ml/min/kg (mean +/- S.E.M.). Although this is slightly higher than the combined renal hepatic plasma flow of 46.8 ml/min/kg calculatedby Altman and Dittmer (1), the experimental value would be expected to be high because of the shortage of early time points and an underestimation of the maximum plasma values.

The pharmacokinetics of THC appear to be typical for that of a lipophilic drug. The long terminal half-life and high volume of distribution implies extensive uptake into tissues, of which fat would appear to be most likely depot, as indicated by the work of Kreuz and Axelrod (15). Levels of THC in

FIGURE 3. THC levels in rabbit plasma after a single dose of 0.1 mg/kg, 8 daily doses of 0.1 mg/kg, and 22 daily doses of 1 mg/kg. Reprinted from reference 10 with permission.

various tissues of rabbits killed at different times after both single and 8 daily treatments with THC were therefore measured in several tissues including fat (renal and peritoneal), brain, heart, lung, and spleen. For the measurement of THC levels in these tissues, the work-up procedure had to be modified from that used for plasma in order to remove the considerable amount of lipid material extracted by hexane. Chromatography of the extracted material on Sephadex LH-20 in chloroform reduced the lipid levels to acceptable values although in the case of fat, two passes over the column were necessary. The method adopted was similar to that used for separating THC and its metabolites from liver (11) but the volume collected for THC had to be increased in order to collect all of the [$^2H_4$]CBN. This resulted in most of the extracted fatty acids being eluted with the cannabinoids, but these were not present in amounts too large to be handled by the subsequent methylation stage.

Values found for the concentrations of THC in the tissues studied after treatment with the drug for 8 days are shown in Fig. 4. Similar ratios were found between the levels in the tissues of the singly treated rabbits although the levels were lower. All animals were killed after the terminal pharmacokinetic phase had been reached, and the ratio of the drug levels in both plasma and the various tissues were reasonably constant, reflecting the equilibrium of the drug with the tissues. As expected, highest levels were found in fat with the concentration in the two samples (renal and peritoneal) examined being very similar and being some 10^3-10^4 times the plasma levels. Of the tissues studied, brain had the lowest levels of the drug in agreement with earlier studies reviewed by Burstein (2) and by King et al. (14). Lung and spleen levels were somewhat higher but much larger values were found for heart; these were around 100 times the plasma values. Again, this pattern of THC distribution between the tissues appears to be typical for lipophilic drugs and reflects no specific abnormality for THC. Domino et al. (3) for example have found a very similar tissue distribution for the unrelated compound 2,2',4,4',5,5'-hexabromobiphenyl in the rat suggesting that the distribution of THC into the tissues studied is governed solely by its lipophilicity and not by any active transport processes or by exclusion from tissues by specific barriers.

B. Pharmacokinetics of THC in Mice

Levels of THC in the pooled plasma and brains of groups of 4 mice killed at various times after drug administration at a dose of 10 mg/kg were measured as for the rabbit study. Brain

TABLE I. Half lives (mins) Calculated by NONLIN Analysis Using a Triexponential Fit for delta-9-THC in Rabbit Plasma following a Single Dose of 1.0 mg/kg*

Rabbit	Phase 1	Phase 2	Phase 3	Phase 4
2		31.86	492.34	2,421.7 (40.36 hrs)
3	2.29	44.67		2,538.4 (42.31 hrs)
4		37.17	711.0	2,049.6 (34.16 hrs)
9		60.0	700.74	3,558.7 (59.3 hrs)
mean				2,642.1 (44.03 hrs)

*Although a triexponential curve gave the best fit in each case, the results would appear to indicate at least four phases with phases 1 and 2 being combined in rabbits, 2, 4 and 9 and phase 3 being combined with either phase 2 or 4 in the other rabbit.

levels were around 5 times the plasma values and both values fell in parallel with time again reflecting the steady state. The drug measured for 72 hours after drug administration to a level of 100 pg/ml. Pharmacokinetic analysis of the data using NONLIN gave a triexponential decay with a terminal half-life of 20.12 hours. The plasma:brain ratio of THC concentration was very similar to that found in the rabbits.

C. Concentrations of THC in Rabbit Ocular Fluids and Tissues

Table II shows the concentrations of THC in the eyes of a single rabbit at 125 min after an intravenous dose of 1 mg/kg THC which resulted in a plasma value of 42.0 ng/ml at the time of death. These studies are not yet complete but results from other rabbits gave values in good agreement with those shown in Table II. The highest levels of THC were found in the uvea; these were some 3-4 times higher than the plasma concentration and correlated well with results obtained by Krupin et al. (16), who showed by means of radiolabelling that the uvea accumulated the drug against a concentration gradient *in vitro*.

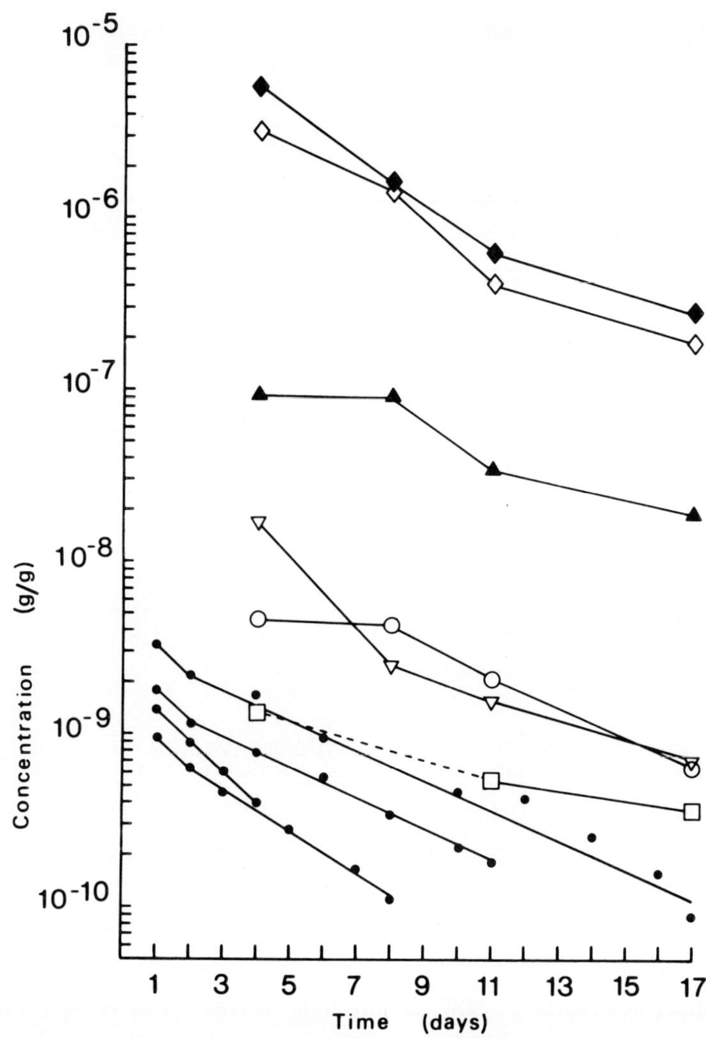

FIGURE 4. Concentrations of THC found in several tissues of four rabbits sacrificed at various times after the last of 8 daily doses of THC at a dose of 1 mg/kg. The plasma curves for each rabbit are also shown, the last point being recorded immediately before death. Legend: closed circle, plasma; open circle, spleen; closed diamond, fat (renal); open diamond, fat (peritoneal); closed triangle, heart; open triangle, lung; square, brain.

D. Measurement of THC in Mouse Erythrocytes

It has been proposed that the cell membrane is one of the major sites of action of THC and that the drug exerts its effect by disordering the molecular structure of the lipid bilayer in a manner qualitatively similar to that of general anaesthetics. Because of saturation effects, THC is not able to achieve levels comparable to those needed to produce clinical anaesthesia and this has led to the concept of THC being classed as a "partial anaesthetic" (26). Electron-spin resonance studies by Lawrence and Gill (17) using model membrane systems have in fact demonstrated an increased fluidity in the presence of both THC and its 7-hydroxy metabolite but not in membranescontaining an equivalent amount of the non-psychoactive cannabinoids CBD and CBN. Levels of THC reached in membranes _in vivo_ have not been determined. Consequently we have now examined THC levels in erythrocyte membranes using the metastable ion monitoring method and have determined these for 10 hours after drug treatment.

Concentrations of THC in the membranes were around 10 ng/mg protein at 1 hour after drug administration falling to around 300 pg/mg protein at 10 hours. Rapid equilibration of the drug with the membrane was observed with a subsequent parallel fall of the drug level in the two media. Further studies are underway to determine if any changes in membrane fluidity are produced by these levels of THC.

TABLE II. Concentrations of delta-9-THC in Rabbit Eyes 125 min after a Single Dose of 1 mg/kg

Tissue/Fluid	Right Eye	Left Eye	Mean
Aqueous humour[a]	26.3	21.9	24.1
Vitreous humour[a]	4.3	1.0	2.65
Anterior Uvea[b]	98.0	183.3	140.65
Lens[b]	2.6	2.3	2.45
Plasma[a]		42.0	

[a]Units are in ng/ml.
[b]Units are in ng/g.

ACKNOWLEDGMENTS

We thank Dr. R. Bullingham for assistance with the pharmacokinetic analysis, Miss Janet Hughes for expert technical assistance, and NIDA, through the M. R. C., for supplies of THC.

REFERENCES

1. Altman, P. L., and Dittmer, D. S., "Biology Data Book", 2nd Edition. Federation of American Societies for Experimental Biology, 1974.
2. Burstein, S. H., Labelling and metabolism of the cannabinoids, in "Marihuana, Chemistry, Pharmacology and Clinical Effects" (R. Mechoulam, ed.), pp. 167-190. Academic Press, New York, 1973.
3. Domino, L. E., Domino, S. E., and Domino, E. F., Toxicokinetics of 2,2',4,4',5,5'-hexabromobiphenyl in the rat, J. Toxicol. Environmental Health 9:812-833 (1982).
4. Fishbein, L., "Chromatography of Environmental Hazards, Vol. 4: Drugs of Abuse", pp. 394-423. Elsevier, Amsterdam, 1982.
5. Foltz, R. L., Clarke, P. A., Hidy, B. J., Lin, D. C. K., Graffeo, A. P., and Petersen, B. A., Quantitation of delta-9-tetrahydrocannabinol and 11-nor-delta-9-tetrahydrocannabinol-9-carboxylic acid in body fluids by GC/CI-MS, in "Cannabinoid Analysis in Physiological Fluids", ACS. Symp. Ser. No. 98 (J. A. Vinson, ed.), pp. 59-71. American Chemical Society, Washington, D. C., 1979.
6. Gaskell, S. J., and Millington, D. S., Selected metastable peak monitoring: a new specific technique in quantitative gas chromatography mass spectrometry, Biomed. Mass Spectrom. 5:557-558 (1978).
7. Garrett, E. R., and Hunt, C. A., Pharmacokinetics of delta-9-tetrahydrocannabinol in dogs, J. Pharm. Sci. 66:395-407 (1977).
8. Hanaban, D. J., and Ekholm, J. E., The preparation of red cell ghosts (membranes), Methods in Enzymology 31A:168-172 (1974).
9. Harvey, D. J., Leuschner, J. T. A., and Paton, W. D. M., Measurement of delta-9-tetrahydrocannabinol in plasma to the low picogram range by gas chromatography-mass spectrometry using metastable ion detection, J. Chromatogr. 202:83-92 (1980).

10. Harvey, D. J., Leuschner, J. T. A., and Paton, W. D. M., Gas chromatographic and mass spectrometric studies on the metabolism and pharmacokinetics of delta-1-tetrahydrocannabinol in the rabbit, J. Chromatogr. 239:243-250 (1982).
11. Harvey, D. J., Martin, B. R., and Paton, W. D. M., Identification of di- and tri-substituted hydroxy and ketone metabolites of delta-1-tetrahydrocannabinol in mouse liver, J. Pharm. Pharmacol. 29:482-486 (1977).
12. Harvey, D. J., Martin, B. R., and Paton, W. D. M., Identification and measurement of cannabinoids and their _in vivo_ metabolites in liver by gas chromatography-mass spectrometry, in "Marihuana: Biological Effects" (G. G. Nahas and W. D. M. Paton, eds.), pp. 45-62. Pergamon, Oxford, 1979.
13. Harvey, D. J., and Paton, W. D. M., The metabolism of deuterium labelled analogues of delta-1-, delta-6-, and delta-7-tetrahydrocannabinol and the use of deuterium labelling, in "Recent Developments in Mass Spectrometry in Biochemistry and Medicine", Vol. 2 (A. Frigerio, ed.), pp. 127-147. Plenum, New York, 1979.
14. King, L. J., Teal, J. D., and Marks, V., Biochemical aspects of cannabis, in "Cannabis and Health" (J. D. P. Graham, ed.), pp. 77-107. Academic Press, London, 1976.
15. Kreuz, D. A., and Axelrod, J., Delta-9-tetrahydrocannabinol: localization in body fat, Science 179:391-393 (1973).
16. Krupin, T., Fritz, C., Dutton, J. J., and Becker, B., Delta-9-tetrahydrocannabinol transport in rabbit eyes, Exp. Eye Res. 30:345-350 (1980).
17. Lawrence, D. K., and Gill, E. W., The effects of delta-1-tetrahydrocannabinol and other cannabinoids on spin-labelled liposomes and their relationship to mechanisms of general anaesthesia, Biochem. Pharmacol. 11:595-602 (1975).
18. Lee, M. G., and Millard, B. J., A comparison of unlabelled and labelled internal standards for quantification by single and multiple ion monitoring, Biomed. Mass Spectrom. 2:78-81 (1975).
19. Lemberger, L., Silberstein, S. D., Axelrod, J., and Kopin, I. J., Marihuana: studies on the disposition and metabolism of delta-9-tetrahydrocannabinol in man, Science 170:1320-1322 (1970).
20. Lemberger, L., Tamarkin, N. R., Axelrod, J., and Kopin, I. J., Delta-9-tetrahydrocannabinol: metabolism and disposition in long-term marihuana smokers, Science 173:72-73 (1971).
21. Lowry, O. H., Rosebrough, N. J., Farr, A. L., and Randall, R. J., Protein measurement with the Folin phenol reagent, J. Biol. Chem. 193:265-272 (1951).

22. Mechoulam, R., Yagnitinsky, B., and Gaoni, Y., Stereoselective factor in the chloranil dehydrogenation ofcannabinoids, Total synthesis of d,l-cannabichromene, J. Amer. Chem. Soc. 90:2418-2420 (1968).
23. Metzler, C. M., Elfring, G. L., and McEwen, A. J., A package of computer programs for pharmacokinetic modeling, Biometrics 30:562 (1974).
24. Ohlsson, A., Lindgren, J. E., Leander, K., and Agurell, S., Detection and quantification of tetrahydrocannabinol in blood plasma, in "Cannabinoid Assays in Humans", Res. Monogr. Ser. No. 7 (R. E. Willette, ed.), pp. 48-63. NIDA, Rockville, MD, 1976.
25. Ohlsson, A., Lindgren, J. E., Wahlen, A., Agurell, S., Hollister, L. E., and Gillespie, H. K., Single dose kinetics of deuterium labelled delta-1-tetrahydrocannabinol in heavy and light cannabis users, Biomed. Mass Spectrom. 9:6-10 (1982).
26. Paton, W. D. M., Pertwee, R. G., and Temple, D., The general pharmacology of cannabinoids, in "Cannabis and its Derivatives" (W. D. M. Paton and J. Crown, eds.), pp. 50-75. Oxford University Press, London, 1972.
27. Rosenthal, D., Harvey, T. M., Bursey, J. T., Brine, D. R., and Wall, M. E., Comparison of gas chromatography massspectrometry methods for the determination of delta-9-tetrahydrocannabinol in plasma, Biomed. Mass Spectrom. 5:312-316 (1978).
28. Vinson, J. A. (ed.), "Cannabinoid Analysis in Physiological Fluids", A.C.S. Symp. Ser. No. 98. Amer. Chem. Soc., Washington, D. C., 1979.
29. Wall, M. E., and Perez-Reyes, M., The metabolism of delta-9-tetrahydrocannabinol and related compounds in man, J. Clin. Pharmacol., 21:178S-189S (1981).
30. Willette, R. E., (ed.) "Cannabinoid Assays in Humans", NIDA Res. Monogr. Ser. No. 7. NIDA, Rockville, MD, 1976.

DISTRIBUTION AND DISPOSITION OF DELTA-9-TETRAHYDROCANNABINOL (THC) IN DIFFERENT TISSUES OF THE RAT

Maureen Bronson
Colette Latour
Gabriel G. Nahas

College of Physicians and Surgeons
Columbia University
New York, New York

and

Laboratorie de Toxicologie cellulaire
Paris, France

I. INTRODUCTION

Data available in the literature reporting short and long term storage of delta-9-tetrahydrocannabinol (THC) in brain and testis are fragmentary. Garrett, for instance, states that following a single I.V. administration, "less than 1% of THC will reach the brain" (1). Kreuz and Axelrod, who administered tagged THC to rodents every two days for a month, report very small accumulation of the drug in the brain, not exceeding twice the amount present after a single administration (2). Distribution and accumulation of THC in the testis, heart, and spleen has not been reported.

The purpose of the present investigation was to study the kinetics of THC storage in these tissues following acute and chronic administration of tracer amounts of ^{14}C tagged THC. Such information should indicate if the effects of THC on these tissues are exerted on these tissues in micromolar or nanomolar concentrations.

Such information might help to define the dosage required to produce acute and chronic effects observed after cannabis intoxication.

ISBN 0-12-044620-0

II. METHODS

A. Experimental Protocol

Two groups of experiments were performed on male Sprague Dawley rats that weighed 192 +/- 20 gm. The first group of animals was given 2 mcCu of ^{14}C delta-8-THC by intramuscular injection in the thigh. They were sacrificed in lots of three at 1, 2, 3, 4, 6, and 24 hours after drug administration.

In the second series, the animals were sacrificed at regular intervals in groups of three after multiple administration of the same dosage of the drug (2 microCu), given intraperitoneally every two days for 32 days. The animals were sacrificed 24 hours following the last administration, at day 2, 8, 14, 20, 26, and 30. I. P. administration was performed in this second series because it was better tolerated.

The following organs and tissues were sampled: peripheral blood (drawn from cardiac puncture), brain, lung, liver, spleen, testis, and epididymal fat. All organs and tissues were weighed and fast frozen.

B. Preparation of THC

The ^{14}C-tagged THC was provided by Dr.R.Willette from NIDA. It had a specific activity of 30 mCi/mM. It was dissolved in ethanol and kept under nitrogen at $0^{o}C$ in a dark environment.

For its administration, THC was dissolved in ethanol to a final concentration of 0.2 mCu/ml. Ten microliters of this solution, containing 2 microCu, were injected intramuscularly in the thigh of each animal for the acute experiment or intraperitoneally for the chronic study. This amount corresponds to 30 mcg THC or 0.1 mcM.

C. Analysis of Samples

The different tissues were solubilized and extracted according to the method described by Garrett for THC extraction (3). Fragments of liver, lung, epidiymal fat, or the entire heart, brain, spleen and testis were homoginizedin water adjusted to pH 9 to 9.5 with 0.1 N sodium carbonate. For plasma, a 2 ml sample was similarly treated with the alkali and water for a final volume of 2.5 ml. The plasma sample or a 10 ml aliquot of the tissue homogenate was transferred to a silylated glass centrifuge tube to which 40 ml of heptane containing 1.5% isoamylalcohol was added (or 15 ml of the same solution for the plasma sample). The tube was stoppered and shaken for 30 minutes and centrifuged for 10 minutes. An aliquot of the organic layer to be used for thin layer chromatography (TLC) was transferred to a centrifuge tube and a second aliquot transferred to a glass liquid scintillation vial. Both vial and tube contents were dried under a stream of nitrogen in a water bath at 50°C.

A scintillation solution was added to the vial content and the sample was analyzed by liquid scintillation spectroscopy. The aliquot in the tube was analyzed by TLC.

III. RESULTS

A. After a Single Intramuscular Dose (Tables I and II)

Following a single intramuscular administration of 30 mcg of THC, maximum plasma concentration (from mixed venous and arterial blood) was reached at 2 hours and amounted to 4.8 +/- 2.0 ng/g (Table I). After 4 hours, it had fallen to 1.8 +/- ng/g, to rise after 24 hours to a significantly higher concentration of 4 +/- 1.0 ng/g. Concentration in brain reached a maximum level of 6.8 +/- 22.8 to 9.2 +/- 1.4 ng/g between 1 and 4 hours after THC administration. These concentrations were significantly higher than mixed plasma concentration. After 24 hours, brain concentration was 3.0 +/- 0.6 ng/g, not significantly different from that of plasma.

During the first four hours, concentration of THC in testis was 2.2 +/- 0.4 to 3.2 +/- 0.6 ng/g, not significantly different from plasma concentration. After 24 hours THC concentration was 1.0 +/- 0.4 ng/g, significantly lower than plasma.

THC concentration in the spleen was at a maximum after 1 hour (16 +/- 4.4 ng/g), reaching equilibrium with plasma after 24 hours.

THC concentrations in heart and lung were not significantly different and followed a similar course, with a maximum after 1 to 2 hours (12.8 +/- 2.4 to 16.8 +/- 3.2 ng/g) and reaching approximate equilibrium with plasma after 24 hours.

In the spleen, concentration was also high during the first 2 hours (16.0 to 12.6 ng/g). In liver, THC concentration was higher than in plasma for the first 4 hours (7.4 to 5.2 ng/g).

In fat, concentration reached a plateau of 34.0 to 36.6 ng/g after 6 hours, which persisted at that level for 24 hours.

The percentage of THC administered and recovered in brain, testis, heart and spleen is listed on Table II. In the brain

TABLE I. Concentration of THC in Different Tissues (ng/g) Following a Single Intramuscular Injection of 30 mcg of ^{14}C Delta-9-THC

	Time of Sampling after Injection (+/- S.D.)					
Tissue	1 h	2 h	3 h	4 h	6 h	24 h
Plasma	3.6 (1.4)	2.8 (2.0)	3.2 (1.0)	1.8 (0.8)	2.0 (0.9)	4.0 (1.0)
Brain	7.0 (2.8)	9.2 (1.4)	7.6 (1.2)	8.8 (0.8)	4.0 (1.8)	3.0 (0.6)
Testis	3.0 (0.2)	2.9 (0.5)	2.2 (0.4)	3.2 (0.6)	2.8 (0.6)	1.0 (0.4)
Spleen	16.0 (4.4)	12.6 (5.2)	6.6 (0.8)	7.6 (1.8)	7.0 (0.8)	3.9 (0.6)
Heart	12.8 (2.4)	16.8 (3.2)	13.2 (2.6)	8.0 (3.0)	6.6 (1.2)	4.8 (1.0)
Lung	14.8 (4.4)	12.0 (2.8)	10.0 (3.0)	7.6 (2.4)	5.2 (1.2)	5.2 (1.0)
Liver	7.4 (3.4)	7.4 (3.2)	5.2 (1.0)	7.0 (1.2)	4.6 (0.8)	2.8 (0.6)
Fat	12.2 (4.2)	23.4 (4.0)	34.0 (2.2)		36.6 (1.2)	37.0 (5.0)

a maximum percentage was reached in the first 3 hours following THC administration (0.06 +/- 0.07% of the administered dose). A similar fraction of the administered dose was recovered in the heart. In the spleen, percentage was lower. The lowest percentage of the administered dose was recovered in the testis (0.020 to 0.014%).

B. Multiple Doses by the Intraperitoneal Route (Table III)

Concentration of THC in brain increased significantly ($p < 0.05$) at day 14 after 7 injections of the drug (from 2.8 +/- 0.4 to 4.8 +/- 0.6 ng/g). Thereafter brain concentrations reached a plateau.

In the testis, increase of THC concentration reached significance ($p < 0.01$) after 4 injections of the drug at day 8. Thereafter, no further increase was observed.

Accumulation of THC was more marked in some of the other organs studied: from day 2 to day 34, THC concentration rose from 3.4 +/- 0.2 to 14 +/- 1.2 ng/g in the spleen, and from 5.4 +/- 0.6 to 11.2 +/- 2.6 ($p < 0.01$) in the heart.

Accumulation of THC was also observed in the lung, liver and mostly in fat, where it reached a concentration of 432 +/- 112 ng/g at day 34.

TABLE II. Percentage of THC Recovered in Brain and Testis of Rats Following a Single Administration of 30 mcg of ^{14}C Delta-8-THC (10 mcCuries/kg)

		Time after administration (in hours)					
Tissue	Wt. (g)	1	2	3	4	6	24
Brain	1.8	0.043	0.056	0.046	0.054	0.015	0.018
Testis	1.8	0.018	0.016	0.014	0.019	0.017	0.006
Heart	1.2	0.052	0.068	0.054	0.033	0.027	0.016
Spleen	0.9	0.050	0.041	0.024	0.026	0.016	0.012

IV. DISCUSSION

The present data indicate that after a single intramuscular dose of ^{14}C delta-8-THC, maximum concentration of this drug in the brain is reached 2 to 4 hours after its administration, and that it is significantly higher than in peripheral blood during the same period. This observation is consistent with that of Ohlsson et al. who reported that while plasma levels in mice are falling initially, brain concentrations are rising (4). Others have reported that in man, maximal psychoactive effects do not correlate well with plasma THC concentration: there is maximum psychoactive effect ("high") when plasma concentrations are falling (5). These authors stated, "It is probable that brain concentration of THC as judged by the psychoactive effects were higher than plasma concentrations much of the time of the 'high'." Similar observations were made by Hollister et al. who reported a temporal lag between maximum plasma concentration and peak psychoactive effect (6).

The maximum fraction of THC recovered in the brain after a single administration was one sixthousandth of the administered dose, much less than previously reported (1). And after 34 days and 16 injections, the amount of THC stored in the brain had not quite doubled (from 2.8 +/- 0.4 to 5.2 +/- 0.2 ng/g).

The amount of THC stored in the testis after a single administration of the drug was also quite low, amounting to less than two ten thousandths of the administered dose. Following multiple administration, accumulation in the testis was limited after 34 days to the double of the amount observed after a single dose.

Storage of THC in liver, lung and mostly in fat, reported by previous authors, was also observed in the present experiments.

Accumulation in heart and spleen deserves special mention. In the heart, after a single administration, THC concentration was higher than in the lungs, and peak concentration was observed at the same time as it was in the brain (2 hours after administration) but it was 3.5 times higher (16.00 +/- 3.2 ng/g) than in brain.

THC-induced chronotropic changes in the heart are a good index of its psychoactivity, but its mechanism is not clear. The present observation would indicate that such changes are associated with sustained and relatively high THC concentration in the heart.

After multiple administration, THC concentration (11.2 ng/g) in the heart was more than twice the concentration present 24 hours after the first injection (5.4 ng/g).

TABLE III. Concentration of THC (ng/g) in Different Tissues Following Multiple Administration of 1 to 14 Doses of 30 mcg ^{14}C Delta-9-THC (+/- S.D.)

Day sacrificed	2	8	14	20	26	34
No. of doses	1	4	7	10	13	16
Plasma	1.2 (0.4)	3.0 (0.4)	1.6 (0.3)	1.6 (0.3)	3.6 (0.8)[a]	7.0 (1.2)[b]
Brain	2.8 (0.6)	3.8 (0.8)	4.8 (0.6)[a]	4.2 (0.2)[a]	4.2 (0.6)[a]	5.2 (0.6)[b]
Testis	0.8 (0.4)	2.7 (0.8)[a]	1.6 (0.4)[a]	1.7 (0.8)[a]	1.4 (0.6)	1.7 (0.4)[a]
Spleen	3.4 (0.2)	18.3 (4.2)[b]	11.6 (0.8)[b]	11.0 (0.7)[b]	11.8 (0.6)[b]	14.2 (1.2)[b]
Heart	5.4 (0.6)	5.2 (0.5)	10.2 (2.0)[b]	9.4 (2.2)[a]	11.6 (2.0)[a]	11.2 (2.6)[b]
Lung	6.2 (2.4)	14.0 (2.6)[b]	16.4 (3.0)[b]	8.0 (1.4)	8.0 (1.4)	17.2 (2.8)
Liver	1.6 (0.4)	9.4 (0.8)[b]	5.0 (0.8)[b]	6.6 (0.6)[b]	6.6 (0.6)[b]	5.8 (0.6)
Fat	36.0 (6.0)	319.0 (92)[b]	315.0 (92)	354.0 (112)[c]	327.0 (54)[c]	432.0 (112)[c]

[a]Significantly different from day 2: $p < 0.05$.
[b]Significantly different from day 2: $p < 0.01$.
[c]Significantly different from day 2: $p < 0.001$.
NOTE: Animals were sacrificed 24 hours after the last administration of the drug.

The concentration of THC in the spleen (16 +/- 4.4 ng/g), one hour after administration of the drug, was higher than in any other tissue studied except fat. It decreased thereafter, reaching equilibrium with plasma after 24 hours. Affinity of the spleen for THC was further documented after multiple administration of the drug: the concentrations of THC after 6 doses was 14.2 ng/g, 6 times that observed 24 hours following the first injection (2.4 ng/g). These data are of interest in view of the reported effect of cannabis on lymphocyte function (7,8).

Our data indicate that the acute and chronic effects produced by cannabis on brain and testis will result from nanomolar concentration of this drug in these tissues. Such concentrations usually act on or close to receptor sites. Specific sites for THC have not been identified.

The interaction of THC with beta-adrenergic receptors in the brain has been described by Bloom (9). No such interactions with receptors have been described in the testis where THC depresses sperm production and alters sperm morphology (10,11).

This data also illustrates the efficiency of the blood brain barrier and of the blood testicular barrier in limiting the deposition of THC in brain and testis to nanomolar concentrations. The mechanisms which limit the storage of such a highly lipophilic substance in these organs deserves additional investigation.

REFERENCES

1. Garrett, E. R., Pharmacokinetics and disposition of delta-9-THC and its metabolites, in "Marihuana, Biological Effects" (G. G. Nahas, and W. D. M. Paton, eds.), pp. 105-21. Pergamon Press, Oxford, 1979.
2. Kreuz, D. S., and Axelrod, J., Delta-9-tetrahydrocannabinol: Localization in body fat, Science 179:391-393 (1973).
3. Garrett, E. R., Hunt, C. A., Separation and analysis of delta-9-THC in biological fluids by high pressure liquid chromatography and GLC., J. Pharm. Sci. 66:20-26 (1977).
4. Ohlsson, A., Widman, M., Carlsson, S., Ryman, T., and Steed, C., Plasma and brain levels of delta-6-tetrahydrocannabinol and seven monooxygenated metabolites correlated to the cataleptic effect in the mouse, Acta Pharmacol. Toxicol. 47:308-17 (1980).
5. Ohlsson, A., Lindgren, J. E., Wahlen, A., Agurell, S., Hollister, L. E., and Gillespie, H. K., Plasma delta-9-tetrahydrocannabinol concentrations and clinical effects

after oral and intravenous administration and smoking, Clin. Pharmacol. Ther. 28:409-16 (1980).
6. Hollister, L. E., Gillespie, H. K., Ohlsson, A., Lindgren, J. E., Wahlen, A., and Agurell, S., Do plasma concentrations of delta-9-THC reflect the degree of intoxication? J. Clin. Pharmacol. 21:171-77 (1981).
7. Rosenkrantz, H., The immune response and marijuana, in "Marihuana: Chemistry, Biochemistry and Cellular Effects" (G. G. Nahas, ed.), pp. 441-56. Springer Verlag, New York, 1976.
8. Nahas, G. G., Morishima, A., and Desoize, B., Effects of cannabinoids on macromolecular synthesis replication of cultured lymphocytes, Fed. Proc. 36:1746-52 (1977).
9. Bloom, A. S., Effects of cannabinoids on neurotransmitters in the brain, This volume.
10. Dalterio, S., Steger, R., and Bartke, A., Effects of psychoactive or non psychoactive cannabinoids on reproductive functions in male offspring, This volume.

SUPEROXIDE RADICAL GENERATION AND NITRO BLUE TETRAZOLIUM REDUCTION BY ETHANOL IN THE PRESENCE OF ULTRAVIOLET LIGHT AND ITS INHIBITION BY SUPEROXIDE DISMUTASE AND DELTA-9-TETRAHYDROCANNABINOL

Charles N. Gutierrez

Division of Microbiology
Veterans Administration
Mountain Home, Tennessee

R. D. Blevins

Department of Biological Sciences
Health Sciences Division
East Tennessee State University
Johnson City, Tennessee

I. INTRODUCTION

The superoxide radical is a highly reactive compound produced when oxygen is reduced by a single electron ($O_2 + 1e^- \rightarrow O_2^-$). The superoxide radicals are important agents in the toxicity of oxygen and are partially hazardous to living matter (1). This reduction may occur by several different mechanisms in biological systems. Superoxide radicals may be generated during the normal catalytic function of a number of enzymes, including xanthine oxidase, the enzyme responsible for uric acid production (2), and cytochrome P-450, a component of one of the drug detoxifying systems of liver (3); it can also be formed during the oxidation of hemoglobin to methemoglobin (4).

The short-lived superoxide radical can also be produced by non-enzymatic reactions. It can be generated in a secondary reaction after the passage of ionizing radiation through water (5) thus making possible production of the O_2^- in tissues exposed to ionizing radiation. Ionization radiation,

ISBN 0-12-044620-0

especially the technique of pulse radiolysis, is claimed by Rabini to be one of the better methods of generating high concentrations of O_2^- (6).

Exposure of aerated aqueous solutions to ultraviolet light (UV) with wavelengths below 200 nm generates H^- and OH· radicals with the subsequent formation of superoxide radicals. They can also be produced by electrochemical reduction of oxygen resulting in O_2^- diffusion from a cathode surface (7).

The implication of tissue damage due to products or by-products formed by the oxidation of ethanol has recently been of interest. The literature reveals that superoxide radicals (O_2^-) may be involved in tissue damage. The purpose of this research is to ascertain if ethanol could form O_2^- and whether these radicals could be monitored by an assay system; and if so, whether superoxide dismutase could inhibit O_2^- formation. Findings in this laboratory using a photoillumination system of O_2^- production have shown superoxide radicals to interact with delta-9-tetrahydrocannabinol (THC) in the presence of ethanol as a solvent. The use of ultraviolet light, however, showed ethanol to be a source of O_2^- radicals. The use of THC, having shown to interact with the O_2^-, offered an alternative method to confirm the production of O_2^- from UV-irradiated ethanol.

II. METHODS

A. Superoxide Radical Generation and Nitro Blue Tetrazolium Reduction by Ethanol in the Presence of Ultraviolet Light

Three reaction mixtures (Table I) were prepared containing 1.8 ml absolute ethanol, plus 1.2 ml of 5.6×10^{-5} <u>M</u> nitro blue tetrazolium (NBT). Each was irradiated for 60 minutes

TABLE I. Superoxide Radical Generation and Nitro Blue Tetrazolium (NBT) Reduction by Ethanol in the Presence of UV Light*

Cuvette	I (UV Exposed)	II (Shielded)	III (Fluor. Light)
Absolute Ethanol	1.8	1.8	1.8
NBT (5.6×10^{-5}M)	1.2	1.2	1.2
Total Volume	3.0	3.0	3.0

*Units are in ml.

with 254 nm shortwave ultraviolet lamp in a closed aluminum lined box at a distance of 17.5 cm. Absorbance readings were taken every 5 minutes and recorded. The first cuvette was exposed to the UV light; whereas, the second cuvette was covered with parafilm and aluminum foil to shield it from the UV light. The third cuvette was irradiated with two 15 watt fluorescent lamps, and its absorbance was read every 5 minutes for 60 minutes.

B. Inhibition of NBT Reduction by SOD and THC During Irradiation of Ethanol by Ultraviolet Light

The reduction of NBT was further investigated to determine if NBT reduction was a direct reduction by ethanol or if the reduction of NBT involved an indirect pathway using the superoxide radical.

The UV stimulated reduction of NBT would involve the transfer of two hydrogen atoms to NBT from ethanol. Ethanol in turn would be converted into acetaldehyde. Ethanol has a negative standard potential relative to hydrogen and thus has a greater tendency to lose its two electrons. If these electrons derived from ethanol were transferred to oxygen to form the superoxide radical, the addition of superoxide dismutase should inhibit the reaction. If there was a direct reaction between ethanol and NBT, the enzyme would not be expected to inhibit the rate of NBT reduction. To test this the following experiment was prepared (Table II). One cuvette contained 1.8 ml ETOH, 1.1 ml NBT, and 0.1 ml distilled water. A second cuvette substituted the 0.1 ml of water with 0.1 ml (20 units) of superoxide dismutase prepared in this laboratory. A third cuvette contained 1.8 ml ETOH, 1.1 ml NBT, 0.1 ml water and

TABLE II. Inhibition of Nitro Blue Tetrazolium (NBT) Reduction by Superoxide Dismutase (SOD) and THC during Irradiation of Ethanol by Ultraviolet Light

Cuvette	I	II	III
Absolute Ethanol	1.8 ml	1.8 ml	1.8 ml
NBT (5.6 x 10^{-5}M)	1.1 ml	1.1 ml	1.1 ml
Distilled Water	0.1 ml	0.1 ml	0.1 ml
SOD	-	20 units	-
THC	-	-	6.3 mcg/ml
Total Volume	3.0 ml	3.0 ml	3.0 ml

6.3 mcg/ml THC. The pH was approximately 8.7 in the three cuvettes. The SOD was used to test for inhibition of NBT reduction caused by O_2^{-}·. The THC was examined with respect to its potential for contributing to NBT reduction when exposed to UV light for 60 minutes, and the absorbance of the contents of the cuvettes were read every five minutes. After monitoring the absorbance for one hour, the cuvettes were then irradiated 11 additional hours with short wavelength UV light with absorbance readings being taken at the end of that time.

III. RESULTS

A. Superoxide Radical Generation and NBT Reduction by Ethanol in the Presence of Ultraviolet Light

Figure 1 illustrates the results of ultraviolet and fluorescent light irradiation of cuvettes one and three. Cuvette one showed a definite increase in blue formazan production in the presence of UV light, while cuvette three showed a minimal increase with fluorescent light. The second cuvette shielded from UV light showed no increase in absorption after 60 minutes and remained at zero. Twelve hours of UV irradiation gave a final absorbance of 0.350 units; whereas, a control using 1.8 ml water and 1.2 ml NBT showed an absorbance increase of only 0.023 units after 12 hours of UV exposure.

B. Inhibition of NBT Reduction by SOD and THC during Irradiation of Ethanol by Ultraviolet Light

Figure 2 illustrates the results from the irradiation of the cuvettes with UV light for 60 minutes. Superoxide dismutase inhibited NBT reduction by 59% and 6.3 mcg/ml THC inhibited NBT reduction by 50%. After 50 minutes a sharp increase in NBT reduction in the presence of THC was noted; whereas, in the presence of superoxide dismutase there is a slow and steady increase in NBT reduction.

The results after 12 hours of UV irradiation of the contents of the three cuvettes are shown in Table III. The large inhibition (76%) by superoxide dismutase of NBT reduction to blue formazan in the presence of UV light, demonstrated that the superoxide radical was an intermediate in the oxidation of ethanol to acetaldehyde.

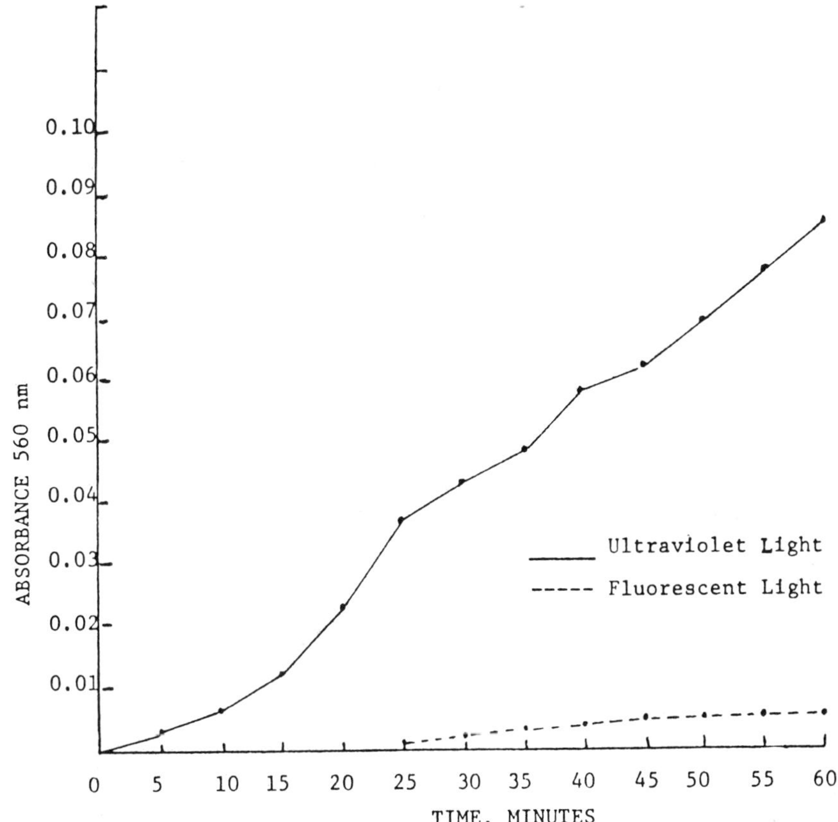

FIGURE 1. NBT reduction by absolute ethanol irradiated with UV (solid line) and fluorescent light (dashed line) at 33°C, pH 8.5.

IV. DISCUSSION

The assay for NBT reduction by O_2^- was primarily developed to measure superoxide dismutase activity 98). The role of superoxide radicals in oxidation-reduction reactions involving water soluble compounds is being observed in both biological and chemical systems (9-11). This investigation using the system of NBT reduction in ethanol provides a method in which the role of superoxide radicals in oxidation-reduction reactions, involving water insoluble compounds, may be investigated.

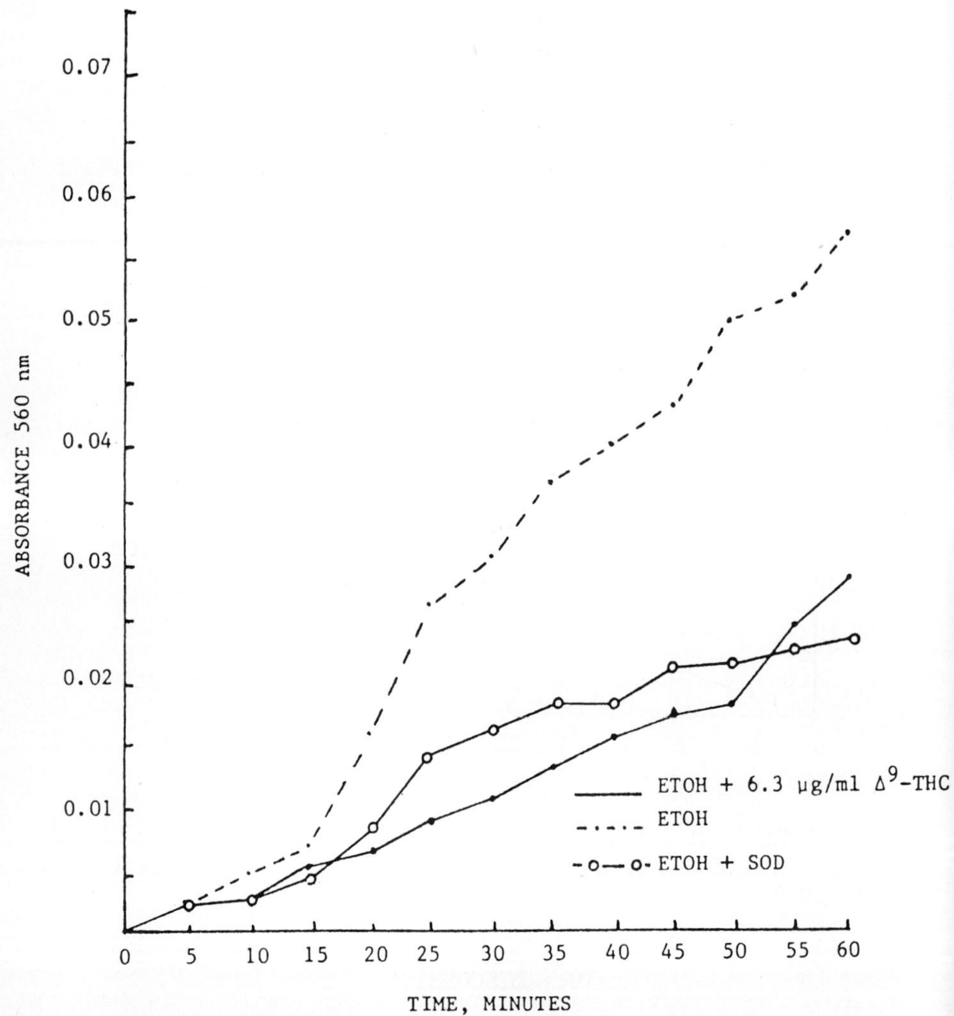

FIGURE 2. NBT reduction by 95% ethanol irradiated with UV light (control, dashed line) in the presence of 20 units SOD/ml (circles) and 6.3 mcg/ml THC (dots) at 33°C.

The oxidation of ethanol by oxygen and the formation of the superoxide radical suggest that the enzymatic oxidation of ethanol to acetaldehyde by alcohol dehydrogenase, could involve superoxide radical production. It has been shown that ethanol can be oxidized by a free radical chain reaction. Heberling and McCormack (12) showed that, in the formation of

TABLE III. Effects of Superoxide Dismutase (SOD) and THC on Nitro Blue Tetrazolium (NBT) Reduction in Ethanol Irradiated by Ultraviolet Light after 12 Hour

Assay + NBT	Absorbance at 12 hr, 560 nm	Color	% Inhibition
95% Ethanol	0.360	Purple	-
Ethanol + 20 units SOD	0.086	Lt. Pink	76.12
Ethanol + 6.3 mcg/ml THC	0.287	Purple	20.28

silver halide, ethanol was oxidized and various polyhalomethanes were reduced, when bromoform or methylene iodide was treated with ethanolic silver nitrate. He postulated a free radical chain involving ethanol. Razuvaev, et al., (13) showed that primary and secondary alcohols are oxidized by carbon tetrachloride when the reaction is initiated chemically, photochemically or thermally (200°C). He suggested that these oxidations proceeded by free radical formation. No mention of superoxide radical formation was made in Heberlings (12) and Razuvaev findings (13). Other investigations involving ethanol's oxidation to acetaldehyde in biological systems, do not show superoxide radical formation to be an intermediate step if oxygen is required in the reaction (14,15).

The results in Table II show that superoxide dismutase provided a 76% inhibition of NBT reduction in 57% ethanol when irradiated with UV light. Since 100% inhibition was not obtained, it is possible that ethanol, under the given condition, reacts with NBT directly to form blue formazan. The 20% inhibition of NBT reduction, as shown in Table III, after 12 hours of UV irradiation in the presence of THC and O_2^- would decrease the amount of superoxide radicals available to reduce NBT and thus lower the amount of blue formazan formed in the system.

REFERENCES

1. Gregory, E. M., Goscin, S. A., and Fridovich, I., Superoxide dismutase and oxygen toxicity in a eukaryote, J. Bacteriol. 117:456-460 (1974).
2. Fridovich, I., and Handler, P., Detection of free radicals generated during enzymic oxidation by the initiation

of sulfite oxidation, J. Biol. Chem. 236:1836-1840 (1961).

3. Strobel, H. W., and Coon, M. T., Effects of superoxide generation and dismutation on hydroxylation reactions catalyzed by liver microsomal cytochrome P-450, J. Biol. Chem. 246:7826-7829 (1971).
4. Misra, H. P., and Fridovich, I., The generation of superoxide radical during autoxidation of hemoglobin, J. Biol. Chem. 274:6960-6966 (1972).
5. Hart, E. T., Radiation chemistry of aqueous solutions, Ann. Rev. Nucl. Sci. 15:125-150 (1965).
6. Rabini, J., and Nielson, S. O., Absorption spectrum and decay kinetics of O_2^- and HO_2 in aqueous solutions by pulse radiolysis, J. Phys. Chem. 73:3736 (1969).
7. Forman, H. T., and Fridovich, I., Superoxide dismutase: A comparison of rate constants, Arch. Biochem. Biophys. 158:396-400 (1973).
8. Beauchamp, C., and Fridovich, I., Superoxide dismutase: Improved assay and an assay applicable to acrylamide gels, Anal. Biochem, 44:276-287 (1971).
9. Kellogg, E. W., and Fridovich, I., Superoxide, hydrogen peroxide, and singlet oxygen in lipid peroxidation by a xanthine oxidase system, J. Biol. Chem. 250:8812-8817 (1975).
10. Bors, W., Saran, M., Lengfelder, E., Spottl, R., and Michel, C., The relevance of the superoxide anion radical in biological systems, Curr. Top. Radiat. Res. 9:247-309 (1974).
11. Fridovich, I., Superoxide dismutases, in "Annual Reviews Biochemistry", Vol. 44, (E. E. Snell, ed.) pp. 147-159. Annual Reviews Inc., Palo Alto, CA, 1975.
12. Heberling, T. W., and McCormack, W. W., A reaction of some perhalomethanes an alcohol, J. Amer. Chem. Soc. 78:5433 (1955).
13. Razuvaev, G. A., Morganov, B. N., and Korman, H. E., Triggering the reaction between carbon tetrachloride and isopropyl alcohol with benzoyl peroxide, J. Gen. Chem. U.S.S.R. 26:2485 (1956).
14. Li, T. K., Enzymology of human alcohol metabolism, in "Advances in Enzymology", Vol. 45, (A. Meister, ed.), pp. 427-483. John Wiley and Sons, New York, 1977.
15. Roach, M. K., Microsomal ethanol oxidation: Activity _in vitro_ and _in vivo_, in "Biochemical Pharmacology of Ethanol", Vol. 56, (E. Majchrowicz, ed.), pp. 33-55. Plenum Press, New York, 1973.

SUPEROXIDE RADICAL INVOLVEMENT IN THE OXIDATION OF DELTA-9-TETRAHYDROCANNABINOL AND ITS INHIBITION BY SUPEROXIDE DISMUTASE

Charles N. Gutierrez

Division of Microbiology
Veterans Administration
Mountain Home, Tennessee

R. D. Blevins

Department of Biological Sciences
Health Sciences Division
East Tennessee State University
Johnson City, Tennessee

I. INTRODUCTION

The plant Cannabis sativa, commonly called marijuana, is a quite complex plant when described chemically. The major psychoactive ingredient of this plant is delta-9-tetrahydrocannabinol (THC). Many years of research have resulted in the elucidation of the chemistry and biochemistry of cannabis. A review by Mechoulam detailed the recent advances made in this area (1). The chemistry, analytical aspects, biotransformations, and biochemical effects of the cannabinoids are discussed and reviewed thoroughly. Delta-9-tetrahydrocannabinol is capable of undergoing transformations to a large number of compounds. Most of these new compounds formed are oxidative products of the parent compound THC and are non-psychoactive (2).

The stability of THC has been the object of some study. Razdan reported that THC oxidizes to cannabinol (CBN) at a rate of 10% per month when spotted on filter paper and kept at room temperature (3). At 80°C, over 50% of the THC was converted to CBN in four days. Lerner reported that the concen-

The Cannabinoids: Chemical,
Pharmacologic, and Therapeutic Aspects

ISBN 0-12-044620-0

tration of THC in marijuana decreased at a rate of 3-5% per month when stored at a room temperature of 24°C (4). Very little CBN was found in fresh marijuana, and the presence of high concentrations of CBN probably indicated that the hashish or marijuana sample has been stored for some time prior to analysis. Bundled marijuana, when stored, showed greater CBN content on the outer part exposed to air than that located in the center (5). Mechoulam stated that the rate of oxidation of THC in marijuana required further examination since "street users" of marijuana stated that they did not detect noticeable change in the potency of marijuana stored at room temperature for periods to one year (2).

Mechoulam also suggested that THC should be stored in an inert solution, preferably chloroform, ether or in any dilute alcohol or hydrocarbon solvent under nitrogen in order to decrease degradative changes (2). The samples should be refrigerated but not frozen. Storage by this method reduces the rate of oxidative degradation of THC to CBN and also decreases the rate of polymer formation. The main reason for this is that in the presence of oxygen THC is slowly converted into unknown decomposition products (6).

The fact that THC is rapidly inactivated by exposure to oxygen, light, humidity and elevated temperatures suggests that it may be involved in a photochemical reaction with oxygen. The structure of THC is shown in Figure 1. The oxidation of THC to CBN involves the loss of four hydrogen atoms. Figure1 also shows the structure of CBN. It may be possible for THC to be photoexcited by means of light such that it would give off electrons, possibly to oxygen, and in this way lose hydrogen atoms and convert to an oxidized compound in the

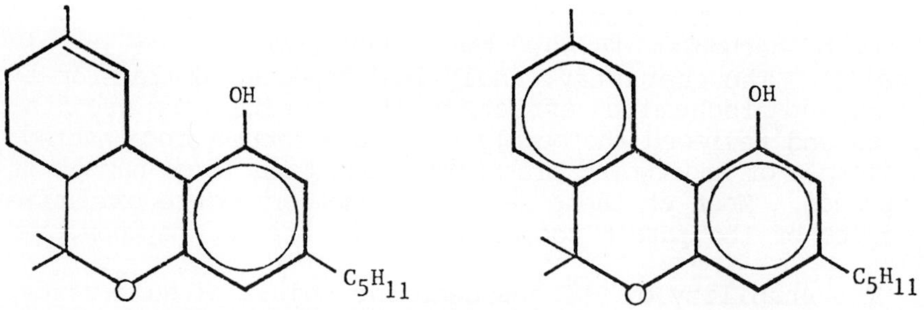

OH C_5H_{11}

Δ^9-THC

OH C_5H_{11}

CBN

FIGURE 1. Structure of delta-9-tetrahydrocannabinol (THC) and cannabinol (CBN).

form of cannabinol. Photoexcited molecules exist in a high energy state, and their chemistry is much more varied than molecules that are not excited. Photons may be released from or taken up by photoexcited molecules and as a result of changes in the pK_a (logarithmic transformation of dissociation constant), dissociate into either ions or radicals. Photo-elimination and photoaddition reactions both occur. Some molecules may carry out photoreduction of another molecule and are themselves oxidized (7).

The superoxide radical O_2^-) is a highly reactive compound produced when oxygen is reduced by a single electron (O_2 + 1 $e^- \longrightarrow O_2^-$). The superoxide radicals are important agents in the toxicity of oxygen and are partially hazardous to living matter (8). This reduction may occur by several different mechanisms in biological systems. Superoxide radicals may be generated during the normal catalytic function of a number of enzymes including xanthine oxidase (the enzyme responsible for uric acid production (9), and cytochrome P-450, a component of one of the drug detoxifying systems of liver (10); it can also be formed during the oxidation of hemoglobin to methemoglobin (11).

The short-lived superoxide radical can also be produced by non-enzymatic reactions. It can be generated in a secondary reaction after the passage of ionizing radiation through water (12) thus making possible production of the O_2^- in tissues exposed to ionizing radiation. Ionization radiation, especially the technique of pulse radiolysis is claimed by Rabini (13) to be one of the better methods of generating high concentrations of O_2^-.

Another method of O_2^- production is photochemical reduction. Several photosensitive dyes, after being reduced by exposure to light, reoxidize in a dark reaction and provide sufficient amounts of O_2^- to initiate O_2^- specific reactions. Among these dyes are methylene blue, flavins (14) and nitro blue tetrazolium chloride (NBT) (15).

Non-enzymatic generation of O_2^- radicals was obtained by fluorescent illumination of a solution containing riboflavin and NBT. The illumination resulted in a linear accumulation of blue formazan in the presence of oxygen. Blue formazan production was followed by increased absorbance at 560 nm. The absorbance increased linearly with time of illumination. Figure 2 shows the general scheme of the reaction. Riboflavin is reduced by illumination in the presence of methionine (hydrogen donor) to the dihydro form of riboflavin. The dihydro form is oxidized to riboflavin in what is called the dark reaction. In the course of this cyclic reduction-oxidation of riboflavin, electrons are given off to oxygen (16) to form the superoxide radicals. The superoxide radical then donates an electron to NBT forming the insoluble formazan blue (17).

Production of O_2^- was followed by monitoring the increased absorbance at 560 nm due to formazan blue formation (NBT reduction) formed with electrons donated by superoxide radicals.

In this study the above method was modified to accommodate the solubility of THC. Ethanol was substituted for water as the solvent. Using this modification the reaction scheme was tested for O_2^- production as well as inhibition of NBT reduction by superoxide dismutase (SOD) upon finding the modified assay workable, THC was substituted for NBT as shown in Figure 2.

Within the wavelength range of 277-290 nm THC in ethanol has a shallow extinction coefficient ($epsilon_{285}$ = 1550 liter mol^{-1} cm^{-1})(1); but when converted to CBN, it has a much larger extinction coefficient ($epsilon_{285}$ = 18,000 liter mol^{-1} cm^{-1}) (1). If THC is converted to CBN in the presence of the O_2^-, the increase absorbance at 285 nm can be monitored with this assay.

Assays involving O_2^- production were performed in the presence and absence of THC. If THC was converted to CBN or another cannabinoid by the O_2^- radicals, a change in absorbance should be detected due to the cumulative presence of CBN or another cannabinoid (newly oxidized THC).

II. METHODS

A. Non-enzymatic Production of O_2^-

Superoxide radicals were produced by photoillumination of glass cuvettes containing 1.17 x 10^{-6} M riboflavin, 5.6 x 10^{-5} M NBT, 0.01 M methionine, and 5.6 x 10^{-5} M potassium phosphate with a pH of 7.8 at 30-33°C. The illumination source consisted of two 15 watt fluorescent lamps set at a distance of 17.5 cm from the top of the cuvettes. All illuminations were performed in an aluminum foil lined box (23 x 55 cm) with a foil lined cardboard lid. A volume of 0.3 ml of each given stock solution was combined and mixed with 1.8 ml ethanol to give the final desired concentrations in a total volume of 3.0 ml. Proper precautions were taken to avoid exposure of riboflavin and NBT to light. Both solutions were covered with aluminum foil and opened only under dim light.

B. Absorption Spectrum of THC in 95% Ethanol

A reference absorption spectrum (200-300 nm) of THC (6.3 mcg/ml) was made in 95% ethanol using a quartz cuvette. The spectrum obtained in ethanol was compared to the spectrum of

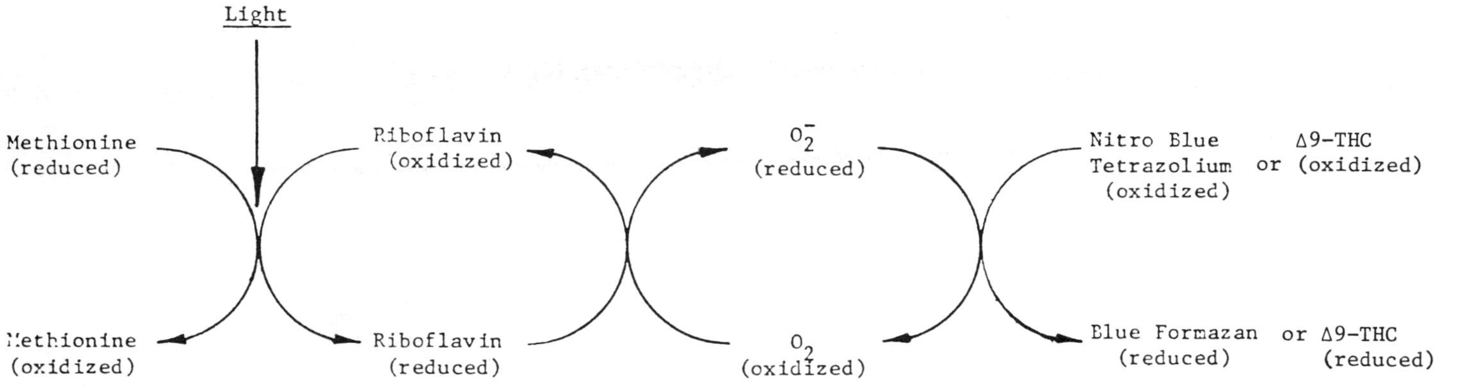

FIGURE 2. Pathway of nitro blue tetrazolium and THC reduction.

THC (6.3 mcg/ml) obtained in the modified reaction mixture. Wavelengths scans of the individual reactants and their combinations with and without THC (6.3 mcg/ml) and light were done under all combinant conditions using the ACTA II spectrophotometer and a Beckman 10" recorder (Figure 3).

C. NBT Reduction Inhibition by SOD in Ethanol

Inhibition of NBT reduction by SOD in the photoreduction system involving ethanol and riboflavin was accomplished by preparing cuvettes containing 1.17 x 10^{-5} M NBT and 0.05 M

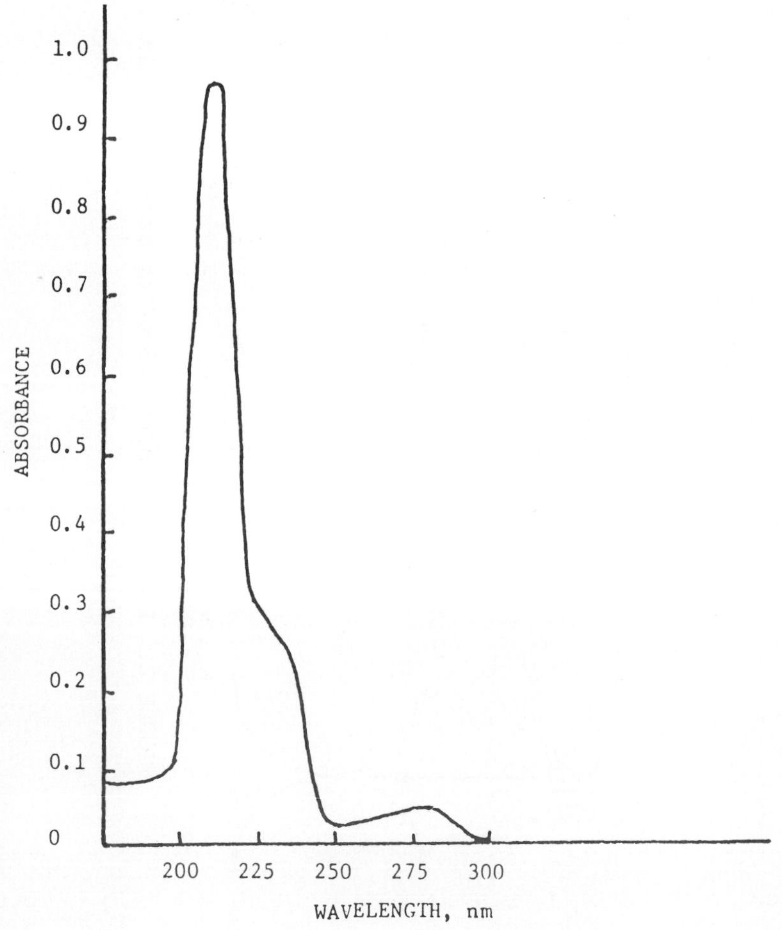

FIGURE 3. Wave length scan of 6.3 mcl/ml THC in 95% ethanol.

potassium phosphate pH 7.8. A volume of 0.3 ml of each stock solution prepared gave the final concentration in a total volume of 3.0 ml. The final concentration of ethanol (EtOH) was adjusted as close as possible to 57% by use of 95% EtOH and absolute EtOH plus water. The following volumes were used for the different concentrations of SOD: No SOD, 1.8 ml 95% EtOH; 0.3 ml SOD, 1.5 ml absolute EtOH; 0.1 ml SOD, 1.70 ml absolute EtOH; 10 mcl SOD, 1.71 ml absolute EtOH, 0.08 ml water; 5 mcl SOD, 1.710 ml absolute EtOH, 0.085 ml water and 1 mcl SOD, 1.710 ml absolute EtOH, 0.089 ml water. The final concentrations of EtOH are given in Table 1. It is important that solutions are added in the following order: EtOH, H_2O, buffer, NBT, methionine, SOD, and riboflavin last. If methionine is added to the alcohol first, it will tend to precipitate out at the high concentrations of ethanol. The superoxide dismutase used in this experiment was isolated, purified, and assayed as to activity in our laboratory.

After addition of riboflavin (shielded from light), the cuvettes were immediately blanked on the spectrophotometer and then illuminated with the two 15 watt fluorescent lamps for 30 minutes with absorbance readings recorded every five minutes. The percent inhibition was calculated from change in absorbance after 15 minutes since the reaction rate declined after 20 minutes.

TABLE I. Inhibition by Superoxide Dismutase (SOD) of Nitro Blue Tetrazolium (NBT) Reduction System Containing Riboflavin and Ethanol*

% Ethanol	SOD (ml)	SOD (mcg)	560 15 min	% Inhibition
57.0	0.000	0	0.174	-
50.0	0.300	3,600	0.001	99.43
56.6	0.100	1,200	0.004	97.71
57.0	0.010	12	0.041	76.94
57.0	0.005	6	0.080	54.03
57.0	0.001	1.2	0.160	8.05

*Reduction of NBT, during 15 min of illumination, was measured in terms of increased absorbancy at 560 nm. Inhibition (%) caused by superoxide dismutase was calculated as function of concentration of this enzyme. Results were calculated on the basis of two separate trials made in a total volume of 3.0 ml at 33°C, pH 7.8 in presence of air.

D. Substitution of NBT with THC (6.3 mcg/ml)

Nitro blue tetrazolium was omitted from the reaction mixture and replaced with 0.3 ml of water and 6.3 mcg/ml of THC in order to direct all the superoxide radicals produced at THC. An absorption spectrum of THC in quartz cuvette, was obtained prior to illumination with fluorescent light and 20 minutes after illumination.

E. Substitution of NBT with THC (6.3 mcg/ml), plus SOD

The above experiment was repeated with the addition of 20 units SOD to each cuvette. The absorption spectrum of 6.3 mcg/ml THC remained the same prior to and after fluorescent illumination (Data not shown).

F. Substitution of Methionine with THC (15.7 mcg/ml) in presence of NBT

The photoreduction reaction of riboflavin was performed in the absence of methionine. Assays were conducted with and without THC. The rational was that since methionine provides the hydrogen atoms necessary for riboflavin reduction; replacing it with THC would test the ability of THC to act as a hydrogen source. In order to provide a sufficient source of hydrogen atoms, the concentration of THC was increased to 15.7 mcg/ml.

One cuvette contained only the reaction mixture (minus methionine), and another cuvette contained the same mixture plus 15.7 mcg/ml THC. A third cuvette also contained 15.7 mcg/ml THC, but it was shielded from light with parafilm and aluminum foil. All three were illuminated for 60 minutes with two 15 watt fluorescent lamps, and 560 nm absorbance reading were taken at 10 minute intervals.

III. RESULTS

A. Non-enzymatic Production

Figure 4 presents a wavelength scan of blue formazan formed as a result of superoxide radicals reducing NBT. The scheme for formation of blue formazan is shown in Figure 2. Blue formazan production was quantitated by monitoring its increase in absorbance at 560 nm. Table I indicates production of blue formazan in ethanol by O_2^- while riboflavin and methionine are illuminated by two 15 watt fluorescent lamps.

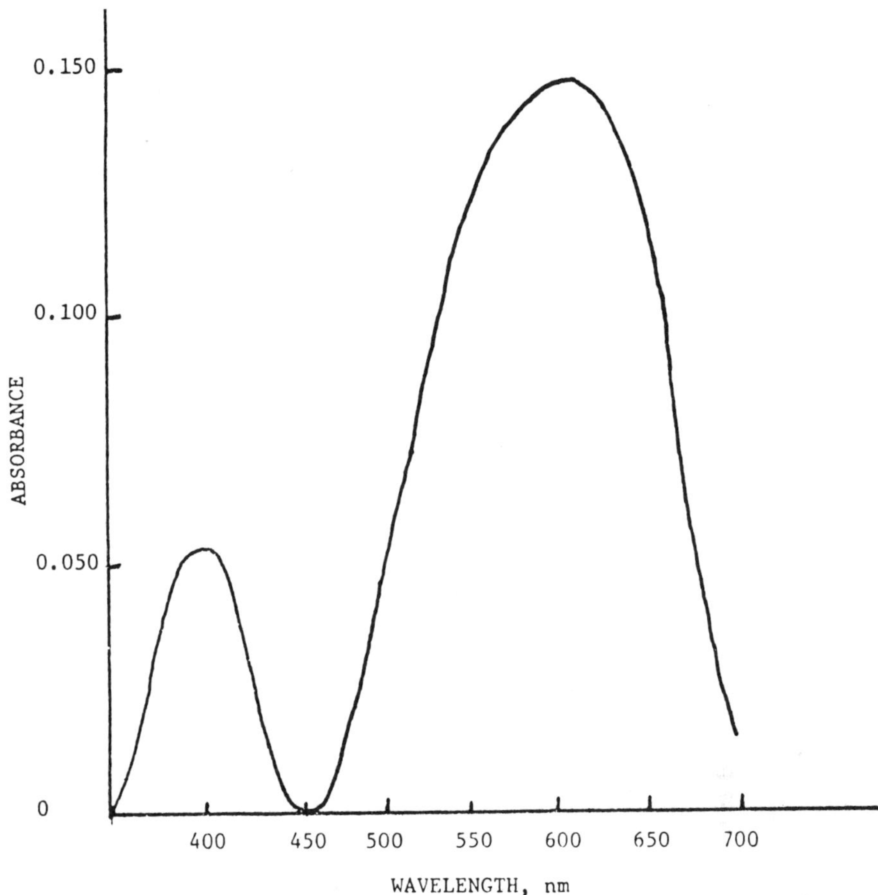

FIGURE 4. Wavelength scan of reduced nitro blue tetrazolium produced by photoreduction of riboflavin.

This method of O_2^- production was first used by Beauchamp and Fridovich as an assay for superoxide dismutase insolution (15). They employed water as the solvent. In this investigation ethanol was substituted for water because of THC's solubility in ethanol and because superoxide radicals could be easily generated from riboflavin using the organic solvent.

B. NBT reduction Inhibition by SOD in Ethanol

Table I shows that superoxide dismutase was actively functional at a concentration of 57% ethanol in the photoilluminated reaction mixture containing riboflavin and methionine. The enzyme was not denatured at this concentration. At the end of 15 minutes the photoilluminated NBT mixture showed an absorbance of 0.174. The system, using ethanol as solvent was assayed for SOD activity in that one unit is defined as that amount of enzyme causing 50% inhibition of the reaction under specified conditions of the assay. This is shown in Table I. One unit of SOD which caused a 50 +/- 4% inhibition under these conditions was equivalent to 2 mcg of bovineerythrocyte enzyme per milliliter (6.0 mcg/3 ml). The inhibition of the NBT reduction system is illustrated in Figure 5. The formation of blue formazan was inhibited by SOD due to SOD scavenging the O_2^- produced.

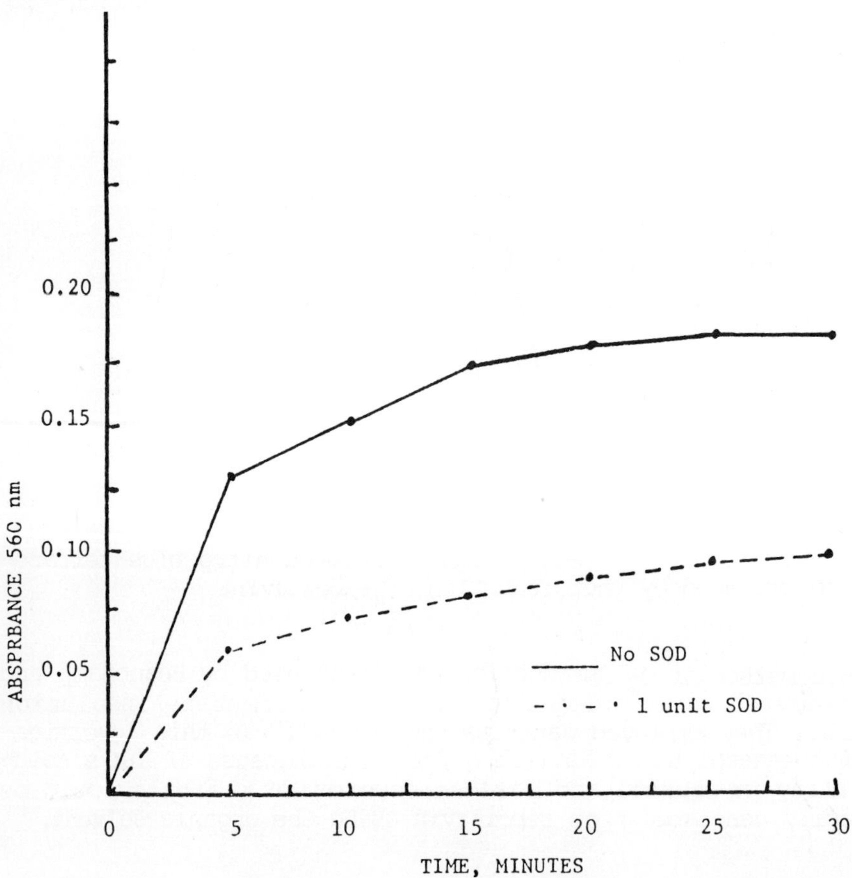

FIGURE 5. Rate of blue formazan production in ethanol (solid line) and inhibition by 1 unit SOD (dashed line) during photoreduction of riboflavin, pH 7.8, 30°C.

C. Substitution of NBT with THC (6.3 mcg/ml)

The resulting scans obtained prior to and after illumination are shown in Figure 6. After exposure to O_2^- (scan B, Figure 6) there is a 42% reduction at the 285 nm peak as compared to the previous scan (scan A, Figure 6) of THC exposed to superoxide radicals. The exposure of THC to O_2^- resulted in formation of a new cannabinoid which was not cannabinol.

Scans A and B of Figure 6 when compared to the absorption spectrum of THC in ethanol alone (Figure 3) showed some marked differences. The ethanol alone THC showed a peak at 210 nm and a shoulder at 225-237 nm. In the photoreduction reaction, prior to and after illumination with fluorescent light, the

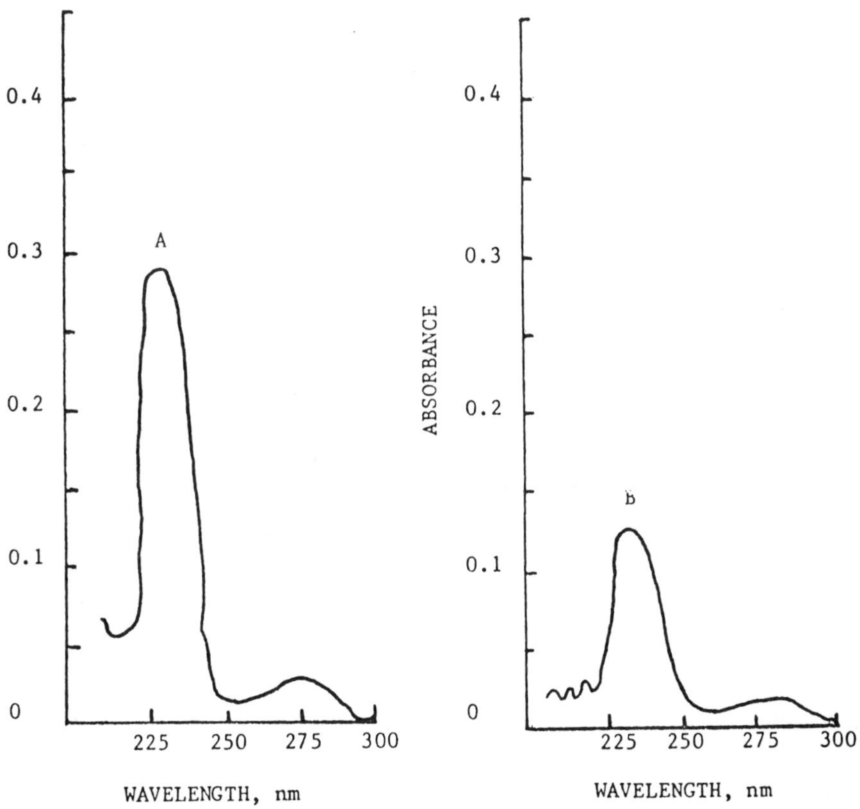

FIGURE 6. Absorption spectrum of THC prior to (A) and after illumination (B) of the photoreduction system in the absence of NBT.

peak of 210 nm is replaced by a peak at 232 nm, and the shoulder is not visible. Some semblance of the peak at 210 nm could be detected in the reaction mixture when a higher dynode voltage on the spectrophotometer was used, but only in ethanol alone was the 210 nm peak readily visible.

The reagents used in the reaction mixture were scanned (data not shown), and only methionine showed a high absorbance peak at 230 to 235 nm. Methionine did not show a peak at 275 to 285 nm. The possibility exists that methionine contributed to the peak at 232 nm because the high concentration of methionine used in the experiments may not be blanked out completely. The 42% decrease in absorbance shown by scan B, as compared to scan A (Figure 6) could be due to methionine's loss of hydrogen atoms to riboflavin. During illumination the configuration of methionine might change from the reduced form to the oxidized form, and be responsible for the decreased absorbance shown. This seems unlikely, since all concentrations of methionine receiving fluorescent illumination were blanked by a reference cuvette.

D. Substitution of NBT with THC (6.3 mcg/ml), plus SOD

No change was noted at 232 nm or 285 nm. These results indicate that O_2^- might be responsible for the decreased absorbance at 232 nm, as seen in the previous results.

E. Substitution of Methionine with THC (15.7 mcg/ml) in the Presence of NBT

After 60 minutes, the cuvette without THC read 0.002 absorbance units. The cuvette containing THC had an absorbance of 0.006; while the one shielded from light still read zero. These were then irradiated with fluorescent light for 11 additional hours. At the end of 12 hours, readings were again taken. The cuvette shielded from light remained at zero, the cuvette with no THC read 0.033, and the illuminated cuvette containing THC read 0.052.

The assays done in the absence of methionine demonstrated to a limited extent that THC was able to act as a hydrogen donor during the illumination of riboflavin. In the absence of light THC did not have the ability to act as a hydrogen donor; although the reaction was slow, it was reproducible.

The ability of THC to donate it's hydrogens was dependent on the presence of riboflavin. Illumination of the reaction mixture in the absence of methionine and riboflavin for 2 hours showed no significant increase in absorbance (data not shown). In a span of 12 hours, THC could not be photoexcited nor could it directly reduce NBT by losing an electron to O_2 or donating its hydrogen directly to NBT.

IV. DISCUSSION

The insolubility problem of THC was overcome by the useof a non-enzymatic system of O_2^- generation. A modification of the system of Beauchamp and Fridovich (15) used ethanol instead of water and had distinct advantages. This modification provides a means of assaying the oxidation or reduction of many water insoluble compounds by superoxide radicals. It also provides a means to study reactions involving oxygen in reference to photochemical reactions involving visible light. Also, the fact that superoxide dismutase remains functional in 57% ethanol fortifies the use of ethanol in the NBT photoreduction system.

The non-enzymatic production of O_2^- in ethanol demonstrated (Figure 6) that THC could be converted to cannabinol by means of the superoxide radical and that formation of this cannabinoid was prevented in the presence of superoxide dismutase.

Modifications of the NBT assay in ethanol can be made to serve several purposes. A chemical may be substituted for methionine (see scheme, Figure 2) to determine whether the chemical can serve as a hydrogen donor for riboflavin when illuminated with fluorescent light. The ability of the chemical to donate hydrogens to riboflavin can be measured spectrophotometrically by the amount of NBT reduced to blue formazan. The different absorbance spectra of the neutral, anion and dihydro forms of riboflavin (7) can also be easily differentiated and may be used to ascertain if riboflavin is reduced by the chemical being tested in the presence of fluorescent light.

Both methionine and riboflavin can also be substituted by the chemical being tested in order to determine if the chemical can donate electrons to NBT directly or indirectly by means of O_2^- when illuminated with fluorescent light.

Another substitution would be to replace NBT alone with the chemical being studied. By doing this, the flux of superoxide radicals generated can be directed to the chemical under study. Any reaction between the O_2^- and the chemical may be monitored using the spectrophotometer.

The assay for NBT reduction by O_2^- was primarily developed to measure superoxide dismutase activity (15). The role of superoxide radicals in oxidation-reduction reactions involving water soluble compounds is being observed in both biological and chemical systems (18-20). This investigation using the system of NBT reduction in ethanol provides a method in which the role of superoxide radicals in oxidation-reduction reactions, involving water insoluble compounds, may be investigated.

Assays applying the NBT reduction system, in either water or ethanol, may provide information in the study of drug detoxification by means of O_2^- generation as it takes place in cells and cytochrome systems - i.e. the P-450 cytochrome system (10). One objective of this investigation was to explore the possibility that THC exposed to superoxide radicals could form a new metabolite, and that this new metabolite could be a non-psychoactive substance. These studies suggest that O_2^- might well be used to detoxify drugs. The results of cannabinol formation from THC indicated that oxidation of THC *in vitro* is a slow process and that more drastic conditions such as increased heat and long term exposure to oxygen are needed to dehydrogenate THC. Due to THC's solubility in lipid components of living cells, the oxidation of THC is probably more easily facilitated *in vivo*.

REFERENCES

1. Mechoulam, R., McCallum, N. K., and Burstein, S., Recent advances in the chemistry and biochemistry of cannabis, Chem. Rev. 76:75-112 (1976).
2. Mechoulam, R., "Marijuana", p. 151. Academic Press, New York, 1973.
3. Razdan, R. K., in "Proceeding of the National Academy of Science Committee on Problems of Drug Dependence: 32nd Meeting", Toronto, 1970.
4. Lerner, N., Marijuana: Tetrahydrocannabinol and related compounds, Science 140:175 (1963).
5. Korte, F., and Sieper, H., Paper chromatographic identification hashish - containing substances, Tetrahedron 10:153 (1960).
6. Allward, W. H., Babcock, P. A., Segelman, A. B., and Cross, T. M., Photochemical studies of marijuana (Cannabis) constituents, J. Pharm. Sci. 61:1995 (1972).
7. Metzler, D. A., "Biochemistry", pp. 766-767. Academic Press, Inc., New York, 1977.
8. Gregory, E. M., Goscin, S. A., and Fridovich, I., Superoxide dismutase and oxygen toxicity in a eukaryote, J. Bacteriol. 117:456-460 (1974).
9. Fridovich, I., and Handler, P., Detection of free radicals generated during enzymatic oxidation by the initiation of sulfite oxidation, J. Biol. Chem. 236:1836-1840 (1961).

10. Strobel, H. W., and Coon, M. T., Effects of superoxide generation and dismutation on hydroxylation reactions catalyzed by liver microsomal cytochrome P-450, J. Biol. Chem. 246:7826-7829 (1971).
11. Misra, H. P. and Fridovich, I., The generation of superoxide radical during autoxidation of hemoglobin, J. Biol. Chem. 247:6960-6966 (1972).
12. Hart, E. T., Radiation chemistry of aqueous solutions, Ann. Rev. Nucl. Sci. 15:125-150 (1965).
13. Rabini, J., and Nielsen, S. O., Absorption spectrum and decay kinetics of O_2^- and HO_2 in aqueous solutions by pulse radiolysis, J. Phys. Chem. 73:3736 (1969).
14. Goscin, S. A., and Fridovich, I., The purification and properties of superoxide dismutase from Saccharomyces cerevisiae, Biochem. Biophys. Acta. 289:276-283 (1972).
15. Beauchamp, C., and Fridovich, I., Superoxide dismutase: Improved assay and an assay applicable to acrylamide gels, Anal. Biochem. 44:276-287 (1971).
16. Massey, V., Strickland, S., Mayhew, S. G., Howell, L. G., Engel, P. C., Matthews, R. G., Shuman, M., and Sulivan, P. A., Production of superoxide anion radicals in the reaction of reduced flavins and flavoproteins with molecular oxygen, Biochem. Biophys. Res. Commun. 36:891 (1969).
17. Rajogopalan, K. V., and Handler, P. J., Hepatic aldehyde oxidase. II. Differential inhibition of electron transfer to various electron acceptors, J. Biol. Chem. 239:2022 (1964).
18. Lavelle, F., Michelson, A. M., and Dimitrijevic, L., Biological protection by superoxide dismutase, Biochem. Biophys. Res. Commun. 55:350-357 (1973).
19. Fridovich, I., Superoxide dismutase, in "Ann. Rev. Biochem.", Vol. 44 (E. E. Small, ed.), pp. 147-159. Annual Reviews Inc., Palo Alto, CA, 1975.
20. Bors, W., Saran, M., Lengelder, E., Spottl, R., and Michel, C., The relevance of the superoxide anion radical in biological systems, Curr. Top. Radiat. Res. 9:247-309 (1974).

Section IV REPRODUCTIVE ASPECTS

THE EFFECTS OF CHRONIC ADMINISTRATION OF DELTA-9-TETRAHYDROCANNABINOL ON THE EARLY EMBRYONIC DEVELOPMENT OF MICE

T. Nogawa, O. Shinohara
R. T. Henrich, A. Morishima

Department of Pediatrics
College of Physicians and Surgeons
Columbia University
New York, New York

I. INTRODUCTION

The effects of cannabis and its principal psychoactive cannabinoid, delta-9-tetrahydrocannabinol (THC), on the reproductive system have been examined by a number of investigators. In males, marijuana smoking or administration of THC has been shown to suppress the circulating levels of follicle-stimulating hormone (FSH) and luteinizing hormone (LH), accompanied by a decrease in the level of testosterone in man, rhesus monkeys and rodents (1-5). Chronic administration of cannabinoids to man, mice and rats have resulted in decreased weights of the testes and the accessory sex organs, in histological changes of the testes, in decreased sperm counts, and in increased incidence of morphologically abnormal sperms (6-12). Although most of these observations can be explained by the suppressive effect of cannabinoids on testosterone, through decreasing the levels of FSH and LH, the available evidence indicates that cannabinoids can also act directly on the testes. In rats, the effects of THC could not be blocked by administration of testosterone (13), and *in vitro* production of testosterone and protein synthesis by isolated Leydig cells were inhibited when THC or other cannabinoids were added to the incubation medium (14). In mice, chromosome aberra-

*Supported, in major part, by NIDA grant DA-02833.

ISBN 0-12-044620-0

tions of the primary spermatocytes were induced by administration of cannabinoids, including THC (12,15).

Less information is available on the effects of cannabis and THC on the female reproductive system. An altered menstrual cycle characterized by anovulatory or shortened luteal phase have been found in women who smoked marijuana frequently (16). In rats and rhesus monkeys administration of THC abolished the pre-ovulatory LH surge, inducing anovulation (17,18). In rodents, chronic treatment with marijuana extract or THC resulted in abolishment of the estrus cycles, a decrease in weights of the ovaries and the uterus, and a decline in the glycogen contents of the uterus (19-21). An acute administration of THC to ovariectomized rhesus monkeys induced a dose-dependent decrease of plasma FSH and LH levels, which could be prevented by administration of LH-releasing hormone (22). This observation suggested that THC acts through the hypothalamic controls of gonadotropins. However, a recent study has shown that THC may affect the ovaries directly. *In vitro* steroidogenesis by isolated rat follicles was inhibited by THC, and the resumption of meiosis, as determined by the germinal vesicle breakdown, was induced without the usual accompaniment of detachment of the cumulus-granulosa cells from the ova (23).

The available teratogenic studies on cannabis and THC have been reviewed by Rosenkrantz (24). There is a general agreement that, when cannabis extract or THC is administered chronically to pregnant animals, there is an increase in *in utero* fetal wastage and a decrease in the birth weight. When non-pregnant adult female rhesus monkeys were chronically treated with THC and mated with untreated males, a similar increase in fetal wastage was observed (25).

Currently, marijuana is widely abused by young females who are sexually immature or in the process of sexual maturation (26). Yet, there is a paucity of information concerning the possible sequela on their reproductive function by a prolonged use of the drug. Unlike sperms and most somatic tissues, *de novo* formation of oogonia does not occur postnatally, oocytes have already reached the dictyate stage at about the time of birth (27). Therefore, damages inflicted on oocytes are more likely to be permanent, and may be detected in the fertilized eggs and embryos. To imitate the abuse of marijuana by sexually immature and adolescent girls, immature female mice were chronically treated with THC and their early embryogenesis was examined in the present study.

II. MATERIALS AND METHODS

Twenty-six-day old female Swiss-Webster mice were obtained from CAMM (New Jersey) and maintained under the condition of a controlled light-dark cycle (lights on 05:00-19:00 h.). The room temperature was maintained at 24°C. Purina chow and water were available _ad libitum_. THC (100 mg/ml in absolute ethanol) was obtained from the National Institute on Drug Abuse. The vial containing THC was kept under nitrogen gas in a refrigerator after it had been opened. The original solution was diluted first with absolute ethanol to obtain a concentration of 5 mg/ml and then further diluted with 10% polysorbate (TWEEN-80) in saline. The final concentration of THC was 0.5 mg/ml and that of ethanol was 10%.

Administration of THC or the vehicle was started when the mice were 30-days old, and was continued daily for a total of 21 days. The vaginal opening generally occurs in the mice on the 35th day of life. The experimental group of mice were injected intraperitoneally with 0.2 ml. of THC solution (0.1 mg THC). The dose of THC was calculated to be approximately 5 mg/kg/day, and roughly equivalent to that absorbed by a man smoking 1 to 2 marijuana cigarettes per day, in accordance with the conversion described by Rosenkrantz (28). The control group received only the vehicle.

The mice were injected intraperitoneally with 5 I.U. of pregnant mare serum (Gestyl, Organon) at noon on the last day of THC injection, and 48 hours later with 5 I. U. of human chorionic gonadotropin (hCG, Pregnyl, Organon) in order to induce superovulation. Pregnant mare serum of 5 I.U. was considered to be the optimum dose after a preliminary studyin which attempts were made to maximize the yield of recoverable ova and minimize the incidence of morphologically abnormal ova. The time of hCG injection was considered as time zero. Females were placed with untreated adult males immediately after hCG injection, and were allowed to mate for 16 hours. At the end of this period, the vagina of each female mouse was checked for the presence of a vaginal plug, and the males were removed from the cages.

Females were sacrificed by cervical dislocation at 49 to 52 hours after hCG injection. From a preliminary study, it had been determined that this timing would approximately correspond to the time for the second cleavage division. The ovaries, oviducts and uterine horns were removed, and were examined for inflammatory signs. The ova were flushed out from the oviduct into the Hank's balanced salt solution, using a 31 gauge needle attached to 1 ml tuberculin syringe under a dissecting microscope. The ova were transferred onto a depression slide by mouth-operated micropipette and were subjected to photomicroscopy with the phase contrast optics. They were then pipetted onto a slide, air-dried, stained with Giemsa solution, and were subjected to photomicroscopy for studies of segregational errors of chromosomes (29). The data were analyzed by the Chi-square test.

III. RESULTS

From 146 control and 158 THC-treated mice, 4384 and 4973 ova were obtained, respectively. The rate of mating (number of mice with vaginal plug/total number of mice) and the rate of fertilization (number of mice that had 2-, 3-, and/or 4-cell stage ova/number of mice with vaginal plug) were 62.6% and 87.1%, respectively, in the control, and 60.8% and 88.4% respectively, in the THC-treated group. The mean number of ovulated ova was 30.1 +/- 18.9 (S.D.) in the control and 31.5 +/- 13.0 in the THC-treated group. These differences were not statistically significant.

Between 49 and 52 hours after hCG injection, the majority of ova were in the 2-cell stage, 62.4% in the control and 59.7% in the THC-treated group (Table I). Three or 4-cell stage ova were seen in 13.1% in the control and 10.9% in the THC-treated group. The incidence of abnormal ova was 14.2% for the controls, and was higher at 20.0% in the THC-treated group. This difference was statistically significant at $p<0.005$.

From the observations made in both the control and the THC-treated groups, morphologically abnormal ova were classified in accordance with the description of Harman and Talbert

TABLE I. Incidence of Morphologically Normal and Abnormal Gestational Products of the Mouse, 49 to 52 hours after Injection of Human Chiorionic Gonadotropin*

	Normal (%) Cell Stage				Abnormal (%)	Total No. of ova
	1	2	3	4		
Control	10.3	62.4	4.7	8.4	14.2	4384
THC	9.4	59.7	3.2	7.7	20.0	4973

*Increase of Abnormal ova in THC group $p < 0.005$

(Fig. 1) (30). Liquifaction degeneration (D) takes an appearance of amorphous material dispersing within the zona pellucida. In fragmentation of ooplasm (E), the ooplasm takes the appearance of numerous fragments of non-uniform sizes. Unequal cleavage (F) has one cytoplasm less than one-half of the diameter of the other. Premature loss of zona pellucida (G) lacks zona around the ooplasm. In addition there were some abnormalities that were not described by Harman and Talbert (30). These abnormalities were defined as follows: Zona only (H) is the zona pellucida without the ooplasm, and premature hatching (I) is an ovum with the ooplasm extruding from the zona pellucida. The latter may be a process leading to a loss of zona pellucida. In morphologically abnormal ova, it was often impossible to determine the exact stage of development of the ova with confidence. Therefore, no attempt was made to assign them into 1- to 4-cell stages.

In both the control and the THC-treated groups, fragmentation of ooplasm and liquifaction degeneration were the main types of abnormalities (Table II). Taken together, 90.4% from the control and 87.5% from the THC-treated group were in these categories. The incidence of the other abnormalities was considerably lower. The distribution of each type of abnormality was not different between the two groups.

The mitotic indices of the ova between the two groups did not differ significantly at 8.1% for the controls and 7.0% for the THC-treated group. A total of 327 ova from the control and 292 from the THC-treated group were found to be in mitosis. The total number of ova undergoing an abnormal segregational process (29) was too small to derive a meaningful anal-

TABLE II. Types and Incidence of Morphologically Abnormal Gestational Products of the Mouse, 49 to 52 hours after Injection of Human Chorionic Gonadotropin

Types of Abnormalities	Percent of Abnormalities: Control 623 ova	Percent of Abnormalities: THC 997 ova
Fragmentation of Ooplasm	46.9	50.6
Liquifaction Degeneration	43.5	36.9
Zona Only	5.9	8.0
Absence of Zona	2.6	3.0
Unequal Cleavage	0.8	1.3
Premature Hatching	0.3	0.2

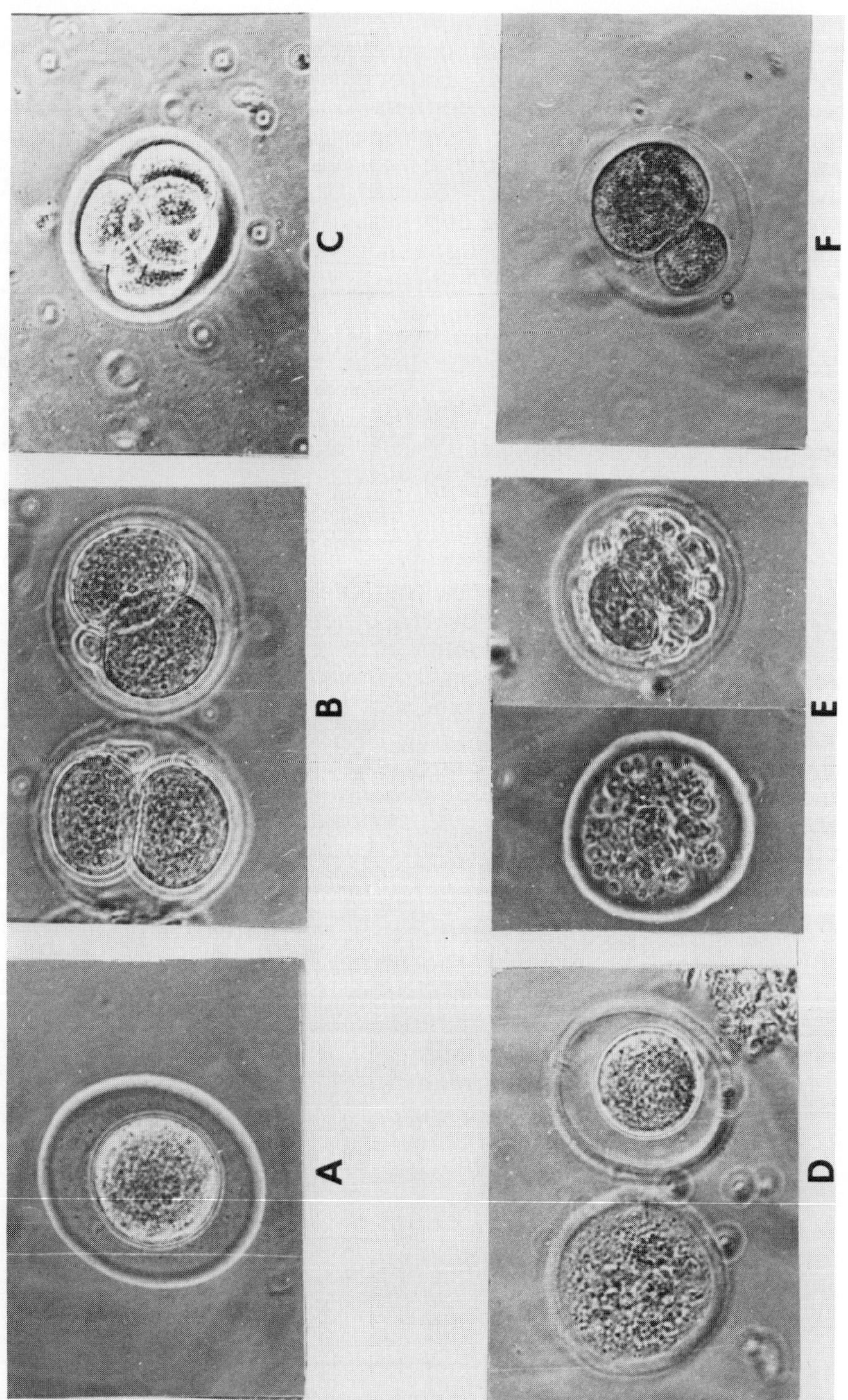
A
B
C
D
E
F

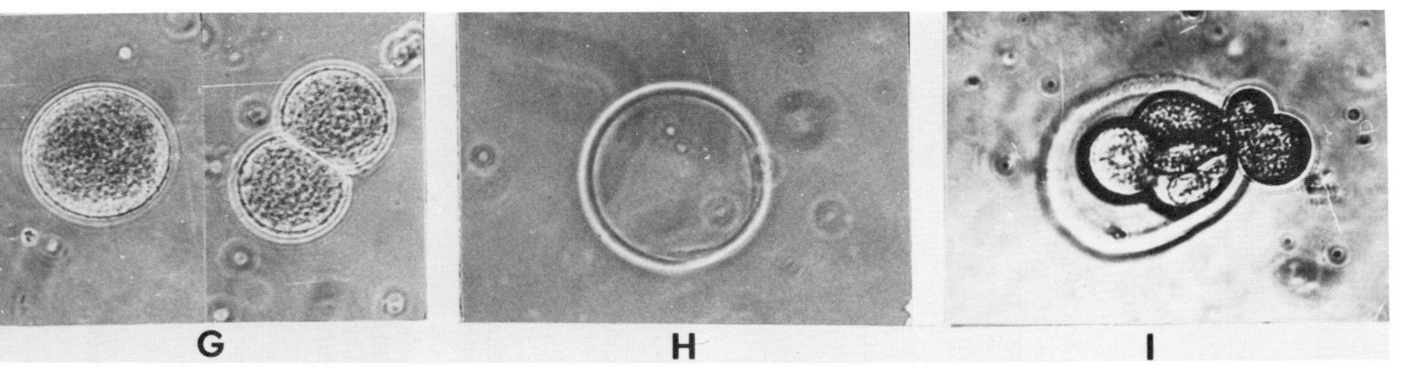

FIGURE 1. A–C: Normal ova. (A) A normal 1-cell stage ovum; (B) Normal 2-cell stage ova with with a polar body in the right ovum; (C) A normal 4-cell stage ovum.

D–I: Abnormal ova of various morphology. (D) Liuification degeneration of the left ovum, and a normal ovum on the right; (E) Fragmentation of ooplasm in 2 ova; (F) Unequal cleavage; (G) Premature loss of zona pellucida in 1-cell and 2-cell stage ova; (H) Zona only; (I) Premature hatching.

ysis, although no obvious difference in the incidence was observed between the two groups.

IV. DISCUSSION

Chronic administration of THC, at a modest dose, to presumably sexually developing mice and continuing through their early adulthood but terminating before mating, induced a significant increase in morphologically abnormal ova. Although the absolute percentage increase was relatively small at 5.8%, the order of magnitude was not greatly different from the induction of abnormal sperms by THC in mice (12,15). Considering the large attrition rate of pre-implantation eggs in both men and mammals (31), this degree of increase in abnormal ova will readily escape clinical detection even if the same phenomenon were to occur in female marijuana abusers.

The abnormality of ova, induced by THC, did not take on a specific morphologic appearance. The ovulation, per se, did not appear to be affected by THC since the mean number of ovulated ova did not differ between the THC-treated animals and the control group.

Although the last dose of THC was injected some 4 days before recovering the ova, the known sequestration of THC in various tissues (32) makes it impossible to eliminate the possibility that the observed induction of abnormal ova was not due to the effect of THC remaining at about the time of superovulation, and did not reflect the imprint of damage inflicted on the ovarian oocytes. A study with a recovery period of 42 days before sacrifice is in progress to eliminate this possibility. Damages induced in sperms (8,9,12,15) and somatic cells (6,21) by cannabis or THC tended to recover after a sufficient period of abstinence. However the ovum, a non-regenerative cell, islikely to differ considerablyfrom other tissues in its ability to repair damages.

Several mechanisms leading to the induction of abnormal ova by THC may be considered. A direct action of THC on the ovarian oocytes appears as a reasonable possibility. THC or its metabolites have been shown to accumulate in relatively high concentrations for a long period of time in the gonadal fat tissue of both male and female mice (33). A direct suppressive effect of THC on testosterone synthesis by the Leydig cells (14), and on the production of ovarian hormones by the follicular cells (23) have been described using in vitro models. Further, THC appears to affect the meiotic resumption of the dictyate oocytes (23).

A direct action of THC may well be mediated through induction of chromosomal abnormalities. Marijuana smoke has induced abnormal amounts of DNA in lung cells cultured in vitro (34,35), and an increased incidence of aneuploidy have been observed in heavy marijuana smokers (36,37). THC has induced segregational errors of chromosomes in cultured human lymphocytes (29). Aneuploidy and structural rearrangements of chromosomes have occurred in primary spermatocytes of miceafter exposure to THC (12,15). Chromosomal aberrations have also been observed in bone marrow mitosis of these mice (38).

The second possible mechanism for the induction of abnormal ova involves an indirect action of THC through its effects on the hypothalmohypophyseal axis. The known suppressive effects of THC on the gonadotropins (2,4,5,16-18,22) could affect the normal growth and/or maturation process of ovarian oocytes in a fashion not clearly understood, thus leading to an apparently normal ovulation but degeneration shortly thereafter. However, there is evidence to suggest that the suppressive effect of cannabis and THC on gonadotropin secretion is not permanent (6,21). Therefore, this hypothesis may be tested by a prolonged recovery period after the administration of THC.

Yet another possible mechanism involves direct or indirect suppression of respiration, ATP content and glucose metabolism of oocytes as was found in sperms exposed to THC (39).

These possible sites of action of THC, singularly or in combination, could lead to degeneration of ovarian oocytes or to an inhibition of fertilization, both of which may result in the observed increase in abnormal ova at the time of the second cleavage division.

ACKNOWLEDGMENTS

The authors thank Dr. Monique C. Braude of NIDA for her advice and assistance in obtaining THC.

REFERENCES

1. Cohen, S., The 94-day cannabis study, Ann. N. Y. Acad. Sci. 282:211 (1976).
2. Smith, C. G., Besch, N. F., and Asch, R. H., Effects of marijuana on the reproductive system, in "Advances in Sex Hormone Research". (J. A. Thomas and R. L. Singhal, eds.), p. 273. Urban and Schwarzenberg, Baltimore, 1980.
3. Kolodny, R. C., Masters, W. H., Kolodner, R. M., and Toro, G., Depression of plasma testosterone levels after

chronic intensive marijuana use, N. Engl. J. Med. 290:872 (1974).

4. Smith, C. G., Moore, C. E., Besch, N. F., and Besch, P. K., The effect of marijuana (delta-9-tetrahydrocannabinol) on the secretion of sex hormones in the mature Rhesus monkey, Clin. Chem. 22:1120 (1976).
5. Harclerode, J., Nyquist, S. E., Nazar, B., and Lowe, D., Effects of cannabis on sex hormones and testicular enzymes of the rodent, in "Marihuana: Biological Effects" (G. G. Nahas and W. D. M. Paton, eds.), p. 395. Pergamon Press, Oxford, 1979.
6. Fujimoto, G. I., Rosenbaum, R. M., Ziegler, D., Rettura, G., and Morrill, G. A., Effects of marijuana extract given orally on male rat reproduction and gonads, 60th Ann. Meeting The Endocrine Soc., 373, 1978.
7. Huang, H. F. S., Nahas, G. G., and Hembree, W. C., III., Effects of marijuana inhalation on spermatogenesis of the rat, in "Marihuana: Biological Effects" (G. G. Nahas and W. D. M. Paton, eds.), p. 419. Pergamon Press, Oxford, 1979.
8. Hembree, W. C., Zeidenberg, P., and Nahas, G. G., Marijuana's effects on human gonadal function, in "Marihuana: Chemistry, Biochemistry and Cellular Effects" (G.G. Nahas, W. D. M. Paton, and J. E. Idänpään-Heikkilä, eds.), p. 521. Pergamon Press, Oxford, 1976.
9. Hembree, W. C., III, Nahas, G. G., Zeidenberg, P., and Huang, H. F. S., Changes in human spermatozoa associated with high dose of marijuana smoking, in "Marihuana: Biological Effects" (G. G. Nahas and W. D. M. Paton, eds.), p. 429, Pergamon Press, Oxford, 1979.
10. Stefanis, C. N., and Issidorides, M. R., Cellular effects of chronic cannabis use in man, in "Marihuana: Chemistry, Biochemistry, and Cellular Effects" (G. G. Nahas, W. D. M. Paton, and J. E. Idänpään-Heikkilä, eds.), p. 533. Springer-Verlag, New York, 1976.
11. Dixit, V. P., Sharma, V. N., and Lohiya, N. Y., The effect of chronically administered cannabis extract on the testicular function of mice, Eur. J. Pharmacol. 26:111 (1974).
12. Zimmerman, A. M., Zimmerman, S., and Yesoda Raj, A., Effects of cannabinoids on spermatogenesis in mice, in "Marihuana: Biological Effects" (G. G. Nahas and W. D. M. Paton, eds.), p. 407. Pergamon Press, Oxford, 1979.
13. Purohit, V., Singh, H. H., and Ahluwalia, B. S., Evidence that the effects of methadone and marijuana on male reproductive organs are mediated at different sites in rats, Biol. Reprod. 20:1039 (1979).
14. Jakubovic, A., McGeer, E. G., and McGeer, P. L., Biochemical alterations induced by cannabinoids in the Leydig

cells of the rat testis*in vitro*: Effects on testosterone and protein synthesis, in "Marihuana: Biological Effects" (G. G. Nahas and W. D. M. Paton, eds.), p. 251. Pergamon Press, Oxford, 1979.

15. Dalterio, S., Badr, F., Bartke, A., and Mayfield, D., Cannabinoids in male mice: Effects on fertility and spermatogenesis, Science 215: 315 (1982).
16. Bauman, J. E., Kolodny, R. C., Dornbush, R. L., and Webster, S. K., Effectos endocrinos del uso cronico de la marijuana en mujeres, in "Simposio Internacional Sobre Actualizacion en Marijuana", Vol. 10, p. 85, Talalpan, Mexico, 1979.
17. Nir, I., Ayalon, D., Tsafriri, A., Cordova, T., and Linder H. R., Suppression of the cyclic surge of luteinizing hormone secretion and of ovulation in the rat by delta-1-tetrahydrocannabinol, Nature 243:470 (1973).
18. Asch, R. H., Smith, C. G., Siler-Knodr, T. M., and Pauerstein, C. J., Effects of delta-9-tetrahydrocannabinol during follicular phase of the Rhesus monkey (*Macaca mulatta*), J. Clin. Endocrinol. Metab. 52:50 (1981).
19. Chakravarty, I., Sengupta, D., Bhattacharyya, P., and Ghosh, J. J., Effect of treatment with cannabis extract on the water and glycogen contents of the uterus in normal and estradiol-treated prepubertal rats, Toxicol. Appl. Pharmacol. 34:513 (1975).
20. Dixit, V. P., Arya, M., and Lohiya, N. K., The effect of chronically administered cannabis extract on the female genital tract of mice and rats, Endokrinologie 66:365 (1975).
21. Fujimoto, G. I., Kostellow, A. B., Rosenbaum, R., Morrill, G. A., and Bloch, E., Effects of cannabinoids on reproductive organs in the female Fisher rat, in "Marihuana: Biological Effects" (G. G. Nahas and W. D. M. Paton, eds.), p. 441. Pergamon Press, Oxford, 1979.
22. Smith, C. G., Smith, M. T., Besch, N. F., Smith R. G., and Asch R. H., Effects of delta-9-tetrahydrocannabinol (THC) on female reproductive function, in "Marihuana: Biological Effects" (G. G. Nahas and W. D. M. Paton, eds.), p. 449. Pergamon Press, Oxford, 1979.
23. Reich, R., Laufer, N., Lewysohn, O., Cordova, T., Ayalon, D., and Tsafriri, A., In vitro effects of cannabinoids on follicular function in the rat, Biol. Reprod. 27:223 (1982).
24. Rosenkrantz, H., Effects of cannabis on fetal development of rodents, in "Marihuana: Biological Effects" (G. G. Nahas and W. D. M. Paton, eds.), p. 479. Pergamon Press, Oxford, 1979.
25. Sassenrath, E. N., Chapman, L. M., and Goo, G. P., Reproduction in rhesus monkey chronically exposed to delta-9-

tetrahydrocannabinol, in "Marihuana: Biological Effects" (G. G. Nahas and W. D. M. Paton, eds.), p. 501. Pergamon Press, Oxford, 1979.

26. Fishburne, P. M., Abelson, H. I., and Cisin, I., National Survey on Drug Abuse: Main Findings: 1979. DHHS Publication No. (ADM) 80-976. Washington, D. C., U.S. Government Printing Office, 1980.
27. Zuckerman, S., The regenerative capacity of ovarian tissue, Ciba Found. Coll. Ageing 2:31 (1956).
28. Rosenkrantz, H., The immune response and marijuana, in "Marihuana: Chemistry, Biochemistry, and Cellular Effects" (G. G. Nahas, W.. D. M. Paton, and J. E. Idänpää-Heikkilä, eds.), p. 441. Springer-Verlag, New York, 1976.
29. Henrich, R. T., Nogawa, T., and Morishima, A., In Vitro induction of segregational errors of chromosomes by natural cannabinoids in normal human lymphocytes, Environmental Mutagenesis 2:139 (1980).
30. Harman, S. M., and Talbert, G. B., Effect of maternal age on synchronization of ovulation and mating and on tubal transport of ova in mice, J. Gerontol. 29:493 (1974).
31. Roberts, C. J., and Lowe, C. R., Where have all the conceptions gone? Lancet i:498 (1975).
32. Hunt, A., and Jones, R. T., Tolerance and disposition of tetrahydrocannabinol in man, J. Pharmacol. Exp. Ther. 215:35 (1980).
33. Rawitch, A. B., Rohrer, R., and Vandaris, R. M., Delta-9-tetrahydrocannabinol uptake by adipose tissue: Preferential accumulation in gonadal fat organs, Gen. Pharmacol. 10:525 (1979).
34. Leuchtenberger, C., Leuchtenberger, R., and Schneider, A., Effects of marijuana and tobacco smoke on human lung physiology, Nature 241:137 (1973).
35. Leuchtenberger, C., Leuchtenberger, R., and Ritter, U., Effects of marijuana and tobacco smoke on DNA and chromosomal complement in human lung explants, Nature, 242:403 (1973).
36. Morishima, A., Milstein, M., Henrich, R. T., and Nahas, G. G., Effects of marijuana smoking, cannabinoids, and olivetol on replication of human lymphocytes: Formation of micronuclei, in "Pharmacology of Marihuana" (M. C. Braude and S. Szara, eds.), p. 711. Raven Press, New York, 1976.
37. Morishima, A., Henrich, R. T., Jayaraman, J., and Nahas, G. G., Hypoploid metaphases in cultured lymphocytes of marijuana smokers, in "Marihuana: Biological Effects" (G. G. Nahas and W. D. M. Paton, eds.), p. 371. Pergamon Press, Oxford, 1979.

38. Zimmerman, A. M., and Raj, A. Y., Influence of cannabinoids on somatic cells in vivo, Pharmacol. 21:277 (1980).
39. Shahar, A., and Bino, T., In vitro effects of delta-9-tetrahydrocannabinol (THC) on bull sperm, Biochem. Pharmacol. 23:1341 (1974).

CYTOLOGICAL OBSERVATIONS ON THE SEMINAL VESICLE, VENTRAL PROSTATE AND ADRENAL OF 39 DAY OLD MALE RATS TREATED NEONATALLY WITH ESTRADIOL BENZOATE AND/OR DELTA-9-TETRAHYDROCANNABINOL

Mary D. Albert
Jolane Solomon

Department of Biology
Boston College
Chestnut Hill, Massachusetts

I. INTRODUCTION

The multiple effects of marijuana and its major psychoactive components, delta-9-tetrahydrocannabinol (THC) and their metabolites on reproduction and development in humans and laboratory animals have been extensively documented (1,2).

The effects of a single injection of Estradiol Benzoate (EB) to neonatal male rats have also been investigated: on becoming adults, the rats are sterile and the testes, prostate, and seminal vesicles are underdeveloped (3-8). It has not been demonstrated whether or not these effects are produced solely by affecting the hypothalamic-pituitary axis.

Since some of the effects of THC in adult male and female humans and rodents are other effects and are not similar to those of EB (1), this study was undertaken in part to determine whether or not the effect of THC administered alone to male neonates were similar to EB. The histological results with EB on seminal vesicle, ventral prostate and adrenals confirmed the results of earlier studies, and administration of THC alone produced results similar to EB with some differences discussed in the results and discussion.

It was also of interest to determine the effect of THC administered simultaneously with EB on these target organs. In this instance the results were striking; combined doses of THC and EB markedly increased the cytological effects observed on the adrenals, ventral prostates and seminal vesicles.

The Cannabinoids: Chemical,
Pharmacologic, and Therapeutic Aspects

ISBN 0-12-044620-0

II. MATERIALS AND METHODS

Two hundred neonatal male rats, four-days old, were obtained from Charles River (Sprague-Dawley strain). THC was obtained from the National Institute on Drug Abuse (NIDA). Uninjected and sesame oil injected control animals were grouped together (n = 37) as no statistical differences were observed between the two control groups.

The experimental groups were as follows: (1) 0.5 mg/kg EB (n = 24); (2) 5.0 mg/kg EB (n = 17); (3) 10 mg/kg EB (n = 29);

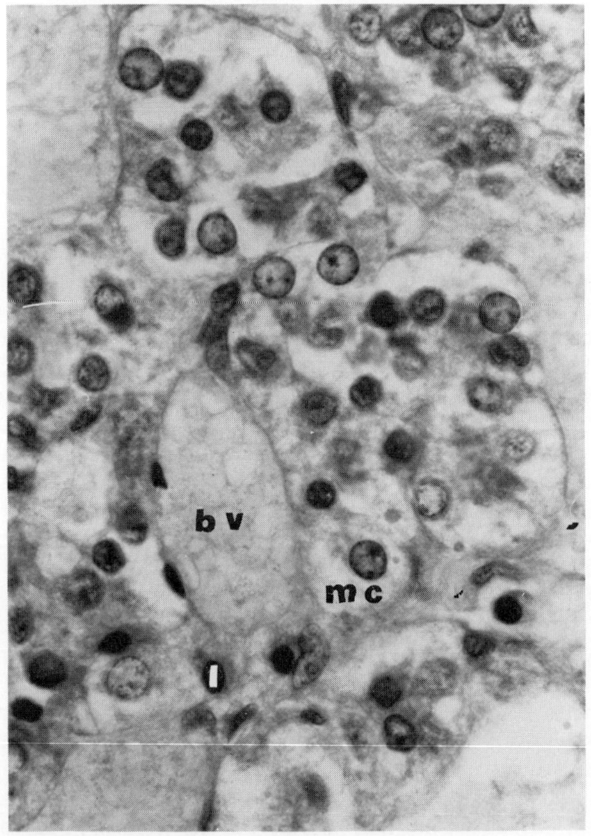

FIGURE 1. Adrenal: Medulla of control rat, 1000X. (Abbreviations used in figures: blood vessel (bv); cellular debris (cd); epithelium (e); lumen (l); matrix (m); medullary cell (mc); muscle (mu); secretory material (sm).

(4) 1 mg/kg THC (n = 17); (5) 10 mg/kg THC (n = 14); (6) 20 mg/kg THC (n = 15); (7) 0.5 mg/kg EB + 20 mg/kg THC (n = 15); (8) 5.0 mg/kg EB + 20 mg/kg THC (n = 10); (9) 10 mg/kg EB + 20 mg/kg THC (n = 10); (10) 10 mg/kg EB + 20 mg/kg THC (n = 21).

The animals were injected subcutaneously at four days of age with the appropriate compound(s) in sesame oil. The animals were sacrificed by chloroform inhalation at 30 days of age. At autopsy, seminal vesicles, prostates and adrenals were excised, weighed, and fixed in Bouin's aqueous fixative. Organs were cut at 5 microns and stained in hematoxylin and eosin (H & E) for histological examination.

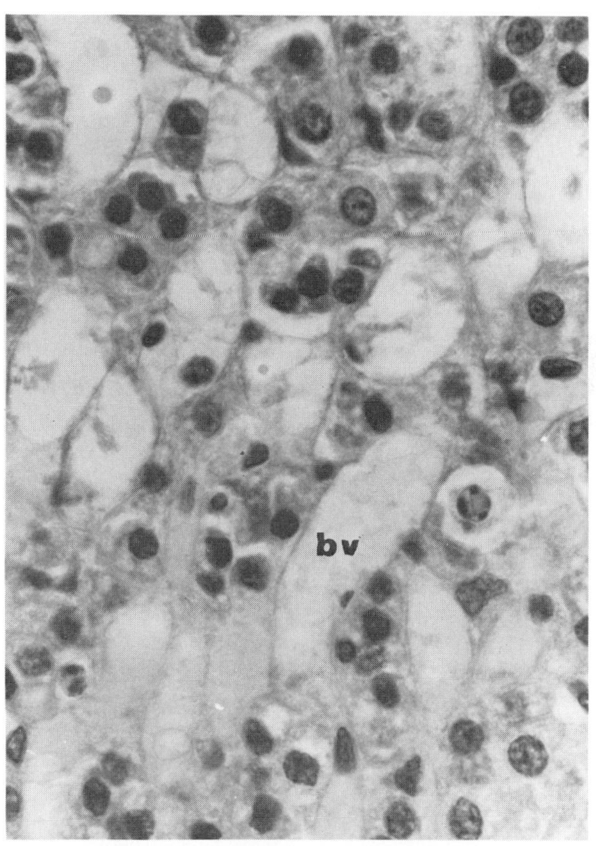

FIGURE 2. Adrenal: Zona reticularis adjacent to medulla of adrenal in Fig. 1. Control rat, 1000X.

III. RESULTS

A. Adrenals

With 0.5 mg/kg of EB there was a noticeable reduction of lymphocytes (9) in the medulla. There appeared to be a slight, stimulatory effect on the zona reticularis but the effect was not seen consistently and differentiating from controls was difficult.

With the largest doses of EB (5 and 10 mg/kg), thereduction in the number of lymphocytes was more apparent; the blood vessels of the medulla were distended. The effect on the zona

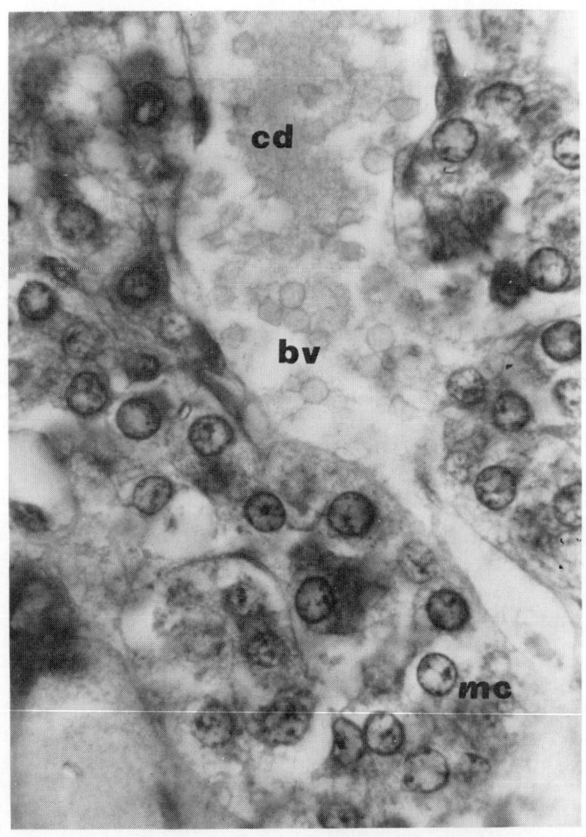

FIGURE 3. Adrenal: Medulla of rat treated with 10 mg/kg EB + 20 mg/kg THC, 1000X. Note sinusoids filled with apparent cellular debris and the decrease in lymphocytes.

reticularis was obvious: the cells appeared highly stimulated, opalescent, transparent, and the blood vessels between these anastomosing cells were widely distended.

With the 1 mg/kg dose of THC the lymphocytes in the medulla were almost entirely eliminated; the same effect was seen at the next two dose levels of THC (10 and 20 mg/kg). In essence, all 3 doses of THC eliminated medullary lymphocytes. The effect of THC on these cells was greater than that seen with any dose level of EB alone. There were few consistent observable effects of THC alone on the cortex, in contrast to the stimulatory effects of EB on the cortex.

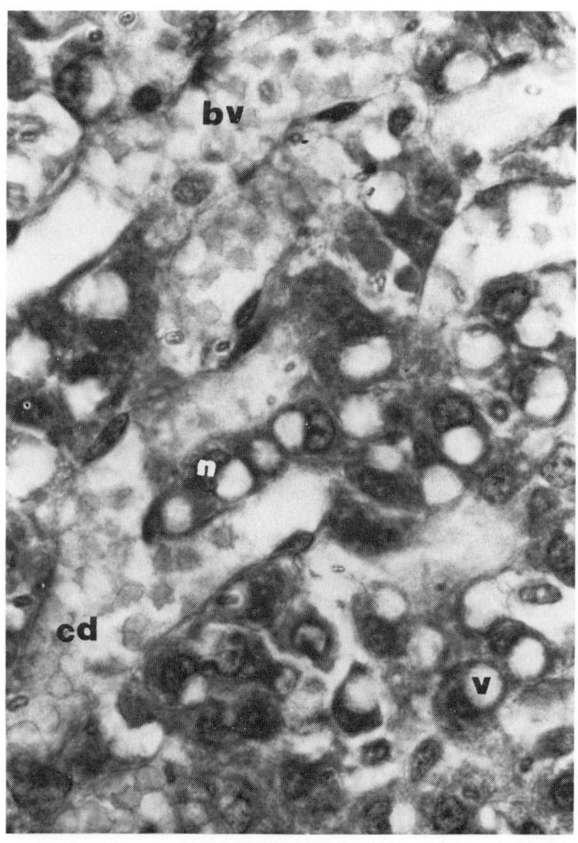

FIGURE 4. Adrenal: Zona reticularis adjacent to medulla of adrenal in Fig. 3. Rat treated with 10 mg/kg EB + 20 mg/kg THC, 1000X. Note vacuolated cells and sinusoids filled with material similar to that found in medulla sinusoids.

When 0.5 mg/kg EB was combined with 20 mg/kg THC, the effects appeared to be additive. The medulla had few if any lymphocytes, but the zona reticularis looked more stimulated than in animals receiving 0.5 mg/kg EB alone or any dose of THC alone, and were easily differentiated from controls.

The result was somewhat different when 5 or 10 mg/kg EB was combined with 20 mg/kg THC. In the medulla the number of lymphocytes continued to be markedly reduced as above, and in addition, the medullary blood vessels were greatly distended with what appeared to be large amounts of cellular debris. In the cortex, the zona reticularis was much more obviously stimulated by THC plus 5 or 10 mg/kg EB than with the same doses

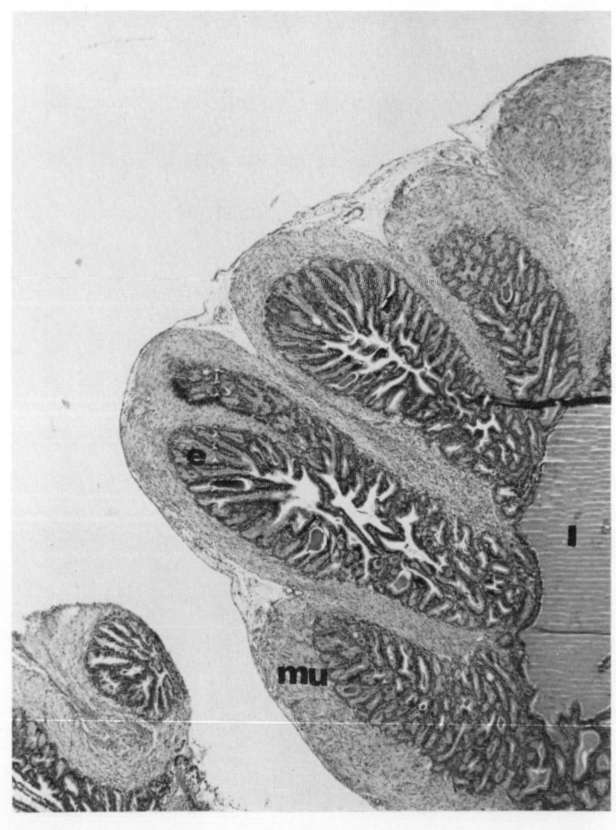

FIGURE 5. Seminal Vesicle: Control rat, 40X. Note highly infolded epithelium with secondary and tertiary folds and large lumen filled with heavily staining secretory material (marked l).

of EB alone. The sinusoids were widely distended and packed with red blood cells and debris. The majority of the cells of the reticularis appeared so vacuolated that the nucleus was displaced to one side of the cell (Figures 1-4). In sum, all doses of THC alone affected medullary lymphocytes but had little if any effect on the adrenal cortex. EB alone affects both the medulla and cortex. When THC and EB are administered simultaneously, THC potentiates the effect of EB on the zona reticularis and possibly the medulla.

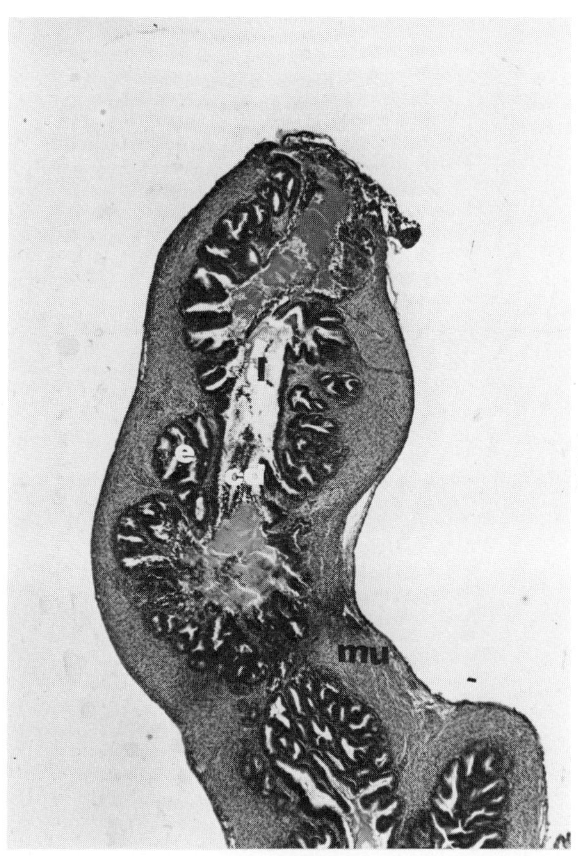

FIGURE 6. Seminal Vesicle: Rat treated with 20 mg/kg THC, 40X. Note change in organization of seminal vesicle. Compared to control, there is a shrinkage of epithelium and large amounts of hemorrhagic cellular debris in the lumen. Secretory material is markedly decreased.

B. Seminal Vesicle

The effect of 0.5 mg/kg EB was not uniform. In the most affected tissues there was less secretory material and less extensive infolding of the epithelium. The height of the epithelium (high columnar) appeared unchanged. There was some disruption of the smooth muscle and connective tissue sheath.

With the increase in dose to 5 or 10 mg/kg EB there was still variation form organ to organ. Those most affected showed a further reduction in the amount of secretory material and infolding of the epithelium. With increasing doses of EB,

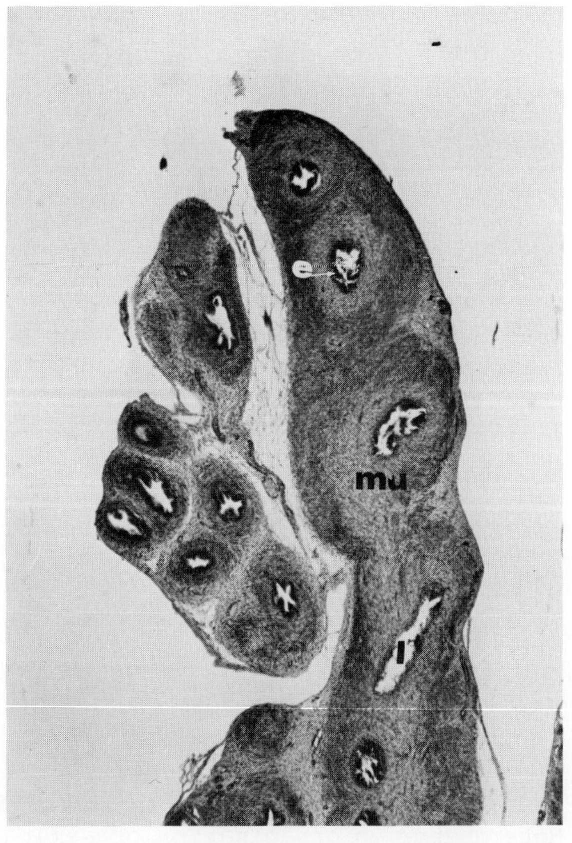

FIGURE 7. Seminal Vesicle: Rat treated with 10 mg/kg EB, 40X. Note dramatic loss of infolding and decrease in size of lumen and loss of secretory material.

there was a further disruption of the smooth muscle and connective tissue sheath and a decided increase in the cellular debris within the lumina (Figures 5,7,9,11).

There was a progressive effect with the three dose levels of THC. With 1 mg/kg THC there was a slight reduction in luminal material, and an infolding of the epithelium. There was more loss at the 10 mg/kg dose level; and at 20 mg/kg THC there was still less secretory material. The epithelium had retracted further. Disruption of the smooth muscle and connective tissue sheath was more apparent, and large amount of cellular debris were seen in the lumina (Figures 6,10).

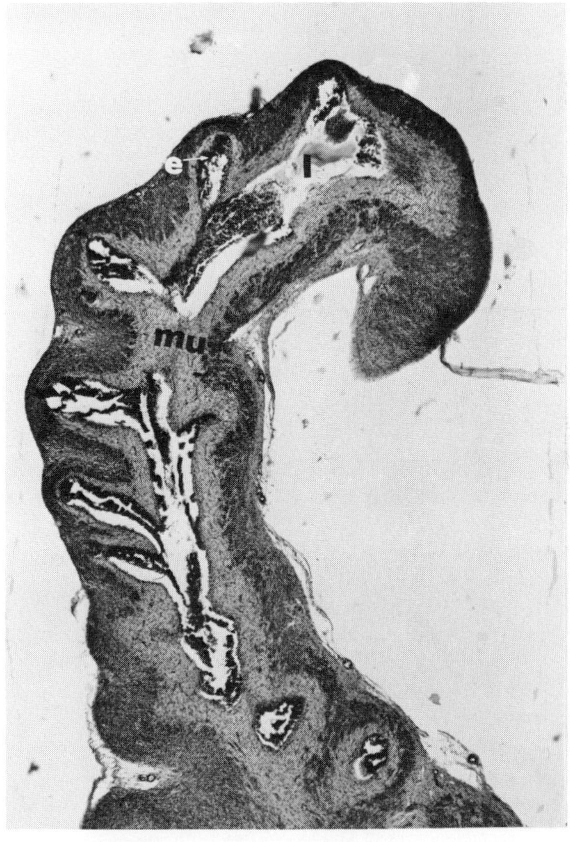

FIGURE 8. Seminal Vesicle: Rat treated with 10 mg/kg EB + 20 mg/kg THC, 40X. Note entire epithelial lining is disintegrating. The fibromuscular layer surrounding the epithelium appears hypertrophized. The connective tissue sheath is disorganized.

When 0.5 of 5 mg/kg EB and 20 mg/kg THC were combined, the effect was much greater than with either substance alone. Some secretory material was present, but markedly decreased from the same doses of THC or EB alone. The epithelium had retracted still more with loss of secondary and tertiary folds. Cells within the epithelium were disrupted.

When 10 mg/kg EB and 20 mg/kg THC were combined the damage was so severe that in only a few of the animals could the seminal vesicle be recognized as the organ observed. The amount of secretory material was negligible. The epithelium was almost non-existent. There were enormous amounts of cellular debris. There were only tiny openings in the areas here and there to indicate where they had originally been large lumina. The smooth muscle and connective tissue sheaths were

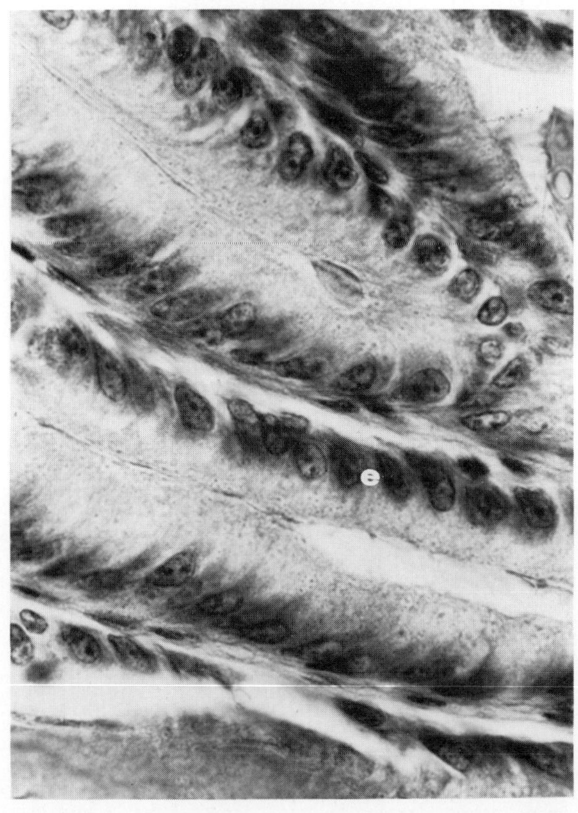

FIGURE 9. Seminal Vesicle: Control rat, 1000X. Note high columnar epithelium and cytoplasm filled with secretory material.

markedly disrupted (Figures 8,12). In sum, both THC and EB alone disrupted seminal vesicle tissue in a dose response manner. When THC and EB were administered simultaneously, the disruptive effect was greatly magnified.

C. Ventral Prostate

With 0.5 mg/kg EB, it was somewhat difficult to make comparisons because the ventral prostate tissue obtained from the controls (Figures 13,17) varied more widely than control adre-

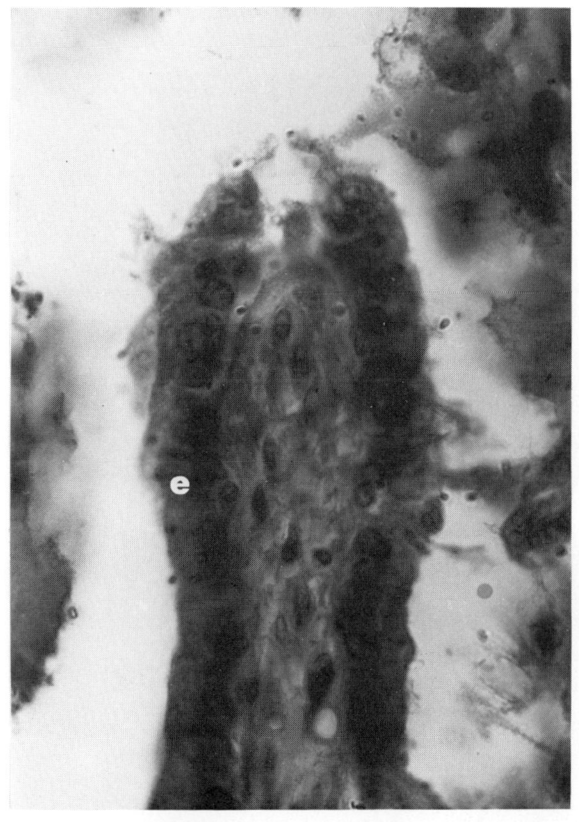

FIGURE 10. Seminal Vesicle: Rat treated with 20 mg/kg THC, 1000X. Note loss of integrity of epithelium and cells sloughing off at tip. Little if any secretory material is present in the compact cytoplasm. Cells low columnar or cuboidal.

nals or seminal vesicles. A few organs from treated animals showed a slight reduction in secretory material, and a loss of interluminal matrix.

However, there was a decided effect when the dose of EB was increased to 5 or 10 mg/kg. The amount of secretion and interluminal matrix was reduced. The orderly arrangement of the organ was disrupted. The epithelium for the most part was cuboidal whereas in controls there was wide variation from squamous to high columnar. In many areas, cells looked moribund with pale nuclei and compact darkly staining cytoplasm (Figures 15,19).

With 1 mg/kg THC there was a reduction in interluminal matrix and a change in the staining characteristics of the

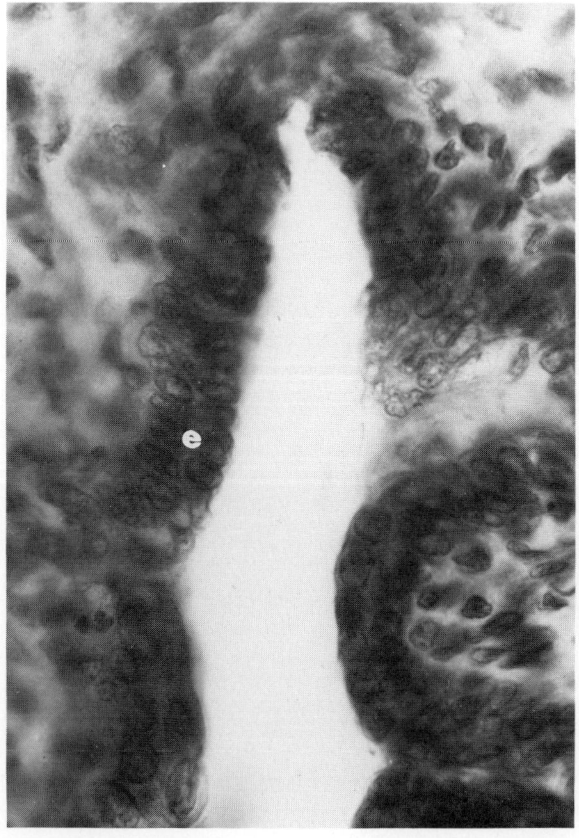

FIGURE 11. Seminal Vesicle: Rat treated with 10 mg/kg EB, 1000X. Note striatified-like appearance of epithelial cells.

secretory material. With increase of the dose to 10 mg/kg THC there was a definite effect. There was increased reduction in interluminal matrix; naked strands of connective tissue fibers stood out between lumina. There was a marked difference in staining of luminal material when compared to controls.

At the highest level, 20 mg/kg THC (Figures 14,18), there was a greater loss of interluminal matrix, and the luminal material was comparable to that seen with 10 mg/kg THC (not shown).

When 0.5 mg/kg EB and 20 mg/kg THC were combined, the effect was striking. Damage was extensive. Only little secretory material was present. The interluminal matrix had

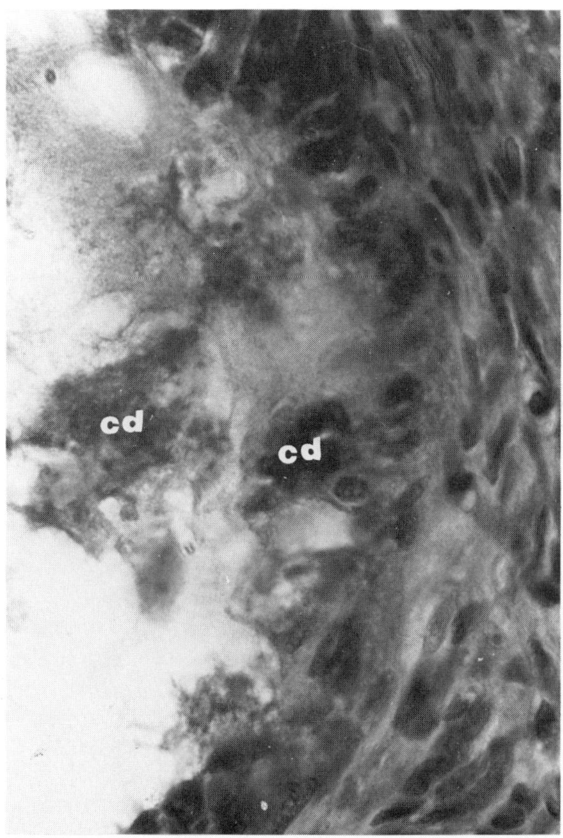

FIGURE 12. Seminal Vesicle: Rat treated with 10 mg/kg EB + 20 mg/kg THC, 1000X. Note lining has disintegrated completely and cells and cellular remnants are spilling out into the lumen.

disappeared in large areas, and the organ was barely held together by the outer connective sheath-membrane.

The damage was more severe in those rats receiving 5 and 10 mg/kg EB and 20 mg/kg THC. The thin layer of smooth muscle surrounding each lumen was all that appeared intact. The matrix was all but gone, leaving the connective tissue fibers naked. There was little secretory material, and the epithelium had disintegrated (Figures 16,20).

In summarizing the effect of EB and THC on the ventral prostate, although EB and THC each affect the secretory material and matrix, EB was more effective in reducingsecretory material, and THC more effective in reducing the matrix, when combined, the cytological effects were much greater thanwith either substance alone.

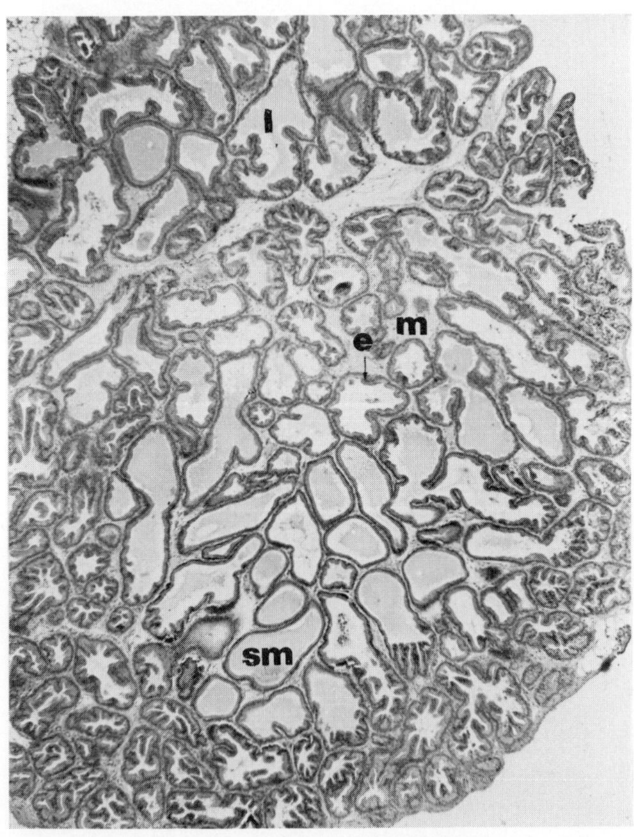

FIGURE 13. Ventral Prostate: Control rat, 40X. Note lumina filled with uniformly stained secretory material. Matrix surrounding lumina is also uniformly stained.

IV. DISCUSSION

There are many reports which suggest that cannabinoids stimulate adrenal cortical activity by increasing ACTH activity (10-19). One site of action appears to be the hypothalamic-pituitary axis, see the review of Block et al. (1). Neto et al. found CME (crude marijuana extract) potentiated estradiol stimulation of adrenal and pituitary weight gain of corticosteroidogenesis (20). Simmons found increased adrenal and pituitary weights when EB alone was administered to neonatal male rats (21). In our study, we find that THC which alone had no observable effect on the cortex, increased the

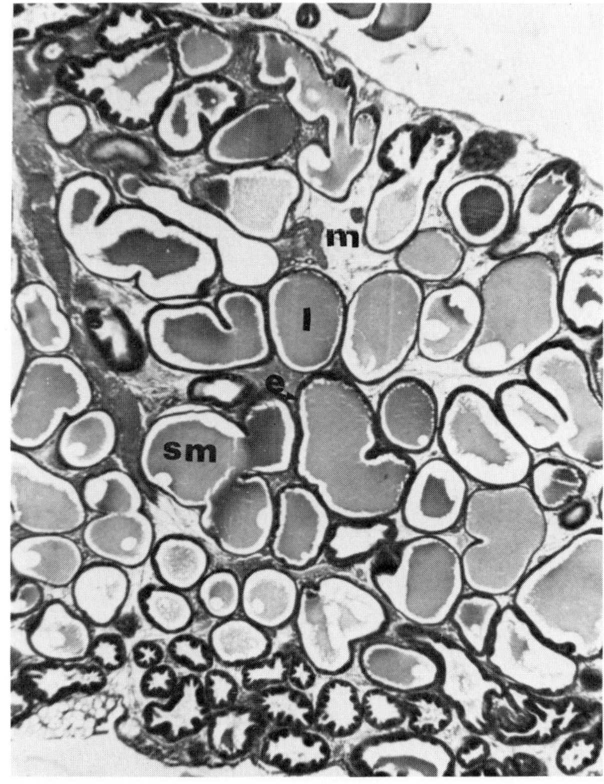

FIGURE 14. Ventral Prostate: Rat treated with 20 mg/kg THC, 40X. Note the intensely dark staining of both the luminal material and the epithelial cells. This is typical of all THC-treated tissues stained with H & E.

stimulatory effect of EB on the cortex, specifically on the zona reticularis. This effect was observed only at the highest dose level for both EB (10 mg/kg) and THC (20 mg/kg).

In this study, high doses of EB alone affected the medulla, causing a reduction in the number of lymphocytes and an increase in sinusoidal material. Again, THC potentiated the effect of EB. THC alone sharply reduced the number of lymphocytes in the medulla. Banchereau et al. found that THC depressed H^3-thymidine and H^3-uridine uptake in vitro in cultured lymphocytes obtained from healthy men (22). Other authors have obtained similar results (23-27). This action may not be specific to the lymphocyte population of the adrenals, for there has been a reported decrease in thymus weights after the use of either THC (28) or CME (29-31).

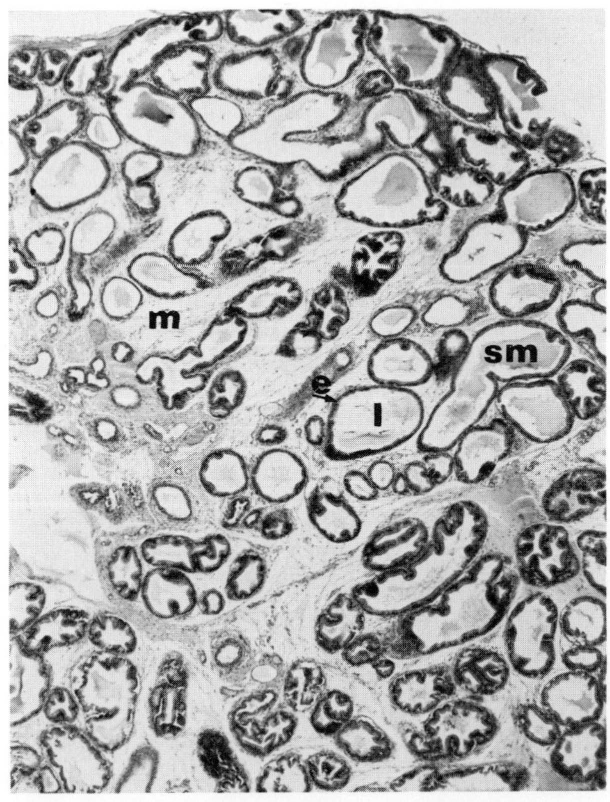

FIGURE 15. Ventral Prostate: Rat treated with 10 mg/kg EB, 40X. Note disintegration and disruption of intercellular matrix, leaving bare reticular fibers, and loss of secretory material.

In the case of the adrenal cortex, THC alone had no observable histological effect. However, Maskarinec et al. using adult male rats, injected THC p.o. for seven days and found dose-dependent elevations of corticosterone and its metabolite, 5-alpha-pregnane-3,11,21-triol-20-one (31). Levels of androgen metabolites also increased although testosterone remained unchanged, except at a dose level of 50 mg/kg.

The lobes of prostate, dorsal, ventral, and lateral, do not react uniformly to treatment with the same compound, e.g., Zn^{65}, prolactin. However, similar tissues of different glands, chiefly, epithelial, muscular, and connective of the prostate and seminal vesicle, respond similarly to EB or testosterone. Belis et al. found that EB _in vivo_ selectively

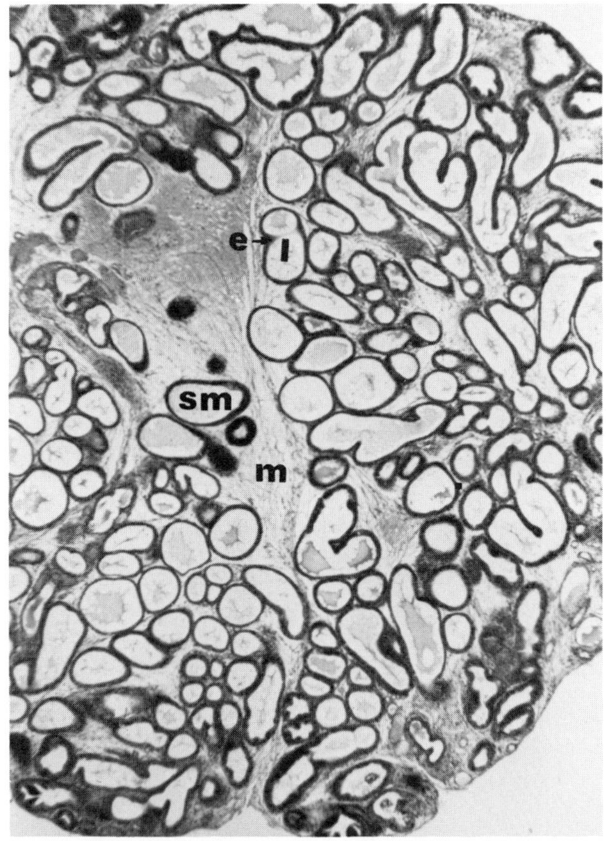

FIGURE 16. Ventral Prostate: Rat treated with 10 mg/kg EB + 20 mg/kg THC, 40X. Note increased loss of secretory material and intercullular matrix as compared to rats treated with THC and EB alone.

caused growth of the fibro-muscular component of both the prostate and seminal vesicle in castrated guinea pigs (37). They raise the possibility that hormonal regulation of the prostate may be primarily estrogenic. Feyel-Cabanes et al., working with explants of the ventral prostate of intact seven- to eight-week old rats, found that fibro-muscular growth appeared to depend on the absolute concentration of testosterone (38,39).

One unified factor in reproductive organ development of male rats is that administration of EB during the critical time of 1 to 5 days postnatally inhibits the growth and maturation of both the ventral prostate and seminal vesicle; spermatogenesis and the usual rise in testosterone levels are

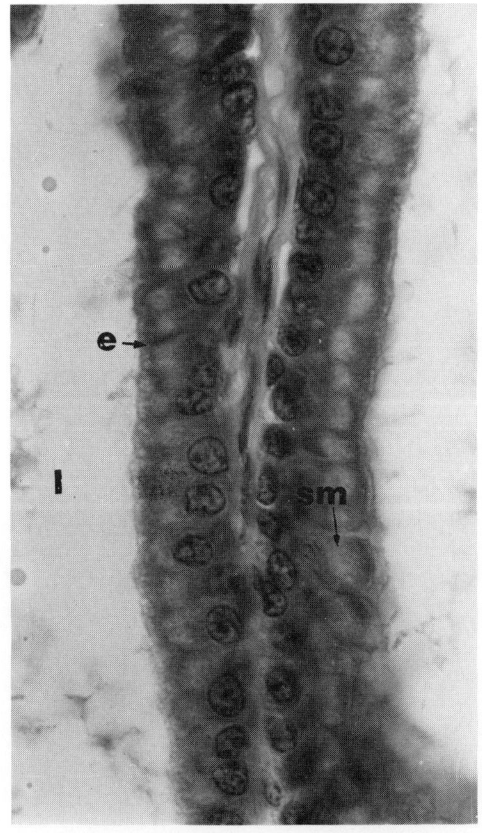

FIGURE 17. Ventral Prostate: Control rat, 1000X. Note high columnar epithelium filled with lightly staining secretory material.

inhibited when these animals are examined at about 39 days of age (3,4,7,40). Our results with EB on the seminal vesicle and ventral prostate corroborate our findings on the testes of rats treated similarly and sacrificed at 39 days of age (see Chapter 26, this volume).

How this action is accomplished is open to question. It has yet to be determined whether is is the result of direct action of EB on the organs themselves or indirect action of gonadotropins on the hypothalamic-pituitary axis. It is possible that a combination of both direct and indirecteffects plays a role. The possibility that both kinds of effects are involved arises again when considering the effects of THC

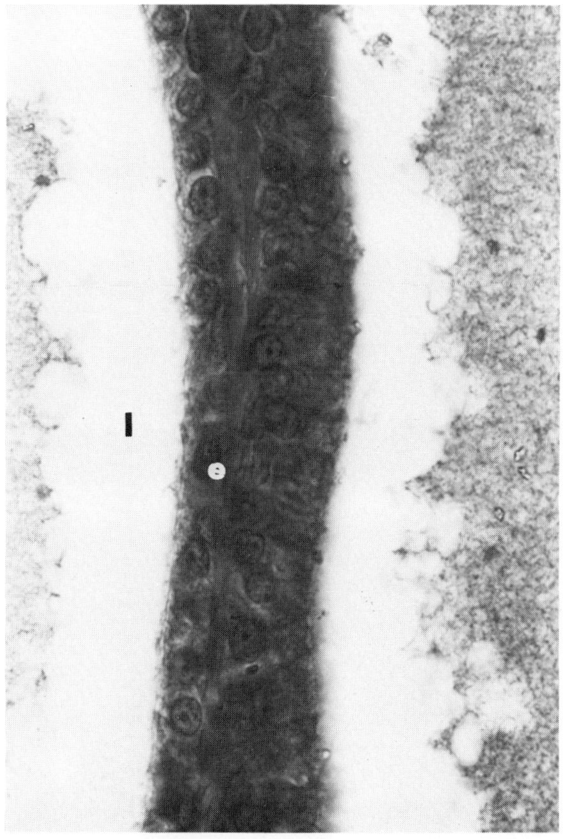

FIGURE 18. Ventral Prostate: Rat treated with 20 mg/kg THC, 1000X. Note the loss of height and marked compactness of epithelial cells. There are two rows of epithelium and a lumen on either side.

alone or combined with EB on the seminal vesicle and ventral prostate. Purochit et al. in a study using castrated and hypophysectomized rats conclude that the antiandrogenic effects of THC on the ventral prostate and seminal vesicle were due to direct effects at the tissue level as well as indirect effects at the hypothalmic-hypophyseal site (41). In a second paper, Purohit et al., using rat prostate cytosol, found that THC and a dozen other metabolites inhibited specific binding of dihydrotestosterone to the androgen receptor (42). They have suggested that both estrogenic and antiandrogenic compounds may be present in marijuana and its metabolites.

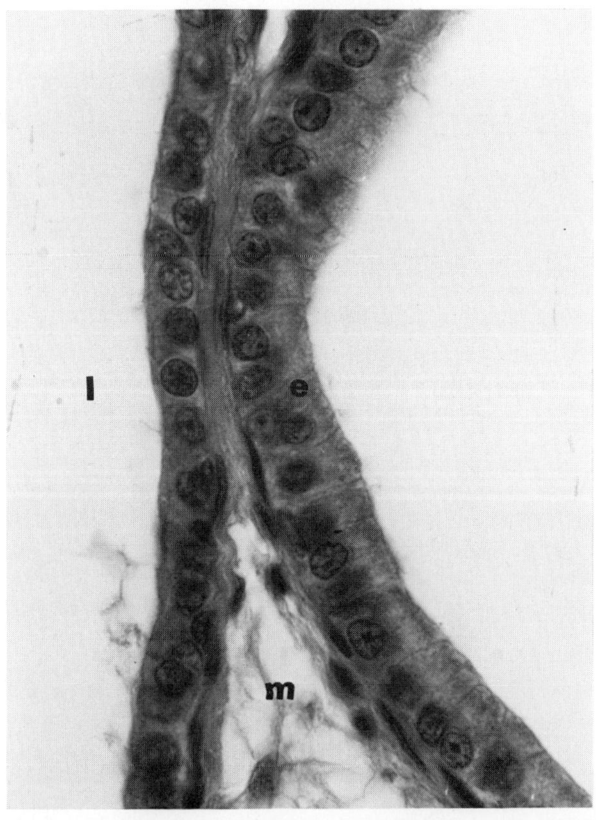

FIGURE 19. Ventral Prostate: Rat treated with 10 mg/kg EB, 1000X. Note lowering in height of cells and decrease in secretory material within cells and loss of interluminal matrix.

When the effect of THC alone or in combination with EB is considered, it is not unlikely that each is acting directly and indirectly.

In summary, this investigation presents a cytological study of the effects of EB and THC alone or combined, on the adrenal, seminalvesicle and ventral prostate of rats treated neonatally. Both THC and EB alone have striking effects on all three organs. Under the conditions of this study, THC increases the effect of EB on all three organs. The mechanism(s) by which THC and EB produce these effects are not yet understood. Cytological observations indicate that THC and EB have similar effects on these organs.

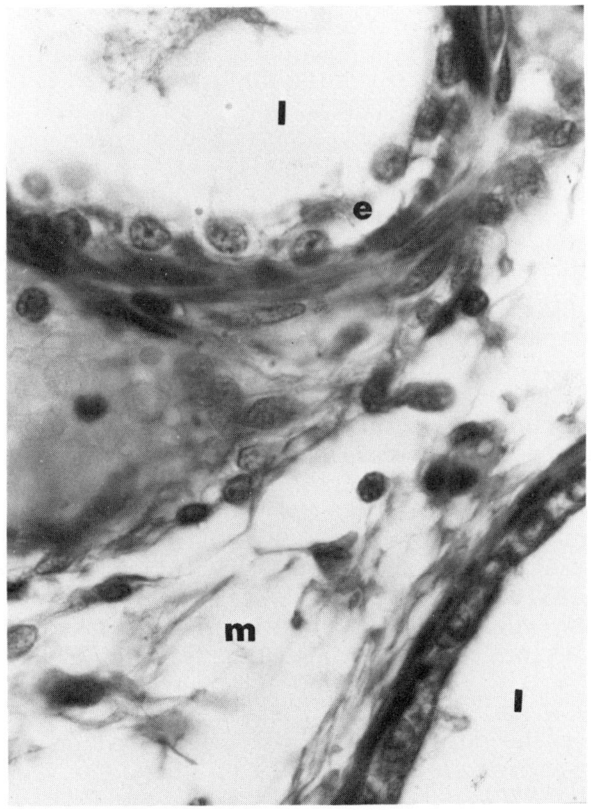

FIGURE 20. Ventral Prostate: Rat treated with 10 mg/kg EB + 20 mg/kg THC, 1000X. Note disintegration of epithelial lining and nuclei free of cellular membranes. The matrix is also markedly disrupted.

ACKNOWLEDGMENTS

The authors wish to express their appreciation to the following for expert technical assistance: R. J. Barry, R. M. Burton, M. C. Dewey, and T. F. Murphy.

REFERENCES

1. Bloch, E., Thysen, B., Morrill, G. A., Gardner, E., and Fujimoto, G., Effects of cannabinoids on reproduction and development, Vitamins and Hormones 36:203 (1978).
2. Nahas, G. G. and Gabriel, G., (eds.), "Marihuana: Chemistry, Biochemistry, and Cellular Effects". Springer-Verlag, Berlin and New York, 1976.
3. Kincl, F. A., Pi, A. F., and Lasso, L. H., Effect of estradiol benzoate treatment in the newborn male rat, Endocrinol. 72:966 (1963).
4. Schiavi, R. C., Adenohypophyseal and serum gonadotropins in male rats treated neonatally with estradiol benzoate, Endocrinol. 82:983 (1968).
5. Frick, J., Chang, C. C., and Kincl, F. A., Testosterone plasma levels in adult male rats injected neonatally with estradiol benzoate or testosterone propionate, Steroids 13:21 (1969).
6. Passquant-Fontaine, T., and Flandre, C., Effects à long terme des oestrogene injectès à la pèriode nèo-natale chex le rat, J. Physiol., Paris 61:423 (1969).
7. Brown-Grant, K., Fink, G., Greig, F., and Murray, M. A. F., Altered sexual development in male rats after estrogen administration during the neonatal period, J. Reprod. Fert. 44:25 (1975).
8. Rajfer, J., and Coffey, D. S., Sex steroid imprinting of the immature prostate long-term effects, Invesigative Urol. 16:186 (1978).
9. Maximow, A., and Bloom, W., in "A Textbook of Histology", 4th Edition, p. 321. W. B. Saunders Co., Philadelphia, 1944.
10. Dewey, W. L., Peng, T. C., and Harris, L. S., The effect of (-)-trans-delta-9-tetrahydrocannabinol on the hypothalamo-hypophyseal-adrenal axis of rats, Eur. J. Pharmacol. 12:382 (1970).
11. Kubena, R. K., Perhach, J. L., Jr., and Barry, H., Corticosterone elevation mediated centrally by delta-1-tetrahydrocannabinol in rats, Eur. J. Pharmacol. 14:89 (1971).
12. Barry, H., Kubena, R. K., and Perhach, J. L., Jr., Pituitary-adrenal activation and related responses to delta-1-

tetrahydrocannabinol, Prog. Brain Res. 39:323 (1972).
13. Drew, W. G., and Slagel, D. E., Delta-9-THC: Selective impairment of corticosterone uptake by limbic structures of the rat, Neuro-pharmacol. 12:909 (1973).
14. Dixit, V. P., Sharma, V. N., and Lohiya, N. K., The effect of chronically administered cannabis extract on the testiular function of mice, Eur. J. Pharmacol. 26:111 (1974).
15. Kokka, N., and Garcia, J. F., Effects of delta-9-THC on growth hormone and ACTH secretion in rats, Life Sci. 15:329 (1974).
16. Biswas, B., Dey, S. K., and Ghosh, J. J., Adrenocortical changes in rats during acute and chronic administration of delta-9-tetrahydrocannabinol, Endocrinol. Exp. 10:139 (1976).
17. Maier, R., and Maitre, L., Steroidogenic and lipolytic effects of cannabinols in the rat and the rabbit, Biochem. Pharmacol. 24:1695 (1975).
18. Bromley, B., and Zimmerman, E., Divergent release of prolactin and corticosterone following delta-9-tetrahydrocannabinol injection in male rats, Fed. Proc., Fed. Amer. Soc. Exp. Bio. 35:220 (1976).
19. Warner, W., Harris, L. S., and Carchman, R. A., Inhibition of corticosteroidogenesis by delta-9-tetrahydrocannabinol, Endocrinol. 101:1815 (1977).
20. Neto, J. P., Nunes, J. F., and Carvalho, F. V., The effects of chronic cannabis treatment upon brain 5-hydroxytryptamine, plasma corticosterone and aggressive behavior in female rats with different hormonal status, Psychopharmacologia 42:195 (1975).
21. Simmons, J. E., Changes in testicular cholesterol associated with estrogen infertility in male mice, J. Exp. Zoology 170:377 (1969).
22. Bancherau, J., Desoize, B., Leger, C., and Nahas, G., Inhibitory effects of delta-9-THC and other psychotropic drugs on cultured lymphocytes, in "Marihuana: Biological Effects" (G. G. Nahas and W. D. M. Paton, eds.), p. 23. Pergamon Press, Oxford, 1979.
23. Nahas, G. G., Suciu-Foca, N., Armand, J. P., and Morishima, A., Inhibition of cellular mediated immunity in marijuana smokers, Science 183:419 (1974).
24. Armand, J. P., Hsu, J. T., and Nahas, G. G., Inhibition of blastogenesis of T-lymphocytes by delta-9-THC, Fed. Proc. 33:539 (1974).
25. Desoize, B. Hsu, J. T., and Nahas, G. G., Inhibition of human lymphocyte transformation _in vitro_ by natural cannabinoids and olivetol, Fed. Proc. 34:783 (1975).
26. Desoize, B., and Nahas, G. G., Effets inhibiteurs du delta-9-THC sur la synthèse des protèins et des acides

nucleiques, C. R. Acad. Sci., Paris 281:475 (1975).
27. Nahas, G. G., Morishima, a., and Desoize, B., Effects of cannabinoids on macromolecular synthesis and replication of cultures lympocytes, Fed. Proc. 36:1748 (1977).
28. Ling, G. M., Thomas, J. A., Usher, D. R., and Singhal, R. L., Effects of Chronically administered delta-1-tetrahydrocannabinol of adrenal and gonadal activity of male rats, Int. J. Clin. Pharmacol. Ther. Toxicol. 7:1 (1973).
29. Dixit, V. P., Arya, M., and Lohiya, N. K., The effect of chronically administered cannabis extract on the female genital tract of mice and rats, Endokrinologie 66:365 (1975).
30. Pertwee, R. G., Tolerance to the effect of delta-1-tetrahydrocannabinol on corticosterone levels in mouse plasma produced by repeated administration of cannabis extract or delta-1-tetrahydrocannabinol, Br. J. Pharmacol. 51:391 (1974).
31. Smith, C. G., Moore, C. E., Besch, N. F., and Besch, P. K., Effect of delta-9-tetrahydrocannabinol (THC) on the secretion of male sex hormone in the Rhesus monkey, Pharmacologist 18:248 (1976).
32. Maskarinec, M. P., Shipley, G., Novotny, M., Brown, D. J., and Forney, R. B., Endocrine effects of cannabis in male rats, Toxicol. Appl. Pharmacol. 45:617 (1978).
33. Gunn, S. A., and Gould, T. C., The relative importance of androgen and estrogen in the selective uptake of ZN^{65} by the dorsolateral prostate of the rat, Endocrinology 58:443 (1956).
34. Moger, W. H., and Geschwind, I. I., The action of prolactin on the sex accessory glands of the male rat, Proc. Exp. Biol. Med. 141:1017 (1972).
35. Lasnitzkik, I., The effect of prolactin on rat prostate glands in organ culture, Fourth Tenovus Workshop: Prolactin and Carcinogenesis, p. 200. Alpha Omega Publishing Company, Cardiff, 1972.
36. Resnick, M. I., and Grayhack, J. T., Effects of 2-bromo-alpha-ergocryptine (CB-154) on estrogen induced growth of the rat prostate, Investigative Urology 15:392 (1978).
37. Belis, J. A., Blume, C. D., and Mawhinney, M. G., Androgen and estrogen binding in male guinea pig accessory sex organs, Endocrinol. 101:726 (1977).
38. Feyel-Cabanes, T., Robel, P., and Baulieu, E. E., Effets conjoints de la testostérone et de l'oestradiol sur le lobe ventral de la prostate de rat en culture organotypique, C. R. Acad. Sci. Paris 285:1119 (1977).
39. Feyel-Cabanes, T., Secchi, J., Robel, P., and Baulieu, E. E., Combined effects of testosterone and estradiol on rat ventral prostate, Cancer Res. 38:4126 (1978).

40. Harris, G. W., and Levine, S., Sexual differentiation of the brain and its experimental control, J. Physiol., London 181:379 (1965).
41. Purochit, V., Singh, H. H., and Ahluwalia, B. S., Evidence that the effects of methadone and marijuana on male reproductive organs are mediated at different sites in rats, Biol. Reprod. 20:1039 (1979).
42. Purochit, V., Ahluwalia, B. S., and Vigersky, R. S., Marijuana inhibits dihydrotestosterone binding to the androgen receptor, Endocrinol. 107:848 (1980).

EFFECTS OF NEONATAL ADMINISTRATION OF DELTA-9-TETRAHYDROCANNABINOL AND/OR ESTRADIOL BENZOATE (EB) ON REPRODUCTIVE DEVELOPMENT AND FUNCTION OF THE MALE RAT

Mary D. Albert
Jolane Solomon

Department of Biology
Boston College
Chestnut Hill, Massachusetts

I. INTRODUCTION

There is continuing contention concerning the roles of delta-9-tetrahydrocannabinol (THC) in female and male mammalian reproductive physiology. Studies on the *in vivo* effects of THC, and other cannabinoids, show that cannabinoids may be antiestrogenic (1-3), or estrogenic (4-18), or have no effect on reproductive physiology (190).

In *in vitro* studies on female tissues it has been found that THC does not (3,20,21) and does (22,23) bind to receptors in the cytosol.

In some *in vivo* studies, THC may be antiestrogenic. In intact prepubertal female rodents, cannabis inhibits estradiol-induced uterine hypertrophy (5) and estradiol-induced increases in monoamine oxidase activity (1). In addition, feeding cannabis resin caused a decrease in uterine weights of immature and adult ovariectomized rats (23).

On the other hand, others have found that THC is estrogenic *in vivo*. In adult ovariectomized-adrenalectomized rats, Gordon et al. report that THC induces lordosis (11). Solomon et al. found that THC induces vaginal mucification and incipient cornification, as well as uterine hypertrophy and hyperplasia in adult ovariectomized rats (33).

There are others who find that THC has no effect in female mice. Virgo (19) reports that THC neither blocks nor induces implantation in mated female mice treated with THC alone or with THC plus progesterone.

ISBN 0-12-044620-0

In a review article, Block et al. discuss similarities in responses to estrogens and cannabinoids in men and male and female rodents (24). In men and male rodents, heavy chronic marijuana use or THC administration have the following estrogenic effects:

In men, marijuana use elicits gynecomastia (25), oligospermia and transient depression in plasma testosterone levels (24,26,10), which may be accompanied by depressed plasma LH levels (24). Depressed testosterone and gonadotropin levels, gynecomastia (27), anti-androgenic effects on secondary sex glands (18,19) and azoospermia (30) are also seen as a result of estrogen administration in men.

In male mice, chronic administration of THC induces arrest of spermatogenesis, regression of Leydig cell tissue and accessory sex glands (7). Chronic THC is found to depress LH secretion (4), stimulate development of male rat breast tissue (9,24) decrease sexual performance (31), increase adrenal weights (11), depress seminal vesicle weights and somatic growth (15) in male rats. Depressed somatic growth (32,33), increased adrenal weight (34), decreased gonadotropin secretion (35), and depressed seminal vesicle weights (36) are also seen in estrogen-treated male rats. These findings lend further support to the possibility that THC administration may have an estrogen-like action in adult male rodents.

In vivo responses to THC depend on several factors, including age and sex of the animal model. Since the effect on the development of reproductive structures and behavior of males treated neonatally with estradiol is well established, we used this model to examine the response of male neonates to THC and estradiol benzoate (EB) alone and in combination.

II. MATERIALS AND METHODS

Two hundred Sprague-Dawley male pups obtained from Charles River were treated neonatally at 4 days of age with a single subcutaneous (s.c.) dose of either: (a) vehicle alone, (b) estradiol benzoate (EB) alone (0.5, 5.0, 10.0 mg/kg), (c) THC alone (20 mg/kg), or (d) EB plus THC (each dose of EB plus 20 mg/kg THC). Delta-9-THC was kindly supplied by the National Institute on Drug Abuse (NIDA). These animals were placed in one of 3 groups.

Group 1: At 39 days of age, 100 rats were autopsied after chloroform inhalation to examine the effects of treatment on body and reproductive organ weights, and on organ histology of prepubertalmales. Testes and seminal vesicles were excised and weighed at autopsy and immediately placed in modified Bouins solution and cut at 6 microns and stained with hematoxylin and eosin. The degree of damage to the seminiferous tubules was assessed using a modification of the method of Maqueo and Kincl (37). Because of the sexual immaturity of rats at 30 days of age, those tubules having spermatids, rather than free spermatozoa in the lumen, were counted. Approximately 1000-15000 tubules from each group were examined.

Group 2: Several animals from each treatment regimen were retained and autopsied at 60 days of age to examine body and reproductive weights and organ histology. When we found that the testes of 60 day old rats appeared to be near normal, we did a continuation study (Group 3).

Group 3: Several rats from each treatment group were retained and injected subcutaneously for 6 consecutive days (96-102 days of age) with the same substance(s) they received at 4 days of age. Three to 6 weeks after the last injection, these animals were examined for mating abilities from days 117-138. Each male rat was placed with proven female breeders. After each successful mating, the number of the pups were weighed and sexed at 21 days of age.

III. RESULTS

In testes from vehicle-injected controls autopsied at 39 days of age, the seminiferous tubules have intact germinal epithelia. Spermatogonia are abundant, as are the more advanced stages of spermatogenesis. Spermatids are present in the majority of tubules and nearing the last stages of maturation. Interstitial connective tissue completely fills the spaces between seminiferous tubules, and Leydig cells for the most part, are present in small clusters of 3-8 cells between tubules. Histology is seen in Figure 1, weights of the testes and seminal vesicles are shown in Table I.

Compared to controls (Table I, Figures 1) testes removed from animals treated with graded doses of EB alone and sacrificed at 39 days of age are atrophied (Table I and Figures 3 and 4). The atrophied testicular germinal epithelium and interstitial tissue is accompanied by decrease diameter and spermatid content of the seminiferous tubules.

In testes removed from rats treated with EB the diameters of the germinal epithelium appear to narrow as the doses of EB are increased. Concomitant with the decreasing diameter is an increase in interstitial spaces. The amount of loose areolar connective tissue normally filling the interstitial space is reduced. Although the interstitial connective tissue has atrophied, Leydig cells seem comparable to the controls. As seen in Table II, there is a dose-response decrease in testes and seminal vesicle weights in CB-treated rats.

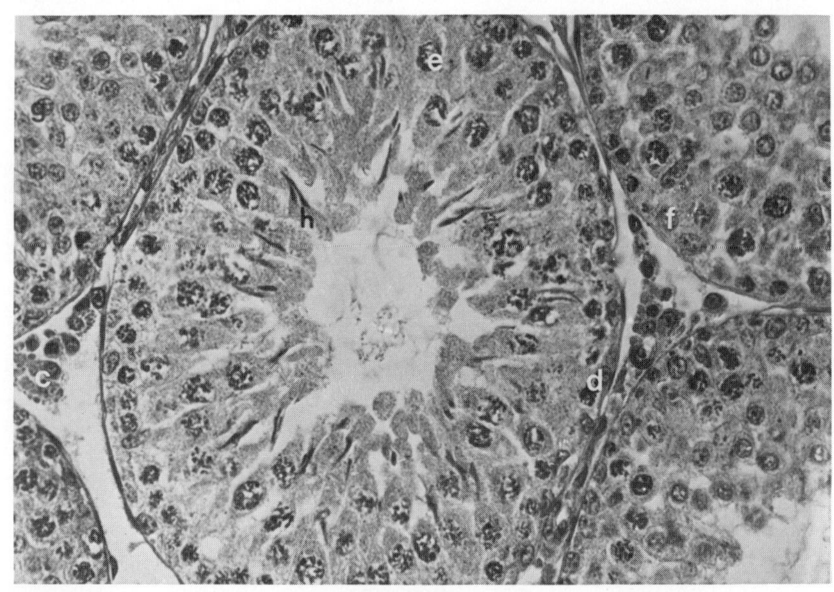

FIGURE 1. Testis: Control rat; labels: Leydig cells (c), spermatogonia (d), primary spermatocytes (e), Sertoli cells (f), spermatids (g), and spermatozoa (h) (400 X).

On the level of the light microscope, testes from 39 day old males treated with 20 mg/kg THC alone (Figure 2) are found to differ from controls only in the diameter of the seminiferous tubules. The germinal epithelium and the interstitial connective tissue all appeared similar to that of control animals. As seen in Table I, the testes and seminal vesicle weights of the THC-treated animals do not differ from those of controls. The testes of animals treated with combined doses of EB plus 20 mg/kg THC were more markedly affected than those treated with EB alone (Figures 5,6). In these doubly-injected rats, there was a sharp reduction in tubular diameters with an increasing amount of empty spaces between tubules. There was, primarily, a reduction in maturing spermatids (Figure 5). With the largest dose of EB (10 mg/kg) and THC, the entire organization of the testes is disrupted. Debris from degenerating germinal epithelium accumulates in the lumen of a large number of the tubules, and the outer periphery of many tubules lose their outlines (Figure 6). It appears that the majority of the cells at this dose level are moribund. However, spermatogenesis was observed in tubules from all groups, even those tubules with the most damage although in these there were no maturing spermatids.

TABLE I. Body and Organ Weights, and Number of Spermatid-Containing Seminiferous Tubules in Male Neonates Treated at 4 Days of Age and Sacrificed at 39 Days of Age

Dose (mg/kg)	Mean[a]			Tubules with Spermatids[b]		
	Body Weight (g)	Testes Weight[c]	Seminal Vesicle Weight[c]	Total Tubules Counted	%	% of Control
Control	182.1 (3.29) (10)	961.11 (38.44) (10)	100.38 (12.34) (10)	690/1079	63.95	100.0
0.5 EB	181.59 (6.76)+ (10)	767.46 (42.01)* (10)	67.76 (6.7)* (10)	1010/1546	65.33	102.12
5.0 EB	188.48 (4.11)++ (10)	607.0 (45.63)** (10)	52.80 (12.09)** (10)	144/1314	10.96	17.14
10.0 EB	170.57 (3.76)++ (10)	552.06 (24.11)++ (10)	40.7 (8.26)++ (10)	42/1024	4.1	6.41
0.5 EB + 20.0 THC	168.53 (4.62)* (10)	849.58 (32.19)* (8)	62.11 (7.8)** (9)	383/1043	36.72	57.42
5.0 EB + 20.0 THC	161.22 (8.1)# (9)	506.46 (40.30)++ (8)	53.0 (6.97)+ (8)	272/1584	17.17	26.85
10.0 EB + 20.0 THC	151.16 (9.75)*** (10)	477.92 (57.50)++ (9)	49.41 (8.98)*** (8)	52/1440	3.61	5.65
20 THC	190.42 (4.39) (10)	902.64 (27.62) (10)	103.4 (7.33) (10)	832/1291	64.45	100.78

[a]Values represent means (+/- S.E.M.) The number below in ( ) represents the nubber of animals per group. Means were tested for significant differences using Student t's test. The symbols represent the following: * = $p < 0.05$; ** = $p < 0.25$; *** = $p < 0.01$; + = $p < 0.005$; ++ = $p < 0.001$; # = $p < 0.1$. Compared to controls, In only one dose 5.0 EB + the mean significantly different ($p < 0.01$) from the corresponding EB dose alone (5.0 EB).

[b]At least three animals per dose were examined. Approximately 1000-1500 tubules from each animal were assessed. [c]Units are in mg/100 g b.w.

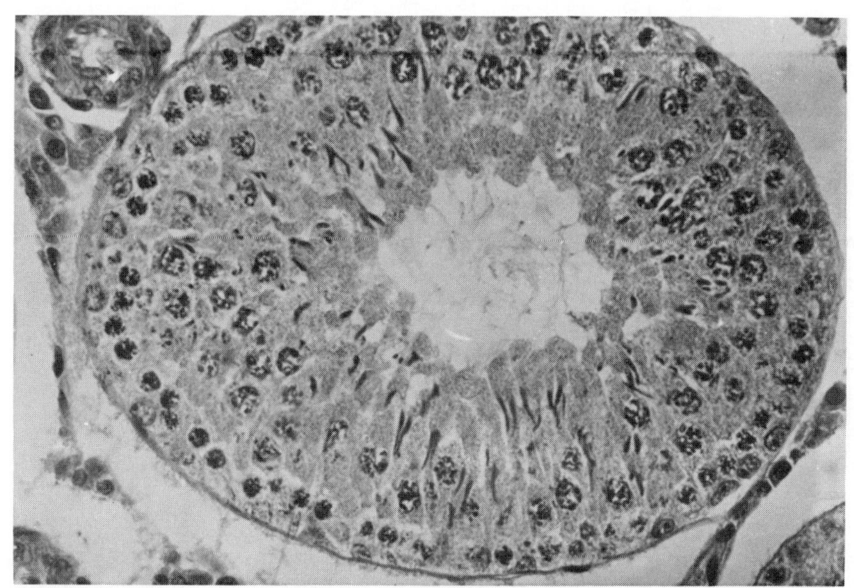

FIGURE 2. Testis: Rat treated with 20 mg/kg THC (400X).

The testes, seminal vesicles, and body weights (Table I), of 39 day old males are, with two exceptions, consistently less when THC and EB are administered simultaneously (See testes weights of 0.5 EB + 20 THC and seminal vesicle weights of 10.0 EB and 20 mg/kg THC). When animals are treated with EB plus THC, the testes are more adversely affected then when compared to animals treated with EB alone. In essence, as with the histological results, THC augments the response to EB.

Despite the normal appearance of the testes in light microscopic studies of 60-75 day old male rats treated neonatally with all doses of estrogen, there is a difference in their mating capacities when examined at 4 months of age after treatment. These four-month old rats were treated again at 96-102 days of age with the same substances they received at 4 days of age (See Materials and Methods, Group 3).

When rats are injected neonatally and at 4 months of age with low doses of EB (0.5 mg/kg) alone and 0.5 mg/kg EB in combination with THC (See Table II), the males sire litters (3/4 and 2/3 respectively), when mated three to six weeks after the last injection. On the other hand, when similarly treated animals are injected with larger doses of EB, 5 and 10 mg/kg, alone or in combination with THC, the males are unable to sire litters (Table II). Kincl et al. found that rats

TABLE II. Effect of Graded Doses of EB Alone or in Combination with 20 mg/kg THC on Mating Proficiency of Treated Males 2-6 Weeks After the Last of the Chronic Injections. (Group 3)

Group	Male Treatment mg/kg Body Weight	Number of Males Mated	Females Giving Birth	Total Number In Litter	Average Weight Of Litter[a]	Number of Females In Litter	Average Weight of Females in Litter	Number of Males In Litter	Average Weight Of Males In Litter[a]
1	Vehicle control	3	3	12	47.7	7	47.4	5	48.3
				13	38.4	4	36.9	9	39.0
				11	43.3	4	40.2	7	45.2
2	0.5 EB	4	3	12	55.1	4	53.2	8	56.0
				6	80.0	2	77.0	4	81.5
				11	53.2	5	52.0	6	54.2
3	5.0 EB	3	0	-	-	-	-	-	-
4	10.0 EB	3	0	-	-	-	-	-	-
5	0.5 EB + 20 THC	3	2	9	58.1	5	57.8	4	58.4
				2	68.6	1	86.8	1	72.5
6	5.0 EB + 20 THC	3	0	-	-	-	-	-	-
7	10.0 EB +	4	0	-	-	-	-	-	-
8	20 THC	3	3	13	44.5	7	46.7	6	48.5
				13	45.1	5	46.7	8[b]	44.2
				10	54.8	4	51.2	6	57.2

[a]Pups were weighted at 21 days of age; weight in grams.
[b]One male pup was a runt.

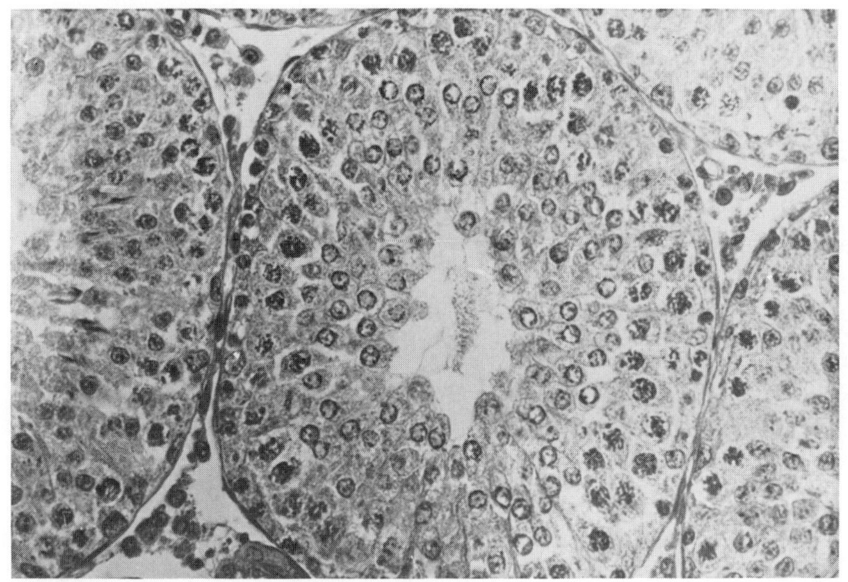

FIGURE 3. Testis: Rat treated with 0.5 mg/kg THC (400 X).

treated perinatally with estrogen were protected from development of testicular atrophy by neonatal administration of progesterone (38).

Brown-Grant et al. tested the fertility of his neonatally estrogen-treated males by placing a single male with a single pro-estrous female overnight (35). We mated our males in a similar fashion with proven female breeders at estrus.

When mating behavior was examined, we found that rats treated with THC alone showed increased mount and ejaculation latencies, and decreased total number of mounts and intromissions, and ejaculations.

IV. DISCUSSION

The effects of estradiol benzoate on the maturation of the testis of neonatally-treated rats have been documented (35,37,39). The results of the present study are in agreement with these previous studies and indicate that the degree of abnormality in testis and seminal vesicle weights and testis histology is dependent on estrogen dose and age of animal at autopsy.

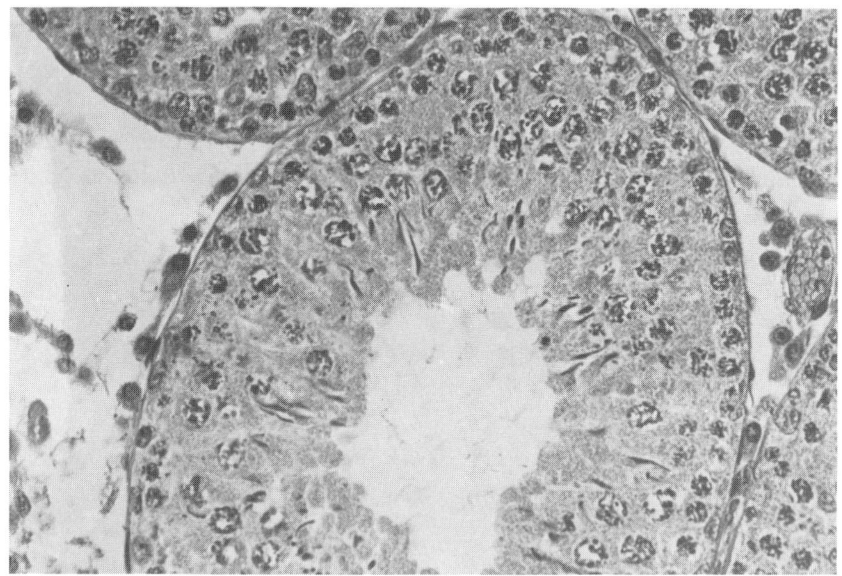

FIGURE 4. Rat treated with 10 mg/kg EB (400 X).

Maqueo and Kincl injected 5 day old animals with 6 to 24 mg/kg EB, autopsied the rats at 45-60 days of age and observed a dose-dependent pathology of the testis (37). Six mg/kg EB produced only slight changes, administration of 24 mg/kg EB caused a nearly complete degeneration of the germinal epithelium in 100% of the seminiferous tubules examined. Less severe atrophy was noted when EB was injected into rats 10 and 20 days old.

Brown-Grant et al. using a similar experimental design, also found degenerated tubules and decreased testes weights (35). When compared to controls, seminiferous epithelium had atrophied and testes and seminal vesicle weights were significantly reduced in EB-treated (25 mg/kg) animals autopsied at 40 days of age. In our experience, the weights of the seminal vesicles and testes were significantly reduced in rats treated at 4 days of age with 0.5 mg/kg EB, 5.0 mg/kg EB, and 10 mg/kg EB and examined at 39 days of age (Table I). Compared to controls, the number of spermatids in the tubules is decreased only with 5.0 and 10.0 mg/kg EB. The number and percent of tubules with spermatids was similar in controls and animals treated with 0.5 mg/kg EB (Table I). Histological examination shows that compared to control (Figure 1), the testes of animals treated with 0.5 mg/kg EB (Figure 3) appear similar to controls. The testes of animals treated with 5 mg/kg EB (no

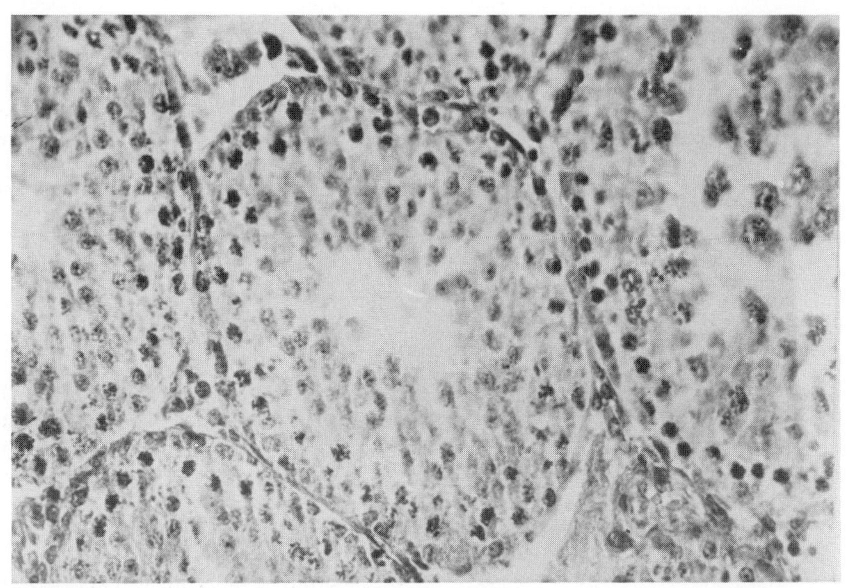

FIGURE 5. Rat treated with 5 mg/kg EB + 20 mg/kg THC (400 X).

figure shown) are less damaged than those treated with 10 mg/kg EB (Figure 4).

Additionally, Brown-Grant et al. observed that three-fourths of the animals sacrificed at 60 days of age had nearly all recovered from their neonatal treatments (35). No differences in the seminiferous epithelium were noted after 75 days. In our experience, 60 day old males treated with EB neonatally appeared to have near normal testes cytology with light microscopy.

The effects of direct THC administration to neonatal males on reproductive development have not been reported. However, Dalterio also found that male mice treated perinatally with THC increased mount latencies, and a decreased number of mounts and intromissions when tested as adults (40). Most studies have dealt with the effects of THC on prepubertal or adult rodents. Numerous reports have appeared indicating that THC caused a depression of testicular endocrine function of adult rats and other mammals (for review, see 24). The evidence, however, is far from conclusive. Cumulative doses greater than 1 gram administered over periods of 28-180 days led to small increases in testes weights (41,42), while with lower cumulative doses testes weights remained the same or were slightly lower than controls (4,43,44).

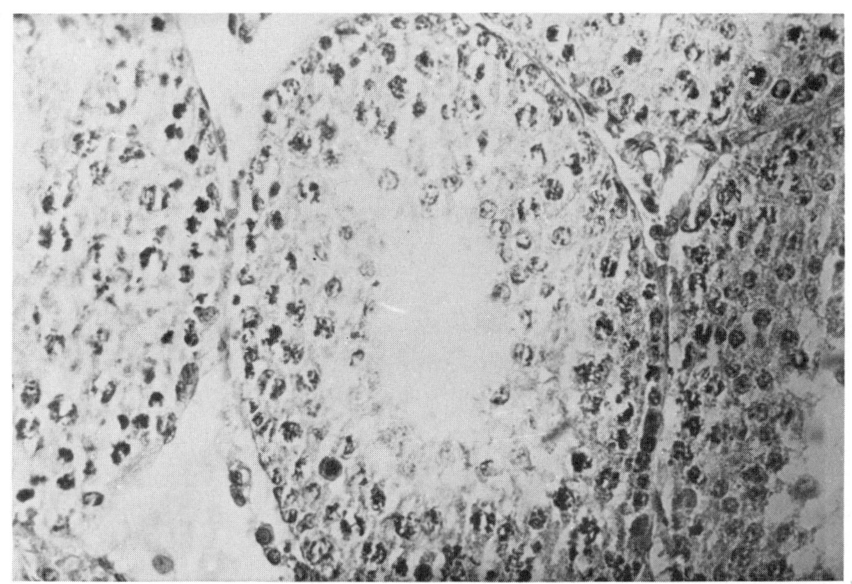

FIGURE 6. Rat treated with 10 mg/kg EB + 20 mg/kg THC (400 X).

In this study, a single injection of THC (20 mg/kg body weight) at 4 days of age reduced the seminiferous tubule diameter (Figure 2) when examined at 39 days of age. However, the histology of the testes of THC-treated rats was comparable to controls: 63.95% of the tubules from the treated rats contained spermatids; this is comparable to the control value of 64.45% (Table I). By day 60, tubule diameters had increased and were indistinguishable from controls. In another study, Dixit et al. administered 2 mg cannabis/day chronicallyto young adult mice and noted a significant decrease in the diameter of the seminiferous tubules (7). However, sixty-three days after the last dose of cannabis, the diameters were comparable to the controls.

The results of the mating studies show that a single dose of THC (20mg/kg at 4 days of age) had no effect on the ability of treated males to sire litters. All males treated with 20 mg/kg THC alone successfully mated with untreated females which became pregnant and gave birth 21-23 days after mating.

Despite the fact that 20 mg/kg THC alone had no observable effect on testes and seminal vesicles, weights and spermatid counts (Table I), or on testes cytology (Figure 4), the cytology of the seminal vesicles was affected by THC (see other paper in this volume). When 20 mg/kg THC, and EB (0.5, 5.0

and 10.0 mg/kg) are administered together, the effect of EB was markedly enhanced in a dose-related manner on both testes weights (Table I), as well as on testes histology (Figures 5,6).

V. SUMMARY

Two hundred male rats were treated neonatally at 4 days of age with a single subcutaneous (s.c.) dose of either: (a) vehicle alone, (b) estradiol benzoate (EB) alone (0.5, 5.0, 10.0 mg/kg), (c) THC alone (20 mg/kg), or (d) EB plus THC (each dose EB plus 20 mg/kg THC). When some of these animals were autopsied at 39 days of age, there was a dose-response decrease in testes and seminal vesicle weights for EB-treated rats. The testes histology also shows a dose-response decrease in architecture to EB administration. Testes obtained from 39-day old rats treated with THC show no changes in weight or cytology when compared to controls. However, testes from animals treated with EB plus THC show that THC augments the effect of EB. By 60 days of age, testes cytology from all groups appeared normal by light microscope examination.

Some members of each group were treated for 6 consecutive days (days 92-106) with the same compound(s) they received at 4 days of age. These retreated rats were studied for reproductive behavior three to six weeks after the last injection. All of the males treated with vehicle alone or THC alone sired litters. However, sexual behavior was affected by administration of THC alone. Some of the animals treated with a low dose of (0.5 mg/kg) of EB alone and in combination with THC sired litters (3/4 and 2/3, respectively). None of the animals treated with higher doses (5.0 and 10.0mg/kg EB alone) or in combination with THC sired litters.

ACKNOWLEDGMENTS

The authors wish to express their appreciation to the following for expert technical assistance: E. E. Smith, J. E. S. Schindler, V. E. Topping and T. F. Murphy.

REFERENCES

1. Chakravarty, I., Sengupta, D., Bhattacharya, P. and Ghosh, J. J., Effect of cannabis extract on the uterine

monoamine oxidase activity of normal and estradiol treated rats, Biochem. Pharmacol. 25:377-378 (1975).
2. Chakravarty, I., Sengupta, D., Bhattacharya, P., and Ghosh, J. J., Effect of treatment with cannabis extract on the water and glycogen content of the uterus in normal and estradiol-treated rats, Toxicol. Applied Pharmacol. 34:513-516 (1975).
3. Okey, A. B., and Truant, G. S., Cannabis demasculinizes rats but is not estrogenic, Life Sciences 17:1111-1118 (1975).
4. Collu, R., Letarte, J., Leboeuf, G., and Ducharme, J. R., Endocrine effects of chronic administration of psychoactive drugs to prepubertal male rats. I: Delta-9-tetrahydrocannabinol, Life Sciences 16(4):533-542 (1975).
5. Dalterio, S., and Bartke, A., Perinatal exposure to cannabinoids alters male reproductive function in mice, Science 205:1420-1422 (1979).
6. Dixit, V. P., Arya, M., and Lottiya, N. K., The effect of chronically administered cannabis extract on the female genital tract of mice and rats, Endocrinologie 66:365-368 (1975).
7. Dixit, V. P., Sharma, V. N., and Lohiya, N. K., The effect of chronically administered cannabis extract on the testicular function of mice, Eur. Pharmacol. 26:111-114 (1974).
8. Gordon, J. H., Bromley, G. L. Gorski, R. A., and Zimmerman, E., Delta-9-tetrahydrocannabinol enhancement of lordosis behavior in estrogen-treated female rats, Pharmacol. Biochem. Behav. 8: 603-708 (1978).
9. Harmon, J. W., and Aliopoulios, M. A., Marijuana-induced gynecomastia: clinical and laboratory experience, Surg. Forum 25:423-425 (1974).
10. Kolodny, R.C., Lessin, P., Toro, G., Masters, W. H., and Cohen, S., Depression of plasma testosterone with acute marijuana administration, in "Pharmacology of Marihuana", Vol. 1 (M. C. Braude and S. Szara, eds.), pp. 217-225. Raven Press, New York, 1976.
11. Ling, G. M., Thomas, J. A., Usher, D. R., and Singhal, R. L., Effects of chronically administered delta-1-tetrahydrocannabinol and luteinizing hormone secretion, Prog. Brain Res. 39:331-338 (1973).
12. Marks, B. H., Delta-1-tetrahydrocannabinol and luteinizing hormone secretion, Prog. Brain Res. 39:331-338 (1972).
13. Merari, A., Barak, A., and Plaves, M., Effects of delta-1-tetrahydrocannabinol on copulation in the male rat, Psychopharmacol. (Berl) 28:243-246 (1973).
14. Nir, I., Ayalon, D., Tsafriri, A., Corodova, T., and Linder, H. R., Suppression of cyclic surge of luteinizing

hormone secretion and of ovulation in the rat by delta-9-tetrahydrocannabinol, Nature (London) 244:470-471 (1973).
15. Solomon, J., and Shattuck, D., Marihuana and sex, New Eng. J. Med. 291:309 (1974).
16. Solomon, J. Cocchia, M. A., Gray, R., Shattuck, D., and Vossmer, A., Uterotrophic effect of delta-9-tetrahydrocannabinol in ovariectomized rats, Science 192:559-561 (1976).
17. Solomon, J., and Cocchia, M. A., Is delta-9-tetrahydrocannabinol estrogenic? Science 195:905-906 (1977).
18. Solomon, J., Cocchia, M. A., and DiMarino, R., Effect of delta-9-tetrahydrocannabinol on uterine and vaginal cytology of ovariectomized rats, Science 195:875-877 (1977).
19. Virgo, B. B., The estrogenicity of delta-9-tetrahydrocannabinol (THC): THC neither blocks nor induces ovum implantation, nor does it effect uterine growth, Res. Comm. Chem. Path. Pharmacol. 25:65-77 (1979).
20. Okey, A. B., and Bondy, G. P., Delta-9-tetrahydrocannabinol and 17-beta-estradiol bind to different macromolecules in estrogen target tissue, Science 200:312-314 (1978).
21. Smith, R. G., Besch, N., and Besch, P. K., Inhibition of gonadotropin delta-9-tetrahydrocannabinol: mediation by steroid receptors? Science 204:325-327 (1979).
22. Rawitch, A. B., Schultz, G. S., Ebner, K. E., and Vardaris, R. M., Competition of delta-9-tetrahydrocannabinol with estrogen in rat uterine estrogen receptor binding, Science 197:1189-1191 (1977).
23. Shoemaker, R. H., and Harmon, J. W., Suggested mechanism for demasculinizing effects of marijuana, Fed. Proc. 36:345 (1977).
24. Block, E., Thysen, B., Morril, G., Gardner, E., and Fujimoto, G., Effects of cannabinoids on reproduction and development, Vitamins and Hormones 36:203-258 (1978).
25. Harmon, J. W., and Aliapoulis, M. A., Gynecomastia in marijuana users, N. Eng. J. Med. 287:936 (1972).
26. Kolodny, R. C., Master, W. H., Kolodner, R. M., and Toro, G., Depression of plasma testosterone levels after chronic intensive marijuana use, N. Eng. J.Med. 290:872-874 (1974).
27. Bronstein, I. P., and Shadaksharappa, K. S., Gynecomastia, in "Progress in Clinical Endocrinology" (Soskin, ed.), Greene and Stratton, New York, 1950.
28. Huggins, C., and Clark, P. J., Quantitative studies of prostatic secretions. II, J. Exp. Med. 72:747 (1940).
29. Huggins, C., Control of cancers of man by endocrinological methods, Cancer Res. 16:825-830 (1956).

30. Heckel, J. J., and Steinmetz, C. R., Production of azoospermia in man from use of estradiol benzoate (progynon B), Proc. Soc. Exp. Biol. Med. 46:174 (1941).
31. Merari, A., Barak, A., and Plaves, M., Effects of delta-1-tetrahydrocannabinol on copulation in the male rat, Psychopharmacol. (Berl) 28:243-246 (1973).
32. Bull, L., Hurley, W., Kennett, Tamplin, C., and Williams, W., Effects of sex hormones on feed intake in rats, J. Nutr. 104:968-975 (1974).
33. Shai, F., and Wallach, S., Interactions of estradiol and calcitonin on the rat skeleton, Endocrinol. 73:253-260 (1973).
34. Kitay, J. I., Pituitary-adrenal function in rat after gonadectomy and gonadal function replacement, Endocrinol. 73:253-260 (1963).
35. Brown-Grant, K., Fink, G., Grief, F., and Murray, M. A. F., Altered sexual development in male rats after oestrogen administration during the neonatal period, J. Reprod. Fert. 44:25-42 (1975).
36. Greep, R. O., and Jones, I. C., Steroid control of pituitary function, Rec. Prog. Hormone Res. 5:197-254 (1950).
37. Macque, M., and Kincl, F. A., Testicular histo-morphology of young rats treated with oestradiol-17-benzoate, Acta Endocrinol. Copehn. 46:25-30 (1964).
38. Kincl, F. A., and Maqueo, M., Prevention by progesterone of steroid-induced sterility in neonatal male and female rats, Endocrinol. 77:859-862 (1965).
39. Kincl, F. A., Pi, A. F., and Lasso, L. H., Effect of estradiol benzoate treatment in the newborn male rat, Endocrinol. 72:966-968 (1963).
40. Dalterio, S., Badr, F., Bartke, A., and Mayfield, D., Cannabinoids in male mice: effects on fertility and spermatogenesis, Science 216:315-316 (1982).
41. Rosekrantz, H., and Braude, M. C., Comparative chronic toxicities of delta-9-tetrahydrocannabinol administered orally be inhalation in rat, in "The Pharmacology of Marijuana" (M. C. Braude and S. Szara, eds.), pp. 517-584. Raven Press, New York, 1976.
42. Rosenkrantz, H., Sprague, R. A., Fleishmann, R. W., and Braude M. C., Oral delta-9-tetrahydrocannabinol toxicity in rats treated for periods up to 6 months, Toxicol. Appl. Pharmacol. 32:399-417 (1975).
43. Collu, R., Endocrine effects of chronic intraventricular administration of delta-9-THC to prepubertal and adult male rats, Life Sciences 18:223-230 (1976).
44. Harmon, J. W., Locke, D., Aliapoulious, M. A., and Macimdoe, J. H., Interference with testicular development by delta-9-THC, Surgical Forum 27:350-352 (1976).

EFFECT OF CHRONIC CANNABINOID TREATMENT ON ANDROGENIC STIMULATION OF MALE ACCESSORY SEX ORGANS IN THE RAT*

G. I. Fujimoto
L. C. Krey
L. Macedonia

Department of Biochemistry
Albert Einstein College of Medicine
Bronx, New York
and
The Rockefeller University
New York, New York

I. INTRODUCTION

Several reports have indicated that chronic treatment with crude marijuana extract (CME) and its principle active component delta-9-tetrahydrocannabinol (THC) either suppresses stimulation or causes involution of male accessory sex organs in the intact rat (1). These effects of CME and THC could occur through several possible pathways: 1) inhibiting gonadotropin output by the CNS-hypothalamo-pituitary complex (2,3); 2) suppressing testicular production of androgens (4); 3) inhibiting androgen binding to receptor or other possible local processes in accessory sex organs (5,6); and/or 4) indirectly, by decreasing appetite and food consumption (7). Purohit et al. reported that 10 mg THC/kg body weight given s.c. daily for 10 days to the castrated male rat suppressed testosterone stimulated ventral prostate and seminal vesicle growth (8). This anti-androgenic effect may result, at least in part, from inhibition of androgen action at the target organ receptor level (5,6).

*Supported in part by NIDA grant no. DA-02214.

ISBN 0-12-044620-0

We are investigating chronic cannabinoid effects on the male reproductive system and their possible sites of action. We wish to report our results from studies on the effects of THC and CME on androgen stimulation of accessory male organs in the intact and castrated rat.

II. MATERIALS AND METHODS

Crude marijuana extract (CME, 33% THC, batch SSC-85077) and delta-9-tetrahydrocannabinol (THC, batch QCD-84924) were obtained from the National Institute on Drug Abuse. To a solution of 1.5 g CME (or 0.5 g THC) in 0.75 g sesame oil was mixed 0.75 g Polysorbate 80, and water was added with thorough shaking to a volume of 100 ml. Both CME and THC suspensions were stored (up to 1 week) at $4^{O}C$ in the dark and shaken well before use. Vehicle medium was similarly prepared. Polydimethylsiloxane (Silastic) tubing, 0.062" I.D., was filled with 2 or 20 mg testosterone propionate (TP) or left empty, and the ends sealed with Dow-Corning Silastic medical adhesive Type A (9). Daily dosages of 25 mg/kg for THC and 75 mg/kg for CME were selected because, in prior dose response studies (10), they produced significant suppression of accessory sex organ weight gain.

Young, adult male Fischer rats were housed at $76-78^{O}C$ with a 12 h lights on, 0700-1900 h, 12 h off-cycle, and given food and water *ad libidum*. After 10 days acclimation to their quarters, they were divided into seven weight matched groups of 8-10 rats each. Group 1 was left untreated. The other 6 groups of animals were intubated daily using 16 gauge, 2 in. needles (Popper & Sons, New Hyde Park, New York), with the following: group 2, Vehicle, 5 ml/kg: group 3) THC, 25 mg/kg: group 4) CME, 75 mg/kg. Animals assigned to groups 5-7 had Silastic implants containing 20 mg TP inserted subdermally in the mid dorsal region under light ether anesthesia the afternoon prior to the start of treatment. They were kept in a separate animal room under similar conditions and were intubated daily thus: group 5, Vehicle, 5 ml/kg: group 6, THC, 25 mg/kg: and group 7, CME,75 mg/kg. On the first 3 days of treatment all intubated animals received only half the above dosages with full dosage starting the 4th day.

After 65 days treatment and 24 h after the last intubation, the rats were decapitated, blood collected, testes, ventral prostate (VP), seminal vesicle (SV), epididymis and adrenals were excised and weighed. SV fluid, when present, was removed prior to weighing. Blood was allowed to clot for about 1 h in an ice bath then centrifuged. Serum was stored at $-14^{O}C$.

In the second experiment male Fischer rats, 7-9 weeks of age, were orchidectomized under light ether anesthesia. Ten days later they were divided into 4 sets of 12 closely weight matched animals in each set and Silastic implants were inserted (as above). Four (1st group) of each set received 20 mg TP implants, 4 (2nd group) received 2 mg TP implants and the third group of 4 received blank implants. On the following day intubations were started as follows: One animal of each group of 4 received no intubations, a second was intubated with vehicle (5 ml/kg) daily, a third received THC, 25 mg/kg, daily and fourth, CME 75 mg/kg daily. After half dosage treatment the first 3 days, full dosages were started on the 4th day. After 64-67 days and 24 h after the last treatment, the animals were decapitated and processed as above.

Serum gonadotropin levels were quantified by RIA using the NIAMD rLH and rFSH kits. Results are expressed as ng NIAMD-RP1 LH and FSH/ml. All samples were monitored in duplicate in single LH and FSH assays with intraassay coefficients of variation of 14.4% and 6.8%, respectively.

Data was analyzed by the Newman-Keuls method for differences between groups and the 't' test.

III. RESULTS

After 65 days intact animals treated with THC or CME showed depressed body weight (BW) gain and accessory sex organ weights when compared with vehicle or untreated controls (Table I), much like previously reported results (10). However, when exogenous androgen was administered (20 mg TP implant) chronic treatment with THC and CME no longer had significant effect on ventral prostate, seminal vesicle, or epididymal weights (Table I). BW gains were slightly less for THC and CME treated animals when compared to TP implanted controls, although this difference was not statistically significant ($p > 0.05$). In addition, androgen treatment suppressed testicular weights uniformly in the 3 groups with implants. Neither THC nor CME had any effect on this suppression.

In castrated animals, 2 mg TP implants stimulated ventral prostate weight gain about 5-6 fold over untreated and vehicle-intubated controls after 64-67 d (Table II). The 20 mg TP implants stimulated this organ 24-30 fold over the same controls (Table II). The ventral prostate of an intact Fischer rat of comparable age weighed 70-130 mg/100 g, or between those of castrated rats treated with 2 and 20 mg TP implants (10). Neither THC nor CME had any significant effect on 2 or 20 mg TP stimulated ventral prostate weight gain

TABLE I. Relative Tissue Wet Weights from Male Fischer Rats with Testosterone Propionate (TP) Implants Intubated with Delta-9-THC or CME Daily for 65 Days

Treatment	N[b]	Boby Weight Gain (g)	Relative Tissue Wet Weights[a] Testis	Ventral Prostate	Seminal Vesicle[c]	Epididymis	Absolute Weight Adrenals (mg)
Untreated Veh	8	159 (11)	871 (17)	73 (8)	124 (19)	169 (5)	52.1 (1.6)
Veh Control	10	134 (9)	915 (24)	94 (10)	184 (13)	188 (8)	57.7 (3.6)
THC 25 mg/kg	10	92 (8)[e,f]	802 (47)	43 (7)[g]	78 (13)[f]	129 (10)[d,g]	54.6 (3.0)
CME 75 mg/kg	10	71 (9)[e,g]	679 (59)[d,g]	29 (8)[e,g]	77 (15)[e]	109 (11)[e,g]	50.4 (2.5)
20 mg TP + Veh	10	125 (9)	490 (23)[e,g]	132 (8)[e,f]	348 (11)[e,g]	160 (6)	57.7 (2.0)
20 mg TP THC	9	103 (10)[e]	464 (36)[e,g]	128 (10)[e]	384 (19)[e,g]	157 (7)[f]	53.5 (2.2)
20 mg TP CME	10	103 (7)[e]	469 (26)[e,g]	124 (6)[e]	368 (20)[e,g]	153 (8)[f]	56.5 (1.2)

[a]Mean mg/100 g final body weight (+/- S.E.M.).
[b]Number of animals.
[c]Without seminal fluid.
[d] $P < .05$.
[e], compared with Untreated Control, Newman-Keuls test.
[f] $P < .05$.
[g] $P < .01$, compared with Vehicle Control, Newman-Keuls test.

TABLE II. Relative Tissue Wet Weights and Body Weight Gains of Castrated Fischer Rats with Testosterone Propionate (TP) Implants after 64-67 Days Intubation with Cannabinoids[a]

Treatment	N[c]	0	2 mg TP[e]	20 mg TP[e]
		Ventral Prostate (mg/100g Final Body Weight)		
Untrtd Control	8-10	6.7 (0.8)	35.1 (4.6)	151.2 (9.9)
Vehicle Control	9-10	5.8 (0.3)	30.7 (3.9)	147.0 (8.7)
THC 25 mg/kg	8-11	5.3 (0.7)	26.1 (3.5)	164.4 (11.2)
CME 75 mg/kg	7-9	5.8 (0.4)	24.7 (2.5)	158.8 (9.0)
		Seminal Vesicle (mg/100g Final Body Weight)		
Untrtd Control	8-10	31.3 (2.4)	67.5 (10.8)	189.2 (14.4)
Vehicle Control	9-10	29.8 (2.6)	51.6 (5.0)	229.9 (12.5)
THC 25 mg/kg	8-11	28.9 (2.7)	63.8 (3.9)	253.0 (26.8)
CME 75 mg/kg	7-9	30.6 (2.8)	58.6 (5.2)	260.1 (16.9)[f]
		Body Weight Gain (g)		
Untrtd Control	8-10	74.0 (12.2)	114.2 (15.9)	134.4 (22.4)[d]
Vehicle Control	9-10	66.4 (14.3)	86.7 (11.7)	105.1 (16.3)
THC 25 mg/kg	8-11	48.4 (11.8)	47.2 (12.4)[g,h]	48.9 (9.8)[g,h]
CME 75 mg/kg	7-9	42.9 (16.4)	77.0 (17.1)	85.4 (12.0)

[a]Mean (+/- S.E.M.).
[b]Without seminal fluid
[c]Number of animals in each implant group.
[d]$P < 0.05$ compared with corresponding 0 TP implant group, 't' test.
[e]$P < 0.01$, compared with corresponding 0 and/or 2 mg TP implant groups, 't' test.
[f]$P < 0.05$
[g]$P < 0.01$, compared with corresponding untreated control, 't' test.
[h]$P < 0.05$, compared with corresponding vehicle control, 't' test.

(Table II). They also did not significantly affect relative VP weights in animals with blank implants. Very similar results were obtained for seminal vesicle weights. Neither THC nor CME treatment for 64-67 days had any significant effect on SV weights in blank or TP implant treated animals when compared with organ weights from respective vehicle intubated controls.

THC (but not CME) appeared to depress androgen-dependent body-weight gains in T treated castrated rats (Table II). The effect of THC alone on body-weight gain appears to be greater than an equivalent amount of THC when in CME. However, this difference is not seen in the growth data of the intact animal experiment above.

The absolute weights of adrenals did not differ significantly in any of the animals in this experiment. Possible stressful effects of oral THC or CME treatment were not significant enough to affect adrenal weights (11).

Circulating LH and FSH levels from the castrated animals are presented in Table III. Serum LH concentrations in castrated rats chronically treated with THC or CME were significantly lower than in control animals. Although serum FSH levels also tended to be suppressed in these cannabinoid-treated rats, differences were not statistically significant ($p > 0.05$). All rats exposed to the 2 mg TP implant displayed reduced LH and FSH levels when compared to the corresponding non-androgen treated groups. Neither THC nor CME had any significant influence on serum gondotropin values following the 2 mg androgen-implant treatment. LH levels in animals with 20 mg TP. THC or CME did not affect FSH levels significantly in these animals ($p > 0.05$).

IV. DISCUSSION

The oral daily dosages of THC (25 mg/kg) and CME (75 mg/kg) employed in this study may be compared to relatively high human usage (6-12 marijuana cigarettes/day) according to calculations and assumptions of Rosenkrantz et al. (12). When given for 9-10 weeks these doses of THC and CME reduced body weight gain and weight gain of accessory sex organs in intact male rats as we have shown previously (10). However, when exogenous androgen is continuously supplied, THC or CME treatment no longer reduced accessory sex-organ weight compared to vehicle-intubated, androgen-treated controls. Therefore, neither THC nor CME appears to inhibit direct androgenic stimulation of accessory sex organs. Since the high dose of exogenous testosterone (20 mg TP implant) added to endogenous androgen present may have overwhelmed possible cannabinoid

TABLE III. Serum Gonadotropin Levels in Castrated Male Fischer Rats Implanted with Testosterone PRopionate (TP) and Intubated with Delta-9-THC or CME for 4-67 Days[a]

Treatment	N[b]	LH (ng/ml)			FSH (mcg/ml)		
		0 TP	2 mg TP	20 mg TP	0 TP	2 mg TP	20 mg TP
Untreated Control	9	786 (82)	413 (98)[c]	<25[d,f]	1.72 (0.51)	1.06 (0.10)[d]	0.23 (0.03)[d,f]
Vehicle Control	9	956 (49)	476 (102)[d]	<25[d,f]	1.92 (0.23)	1.05 (0.11)[d]	0.18 (0.01)[d,f]
THC 25 mg/kg	8	429 (73)[g,h]	268 (81)	<25[d,e]	1.43 (0.43)	0.78 (0.13)[d]	0.15 (0.01)[d,f]
CME 75 mg/kg	8	525 (11)[g,h]	360 (111)	<25[d,e]	1.58 (0.45)	0.80 (0.09)[d]	0.18 (0.01)[d,f]

[a]Mean (+/- S.E.M.).
[b]Number of animals in each implant group.
[c]$P < 0.05$.
[d]$P < 0.01$, compared with corresponding 0 TP group, Newman-Keuls test.
[e]$P < 0.05$.
[f]$P < 0.01$, compared with corresponding 2 mg TP group, Newman-Keuls test.
[g]$P < 0.05$, compared with corresponding untreated control, Newman-Keuls test.
[h]$P < 0.01$, compared with corresponding vehicle control, Newman-Keuls test.

inhibitory action in intact animals, cannabinoid effects on orchidectomized animals treated with lower and identical dosages of androgen were investigated. Results obtained demonstrated that long term THC or CME treatment of castrated rats did not reduce 2 or 20 mg TP implant stimulation of ventral prostate and seminal vesicle weights nor alter the unstimulated tissue weights in animals with blank implants. Thus, chronic THC or CME administration does not appear to affect low or moderately high androgen stimulation of male accessory sex organs.

Chronic THC treatment suppresses body-weight gain in androgen-treated castrated rats as it has been shown to do in intact rats (10). In contrast, CME appears to have much less suppressive effect on growth in castrated animals with TP implants. Since THC content is the same in either treatment, castrates may be more sensitive to possible interactive effects of THC with other constituents of CME than intact animals.

Since chronic THC treatment has been reported to depress serum LH levels (2,3), but not FSH levels (2), in intact animals, we assayed gonadotropins LH and FSH in sera from our castrated animals. As our results indicated, both THC and CME depressed serum LH levels in castrated animals devoid of androgen replacement. FSH levels were not significantly suppressed, nor were serum LH and FSH in androgen treated animals. Reduced body weight gains appear to follow lower LH values. The lesser weight gains in THC-treated animals compared with corresponding vehicle control groups. Thus, LH suppression is very likely due primarily to lesser food consumption in the cannabinoid-treated animals. This relationship would be consistent with our observations in pair-feeding experiments (10). It should be noted that our sera samples were obtained 24 h after last THC or CME treatment. Samples obtained sooner after treatment (during lesser food consumption) may show greater depression in gonadotropin levels. The suppression of LH seen in acute THC studies (3,13,14) may, in part, be due to this reduced feeding effect.

Purohit et al. reported that THC or cannabinol, at 10 mg/kg dosage given subcutaneously daily for 10 days to castrated male rats, suppressed the stimulative effect of 5 mg/kg testosterone daily, s.c., on the ventral prostate and seminal vesicle (8). Since they do not report body weights during this period, effects on relative tissue weights are unknown. In addition, the subcutaneous route of cannabinoid administration and shorter treatment period make comparison with our observations difficult. Our results suggest that the suppressive effects of chronic THC and CME treatment in the male rat reproductive system reflect an action within the CNS-pituitary complex to suppress gonadotropin and, thereby, testicular androgen output rather than an antiandrogenic action on the accessory sex organs. This action in the chronically-treated animal appears to be for the most part a direct one due to reduced food intake. The question of a possible direct effect of cannabinoids on testicular function, as suggested by _in vitro_ studies (4,6), will be the subject of another paper. In conclusion, our results do not demonstrate any inhibition, by chronic THC or CME treatment at the dose level used on testosterone stimulation of ventral prostate or seminal vesicle growth.

ACKNOWLEDGMENTS

The technical assistance of V. Benjamin, R. Chin, K. Kim and M. Teicher is gratefully acknowledged. We thank Drs. M. E. O'Connell and M. C. Braude for their generous counsel.

REFERENCES

1. Bloch, E., Thysen, B., Morrill, G., Gardner, E., and Fujimoto, G., Effects of cannabinoids on reproduction and development, Vitam. Horm. (N.Y.) 36:203-258 (1978).
2. Collu, R., Letarte, J., Leboeuf, G., and Ducharme, J. R., Endocrine effects of chronic administration of psychoactive drugs to prepubertal male rats. I, Delta-9-tetrahydrocannabinol, Life Sci. 16:533-542 (1975).
3. Symons, A. M., Teale, J. D., and Marks, Y., Effect of delta-9-tetrahydrocannabinol on the hypothalamic-pituitary-gonadal system, J. Endocrinol. 68:43P-44P (1976).
4. Dalterio, S., Bartke, A., and Burstein, S., Cannabinoids inhibit testosterone secretion by mouse testes _in vitro_, Science 196:1472-1473 (1977).
5. Purohit, V. D., Ahluwahlia, B. S., and Vigersky, R. A., Marihuana inhibits dihydrotestosterone binding to the androgen receptor, Endocrinol. 107:848-850 (1980).
6. Jakubovic, A., McGeer, E. G., and McGeer, P. L., Effects of cannabinoids on testosterone and protein synthesis in rat testis Leydig cells _in vitro_, Mo. Cell. Endocrinol. 15:41-50 (1979).
7. Abel, E. L., Cannabis: effects on hunger and thirst, Behav. Biol. 15:255-280 (1980).
8. Purohit, V. D., Singh, H. H., and Ahluwahlia, B. S., Evidence that the effect of methadone and marijuana on male reproductive organs are mediated at different sites in rats, Biol. Reprod. 20:1039-1044 (1979).

9. Dzuik, P. J., and Cook, B., Passage of steroids through silicone rubber, Endocrinol. 78:208-211 (1966).
10. Fujimoto, G. I., Morrill, G. A., O'Connell, M. E., Kostellow, A. B., and Retura, G., Effects of cannabinoids given orally and reduced appetite on the male rat reproductive system, Pharmacol. 24:303-313 (1982).
11. O'Connell, M. E., Morrill, G. A., Fujimoto, G. I., and Kostellow, A. B., The effects of chronic ingestion of cannabinoids on adrenocortical activity in female Fischer rats, Fed. Proc. Soc. Exp. Biol. Med. 39:849 (1980).
12. Rosenkrantz, H., and Braude, M. C., Comparative chronic toxicities of delta-9-tetrahydrocannabinol administered orally or by inhalation in rat, in "Pharmacology of Marihuana", Vol. 2 (M. C. Braude and S. Szara, eds.), pp. 571-584. Raven Press, New York, 1976.
13. Besch, N. F., Smith, C. G., Besch, P. K., and Kaufman, P. H., The effect of marijuana (delta-9-tetrahydrocannabinol) on the secretion of luteinizing hormone in the ovariectomized rhesus monkey, Amer. J. Obstet. Gyned. 128:635-640 (1977).
14. Tyrey, L., Delta-9-tetrahydrocannabinol suppression of episodic luteinizing hormone secretion in the ovariectomized rat, Endocrinol 102:1808-1814 (1978).

MATERNAL OR PATERNAL EXPOSURE TO CANNABINOIDS AFFECTS CENTRAL NEUROTRANSMITTER LEVELS AND REPRODUCTIVE FUNCTION IN MALE OFFSPRING

Susan L. Dalterio
Richard W. Steger
Andrzej Bartke

Department of Pharmacology
The University of Texas Health Science Center at San Antonio
San Antonio, Texas

I. INTRODUCTION

Marijuana, and its main psychoactive component delta-9-tetrahydrocannabinol (THC), have been reported to exert a wide range of effects on reproductive performance (1). Association of chronic marijuana use by men with decreased plasma testosterone levels, reduced sperm counts and impotence has been reported (2,3). In adult male mice acute exposure to THC or chronic treatment with CBN, a relatively non-psychoactive cannabinoid, can decrease plasma testosterone, prolactin and gonadotropin levels. While the suppression of prolactin secretion may involve alterations in serotonergic and dopaminergic activity (7), the central mechanisms by which THC alters gonadotropin release are not clear, although direct effects of THC on the hypothalamic-pituitary axis have been suggested (8,9).

In general, the reports on the effects of THC on central nervous system (CNS) neurotransmitters are conflicting, with investigators presenting evidence of increased or decreased levels of norepinephrine (NE) and serotonin (5-HT) after THC treatment (10-13). Recently, low concentrations of THC have been shown to stimulate dopamine (DA) and NE uptake by hypothalamic and striatal synaptosomes whereas higher concentrations inhibited DA and NE uptake (13). In the mouse, THC has been shown to increase synaptosomal DA synthesis in striatum at low doses, but decrease DA synthesis at higher doses (14).

The Cannabinoids: Chemical, Pharmacologic, and Therapeutic Aspects

ISBN 0-12-044620-0

In addition to these effects of cannabinoids on the CNS it is apparent that these compounds can directly affect the steroidogenic and spermatogenic functions of the testes in several species of laboratory animals (1,4,15). Although the mechanisms responsible for cannabinoid-induced alterations in testicular function remain to be elucidate, available evidence suggests that interference with gonadotropic stimulation (15), reduction in testicular synthesis of proteins, lipids, and nucleic acids (17), and prostaglandins (18,19), glucose utilization (20) or activity of cholesterol esterase (21,22) may be involved in the reduction of testicular steroidogenesis.

The testicular hormonal milieu is critical for normal spermatogenesis and at present it cannot be determined whether cannabinoid-induced suppression of spermatogenesis in mice (23), or in humans (24) is secondary to a reduction in testosterone production or due to a direct action on the germinal epithelium. Cannabinoids have been reported to influence acrosomal morphogenesis and condensation of chromatin in sperm heads as well as inhibit sperm maturation (25).

On the basis of these findings it can be concluded that cannabinoids affect adult male reproductive functions. However, the possible implications for male fetal development have been given less attention. We have previously reported that exposure of female mice to either THC or CBN on the last day of gestation and for the first six days post-partum resulted in long term alterations in body weight regulation and reproductive functions in their male offspring (5,6). Effects of perinatal exposure to cannabinoids on the male reproductive system did not become evident until after weaning (21 days of age). During and after sexual maturation male mice exposed to THC had reduced testes weights and elevated levels of plasma luteinizing hormone (LH). In contrast, CBN-exposed males had reduced concentrations of these hormones after sexual maturation. Copulatory behavior was also reduced in adult males exposed to either THC or CBN during the perinatal period of sexual differentiation (5,6). Biochemical changes, including alterations in brain RNA synthesis, in neonatal rats have been induced by THC administration during pregnancy (26) and effects of prenatal cannabinoid exposure on development and learning have been reported (27,28).

The present experiments were designed to further characterize the consequences of perinatal exposure of male mice to THC or CBN, or to the non-psychoactive component cannabidiol (CBD). In particular, we have examined the concentrations of brain amines in adult male mice prenatally exposed to these compounds.

We have previously reported that treatment of adult male mice with THC, CBN or CBD reduced fertility and resulted in chromosomal abnormalities (15). In the present study we have examined the consequences of paternal exposure to cannabinoids on the subsequent fertility of their male offspring.

II. METHODS

Primiparous female mice obtained from our colony of randomly bred animals received a single oral administration of THC, CBN, or CBD at a dose of 50 mg per kg body weight on one of the last four days of gestation. On the first day postpartum litters were culled to five or six male pups; the offspring were weaned at 21 days of age and housed in groups of three until adulthood (60-80 days).

Half of the animals in each treatment group were castrated in connection with ongoing studies on the effects of prenatal cannabinoid exposure on androgen receptor levels in seminal vesicles. Castrations were performed under ether anesthesia and the testes were removed, weighed, homogenized in distilled water (9:1 w/v) and stored frozen for the radioimmunoassay determination of testosterone as described previously (29,30). Two days post-castration the males were sacrificed by cervical dislocation and the brain was quickly removed and stored frozen for measurement of amine concentrations.

Prior to the amine assay, the brains were partially thawed and the hypothalamus was dissected free. The hypothalamus consisted of a tissue block 2.0 mm deep extending from the rostral margin of the mammillary body to the rostral border of the optic chiasm and laterally to the hypothalamic sulci. The hypothalamic block and the remaining brain tissue were weighed and sonicated in 0.1 N $HClO_4$ containing 3-methoxy-4-hydroxyphenethanol (MOPET) as a standard for the indole amine assay, dihydroxybenzylamine (DHBA) as an internal standard for the catecholamine assay and 1.0 mM sodium metabisulfite.

Indolamines were separated by high performance liquid chromatography (HPLC) and quantitated by electrochemistry (29). Standards were run concurrently, and 5-HT and 5-HIAA were calculated by comparison of peak heights with those of the standards. Values were corrected for recovery of the internal standard which averaged 97.3 +/- 1.2%. The intra-assay coefficient of variation was 5.6% for 5-HT, and 7.2% for 5-HIAA.

Catecholamines were prepared for chromatography as previously described (29,30). Norepinephrine, DA and DHBA were separated by HPLC and quantitated by electochemistry. The recovery of DHBA averaged 82.3 +/- 1.1% and the intra-assay coefficient of variation was 6.1% for NE and 6.7% for DA.

For groups and parameters in which no significant differences were found due to the time of prenatal treatment, results from animals exposed to cannabinoids on the different days of gestation were combined for further statistical analysis and presentation.

In studies concerning the effects of paternal exposure to cannabinoids on the subsequent fertility of their male offspring, adult male mice were treated with THC, CBN, or CBD (50 mg/kg) three times a week for five weeks, using 18 males per group as described previously (15). The males were individually housed with a different adult female each during the third, fourth and fifth week of treatment and during the first and fourth post-treatment weeks. In each treatment group half of the pregnant females were allowed to deliver and raise their pups. The surviving F_1 male offspring were weaned at 21 days of age, and housed in groups of four until adulthood (60-80 days). Each F_1 male was given the opportunity (duringa one week cohabitation period) to mate with at least three different females. Females were sacrificed between days 15 and 19 of gestation for determination of the number of corpora lutea, resorptions, dead fetuses, live and still births, and postnatal deaths. The overall percentage of females impregnated was also recorded. Female mice who failed to become pregnant were remated to known fertile males to verify their fertility.

III. RESULTS

A. Maternal Exposure

At two days post-castration the concentrations of NE in hypothalamus and NE and DA in the remaining brain were slightly reduced in CBN- and CBD-exposed animals in comparison to castrate controls. In contrast, levels of 5-HT and 5-HIAA were significantly elevated in both the hypothalamus and the remaining brain in these mice (Tables I and II). Exposure to THC during the latter part of gestation did not significantly affect brain amine concentrations. There were no significant differences in the weights of the brain or hypothalamic tissue blocks or in body weight among the animals in the different treatment groups.

Testicular testosterone concentrations were reduced in adult male mice exposed to CBN, although testes weights were not affected. The weights of the seminal vesicles were increased by CBD exposure, but were significantly reduced by CBN exposure (Table III). Exposure to THC did not influence these parameters.

TABLE I. Brain Amine Concentrations[a]

	NE	DA	5-HT	5-HIAA
Oil	398 +/- 12 (12)	1288 +/- 81 (12)	579 +/- 21 (11)	181 +/- 6 (11)
THC	398 +/- 12 (18)	1345 +/- 39 (18)	583 +/- 46 (18)	194 +/- 6 (11)
CBN	254 +/- 29[b] (14)	793 +/- 97[b] (14)	1024 +/- 60[b] (14)	267 +/- 9[b] (14)
CBD	247 +/- 20[b] (14)	748 +/- 60[b] (14)	1010 +/- 28[b] (14)	249 +/- 4[b] (14)

[a]Units are in ng/g (N).

[b]Significantly different from controls ($p < 0.05$) by analysis of variance and Duncan's test.

N.B. All animals were castrated 2 days prior to sacrifice. In addition, the brain consisted of the remaining tissue after the removal of the hypothalamic block.

TABLE II. Hypothalamic Amine Concentrations[a]

	NE	DA	5-HT	5-HIAA
Oil	1371 +/- 101 (12)	1244 +/- 189 (12)	1308 +/- 52 (12)	359 +/- 17 (12)
THC	1302 +/- 54 (18)	1161 +/- 83 (18)	1274 +/- 54 (18)	377 +/- 13 (18)
CBN	849 +/- 76[b] (13)	1006 +/- 103 (14)	2247 +/- 206[b] (14)	506 +/- 45[b] (14)
CBD		1134 +/- 130 (14)	2191 +/- 144[b] (14)	477 +/- 33[b] (14)
Day 2	800 +/- 72[b] (9)			
Day 3	1225 +/- 256 (5)			

[a]Units are in ng/g (N).
[b]Significantly different from controls ($p < 0.05$) by analysis of variance and Duncan's test.
N.B. All animals were castrated 2 days prior to sacrifice.

B. Paternal Exposure

The F_1 male offspring of the CBD-treated male mice successfully impregnated all the females with whom they were paired, as did the offspring of the oil-treated control mice. However, the F_1 male offspring of the THC and CBN-treated animals had significantly reduced reproductive performance.

For the analysis of results on F_1 male fertility, offspring from each treatment group were classified into three categories. The first included the males which had successfully impregnated all the females with whom they were paired, with all the resulting litters being normal by the standards of our breeding colony, that is litter size of at least 10 pups and less than 10% pre- or post-natal mortality. The second category consisted of those males in which one out of three matings deviated from these criteria. Finally, the third category consisted of those males whom did not produce a single pregnancy that met our criterion of normalcy.

Among the THC and CBN-exposed offspring, a significant percentage, 36% of the THC and 21% of the CBN-F_1 males, fell into the third category (Fig. 1). In addition, in two litters sired by F_1 males from THC-treated fathers, one contained an exencephalic fetus, while another pup (delivered alive at autopsy on day 19) exhibited exencephaly, spina bifida, and exteriorized intestines (Fig. 2). Testes from the most severely affected group of males were examined cytogenetically and, in testes obtained from two out of eight animals, chromosomal abnormalities (as indicated in a representative sample in Fig. 3) in the form of ring and chain translocations, nondisjunction and aneuploidy were observed, as was a reduction in testicular weights.

TABLE III. Hormone Levels and Organ Weights

	Testicular Testosterone Concentrations (ng/ml)	Testes Weights (mg)	Seminal Vesicles (mg)
Oil	138 +/- 22 (12)	278 +/- 7 (12)	258 +/- 13 (12)
THC	112 +/- 15 (17)	296 +/- 9 (18)	219 +/- 28 (18)
CBN	69 +/- 17* (14)	268 +/- 12 (14)	164 +/- 16* (14)
CBD	126 +/- 21 (14)	310 +/- 8 (14)	308 +/- 12* (14)

*Significantly different from controls ($p < 0.05$) by analysis of variance and Duncan's test. Number of animals = (N).

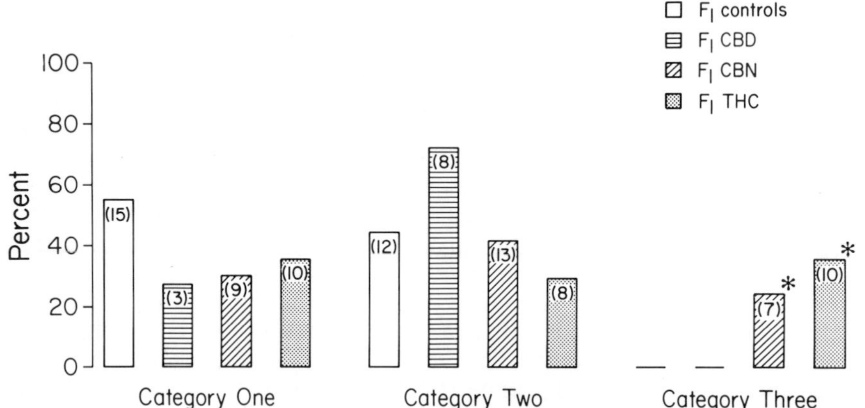

FIGURE 1. Reproductive performance in adult F_1 male offspring of cannabinoid-treated male mice. * = Significantly different from control males in category three; Chi-square = 18.05, df = 3, $p < 0.001$.

IV. DISCUSSION

The present findings indicate that alterations in brain amine levels in adulthood may result from prenatal exposure to cannabinoids. The relatively non-psychoactive CBN and CBD altered brain and hypothalamic concentrations of NE, DA, 5-HT and 5-HIAA as well as testicular testosterone concentrations and seminal vesicles weights, while prenatal THC exposure during late gestation did not appear to influence these parameters. However, we have recently observed that exposure to THC during the mid-portion of gestation did result in altered brain amine levels in adult mice (Dalterio and Steger, unpublished observation). In view of our earlier findings of long-term alterations in other parameters of endocrine and behavioral function in male mice exposed to THC during the perinatal period (5,6) it is possible that critical time periods exist for cannabinoid-induced alterations in developmental processes. We are currently investigating this issue as well as planning experiments to determine effects of perinatal cannabinoid exposure on amine uptake and turnover.

Although we do not know the precise mechanism by which castration differentially affected cannabinoid-exposed animals, it is known that castration stimulates amine turnover in normal animals (31). It is possible that cannabinoid exposure resulted in a differential responsiveness to the surgical stress associated with castration. We have previously reported that adult male mice treated with cannabinoids exhibit a differential hormonal response to stressful stimuli (32). However, we have also reported that the release of pituitary gonadotropins three weeks post-castration is altered in animals perinatally exposed to THC (33) and it is doubtful that surgical stress could be a factor in these observations. It is possible that alterations in catecholamines, which are known to have a role in the regulation of gonadotropin release (34), may be involved. We have also reported that perinatal, but not pre-pubertal, exposure to THC reduces responsiveness of the vas deferens in vitro to NE and D-Ala^2-Met-enkephalin (35).

It is conceivable that the reported effects of prenatal cannabinoid exposure on development and learning are also related to cannabinoid-induced changes in concentrations of these neurotransmitters (27,28). We have previously reported that adult copulatory behavior was reduced differentially by THC or CBN (5,6). Although the influences of neurotransmitters on sexual behavior are not clear (36), it is conceivable

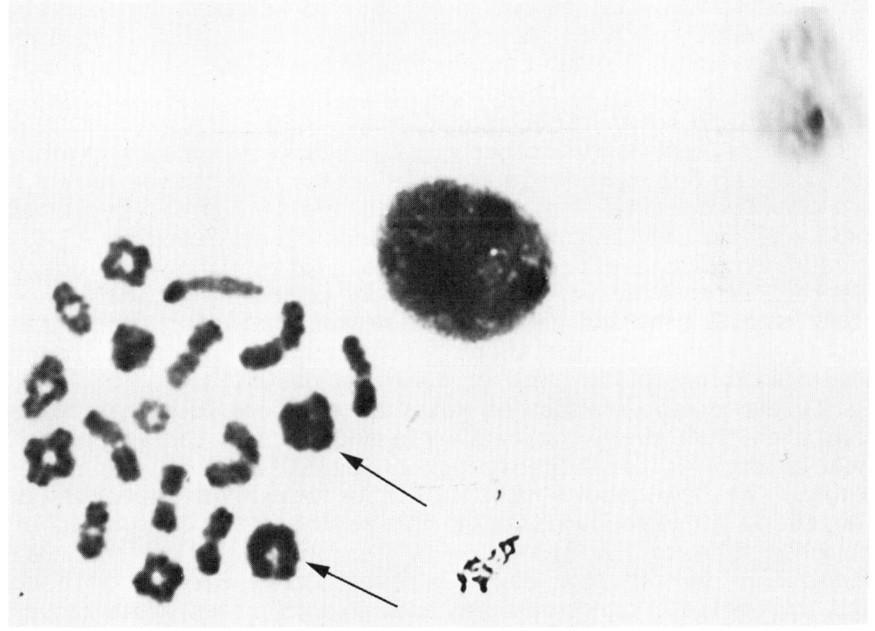

FIGURE 2. Chromasomal abnormalities observed in testes obtained from F_1 offspring of THC-treated adult male mice. N.B. A diakenesis-metaphase 1 plate with 2 ring configurations (indicated by arrows) and 16 bivalents in a spermatocyte from a testis obtained from an F_1 offspring of a THC-treated male.

that changes in behavioral responsivity to stimuli from conspecifics may result from cannabinoid-induced alterations in brain catecholamines during critical periods of sexual differentiation.

Another factor which may be related to the observation that castration brought out an effect of prenatal cannabinoid exposure that was not otherwise observed concerns the presence of gonadal steroids, which can modulate amine levels (37). We have shown that the gonadal steroids modulate the acute hormonal responses to THC administration in adult mice (38). In addition to the possible influences of surgical stress or the presence of gonadal steroids we have also demonstrated that environmental factors such as the presence of female conspecifics can interact with the effects of perinatal cannabinoid exposure. In an earlier study we noted that pre-pubertal cannabinoid-exposed males responded to housing with an immature female as a stressful situation, as suggested by increased adrenal weights and reductions in the weights of the testes and seminal vesicles 95). Thus, although the precise mechanism by which castration appears to reveal effects of prenatal cannabinoid exposure on CNS neurotransmitter levels is at present unclear. However, based on our earlier studies these findings appear to be consistent with cannabinoid-induced alterations in physiological responsivity to events which disturb homeostatic conditions.

In mice, maternal exposure to cannabinoids appears capable of inducing teratogenesis in male offspring. These effects are observed after a single prenatal exposure or repeated exposure during the perinatal periods of development (5,6). In addition, the effects on the male offspring, including alterations in body weight regulation, pituitary-gonadal function, sexual behavior and central neurotransmitter concentrations, are not inconsistent with results of cannabinoid administration to immature or adult males (1).

Evidence from studies of paternal exposure to cannabinoids indicates that these compounds, in addition to their reported embryocidal or teratogenic potential (1) also may be mutagenic. We have shown that brief or repeated exposure in adulthood to psychoactive or non-psychoactive components of cannabis affects the endocrine system and fertility and that these effects were not rapidly reversible, were associated with chromosomal abnormalities and, in some cases, with reductions in testicular weights and alterations in plasma hormone concentrations (15). Although the mechanisms by which cannabinoids influence the genetic apparatus are unclear, we observed that the F_1 male offspring of cannabinoid-treated male mice exhibited reductions in reproductive performance, as well as cytogenetic abnormalities similar in type and frequency to those observed in their treated sires (15). This

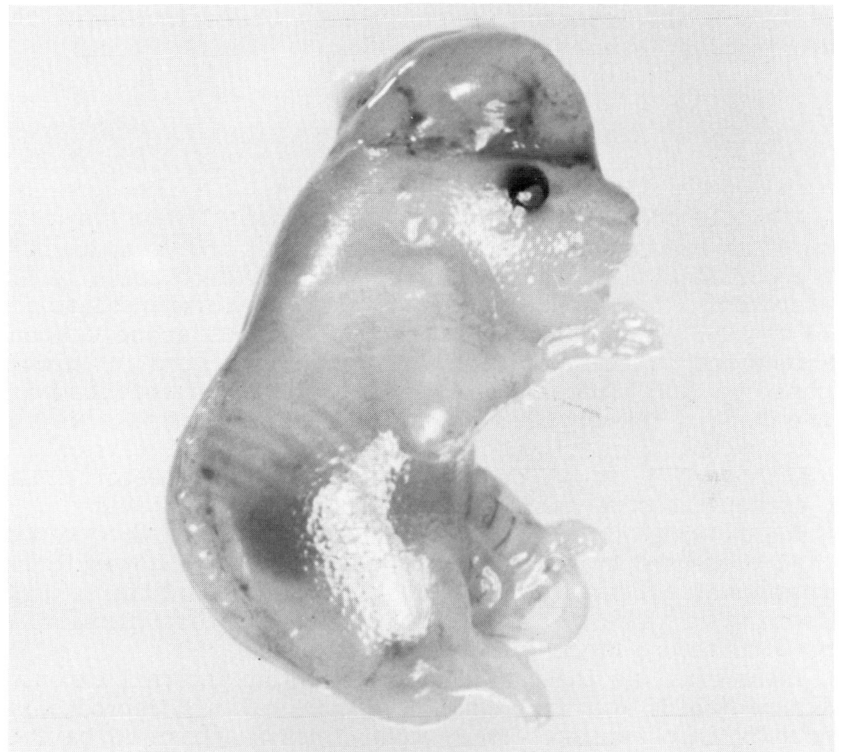

FIGURE 3. Congenital malformations observed in the F_2 generation of THC-treated male mice.

strongly suggests that cannabinoid effects on fertility can be transmitted from one generation to the next. in addition, it must be stressed that these F_1 males were survivors of matings in which indications of subfertility and perinatal loss had been observed, and therefore these animals do not represent the most seriously affected offspring of the cannabinoid-treated males. The observation of severe congenital defects in F_2 offspring of THC-treated males suggests that cannabinoids may affect polygenetic systems involved, not only in reproductive functions, but with a wide range of developmental processes as well.

It is evident that either maternal or paternal exposure to cannabinoids, whether psychoactive or non-psychoactive, are capable of producing long-term alterations in reproductive functions in their male offspring. Furthermore, it is evident that in either situation, that is, pre-gestational orgestational exposure, the effects of cannabinoids may not become apparent until maturational or environmental factors require physiological responses, particularly those involving the endocrine system.

V. SUMMARY

A single prenatal exposure to cannabinol (CBN) or cannabidiol (CBD) reduced brain norepinephrine (NE) and dopamine (DA) and hypothalamic NE concentrations, but increased brain levels of serotonin (5-HT) and its metabolite, 5-hydroxyindoleacetic acid (5-HIAA). In addition, testicular testosterone concentrations and seminal vesicles weights were reduced in animals exposed to CBN. In contrast, seminal vesicles weights were increased in CBD-exposed males. Prenatal exposure to the major psychoactive component of marijuana, delta-9-tetrahydrocannabinol (THC) on one of the last four days of gestation did not affect these parameters.

The F_1 male offspring of male mice treated with CBN, CBD or THC presented evidence of reduced fertility and testicular chromosomal abnormalities. In addition, two of the F_1 male offspring of the THC-treated mice sired litters containing pups with severe congenital malformations.

These findings indicate that maternal or paternal exposure to cannabinoids can influence developmental and reproductive functions in offspring. Thus, cannabinoids appear to be both mutagenic and teratogenic in mice.

REFERENCES

1. Bloch, E., Thysen, B., Morrill, G. a., Gardner, E., and Fujimoto, G., Effects of cannabinoids on reproduction and development, Vitam. Horm. 36:203-258 (1978).
2. Kolodny, R. C., Lessin, P., Toro, G., Masters, W. H., and Cohen, S., Depression of plasma testosterone with acute marijuana administration, in "The Pharmacology of Marihuana" (M. C. Braude and S. Szara, eds.), pp. 217-225. Raven Press, New York, 1976.
3. Kolodny, R. C., Masters, W. H., Kolodner, R. M., and Toro, G., Depression of plasma testosterone levels after chronic intensive marijuana use, New Engl. J. Med. 290:872-874 (1974).
4. Dalterio, S., Bartke, A., Roberson, C., Watson, D., and Burstein, S., Direct and pituitary-mediated effects of delta-9-THC and cannabinol on the testis, Pharmac. Biochem. Behav. 8:673-678 (1978).

5. Dalterio, S. L., Perinatal or adult exposure to cannabinoids alters male reproductive functions in mice, Pharmac. Biochem. Behav. 12:143-153 (1980).
6. Dalterio, S., and Bartke, A., Perinatal exposure to cannabinoids alters male reproductive function in mice, Science 205:1420-1422 (1979).
7. Kramer, J., and Ben-David, M., Prolactin suppression by (-)-delta-9-tetrahydrocannabinol (THC): Involvement of serotonergic and dopaminergic pathways, Endocrinology 103:452-457 (1978).
8. Smith, C. G., Besch, N. F., Smith, R. G., and Besch, P. K., Effect of tetrahydrocannabinol on the hypothalamic-pituitary axis in the ovariectomized Rhesus monkey, Fertil. Steril. 31:335-339, (1979).
9. Asch, R. H., Smith, C. G., Siler-Knodr, T. M., and Pauerstein, C. J., Effects of delta-9-tetrahydrocannabinol on gonadal steroidogenic activity in vivo, Fertil. Steril. 32:576-582 (1979).
10. Fuxe, K., and Johnson, G., The effect of tetrahydrocannabinol on central monoamine neurons, Acta. Pharm. Suec. 8:695-701 (1971).
11. Ho, B. T., Taylor, D. V., Fritchie, G. E., Englert, G. E., and McIsaac, W. M., Neuropharmacological study of delta-9-tetrahydrocannabinol in monkeys and mice, Brain Res. 38:163-170 (1973).
12. Harris, L. S., Dewey, W. L. and Razdan, R., Cannabis: It's chemistry, pharmacology, and toxicology, in "Drug Addiction II" (W. R. Martin, ed.), Handbook of Experimental Pharmacology 45:371-429 (1972).
13. Dewey, W. L., Poddar, M. K., and Johnson, K. M., The effects of cannabinoids on rat brain synaptosomes, in "Marijuana: Biological Effects" (G. G. Nahas and W. D. M. Paton, eds.), p. 343. Pergamon Press, Oxford, 1979.
14. Bloom, A. S., Effect of delta-9-tetrahydrocannabinol on the synthesis of dopamine and norepinephrine in mouse brain synaptosomes, J. Pharmacol. Exp. Ther. 221:97-103 (1982).
15. Dalterio, S., Badr, F., Bartke, A., and Mayfield, D., Cannabinoids in male mice: Effects on fertility and spermatogensis, Science 216:315-316 (1982).
16. Tyrey, L., delta-9-tetrahydrocannabinol: A potent inhibitor of episodic luteinizing hormone secretion, J. Pharmacol. Exp. Ther. 213:300-308 (1980).
17. Jakubovic, A., McGeer, E. G., and McGeer, P. L., Effects of cannabinoids on testosterone and protein synthesis in rat testis Leydig cells in vitro, Molec. Cell. Endocrinol. 15:41-50 (1979).
18. Burstein, S., Levin, E., and Varanelli, C., Prostaglandins and cannabis. II. Inhibition of biosynthesis by

the naturally occuring cannabinoids, Biochem. Pharmacol. 22:2905-2910 (1973).
19. Dalterio, S., Bartke, A., Harper, M. J. K., Huffman, R., and Sweeney, C., Effects of cannabinoids and female exposure on the pituitary-testicular axis in mice: Possible involvement of prostaglandins, Biol. Reprod. 24:315-322 (1981).
20. Husain, S., and Lame, M. W., Inhibitory effects of delta-9-tetrahydrocannabinol on glycolytic substrates in the rat testis, Pharmacology 23:102-112 (1981).
21. Shoupe, T. S., Hunter, S. A., Burstein, S. H., and Hubbard, C. D., Nature of the inhibition of cholesterol esterase by delta-1-tetrahydrocannabinol, Enzyme 25:87-91 (1980).
22. Burstein, S., Hunter, S. A., and Shoupe, T. S., Site of inhibition of Leydig cell testosterone by delta-1-tetrahydrocannabinol, Molec. Pharmacol. 15:663-640 (1979).
23. Dixit, V. P., Sharma, V. N., and Lohiya, N. K., The effect of chronically administered cannabis extract on the testicular function in mice, Eur. J. Pharmacol. 26:111-114 (1974).
24. Hembree, W. C., Nahas, G. G., Zeidenberg, P., and Dyrenfurth, I, Marijuana effects of the human testis, Clin. Res. 24:272A (1976).
25. Issidorides, M. R., Observations in chronic marijuana users: Nuclear aberrations in blood and sperm and abnormal acrosomes in spermatozoa, in "Marijuana: Biological Effects" (G. G. Nahas and W. D. M. Paton, eds.), p. 377. Pergamon Press, Oxford, 1979.
26. Luthra, Y. K., Brain biochemical alterations in neonates of dams treated orally with delta-9-tetrahydrocannabinol during gestation lactation, in "Marihuana: Biological Effects (G. G. Nahas and W. D. M. Paton, eds.), p. 531. Pergamon Press, Oxford, 1979.
27. Fried, P. A., Short and long term effects of prenatal cannabis inhalation upon rat offspring, Psychopharmacology 50:285-291 (1976).
28. Raduoco-Thomas, S., Magnan, F., Grove, R. N., Singh, P., Garcon, F., and Raduoco-Thomas, C., Effect of chronic administration of delta-9-THC on learning and memory in developing mice, in "The Pharmacology of Marihuana" (M. C. Braude and S. Szara, eds.), p. 487. Raven Press, New York, 1976.
29. Steger, R. W., DePaolo, L., Asch, R. H., and Silverman, A. V., Interactions of delta-9-tetrahydrocannabinol (THC) with hypothalamic neurotransmitters controlling luteinizing hormone and prolactin release, Neuroendocrinology, submitted (1982).

30. Steger, R. W., Bartke, A., and Goldman, B. D., Alterations in neuroendocrine function during photoperiod-induced testicular atrophy and recrudiscence in the golden hamster, Biol. Reprod. 26:437-444 (1982).
31. Bapna, J., Neff, N. H., and Costa, E., A method for studying norepinephrine and serotonin metabolism in small regions of the brain: Effect of ovariectomy on amine metabolism in anterior and posterior hypothalamus, Endocrinology 89:1345-1349 (1971).
32. Dalterio, S. L., Michael, S. D., Macmillan, B. T., and Barke, A., Differential effects cannabinoid exposure and stress on plasma prolactin, growth hormone and corticosterone levels in male mice, Life Sci. 28:761-766 (1981).
33. Dalterio, S., Bartke, A., and Sweeney, C., Interactive effects of ethanol and delta-9-tetrahydrocannabinol on endocrine functions in male mice, J. Androl. 2:87-93 (1981).
34. Barraclough, C. A., and Wise, P. M., The role of catecholamines in the regulation of pituitary luteinizing hormone and follicle-stimulating hormone secretion, Endocrinol. Rev. 3:91-119 (1982).
35. Dalterio, S., Blum, K., Dellalo, L., Sweeney, C., Briggs, A., and Barke, A., Perinatal exposure to delta-9-THC in mice: Altered enkephalin and norepinephrine sensitivity in vas deferens, Subs.AlcoholActions/Misuse 1:467-478 (1980).
36. Gessa, G. L., and Tagliamonte, A., Role of brain serotonin and dopamine in male sexual behavior, in "Sexual Behavior: Pharmacology and Biochemistry", p. 117. Raven Press, New York, 1975.
37. Wise, P. M., Rance, N., and Barraclough, C. A., Effects of estradiol and progesterone on catecholamine turnover in discrete hypothalamic regions on ovariectomized rats, Endocrinol. 108:2186-2193 (1981).
38. Dalterio, S., Bartke, A., Michael, S., and Macmillan, B., Gonadal steroids influence the effects of delta-9-tetrahydrocannabinol in male mice, Biol. Reprod. 22:117A (1980).

EFFECTS OF CANNABINOIDS ON SPERMATOGENESIS IN MICE: *IN VIVO* AND *IN VITRO* STUDIES

S. K. Tilak[1]
A. M. Zimmerman[2]

Department of Zoology
University of Toronto
Toronto, Ontario

I. INTRODUCTION

The mechanism of action of marijuana on somatic and germinal cells is controversial. An area of concern is whether cannabinoids act directly or indirectly on the cellular system. A direct effect may involve interaction with cell membranes (10,11), macromolecular synthesis (1,12,15,18,22), DNA replication (2) and the mitotic mechanism (13,14). An indirect effect on these systems may be mediated via metabolites of the cannabinoids as well as via alterations of hormonal levels.

Numerous studies have revealed the potential adverse effects of marijuana on reproductive function. Reduced fertility, aberrations of the repertoire of reproductive behaviors and altered hormonal levels have been reported in rodents and primates. There is increasing evidence that cannabinoids can interfere, either directly or indirectly, with testicular function. Our laboratory is interested in determining the effects of marijuana on spermatogenesis. Spermatogenic differentiation is an intricate process involving neurohormonal control and an as yet undefined control of gene expression in the seminiferous tubule. Cannabinoids may interfere with the hormonal regulation of spermatogenesis at the hypothalamic, pituitary or testicular level. Alternatively, cannabinoids

---

[1]Supported by a NSERC Postgraduate Scholarship.
[2]Supported by a grant from the NSER Council, Canada.

ISBN 0-12-044620-0

may exert some of their effects directly of the differentiating spermatogenic cells. Thus a brief review of the effects of cannabinoids on spermatogenesis and macromolecular synthesis in somatic and germinal cells is pertinent.

A. In Vivo Effects of Cannabinoids on Spermatogenesis

1. Cytogenetic Studies. Treatment of hybrid male mice genotype (C57BL X C3H)F_1 with cannabinol (CBN; 10 mg/kg), cannabidiol (CBD; 10 mg/kg) and delta-9-tetrahydrocannabinol (THC; 10 mg/kg) for 5 days led to an increased incidence of ring and chain translocations in pachytene spermatocytes (25). The animals were sacrificed 16 days after the last treatment and, thus, pachytene spermatocytes scored were assumed to be at the spermatogonium stage when exposed to the cannabinoids.

Exposure of male mice to cannabinoids has been reported to lead to a reduction in fertility and an increased incidence of chromosomal abnormalities (3). Treatment of mice orally with THC (50 mg/kg), CBN (50 mg/kg) or crude marijuana extract (CME; 25 mg/kg) daily for 5 days led to an increase of chromosomal abnormalities in pachytene spermatocytes 50 to 60 days later. The abnormalities included ring and chain translocations, aneuploidy (THC, CBN or CME treatment), univalent chromosomes (THC treatment) and polyploidy (CME or THC treatment). Treatment of mice with a single dose of THC or CBN (100 mg/kg) or CME (50 mg/kg) led to a reduction of cells in diakinesis or metaphase I. Thus it appears that exposure of spermatogonia to cannabinoids *in vivo* can lead to chromosomal abnormalities, while exposure to primary spermatocytes may retard their progression to metaphase I and diakinesis.

2. Sperm Morphology. The induction of abnormal sperm head morphology by cannabinoid treatment has been reported by Zimmerman and co-workers (24). Treatment of hybrid male mice genotype (C57BL X C3H)F_1 for 5 consecutive days with THC (5 and 10 mg/kg) and CBN (10 and 25 mg/kg) led to a statistically higher incidence of abnormal sperm than the vehicle (dimethylsulfoxide; DMSO) treated controls. Since the mice were sacrificed 35 days after the last treatment, sperm scored were assumed to be in the primary spermatocyte stage when exposed to the cannabinoids.

Hembree and co-workers (5) reported that heavy use of marijuana caused a reduction of total sperm count and of concentration of sperm in the ejaculate of human subjects but did not significantly affect the percentage of sperm displaying normal morphology. However, in a later study (6), they reported a reduction of total sperm count and concentration which was accompanied by a decrease in the number of sperm with normal morphology. No evidence for a hormonal effect was observed and their studies suggested a direct effect of marijuana on the germinal epithelium during spermiogenesis. Similar conclusions were drawn from studies (7) using rats, in which cauda epididymal sperm from rats exposed to marijuana smoke displayed a higher incidence of dissociated heads and tails. This study also reported a reduction of epididymal sperm count and histological abnormalities of the seminiferous tubules, including aberrant cellular associations andearly release of spermatocytes and spermatids.

Incomplete or absent acrosomal differentiation has been reported in sperm from chronic hashish users (8). In the same study, forms of sperm were found in the ejaculates that suggested the occurrence of spermatidic maturation arrest in these chronic hashish users.

The results of these various studies suggest that *in vivo* exposure to cannabinoids may interfere with spermatogenic differentiation during the primary spermatocyte or spermatid stages. It has been suggested that the occurrence of abnormal sperm head morphology may serve as an assay method for screening potentially mutagenic agents (20). However, other studies have shown that abnormal sperm morphology in mice does not result from chromosome translocation nor from chromosomal imbalance within the haploid cell (21). The mechanism of induction of abnormal sperm head morphology remains to be elucidated.

B. In Vitro Effects of Cannabinoids on Macromolecular Synthesis

Several studies have suggested that cannabinoid effects on macromolecular synthesis are mediated by the availability of macromolecular precursors. A cannabinoid-induced reduction of the intracellular pool of particular precursors (eg., thymidine or uridine or their nucleotide forms) can lead to a quantitatively similar reduction of incorporation of these precursors into macromolecules (eg., DNA or RNA). This has been demonstrated in HeLa cells (15,18), human lymphocytes (4), rat testicular slices and cell suspensions (9) and in *Tetrahymena pyriformis* (23). It has been suggested that micromolar concentrations of cannabinoids may inhibit intracellular precursor pools by dissolving into membranes, altering their conformation and as a consequence, inhibiting membrane-bound transport systems (4).

II. *IN VITRO* AND *IN VIVO* EFFECTS OF CANNABINOIDS ON URIDINE METABOLISM IN PURIFIED SPERMATOGENIC CELLS

The present studies are part of a program to investigate the effects of specific cannabinoids on spermatogenic differentiation. In view of the reports on the effects of cannabinoids on spermatogenic differentiation and macromolecular synthesis in somatic cells and in mixed rat testicular cells, we decided to investigate whether cannabinoids affect macromolecular synthesis in purified populations of spermatogenic cells. Spermatogenic cells were obtained from mice and homogeneous populations of pachytene primary spermatocytes and round spermatids were obtained by sedimentation at unit gravity. The ability of cells from cannabinoid-treated miceto incorporate uridine in culture into the acid-insoluble fraction was compared to incorporation by cells isolated from vehicle-treated mice to access *in vivo* cannabinoid effects. *In vitro* cannabinoid effects were investigated by studying the metabolism of uridine by pachytene spermatocytes and round spermatids (isolated from untreated mice) exposed to cannabinoids in culture.

A. General Methodology

1. *Spermatogenic Cell Separation and Culture.* Asingle-cell spermatogenic cell suspension was prepared from the testes of mice following the methodology of Bellvè and co-workers (17). An enriched Krebs-Ringer buffer was used for all cell manipulations. Male CD-1 mice were obtained from Canadian Breeding Laboratories, Montreal, at 8-10 weeks of age. Spermatogenic cell suspensions were obtained by sequential collagenase (CLS; Worthington Biochemicals, Mississauga, Ont.) and trypsin (Bovine pancreas, type III, Sigma Chemical Co.,St. Louis, MO) digestion of decapsulated testes. Following gentle pipetting and filtration through Nitex monofilament nylon cloth (80 mcm mesh;Tet Kressilk) and Sephadex G-25 (Pharmacia Fine Chemicals, Dorval, Que.), the cells were fractionated by sedimentation at unit gravity on the basis of size using a STA-PUT apparatus (SP-240, Johns Scientific, Toronto, Ont.). Cells were sedimented for 90 minutes at room temperature (22°C) into a gradient of 2-6% Percoll (Pharmacia Fine Chemicals, Dorval, Que.) in 1% bovine serum albumin (Fraction V; Sigma Chemical Co., St. Louis, MO). Subsequently, 12 ml fractions were collected and fractions containing the desired cell types (as judged by morphology under Nomarski differential interference contrast optics) were pooled. Population of

round spermatids contained 85-90% round spermatids; cell populations were ready for culture within 6 hours of sacrifice.

Cells were cultured in Eagle's minimum essential medium with Earle's balanced salt solution, supplemented with 0.1 mM non-essential amino acids, 1mM sodium pyruvate, 2 mM glutamine, 50 U/ml penicillin base and 50 U/ml streptomycin base. Culturing was carried out in an atmosphere of 5% CO_2 in air at 33°C in Falcon plastic petri dishes in a volume of 2-3 ml; cell concentrations were 2 X 10^4 cells/ml and 4 X 10^4 cells/ml for pachytene spermatocytes and round spermatids respectively. The viability of cells in culture was determined by trypan blue dye exclusion and by the ability of cells to incorporate [^{3}H]-uridine into the acid-soluble fraction. Cells treated with drug vehicle (DMSO) or 5 mcM THC excluded trypan bluefor over 4 hours (viability > 85%) and vehicle-treated cells continued to incorporate [^{3}H]-uridine after 6 hours of culture.

2. Cannabinoids. All cannabinoids were provided byThe National Institute on Drug Abuse, U. S. A., through the Health and Welfare Canada, Health Protection Branch, Ottawa, Ontario.

For *in vivo* studies, THC, supplied dissolved in dehydrated ethanol (200 mg/ml), was suspended in a propylene glycol:Tween 80:saline (10:1:89) vehicle and 0.1 ml was administered i.p.. Vehicle treatment contained 95% ethanol instead of the THC solution. In multiple treatment experiments, the THC treatments were spaced 24 hours apart and the mice were sacrificed 2 hours after the final treatment.

For *in vitro* studies, the cannabinoids, dissolved in ethanol (200 mg/ml), were diluted in DMSO before addition to the culture medium. Control cells received an identical volume of DMSO, the final concentration of DMSO never exceeding 0.35%.

3. Acid-insoluble incorporation of [^{3}H]-uridine. Cells were incubated in the presence of 10mcCi/ml [5-^{3}H]-uridine (25-30 Ci/mmol; NET 174, New England Nuclear, Lachine, Que.) for 2 hours. The incubation was stopped by placing the cells on ice and then precipitated overnight in ice-cold 10% trichloroacetic acid. The acid-insoluble fraction was collected on glass fiber filters and radioactivity was determined by liquid scintillation spectrometry.

4. Acid-soluble incorporation of [^{3}H]-uridine. Cells were incubatedin the presence of 10 mcCi/ml [5-^{3}H]-uridine (25-30 Ci/mmol; NET 174, New England Nuclear, Lachine, Que.) for 2 hours. The incubation was stopped by adding an equal volume of ice-cold phosphate-buffered saline. The cells were collected onto glass fiber filters and washed by gentle suction and then precipitated for 45 minutes in ice-cold 0.5 N perchloric acid. The acid-soluble and acid-insoluble pools were

then collected by filtration through another glass fiber filter. An aliquot or the soluble pool was counted by liquid scintillation spectrometry to determine the total radioactivity in the soluble pool. The rest of the soluble pool was neutralized with alamine-chloroform and fractionated on a DEAE-cellulose anion-exchange column. The column was eluted with an increasing linear gradient of ammonium bicarbonate (0.002 M, pH 8.3 to 0.15 M, pH 8.6) and collected using a peristaltic pump and an automatic fraction collector with a drop counter. Uridine, uridine monophosphate (UMP), uridine diphosphate (UDP) and uridine and uridine triposphate (UTP) standards were used to ascertain the separation as determined by the optical density (lambda = 260 nm). Radioactivity in the nucleoside and nucleotide pools of labelled cells was determined by liquid scintillation spectrometry.

B. *In Vitro* Cannabinoid Effects: Acid-insoluble Incorporation of [^{3}H]-Uridine

In order to determine the effects of *in vitro* cannabinoid treatment on macromolecular synthesis, cells were incubated in the presence of [^{3}H]-uridine and 1, 3 or 5 mcM THC, CBN or CBD for 2 hours. Acid-insoluble incorporation of radioactivity was then determined following overnight precipitation. *In vitro* cannabinoid treatment suppressed the incorporation of radioactivity by pachytene spermatocytes and round spermatids isolated from untreated mice. Acid-insoluble incorporation of radioactivity was significantly suppressed in pachytene spermatocytes by treatments of THC (3 and 5 mcM; 67% and 79% suppressions, respectively), CBN (5 mcM; 85% suppression) and CBD (5 mcM; 67% suppression) (Fig. 1a). In round spermatids, acid-insoluble incorporation of radioactivity was significantly suppressed by treatments of THC (1, 3 and 5 mcM; 39%, 72% and 58% suppressions, respectively), CBN (3 and 5 mcM; 46% and 72% suppressions, respectively) and CBD (3 and 5 mcM; 44% and 67% suppressions, respectively) (Fig. 1b).

C. *In Vitro* THC Effects: Acid-soluble Incorporation of [^{3}H]--Uridine

1. Total Soluble Incorporation of Radioactivity. Soluble incorporation of radioactivity was assessed by culturing cells isolated from untreated mice for 2 hours in the presence of [^{3}H]-uridine and 5 mcM THC. Acid-soluble radioactivity in 5 mcM THC-treated pachytene spermatocytes was reduced in 4 experiments by 37, 44, 10 and 38% (mean = 32%) as compared to vehicle (DMSO) treated cells. In 3 experiments, acid-soluble radioactivity in 5 mcM THC-treated spermatids was reduced by 32, 13 and 58% (mean = 34%) as compared to vehicle (DMSO) treated cells.

2. Fractionation of Uridine Nucleoside and Nucleotide Radioactivity. The soluble pool of radioactivity was fractionated into uridine nucleoside and nucleotide radioactivity by DEAD-cellulose anion-exchange chromatography. In general, 2 hour treatment of pachytene spermatocytes and round spermatids with 5 mcM THC led to reductions in the nucleoside and nucleotide pools as compared to pools from vehicle (DMSO) treated cells (Table I). The amount of radioactivity in the UDP and UTP pools of both cell types was low, being undetectable in most cases. The data suggest a reduction in the uptake of exogenous [^{3}H]-uridine and a suppression of subsequent [^{3}H]-uridine phosphorylation by THC-treated cells.

D. *In Vivo* THC Effects: Acid-insoluble Incorporation of [^{3}H]-Uridine

The ability of cells isolated from mice two hours after the last THC treatment to incorporate [^{3}H]-uridine *in vitro*

TABLE I. Acid-soluble Radioactivity in Pachytene Spermatocytes and Round Spermatids

	CPM/10^4 CELLS	
	Uridine	Nucleotides
Pachytene Spermatocytes		
CONTROL	7406	189
5 mcM THC	4920	-
CONTROL	3719	361
5 mcM THC	2543	42
CONTROL	3933	212
5 mcM THC	3215	-
Round Spermatids		
CONTROL	5801	39
5 mcM THC	5100	-
CONTROL	5170	579
5 mcM THC	5113	167

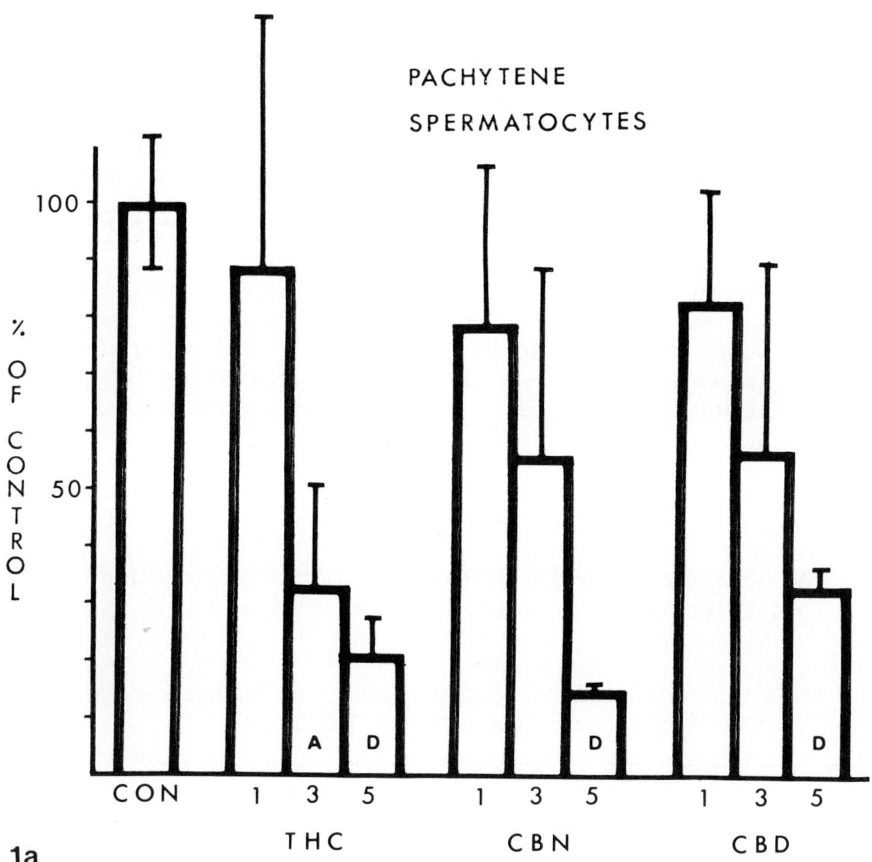

was used as an indicator of _in vivo_ THC-treatment effects. Mice were treated with a single THC dosage of 10 or 20 mg/kg, or dosages of 10 mg/kg on 5 consecutive days. None of the treatment schedules induced a reduction in the acid-insoluble incorporation of radioactivity by pachytene spermatocytes and round spermatids isolated from THC-treated mice as compared to cells isolated from vehicle-treated mice.

III. CONCLUDING REMARKS

In general, these studies have demonstrated that _in vitro_ treatment of isolated pachytene spermatocytes and round spermatids with THC, CBN, or CBD (1, 3 or 5 mcM) interferes with uridine metabolism in these cells. The concomitant reduction

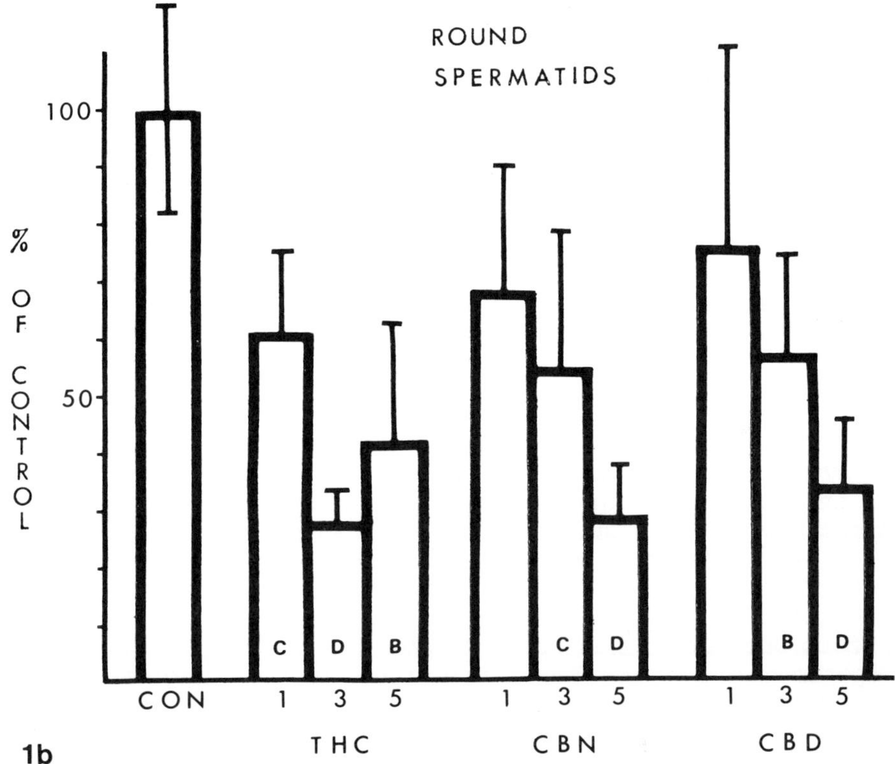

FIGURE 1. Acid-insoluble incorporation of radioactivity (+/- standard error of the mean, n = 3) by a: pachytene spermatocytes, and b: round spermatids treated _in vivo_ with [^{3}H]-uridine and 1, 3 or 5 mcM THC, CBN or CBD for 2 hours. (Student's t-test, one-tail: A: $p < 0.05$; B: $p < 0.01$; C: $p < 0.025$; D: $p < 0.005$.)

of acid-insoluble incorporation of uridine and of the uptake and phosphorylation of uridine, suggests that cannabinoid inhibition of macromolecular synthesis may be a secondary consequence of a reduction of the intracellular pool of macromolecular precursors. Such "non-specific" inhibitions of macromolecular synthesis by psychoactive (THC) as well as non-psychoactive (CBN and CBD) cannabinoids have been demonstrated in HeLa cells (15), rat testicular cells (9) and _Tetrahymena pyriformis_ (23). The significance of these results in relation to spermatogenic differentiation is unclear. Since spermatogenic differentiation has not been demonstrated _in vitro_, a direct cannabinoid effect on the differentiation has not been demonstrated *in vitro*, a direct cannabinoid effect on the differentiation of spermatogenic cells is difficult to ascertain. *In vivo*, pachytene spermatocytes and round spermatids are the stages most active in RNA and protein synthesis during spermatogenesis (16). Interference with these processes could lead to changes in the kinetics, efficiency or fidelity of the orderly processes of spermatogenic differentiation and gene expression. The results of the present *in vitro* studies are consistent with the hypothesis (19) that cannabinoid interference with spermatogenic differentiation, leading to morphologically or chromosomally abnormal sperm, may be partially mediated by interference with macromolecular synthesis.

In vivo treatment of mice with THC in the present studies did not inhibit the incorporation of [^{3}H]-uridine by isolated pachytene spermatocytes and round spermatids. Similar dosages of THC (10 mg/kg for 5 consecutive days) have been shown to lead to the induction of morphologically abnormal sperm when pachytene spermatocytes were exposed to the drug *in vivo* and to an increase of ring and chain translocations in pachytene spermatocytes when spermatogonia were exposed to the drug *in vivo* (25). While it is possible that *in vivo* THC treatment has no effect on uridine metabolism in pachytene spermatocytes and round spermatids *in situ*, it is possible that such an effect does occur but could not be measured by the present experimental design. The suppressive effect on uridine incorporation might be short-lived and may have been dissipated during the cell separation procedure; 5 to 6 hour elapsed between sacrifice and cell culture. An alternative hypothesis is that *in vivo* THC treatment does not lead to a gross alteration of uridine metabolism, but does suppress the synthesis or processing of specific RNA or protein molecules.

In conclusion, it should be noted that the lack of a demonstrable *in vivo* THC effect in the present study requires us to be extremely cautious in the interpretation of our *in vitro* results. Further studies are required to determine whether a cannabinoid-induced inhibition of overall macromolecular synthesis or an inhibition of the synthesis of specific macromolecules may interfere with spermatogenic differentiation. We propose that analysis of macromolecules labelled *in situ* in spermatogenic, Sertoli and Leydig cells from cannabinoid-treated mice is required.

REFERENCES

1. Blevins, R. D., and Regan, J. D., delta-9-Tetrahydrocannabinol. Effect on macromolecular synthesis in humans

and other mammalian cells, Arch. Toxicol. 35:127-135 (1976).

2. Carchman, R. A., Harris, L. S., and Munson, A. E., The inhibition of DNA synthesis by cannabinoids, Cancer Res. 36:95-100 (1976).
3. Dalterio, S., Badr, F., Bartke, A., and Mayfield, D., Cannabinoids in male mice: Effects on fertility and spermatogenesis, Science 216:315-316 (1982).
4. Desoize, B., Leger, C., Jardillier, J-C., and Nahas, G., Inhibition by THC of thymidine transport: A plasma membrane effect, in "Marihuana: Biological Effects" (G. G. Nahas and W. D. M. Paton, eds.), pp. 145-159. Pergamon Press, New York, 1979.
5. Hembree, W. C., Zeidenberg, P., and Nahas, G. G., Marijuana's effects on human gonadal function, in "Marihuana: Chemistry, Biochemistry and Cellular Effects" (G.G. Nahas, ed.), pp. 521-532. Springer-Verlag, New York, 1976.
6. Hembree, W. C., Nahas, G. G., Zeidenberg, P., and Huang, H. F. S., Changes in human spermatozoa associated with high dose marijuana smoking, in "Marihuana: Biological Effects" (G. G. Nahas and W. D. M. Paton, eds.), pp. 429-439. Pergamon Press, New York, 1979.
7. Huang, H. F. S., Nahas, G. G., and Hembree, W. C., Effects of marijuana inhalation on spermatogenesis of the rat, in "Marihuana: Biological Effects" (G. G. Nahas and W. D. M. Paton, eds.), pp. 419-427. Pergamon Press, New York, 1979.
8. Issidorides, M. R., Observations in chronic hashish users, Nuclear aberrations in blood and sperm and abnormal acrosomes in spermatozoa, in "Marihuana: Biological Effects" (G. G. Nahas and W. D. M. Paton, eds.), pp. 377-388. Pergamon Press, New York, 1979.
9. Jakubovic, A., and McGeer, P. L., Biochemical changes in rat testicular cells *in vitro* produced by cannabinoids and alcohol: Metabolism and incorporation of labelled glucose, amino acids and nucleic acid precursors, Toxicol. Appl. Pharmacol. 41:473-486 (1977).
10. Mellors, A., Cannabinoids: Effects on lysosomes and lymphocytes, in "Marihuana: Chemistry, Biochemistry and Cellular Effects" (G. G. Nahas, ed.), pp. 283-298. Springer-Verlag, New York, 1976.
11. Mellors, A., Cannabinoids and membrane-bound enzymes, in "Marihuana: Biological Effects" (G. G. Nahas and W. D. M. Paton, eds.), pp. 329-342. Pergamon Press, New York, 1979.
12. McLean, D. K., and Zimmerman, A. M., Action of delta-9-tetrahydrocannabinol on cell division and macromolecular

synthesis in division-synchronized protozoa, Pharmacol. 14:307-321 (1976).

13. Morishima, A., Henrish, R. T., Jou, S., and Nahas, G. G., Errors of chromosome segregation induced by olivetol, a compound with the structure of the C-ring common to cannabinoids: Formation of bridges and multipolar divisions, in "Marihuana: Chemistry, Biochemistry and Cellular Effects" (G. G. Nahas, ed.), pp. 265-271. Springer-Verlag, New York, 1976.
14. Morishima, A., Milstein, M. M., Henrich, R. T., and Nahas, G. G., Effects of marijuana smoking, cannabinoids and olivetol on replication of human lymphocytes: Formation of micronuclei in "Pharmacology of Marihuana", Vol. 2 (M. C. Braude and S. Szara, eds.), pp. 711-722. Raven Press, New York, 1976.
15. Mon, M. J., Haas, A. E., Stein, J. L. and Stein, G. S., Influence of psychoactive and nonpsychoactive cannabinoids on cell proliferation and macromolecular biosynthesis in human cells, Biochem. Pharmacol. 30:31-43 (1981).
16. Monesi, V., Geremia, R., D'Agostino, A., and Boitani, C., Biochemistry of male germ cell differentiation in mammals: RNA synthesis in meiotic and postmeiotic cells, Curr. Top. Dev. Biol. 12:11-36 (1978).
17. Romrell, L. J., Bellvè, A. R. and Fawcett, D. W.: Separation of spermatogenic cells by sedimentation velocity, Dev. Biol. 49:119-131 (1976).
18. Stein, G. S., Mon, M. J., Haas, A. E., Jansing, R. L., and Stein, J. L., Cannabinoids: The influence on cell proliferation and macromolecular biosynthesis, in "Marihuana: Biological Effects" (G. G. Nahas and W. D. M. Paton, eds.), pp. 171-208. Pergamon Press, New York, 1979.
19. Tilak, S. K., and Zimmerman, A. M., The effects of delta-9-tetrahydrocannabinol on spermatogenesis, J. Cell Biol. 87:148a (1980).
20. Wyrobek, J. A., and Bruce, W. R., Chemical induction of sperm abnormalities in mice, Proc. Nat. Acad. Sci. U.S.A. 72:4425-4429 (1975).
21. Wyrobek, A. J., Heddle, J. A., and Bruce, W. R., Chromosomal abnormalities and the morphology of mouse sperm heads, Can. J. Genet. Cytol. 17:675-681 (1975).
22. Zimmerman, A. M., and McLean, D. K., Action of Narcotic and hallucinogenic agents on the cell cycle, in "Drugs and the Cell Cycle" (A. M. Zimmerman, G. M. Padilla and I. L. Cameron, eds.), pp. 67-94. Academic Press, New York, 1973.
23. Zimmerman, A. M., and Zimmerman, S. B., The influence of marijuana on eukaryote cell growth and development, in "Marihuana: Chemistry, Biochemistry and Cellular Effects"

(G. G. Nahas, ed.), pp. 195-205. Springer-Verlag, New York, 1976.

24. Zimmerman, A. M., Bruce, W. R., and Zimmerman, S., Effects of cannabinoids on sperm morphology, Pharmacol. 18:143-148 (1979).

25. Zimmerman, A. M., Zimmerman, S., and Ray, A. Y., Effects of cannabinoids on spermatogenesis in mice, in "Marihuana: Biological Effects" (G. G. Nahas and W. D. M. Paton, eds.), pp. 407-418. Pergamon Press, New York, 1979.

SEX HORMONE LEVELS IN ADULT RATS INJECTED WITH DELTA-9-TETRAHYDROCANNABINOL AND PHENCYCLIDINE

Jack Harclerode, Lynne Bird
Heather Sawyer, Vickie Berger
Robert Mooney, Richard Smith

Department of Biology
Bucknell University
Lewisburg, Pennsylvania

I. INTRODUCTION

Delta-9-tetrahydrocannabinol (THC), the main psychoactive ingredient in marijuana, has been reported to reduce serum testosterone and gonadotropin levels (1-5), suppress spermatogenesis, and reduce testicular and secondary sex organ weights (1,6). Some of these testicular changes may occur through a direct action of THC on the testis (7-9), while others probably come about through an indirect action on the hypothalamus to suppress gonadotropin releasing hormone (GnRH) (7).

Phencyclidine hydrochloride (PCP or angel dust) has diverse neuropharmacological effects including producing decreased norepinephrine and increased serotonin levels in the brain (10,11), as well as inhibition of dopamine uptake (12,13). It also causes neuroendocrine effects such as lowered growth hormone levels (1) and increased plasma cortisol levels in Rhesus monkeys.

PCP is frequently taken in conjunction with marijuana since the two are often mixed together and smoked in a cigarette. Thus these two neuroendocrine active substances have a chance to interact in certain individuals. This study examined the effects of THC and PCP given singly and in combination on serum testosterone and LH levels in adult rats.

---

*Supported in part by NIDA grant no. DA-02372 and the R. P. Vidinghoff Memorial Fund.

ISBN 0-12-044620-0

II. MATERIALS AND METHODS

A. Drug Administration

THC and PCP were obtained from the Research Technology Branch of the National Institute on Drug Abuse. Ethanolic solutions of THC were evaporated to dryness under a stream of dry nitrogen, and the residue was resuspended in an injection vehicle consisting of 4% Tween 80, 10% propylene glycol, and 86% physiological saline at a final drug concentration of 2.5 mg/ml. A PCP solution of the same concentration and a solution containing 2.5 mg/ml of both THC and PCP were also prepared. Drug treated animals received the drugs at a dosage of 2 mg/kg body weight of each drug by intraperitoneal injection.

B. Animals

Five groups of sexually mature male Wistar rats, weighing approximately 250 g, were maintained on a 14 hr light-10 hr dark schedule at constant temperature with food and water *ad libitum*. Each drug treatment group in all studies contained six animals that received either injection vehicle (VEH), THC, PCP, or both THC and PCP (COM). The rats involved in the two-hour acute study received a single intraperitoneal injection

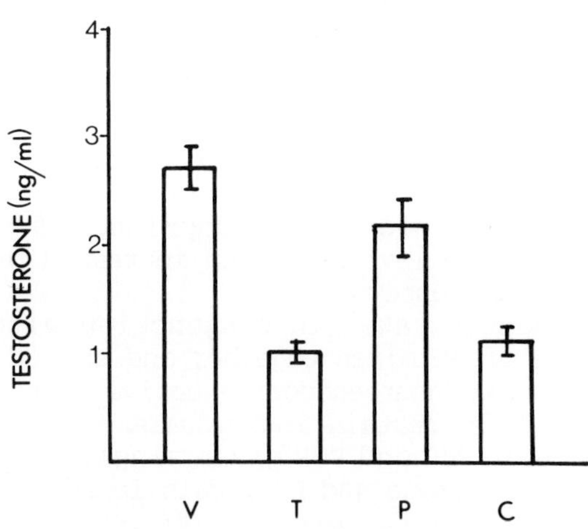

FIGURE 1. Testosterone levels 2 hours after a single drug injection. V = drug solubilizing vehicle; T = 2 mg THC/kg; P = 2 mg PCP/kg; C = both THC and PCP at 2 mg/kg each drug. Values given are mean +/- SEM. Values of P are given in text.

and were sacrificed two hours later. Each animal in the other four recovery studies received one drug injection daily for 9 days and was killed 2 hours later, or after 10, 30, or 60 days following cessation of drug treatment. All animals were sacrificed by decapitation two hours into the light cycle on the final day of their recovery period. Trunk blood was collected and serum testosterone and luteinizing hormone levels were quantified by radioimmunoassay with kits purchased from Amersham and components supplied by National Pituitary Agency, respectively.

Student's t-test was used to test for significant differences ($p < 0.05$) between sets of experimental data.

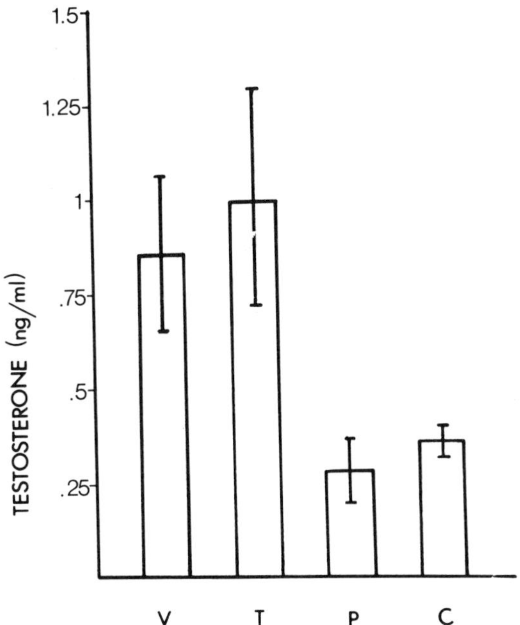

FIGURE 2. Testosterone levels 2 hours after the last of 9 daily drug injections. Daily drug dosage and other conditions as in Fig. 1.

III. RESULTS

A. Testosterone

Animals in all drug treatment groups exhibited significantly reduced serum testosterone two hours after a single injection. While those rats treated with PCP showed only a mild depression (PCP = 80% of VEH) ($p < 0.05$), those treated with either THC or the THC/PCP combination tended toward a more severe depression (THC = 37% of VEH, $p < 0.01$; COM = 41% of VEH, $p < 0.01$), indicating the effects on serum testosterone in the combination-treated group stem primarily from the THC (Fig. 1).

In the animals treated for 9 days, those given PCP showed significantly reduced serum testosterone two hours afterthe last injection ($p < 0.05$). There was a highly suggestive, nonsignificant, trend toward lowered serum testosterone in the animals treated with the THC/PCP combination (Fig. 2), indicating that it was the PCP in the drug combination that maintained the depressed testosterone levels during chronic treatment, while after acute treatment it appeared to be due to the effect of THC (Fig. 1). We note that after 9 days of drug treatment, THC treated animals had returned to control levels with respect to circulating testosterone, suggesting the possible development of tolerance to the drug with prolonged treatment.

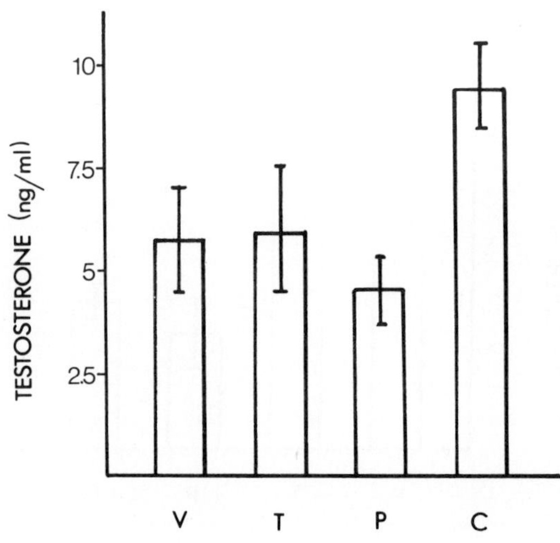

FIGURE 3. Testosterone levels 10 days after 9 daily injections. Daily drug dosage and other conditions as in Fig. 1.

In the rats which recovered for 10 days after the 9 day of drug treatment, there were no significant changes in serum testosterone compared to control values. However, the THC/PCP combination-treated group exhibited a suggestive increase in serum testosterone over vehicle controls (Fig. 3).

After 30 days of recovery following 9 days of drug treatment, this tendency toward elevated serum testosterone in the COM group was highly significant ($p < 0.01$). Circulating testosterone levels in those animals treated with PCP were also significantly higher at this time ($p < 0.005$). It is possible that the elevated testosterone in the serum could be the result of an overcompensation of the testis for the period of reduced testosterone levels at two hours and 9 days, and again seems to be caused by the PCP in the combination since the THC-treated group remained at control values (Fig. 4).

A recovery period of 60 days post-injections was sufficient time for all drug treatment groups to return to control testosterone concentrations (Fig. 5).

B. Organ Weights

Even though testosterone and LH had returned to control levels by 60 days following cessation of drug treatment there were changes in the weights of both the testis and prostate. Testicular weights of the drug combination rats were lighter

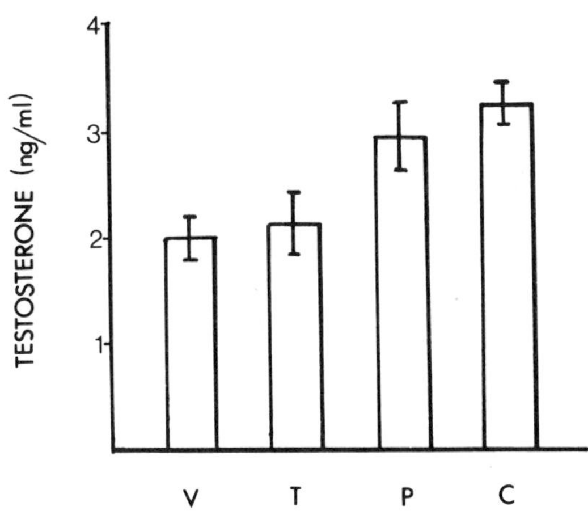

FIGURE 4. Testosterone levels 30 days following the last of 9 daily injections. Daily drug dosage and other conditions as in Fig. 1.

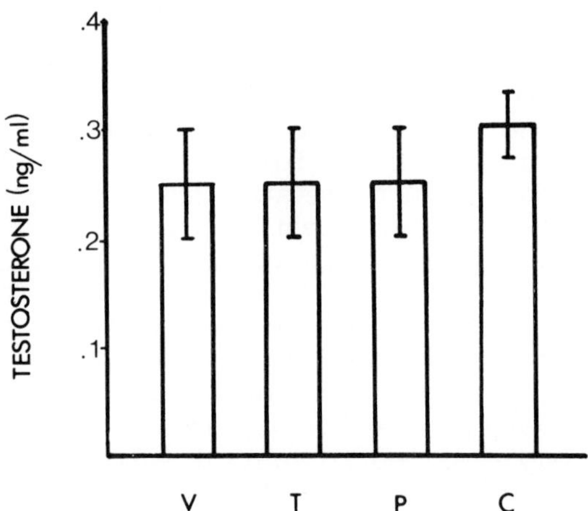

FIGURE 5. Testosterone levels 60 days following the last of 9 daily injections. Daily drug dosage and other conditions as in Fig. 1.

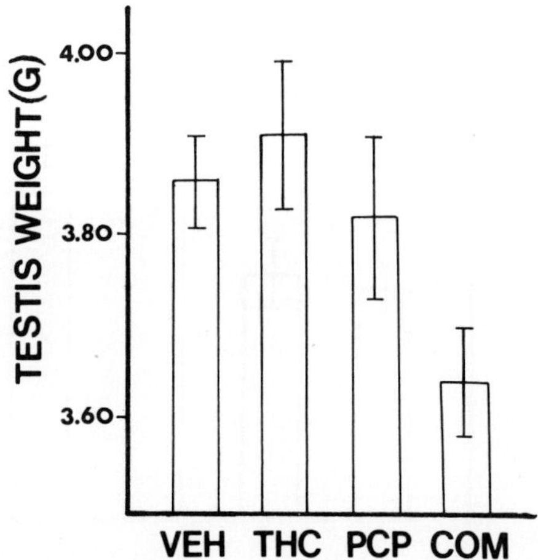

FIGURE 6. Testes weights of rats 60 days after the last of 9 daily drug injections. Daily drug dosage and other conditions as in Fig. 1.

than vehicle injected controls ($p < 0.02$) and THC treated rats ($p < 0.05$) (Fig. 6). Similarly, prostate weights of drug combination rats were lighter than vehicle injected controls ($p < 0.01$) and PCP treated rats ($p < 0.02$) (Fig. 7).

C. Luteinizing Hormone

Two hours following a single drug injection, the serum of rats treated with PCP had less LH than did the serum of the vehicle injected rats ($p < 0.05$). The serum of rats that received both THC and PCP had more LH than animals injected

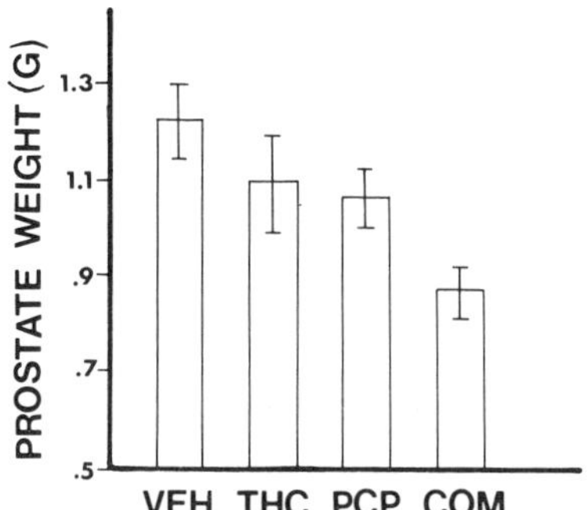

FIGURE 7. Prostate weights of rats 60 days after the last of 9 daily drug injections. Daily drug dosage and other conditions as in Fig. 1.

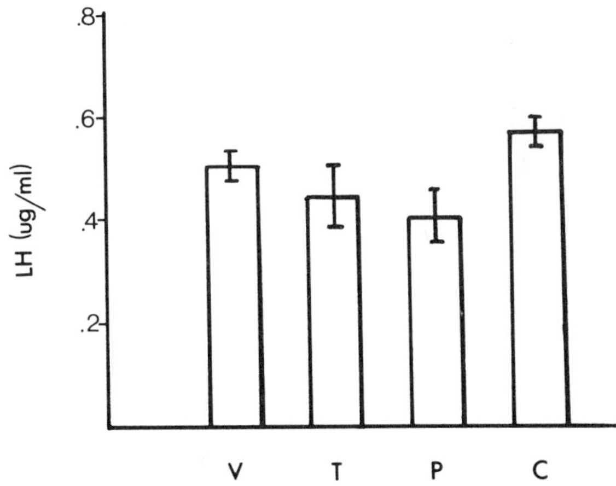

FIGURE 8. LH levels 2 hours after a single drug injection. Daily drug dosage and other conditions as in Fig. 1.

with either THC ($p < 0.05$) or PCP ($p < 0.01$) (Fig. 8). After nine days of drug treatment only the rats that received THC had less LH than those that received PCP (Fig. 9). There were no significant differences from vehicle control LH in any drug treatment groups 10 days after the period of drug treatments was ended (Fig. 10). However, after 30 days the drug combination treated rats had significantly elevated LH above vehicle ($p < 0.001$), THC ($p < 0.001$), and PCP ($p < 0.01$) and the PCP treated rats had more LH in their serum than vehicle ($p < 0.05$) (Fig. 11). By 60 days all drug treated animals had serum LH at control levels.

IV. DISCUSSION

The effect of THC to decrease both testosterone and LH in the serum of rats appears to be temporary, for after continued drug treatment hormone levels returned to control values, suggesting the possible development of tolerance. In contrast, PCP depressed testosterone and LH only after prolonged treatment. Although the depression was reversible with time, following cessation of treatment with PCP or the combination there was a period of increased LH and testosterone, effects probably due to PCP. THC appeared to potentiate the heightened testosterone during this period.

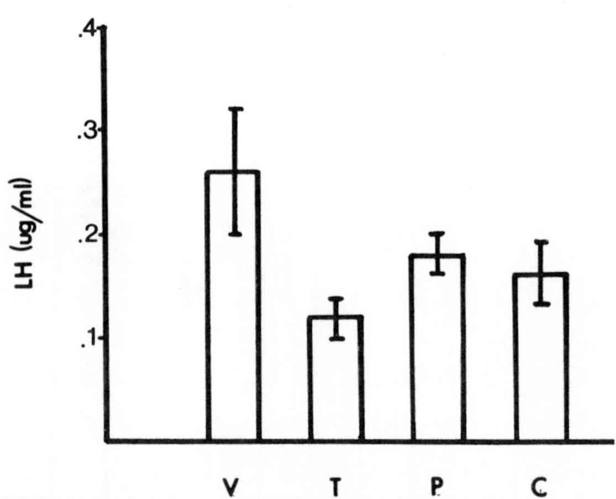

FIGURE 9. LH levels 2 hours after the last of 9 daily drug injection. Daily drug dosage and other conditions as in Fig. 1.

The initial THC-induced reduction of testosterone and luteinizing hormone levels has been well documented (1-5). There is no evidence to indicate that some of the effect is due to a direct action of the drug on the testis (7-9), while others have suggested that THC acts on the hypothalamus to decrease output of GnRH and that the subsequent defects are due to decreased testosterone production. One of the ways that reduced GnRH may occur is through changes in hypothalamic activity due to drug-induced variations inneurotransmitter levels. There is evidence that hypothalamic neurons that release GnRH are regulated by biogenic amines (1,14). Norepinephrine and perhaps dopamine may be involved. THC has often been implicated in alteration of serotonin turnover (14-17), but whether serotoninergic mechanisms are ultimately responsible for the alterations produced in gonadotropin and androgen levels is unknown. THC affects synaptosomal uptake of dopamine and norepinephrine to result in a decreased content of these catecholamines in certain brain areas (14), although this finding is not always corroborated (1).

Perhaps the depressed LH and testosterone observed in this study after prolonged treatment with PCP and the subsequent period of elevated serum hormonal levels seen after cessation of drug treatment are caused by alteration of brain neurotransmitter levels. Behavioral pharmacological studies indicate PCP may act as an indirect dopaminergic agonist similar to amphetamine and/or as a cholinergic antagonist (17). PCP has been reported to elevate whole brain serotonin levels,

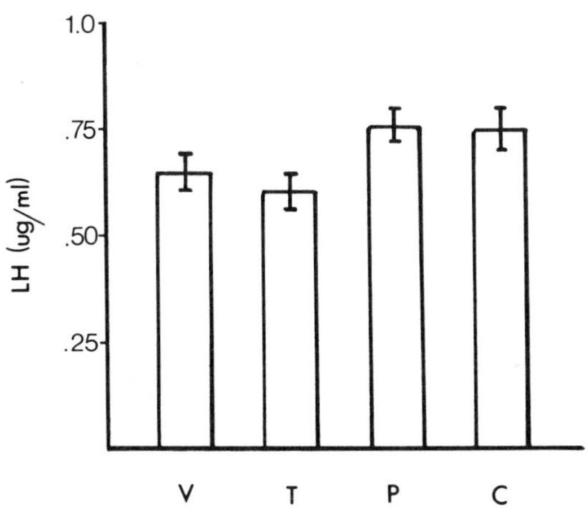

FIGURE 10. LH levels 10 days after 9 daily drug injection. Daily drug dosage and other conditions as in Fig. 1.

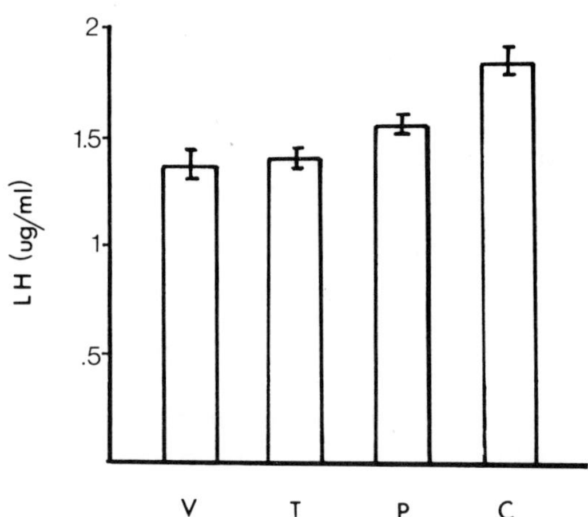

FIGURE 11. LH levels 30 days after 9 daily drug injection. Daily drug dosage and other conditions as in Fig. 1.

decrease serotonin turnover, decrease norepinephrine (NE) levels in the brain, and inhibit uptake of dopamine, NE, and serotonin (18). However, PCP probably acts primarily through an indirect dopamine agonist mechanism rather than an anticholinergic mechanism (13). Little information exists on the effects of both THC and PCP on levels of brain biogenic amines.

Drug induced alteration of normal hormonal balance could also result from changes in hormone receptors on target cells. Thus, the drugs might act directly on the receptor sites themselves or they may have a secondary effect whereby their induced hormonal changes affect receptor populations on the target tissue. However, other researchers have found that THC does not bind to any of the intracellular receptors for steroid hormones (6). Perhaps THC and PCP interact with or alter membrane receptors of the pituitary or hypothalamus, which then could affect the secretion of GnRH or gonadotropins themselves.

Finally, testicular receptor sites for luteinizing hormone are regulated by the concentrations of GnRH. Administration of GnRH reduces the number of testicular LH receptors and androgen production. The decrease in LH receptors appears to result from increased LH secretion and is not direct effect of GnRH (19), suggesting that hormonal imbalances initiated by drug injections could have effects on the receptor modulation of androgen synthesis.

REFERENCES

1. Collu, R., Letarte, J., LeBoeuf, G., and Ducharme, J. R., Endocrine effects of chronic administration of psychoactive drugs to pre-pubertal male rats, Life Sci. 16:533-542 (1975).
2. Smith, C. G., Besch, N. F., and Asch, R. H., Effects of marijuana on the reproductive system, in "Advances in Sex Hormone Research", Vol. 4 (J. A. Thomas and R. L. Singhal, eds.), p. 273. Urban and Schwarzenberg, Baltimore, 1980.
3. Symons, A. M., Teale, J. D., and Marks, V., Proceedings: Effect of delta-9-tetrahydrocannabinol on the hypothalamic-pituitary-gonadal system in maturing male rat, J. Endocrinol. 68(3):33P (1976).
4. Tyrey, L., Delta-9-tetrahydrocannabinol: suppression of episodic luteinizing hormone secretion in the ovariectomized rat, Endocrinology 102:1808-1814 (1978).
5. Tyrey, L., Delta-9-tetrahydrocannabinol: a potent inhibitor of episodic luteinizing hormone secretion, J. Pharmacol. Exp. Ther. 213:306-308 (1980).
6. Smith, R. G., Besch, N. F., Besch, P. K., and Smith, C. G., Inhibition of gonadotropin by delta-9-tetrahydrocannabinol: mediation be steroid receptors? Science 204:325-327 (1979).
7. Dalterio, S., Bartke, A., Roberson, C., Watson, D., and Burstein, S., Direct and pituitary-mediated effects of THC and cannabinol on the testis, Pharm. Biochem. Behav. 8:673-678 (1978).
8. Harclerode, J., Nyquist, S. E., Nazar, B., and Lowe, D., Effects of cannabis on sex hormones and testicular enzymes of the rodent, in "Marihuana: Biological Effects" (G. G. Nahas and W. D. M. Paton, eds.), pp. 395-405. Pergamon Press, New York, 1979.
9. Dalterio, S., Bartke, A., and Burstein, S., Cannabinoids inhibit testosterone secretion by mouse testes in vitro, Science 196:1472-1473 (1977).
10. Weinstein, H., Maayani, S., Glick, S. D., and Meibach, R. C., Integrated studies on the biochemical, behavioral, and molecular pharmacology of phencyclidine: a progress report, in "PCP (Phencyclidine): Historical and Current Perspectives" (E. F. Domino, ed.), pp. 131-176. NPP Books, Ann Arbor, 1981.
11. Vincent, J. P., Vignon, J., Kartalovski, B., and Lazduski, M., Receptor sites for phencyclidine in mammalian brain and peripheral organs, in "PCP (Phencyclidine): Historical and Current Perspectives" (E. F. Domino, ed.), pp. 191-206. NPP Books, Ann Arbor, 1981.

12. Johnson, K. M., and Vickroy, T. W., The effects of phencyclidine and two metabolites on synaptosomal dopamine synthesis, uptake, and release, in "PCP (Phencyclidine): Historical and Current Perspectives" (E. F. Domino, ed.), pp. 191-206. NPP Books, Ann Arbor, 1981.
13. Meltzer, H. Y., Sturgeon, R. D., Simonovic, M., and Fessler, R. G., Phencyclidine as an indirect dopamine agonist, in "PCP (Phencyclidine): Historical and Current Perspectives" (E. F. Domino, ed.), pp. 207-242. NPP Books, Ann Arbor, 1981.
14. Smith, C. G., Effects of marijuana on neuroendocrine function, Natl. Inst. Drug Abuse Res. Monogr. Ser. (31):137-166 (1980).
15. Johnson, K. M., Dewey, W. L., and Bloom, A. S., Adrenalectomy reverses the effects of delta-9-THC on mouse brain 5-hydroxytryptamine turnover, Pharmacol. 23:223-229 (1981).
16. Welch, B. L., Welch, A. S., Messina, F. S., and Berger, H. J., Rapid depletion of adrenal epinephrine and elevation of telencephalic serotonin by (-)-trans-delta-9-tetrahydrocannabinol in mice, Res. Comm. Chem. Path. Pharmacol. 2:382-391 (1971).
17. Miczek, K. A., and Dixit, B. N., Behavioral and biochemical effects of chronic delta-9-tetrahydrocannabinol in rats, Psychopharmacol. 67:195-202 (1980).
18. Zukin, S. R., and Zukin, R. S., Identification and characterization of [^{3}H]phencyclidine binding to specific brain receptor sites, in "PCP (Phencyclidine): Historical and Current Perspectives" (E. F. Domino, ed.), pp. 105-130. NPP Books, Ann Arbor, 1981.
19. Boune, G., Dockhill, M., Marshall, J., Regioni, S., and Payne A., Induction of testicular gonadotropin-releasing hormone (GnRH) receptors by GnRH: effects of pituitary hormones and relationship to inhibition of testosterone production, Endocrinology 110(3):727-732 (1981).

POSSIBLE MECHANISM FOR THE CELLULAR EFFECTS OF MARIJUANA ON MALE REPRODUCTIVE FUNCTION*

Syed Husain
Michael W. Lamè

Department of Pharmacology
University of North Dakota School of Medicine
Grand Forks, North Dakota

I. INTRODUCTION

In the years since the effects of marijuana on male reproductive functions were first reported, initial studies were focused on documenting these changes. More recently, attempts are being made to determine the endocrine and/or biochemical bases of these changes. Kolodny et al. (21,22) reported that acute and chronic administration of delta-9-tetrahydrocannabinol (THC) decreases plasma testosterone level, reduces sperm counts and impairs potency in humans. Later, these observations were confirmed by many other laboratories in different species (1,3,4,20). Similarly, Dixit et al. (8,9), Zimmerman et al. (36), and Dalterio et al. (5) noted that exposure of mice, rats and dogs to THC or marijuana extract decreases size of the testis and other reproductive organs, causes Leydig cell regression, arrests spermatogenesis and results in a decrease level of testosterone. Studies of Smith et al. (32) in rhesus monkey and observations of Symons et al. (33) in rodents implicated the hypothalamic-pituitary gonadal axis for these effects of THC on testicular integrity. In these studies, the observed decreases in testosterone were found to correlate with a reduction in luteinizing hormone (LH) and the follicle stimulating hormone levels. Beside these endocrine effects, argument for the indirect effect of THC on testicular androgen comes from studies of Harclerode et al. (13), which

---

*Supported in part by NIDA grant DA-02655.

ISBN 0-12-044620-0

suggest an inhibition of cytochrome P-450 in the testis. Also, Schwartz et al. (30) noted that injection of either THC or cannabidiol (CBD) to rats not only causes a decrease in cytochrome P-450 from Leydig cells but also reduces gamma-glutamyl transpeptidase, a marker protein for Sartoli cells.

Other studies have also been reported which show a direct effect rather than a pituitary medicated effect of marijuana on the testis. Observations of Jakubovic and McGeer (18) indicated that different constituents of marijuana directly act on rat Leydig cells in vitro, whereby causing a significant decrease in the synthesis of nucleic acids and proteins in these cells. These effects were observed in non-stimulated Leydig cells as well as cells which were stimulated either with human chorionic gonadotropin or by dibutyryl c-AMP (19). Similarly, decapsulated mouse testis grown in culture and exposed to THC or cannabinol (CBN) were less able to release testosterone in the incubation medium than were controls (4). In another study, Huang et al. (15) reported that apart from changing the normal morphology of the sperm, THC also reduces the number of spermatozoa in marijuana smokers. Hembree et al. (14) examined the semen of 16 healthy chronic marijuana smokers under controlled research ward setting. They found no direct evidence for the involvement of gonadotropins inthis oligospermia and suggested this to be a direct effect of THC on the germinal epithelium of the testis.

The site of action and the mechanism by which THC or marijuana disrupts testicular morphology, metabolism and function remains unresolved. Various cellular processes including testosterone synthesis, nucleic acid synthesis, protein synthesis, spermatogenesis and sperm motility have been shown to be inhibited by THC and other cannabinoids. Since these cellular activities require energy for their successful completion, it was planned to examine the effects of THC on the utilization of energy rich substrates such as glucose, fructose and pyruvate in the rat testis. In addition, different experiments were conducted to delineate the site(s) at which THC may act to alter the metabolism of these substances in the testis.

II. MATERIALS AND METHODS

A. Animals and Chemicals

In all phases of this study, Sprague Dawley male rats (250 +/- 50 g) were used. Radiolabeled glucose and fructose were obtained from Amersham/Searle Corp., Arlington Heights, Il. (Specific activities 3/mCi/m mol each). New England Nuclear Corp., Boston, MA, supplied the radiolabeled pyruvate (specific activity 6.5 mCi/mmol) and 2-deoxy-D-glucose (specific activity 337 mCi/m mol). Scintillation cocktails (Instagel and Permaflour II), thixotropic gelling agent (Cab-o-Sil) and tissue solublizer (Soluene-350) were purchased from Packard Instrument Co., Downers Grove, IL. Other chemicals were of analytical grade. The National Institute on Drug Abuse kindly provided the THC, which was greater than 95% pure. Glycerol-3-phosphate dehydrogenase (EC 1.1.1.8), triosphosphate isomerase (EC 5.3.1.1.), aldolase (EC 4.1.2.13), glucose-6-phosphate dehydrogenase (EC 1.1.1.49), phosphoglucose isomerase (EC 5.3.1.9), beta-NADH, beta-$NADP^+$, EDTA and triethanolamine were ordered from Sigma Chemical Co., St. Louis, Mo.

B. Procedures

1. Radiorespirometric Experiments. Rats were decapitated, their testes rapidly removed, and each testis was stripped of its tunica and sectioned into several small pieces. These tissues were divided into control and experimental groups and incubated in separate Warburg flasks containing 2 ml of Tris-buffered medium of the following composition (mM): NaCl, 145.3; KCl, 4.8; KH_2PO_4, 1.2; $MgSO_4$, 0.7; H_2O, 1.33; $CaCl_2$, 0.2 H_2O, 1.22; and Tris 25.0. Depending upon the type of experiment, the medium also contained different concentrations ofglucose, fructose, or pyruvate as the substrate and 6-^{14}C glucose, U-^{14}C fructose, or 2-^{14}C pyruvate as the tracer. The center well and the side arm of the flasks contained 0.2 ml of 3.5 N KOH and 0.2 ml of 70% $HClO_4$ (w/v), respectively. The medium was aerated for 30 minutes with 100% O_2 and maintained at 37°C. THC was dissolved in ethanol and added to the experimental tissue medium prior to incubation in one of the following concentrations: 0.1 mM (3 mcl), 0.2 mM (6 mcl), 0.3 mM (9 mcl), or 0.4 mM (12 mcl). Control tissues received equal volumes of ethanol. Incubations were carried out for 100 minutes and the reaction was terminated by acidifying the medium with $HClO_4$ from the side arm of the Warburg flask. The $^{14}CO_2$ produced from glucose, fructose, or pyruvate in control and THC-exposed tissues were trapped for 60 minutes in KOH of the center well and counted in a Packard Model 3255 Scintillation Counter. Dry weights of the testicular tissues were determined, and the rates of $^{14}CO_2$ production in control and experimental tissues were expressed as mcMoles of CO_2 produced per g dry tissue/100 min incubation by the method of Husain and Paradise (16).

2. Determination of Glycolytic Intermediates.

a. Analysis of D-fructose-1,6-diphosphate (F-1,6-P_2), and dihydroxyacetone phosphate (DAP). Two rats were used for each control and experimental protocol. Testes were sectioned into small pieces and divided into two groups. Each group was washed with Tris-buffered, modified Krebs-Ringer's medium (described earlier) and placed in an Erlenmeyer flask containing 44.4 ml of the same medium kept at 37°C and aerated with 100% O_2 for 30 minutes. Before incubation, the experimental flasks received 0.3 mM THC dissolved in 0.2 ml of ethanol and the control flasks received equal volumes of ethanol. At the end of the 100 minute incubation, tissues were removed from flasks, rinsed several times with ice-cold medium, and freeze-dried in pre-cooled mortars. The control and THC-exposed tissues were then ground to a fine powder, weighed, transferred to separate tubes, and deproteinized with 5 ml $HClO_4$ (6%, w/v). All preparations were centrifuged for 15 min at 3000 x g. The supernatant and the washings of the precipitate, which were also spun, were transferred to calibrated conical tubes and the pH of both control and experimental samples were adjusted to 3.5 with 5 M K_2CO_3. After pH adjustment, both control and experimental supernatants were brought up to a final volume of 8 ml and allowed to stand for 15 minutes before spectrophotometric determination of the intermediates by the method of Michal and Beutler (25).

b. Analysis of D-glucose-6-phosphate (G-6-P). Determination of this glycolytic intermediate was done by the method of Lang and Michal (23). Incubation procedures and tissue preparations were similar to those performed for the analysis of F-1,6-P_2 and DAP.

C. Glucose Uptake Experiments with 2-Deoxy-D-Glucose

To study the effects of THC on glucose uptake, tissues were prepared similar to as in the respirometric experiments. The incubation medium was also identical except for substrate. In these studies, 5.5 mM 2-deoxy-D-glucose was used with ^{14}C-2-deoxy-D-glucose as the tracer. Tissues were transferred to Erlenmeyer flasks containing 2 ml of the aerated incubation medium. Prior to incubation, experimental flasks received 0.033 mM (1 mcl), 0.1 mM (3 mcl), 0.2 mM (6 mcl), 0.3 mM (9 mcl), or 0.4 mM (12 mcl) of THC. Control flasks received equal volumes of ethanol. After incubating for 100 minutes at 37°C, the tissues were washed three times with isotonic saline to remove any adhering radioactivity. Wet weights of the tissues were determined after blotting and each tissue (Control and THC-exposed) was digested in a scintillation vial for 4 hours at 55°C with 1.5 ml of toluene-350 tissue solubilizer. Afterwords, all samples were cooled and 10 ml of Instagel was added to each vial and counted. Efficiency constants for converting CPMs to DPMs were determined and the quantity of 2-deoxy-D-glucose in the control and THC-exposed tissue was calculated and expressed on a per gram tissue weight basis.

Data from control and THC-exposed testicular tissues of all experiments was compared using Students' t-test. The level of significance for these comparisons was $p < 0.05$.

III. RESULTS

In initial radiorespirometric experiments, effects of different concentrations of THC on glucose metabolism in rat testicular tissue were studied. Tissue preparations were incubated in a radiolabeled medium containing 5.5 mM glucose. There was a 15% inhibition in the catabolism of radiolabeled glucose to $^{14}CO_2$ in those tissues which were exposed to 0.1 mM THC. Other tissues exposed to 0.2, 0.3 and 0.4 mM THC dissolved in 6, 9, 12 mcl ethanol also showed a significant reduction in $^{14}CO_2$ production when compared to controls. This inhibition was dose-related as it caused an 18, 20, and 25% inhibition respectively (Fig. 1).

TABLE I. Effects of Ethanol on CO_2 Production From Rat Testicular Tissue Incubated in a 5.5 mM Glucose Medium

Group	Control[a]		Ethanol Exposed[b]		Inhibition (%)	P
1	1.1 +/- 0.2[c]	(10)	1.1 +/- 0.3[c]	(10)	0	N.S.
2	7.8 +/- 0.2	(6)	7.4 +/- 0.5	(7)	5.1	N.S.
3	2.4 +/- 0.6	(6)	2.5 +/- 0.6	(8)	4.2	N.S.

[a]Control tissues received no ethanol in the incubation medium which contained 5.5 mM glucose with 6-^{14}C glucose as the tracer.

[b]Ethanol exposed tissues in groups 1,2 and 3 received 6.9 and 12 mcl of ethanol in the medium prior to incubation.

[c]Values are expressed as mean mcMoles CO_2/g dry tissue/100 min incubation +/- SEM for the number of experiment in parentheses.

Since ethanol served as a vehicle for THC, a separate study was conducted to determine the effects of different concentrations of ethanol on $^{14}CO_2$ production from rat testicular tissue incubated in 5.5 mM radiolabeled glucose medium. These experiments revealed no significant effects of 6, 9, or 12 mcl ethanol on glucose metabolism in the testis (Table I).

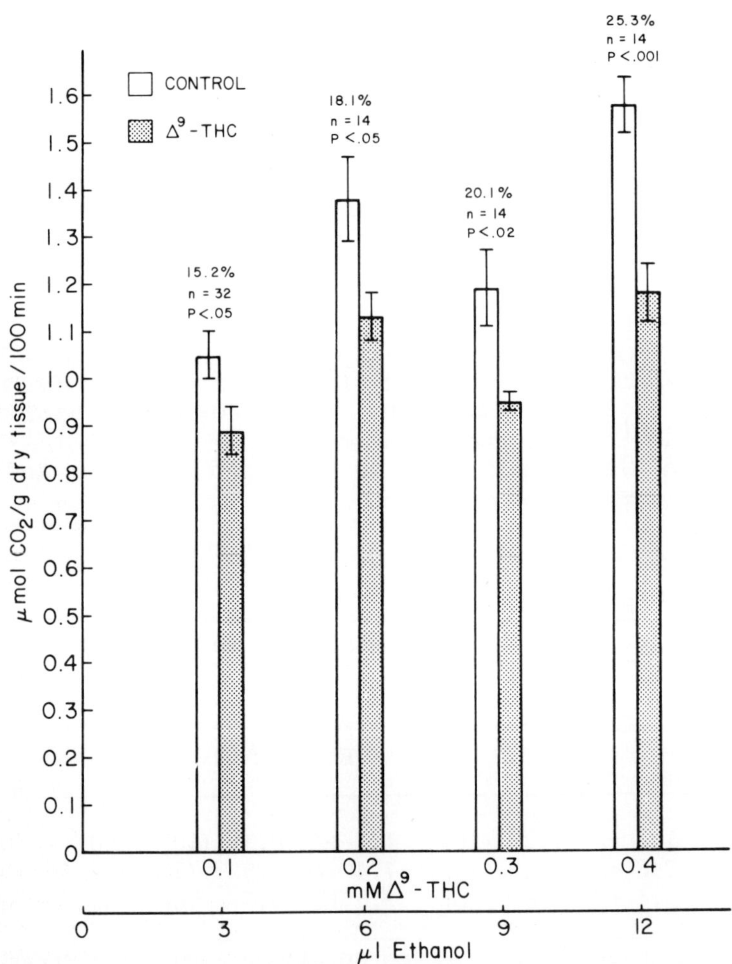

FIGURE 1. Dose-response effects of THC on CO_2 production from rat testicular tissue incubated with 5.5 mM glucose and 6-^{14}C glucose as the tracer. The CO_2 production at each concentration of THC (shaded bars) is the mean of 14 experiments +/- SEM, except at 0.1 mM THC which represents a mean of 32 experiments +/- SEM. Controls = open bars.

In the initial experiments, our observations indicated that above 0.3 mM, THC tends to form a fine suspension and begins to precipitate in the incubation medium. Therefore, in all subsequent experiments, 0.3 mM conc. was chosen to investigate the effects of THC on rat testicular glycolysis. With 1, 3, 5.5 and 10 mM glucose in the medium, exposure of testicular preparations to 0.3 mM THC decreased the output of $^{14}CO_2$. The magnitude of this decrease was 10, 24, 20, and 8%, respectively (Fig. 2). The reductions in $^{14}CO_2$ output with 3.0 and 5.5 mM glucose in the medium were statistically significant.

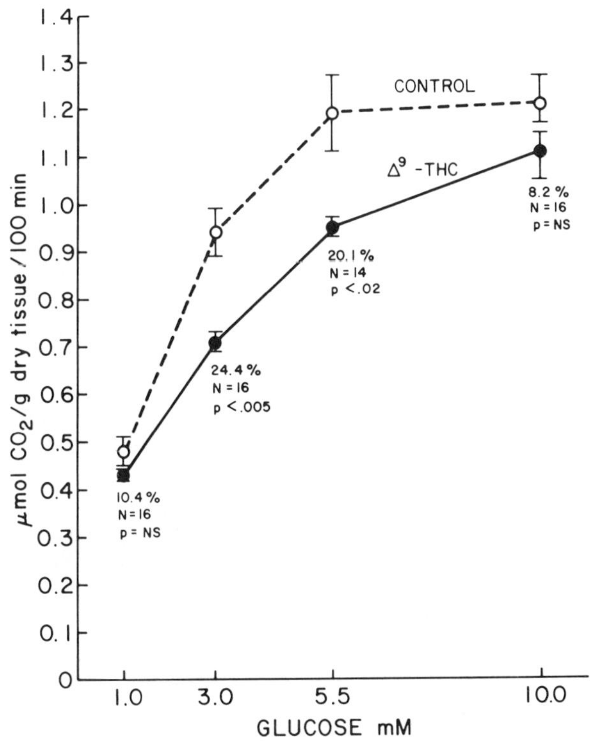

FIGURE 2. Effects of THC on CO_2 production from rat testicular tissue incubated in different concentrations of glucose with 6-^{14}C glucose as the tracer. The CO_2 production is plotted as a function of the concentration of glucose in the presence of 0.3 mM THC in the medium. Each point is a mean of 14 or 16 experiments +/- SEM.

TABLE II. Effects of Delta-9-Tetrahydrocannabinol on CO_2 Production From Rat Testicular Tissue Incubated in Different Concentrations of Pyruvate[a]

Pyruvate (mM)	Control[b]	THC	Inhibition (%)	P
1.0	3.5 +/- 0.2 (8)[c]	3.2 +/- 0.2 (8)	8.6	N.S.
2.5	3.0 +/- 0.1 (8)	2.9 +/- 0.3 (8)	3.3	N.S.
5.5	6.9 +/- 0.4 (8)	6.3 +/- 0.3 (8)	8.7	N.S.
11.0	6.9 +/- 0.5 (8)	7.1 +/- 0.3 (8)	-2.9	N.S

[a]Rat testicular tissues were exposed *in vitro* to 0.3 mM THC with different concentrations of pyruvate and 2-^{14}C-pyruvate (6.5 mCi/mmol) as a tracer in the medium.

[b]Controls received 9 mcl of 95% ethanol per 2 ml of incubation medium.

[c]Values are expressed as mean mcMoles CO_2/gram dry tissue/100 min incubation +/-SEM. The number of experiments is placed in parentheses.

The effects of THC on the ability of testicular tissue to utilize pyruvate as a substrate are presented in Table II. Unlike glucose, testicular tissues incubated with different concentrations of pyruvate and exposed to 0.3 mM THC failed to show any significant differences in $^{14}CO_2$ production when compared to controls.

THC produced a significant decrease in fructose metabolism with all concentrations of this substrate in the medium (Fig. 3). Testicular preparations incubated with 1.0 mM fructose and exposed to 0.3 mM THC exhibited 50% inhibition in $^{14}CO_2$ output compared to controls. Likewise, 2.5, 5.5, and 11.0 mM fructose in the medium showed a decrease in $^{14}CO_2$ production of 43, 39, and 31%, respectively.

The results of the effects of 0.3 mM THC on the concentration of DAP in testicular preparations incubated with 5.5 mM glucose reflected a statistically significant decrease of 23%. In these experiments, the mean control DAP was 163.6 +/- 4.4 nmoles/g frozen tissue/100 min of incubation, whereas the THC-exposed tissue had a mean DAP of 126.5 +/- 3.9 nmoles (Table III). In this experiment, THC also produced a significant reduction in the concentration of F-1,6-P_2 from the control value of 173.0 +/- 8.2 to 120.1 +/- 7.7 nmoles/g frozen tissue/100 min of incubation. This represents a 31% decrease in F-1,6-P_2 in relation to controls ($p < 0.05$). Similarly, tissue concentrations of G-6-P decreased by 29% in the THC-exposed testicular preparations. The mean control value observed for G-6-P was 41.9 +/- 1.5 nmoles, whereas G-6-P in THC-treated tissue showed a mean concentration of 29.6 +/- 1.0 nmoles/g frozen tissue/100 min of incubation.

The uptake of 2-deoxy-D-glucose by testicular tissue incubated in the medium containing 5.5 mM 2-deoxy-D-glucose and

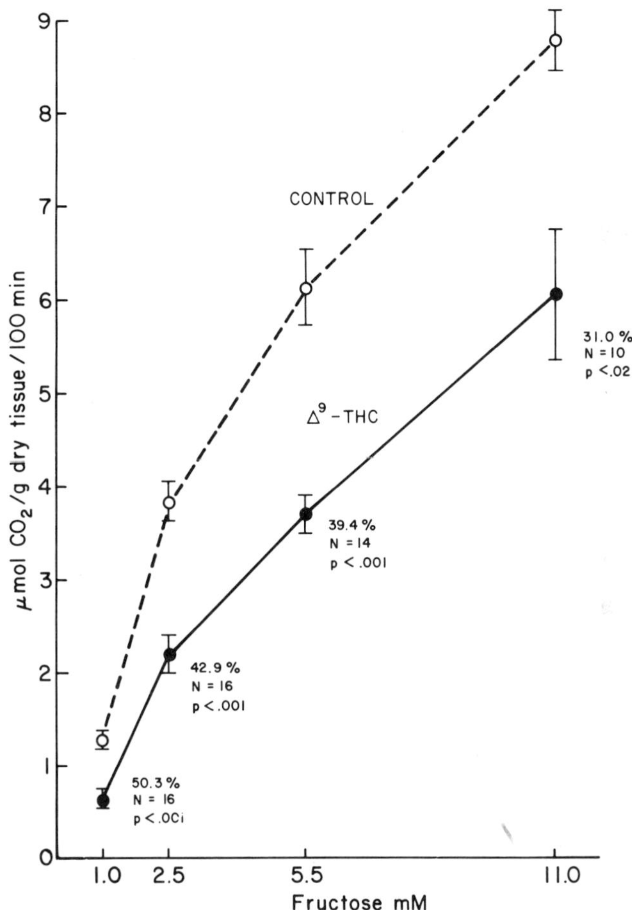

FIGURE 3. Effects of THC on CO_2 production from rat testicular tissue incubated in different concentrations of fructose with U-^{14}C fructose as the tracer. The CO_2 production is plotted as a function of the concentration of fructose in the presence of 0.3 mM THC in the medium. Each point is a mean of 14 or 16 experiments +/- SEM, except for the point with 11.0 mM fructose, which is the mean of 10 experiments +/- SEM.

TABLE III. Levels of Glycolytic Intermediates in Rat Testicular Tissue Exposed to 0.3 mM THC

Glycolytic Intermediates	Control[a]	THC	Inhibition (%)	P
Dihydroxyacetone Phosphate	163.6 +/- 4.4 (6)[b]	126.5 +/- 3.9 (6)	22.7	< 0.001
Fructose-1,6-Diphosphate	173.0 +/- 8.2 (6)	12.01 +/- 7.7 (6)	30.6	< 0.001
Glucose-6-Phosphate	41.9 +/- 1.5 (6)	29.6 +/- 1.0 (6)	29.4	< 0.001

[a]Control tissues received 200 mcl of ethanol (95%) of 44.4 ml of incubation medium which contained 5.5 mM glucose.

[b]Values are mean nmol/gram frozen tissue/100 min incubation +/- SEM for the number of experiments in parentheses.

exposed to THC concentrations ranging from 0.1 through 0.4 mM was significantly reduced. This decrease in uptake ranged from 26 to 46% (Table IV). It was observed that 0.1 mM THC reduced the 2-deoxy-D-glucose tissue concentration from 8.6 +/- 0.4 nmoles to 6.4 +/- 0.2 nmoles/g wet tissue/100 min of incubation. Similarly, 0.2, 0.3, and 0.4 mM THC reduced the concentrations of 2-deoxy-D-glucose in testicular tissue from 7.99 +/- 0.3 to 4.5 +/- 0.1 nmoles, from 8.0 +/- 0.2 mcMoles/g wet tissue/100 min of incubation, respectively. A smaller dose of THC (0.033 mM) had no significant effect on the uptake of 2-deoxy-D-glucose into testicular tissue.

IV. DISCUSSION

Although there are numerous accounts of morphological, metabolic, and functional disruptions of gonadal function by THC or marijuana, the mechanism or mechanisms by which THC produces these effects remain elusive. Data obtained from the experiments reported here and our previous observations that THC inhibits glucose metabolism in rat testicular tissue (17), suggest possible mechanism of THC action. These studies also suggest some sites at which THC may act to produce these gonadal effects. In the initial dose-response experiments, THC showed a definite effect on the evolution of $^{14}CO_2$ from a fixed substrate concentration of 5.5 mM glucose. Two explanations for this action of THC seemed likely. First, THC may be

TABLE IV. Effects of Delta-9-Tetrahydrocannabinol on the Membrane Uptake of 2-Deoxy-D-Glucose By Rat Testicular Tissues[a]

THC (mM)	Control[b]	THC	Inhibition (%)	P
0.033	8.0 +/- 0.3 (8)[c]	7.8 +/- 0.3 (8)	2.5	N.S.
0.1	8.6 +/- 0.4 (8)	6.4 +/- 0.2 (8)	25.6	< 0.001
0.2	7.9 +/- 0.3 (8)	4.5 +/- 0.1 (8)	43.0	< 0.001
0.3	8.0 +/- 0.2(13)	4.6 +/- 0.2(13)	42.5	< 0.001
0.4	8.1 +/- 0.4 (8)	4.4 +/- 0.2 (8)	45.7	< 0.001

[a]The incubation medium contained 5.5 mM 2-deoxy-D-glucose with ^{14}C-2-deoxy-D-glucose (specific activity, 337 mCi/mmol) as a tracer.

[b]Controls received, in each case, an equivalent amount of 95% ethanol used to introduce THC into test flasks. For 0.033, 0.1, 0.2, 0.3 and 0.4 mM doses of THC, the equivalent amounts of ethanol were 1,3,6, 9, and 12 mcl, resp., for 2 ml of incubation medium.

[c]Values are expressed as mean mcMoles 2-deoxy-D-glucose/gram wet tissue/100 min incubation +/- SEM. The number of experiments is placed in parentheses.

inhibiting the uptake of carbohydrate into cellular catabolic cycles by alteration of mitochondrial and/or cytoplasmic membranes. Secondly, it may be inhibiting the enzymes responsible for the breakdown of six carbon sugars, such as enzymes of Embden-Meyerhof pathway, pyruvate dehydrogenase complex, or the citric acid cycle. With these observations, experiments were designed to determine the role of THC in diminishing the supply of energy to the testis by inhibition of carbohydrate catabolism.

In experiments utilizing different concentrations of glucose in the medium, THC caused a significant effect on $^{14}CO_2$ production from 3 and 5.5 mM glucose. A similar inhibition of sugar catabolism was also observed with 1 and 10 mM glucose; however, this decrease in $^{14}CO_2$ production was not significant. Free has reported that glucose uptake in the testis appears to be directly related to the concentration of glucose in the surrounding medium (11). Therefore, if THC inhibited the uptake of glucose in our experiments, it is possible that reduction of $^{14}CO_2$ production with 0.3 mM THC could be overcome by increasing the concentration gradient of glucose across the membrane. Jakubovic and McGeer also observed no significant effects of THC (0.1 mM) on CO_2 production from rat testicular tissue incubated in a Kreb's-Ringer phosphate medium containing 10 mM glucose (19). On the other hand, in case of tissue preparations incubated with 1 mM glucose, the control $^{14}CO_2$ output was only 0.48 micromole/g dry tissue/100 min incubation. It is likely that due to an already low output of $^{14}CO_2$ with 1 mM glucose, THC was unable to depress it any further.

After noticing that THC produces a significant inhibition in glucose utilization, attempts were made to localize the sites of this inhibition. Figure 4 depicts a simplified schematic representation of glycolysis and shows entry points at which different substrates enter this pathway. Thus far, 0.3 mM THC significantly inhibited glucose conversion to $^{14}CO_2$. Pyruvate formation is an intermediate step in this conversion; however, THC failed to inhibit testicular tissue respiration supported by a medium containing different concentrations of pyruvate. This meaningful observation led us to conclude that THC inhibits glucose metabolism at steps above pyruvate entry into glycolytic scheme. Therefore, sites of THC inhibition could be the uptake step and/or the enzymes preceding pyruvate kinase in the pathway. However, if step A is involved, only uptake of glucose and fructose was affected, whereas pyruvate, due to its structural difference was exempt from such a block.

Data obtained from different concentrations of fructose support our observations with glucose since all concentrations of fructose tested had significantly lower $^{14}CO_2$ production from testicular tissues exposed to THC. These results also exclude another step in the glycolytic sequence as a possible site of THC inhibition. Fructose, when taken up by the cell, is phosphorylated by hexokinase to fructose-6-phosphate (Fig. 4) and then further metabolized by subsequent steps in the Embden-Meyerhof pathway. Since fructose-6-phosphate was not derived from glucose, it skipped the phosphoglucose isomerase (PGI) step; however, we still observed inhibition by THC when we used fructose as substrate. Therefore, THC appears not to affect step C in glucose metabolism.

Formation of fructose in the male accessory gland is testosterone-dependent (24); however, testosterone production in itself is inhibited by THC (3,6,21,22,33). Thus, it is possible that THC could presumably affect fructose concentrations in the testis. Fujimoto et al. (12) reported earlier that adult rats, treated chronically with crude marijuana extract, contained a smaller number of sperm in epididymis as well as had a decreased fructose content. Also, in anotherstudy, glucose was found to be a necessary substrate for in vitro capacitation and acrosomal reaction of hamster sperm (10). Our studies showed that THC depressed the energy yielding catabolism of glucose and fructose in the testis. In other words, these combined effects of THC could decrease the energy supply of the testis to the point where it could no longer function normally.

Analysis of the glycolytic intermediates further narrowed the possible sites of THC inhibition. Since concentrations of dihydroxyacetone phosphate (DAP) decreased rather than increased in tissues exposed to THC, it can be concluded that THC inhibition must take place at steps preceding formation of this intermediate. Thus, aside from the Step A, Step E, Step D, and/or Step B were implicated in this inhibition (Fig. 4). However, fructose-1,6-diphosphate (F-1,6-P_2) concentrations of tissue incubated with 0.3 mM THC were also reduced significantly. This observation ruled out the possibility of Step E being a site of THC inhibition since aldolase inhibition should increase F-1,6-P_2 and not decrease it. On the other

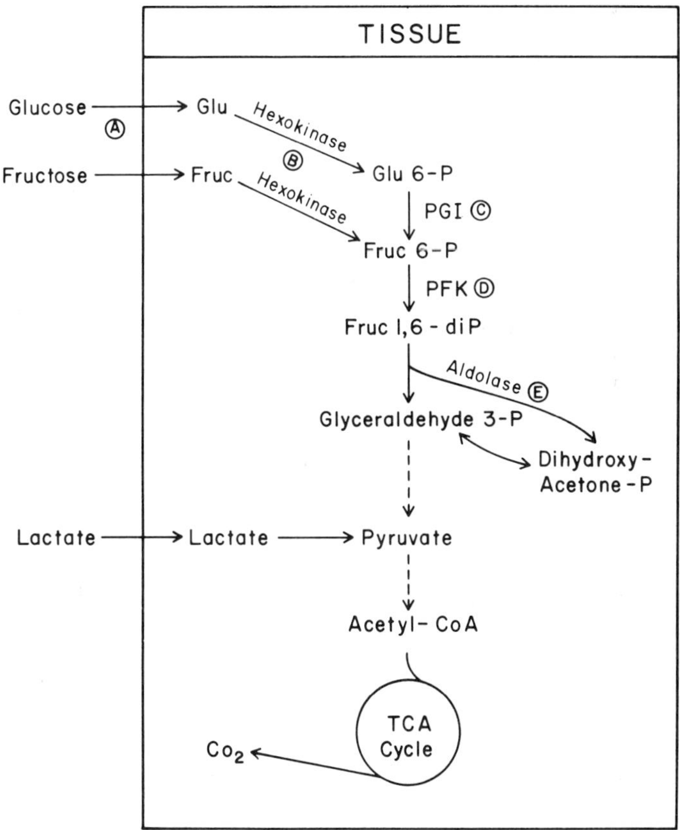

FIGURE 4. A simplified schematic representation of glycolysis in tissue showing entry points at which different substrates enter this pathway.

hand, phosphofructokinase (PFK) inhibition could result in reduction of F-1,6-P_2. Thus, it was anticipated that another glycolytic intermediate, fructose-6-phosphate (F-6-P), would increase; however, its concentration could not be detected by the analytical procedure used in this study.

The last glycolytic intermediate studied was glucose-6-phosphate (G-6-P). The cellular concentration of G-6-P decreased in the presence of 0.3 mM THC, thereby providing support to the data obtained from radiorespirometric experiments using fructose as a substrate. The latter experiments eliminated the possibility that PGI (Step C) as a site of THC action.

The results of the tissue concentrations of glycolytic intermediates suggest that the most likely sites of THC inhibition are the membrane uptake step, hexokinase, and/or possibly the PFK steps. This led to the analysis of the effects of THC on membrane uptake of glucose using uniformly labeled ^{14}C-2-deoxy-D-glucose as the substrate. The biochemical properties of 2-deoxy-D-glucose make it ideal for such studies since it is transported into the cell be the same carrier that transports glucose. However, after phosphorylation, no further metabolism of the compound takes place and it accumulates inside the cell. Results obtained from the 2-deoxy-D-glucose experiments indicated that THC in concentrations ranging from 0.1 to 0.4 mM significantly inhibited uptake of 2-deoxy-D-glucose. These results provide reasonable evidence that in testicular tissue some facets of membrane transport involving six carbon sugars are inhibited by THC. Several earlier studies reported that THC can alter membrane-bound ATPases (2,28,35). Therefore, if sugar transports (glucose and fructose) into the testicular cell is an active process supported by membrane-bound ATPase, inhibition of ATPase by THC could explain reduction in glucose and fructose uptake observed in this study.

THC is a highly lipophilic drug and is sequestered in gonadal fat (29). It is also reported to alter the configurational integrity of cellular membranes (7,31). Membrane active drugs (27) and drugs that interfere with cellular metabolism (34) are known inhibitors of sperm motility. Our in vitro experiments indicate that THC interferes with membrane uptake of glucose in rat testis and inhibits the metabolism of glucose and fructose as well. Observations of Perez et al. (26) with THC in human, rhesus monkey and rabbit sperm, and studies of Dravland and Meizel (4) with hamster sperm lend strong credence to our hypothesis. It is therefore concluded that, in addition to the highly specific hypothalamic-pituitary gonadal effect (32), THC also has an equally important direct effect on the metabolism of energy-yielding substrates in the rat testis. Since marijuana contains a variety of cannabinoids, its effects on gonadal function could be exerted by a single constituent, or could be the result of several constituents. Cannabidiol (CBD) is a cannabinoid which has been shown to exert no effects on gonadotropins (36). Studies with this compound will help to fortify and confirm our hypothesis.

ACKNOWLEDGMENTS

National Institute on Drug Abuse is acknowledged for providing us with delta-9-tetrahydrocannabinol. Thanks are also due to Dr. Elliot Vesell, Editor of Pharmacology, for giving permission to reproduce some of the figures for publication in this paper.

REFERENCES

1. Asch, R. H., Smith, C. G., Siler-Knodr, T. M., and Pauerstein, C. A., Effects of delta-9-tetrahydrocannabinol administration on gonadal steroidogenic activity in vivo, Fertil Steril. 32:576-582 (1979).
2. Bloom, A. S., Huavik, C. O., and Strehlow, D., Effects of delta-9-tetrahydrocannabinol on ATPases in mouse brain subcellular fractions, Life Sci. 23:1399-1404 (1978).
3. Burstein, S., Hunter, S. A., Shoupe, T. S., Taylor, P., Bartke, A., and Dalterio, S., Cannabinoid inhibition of testosterone synthesis by mouse leydig cells, Res. Communs. Chem. Path. Pharmacol. 19:557-560 (1978).
4. Dalterio, S., Bartke, A., and Burstein, S., Cannabinoids inhibit testosterone secretion by mouse testis in-vitro, Science 1976:1472-1473 (1977).
5. Dalterio, S., Bartke, A., Harper, M. J. K., Huffman, R., and Sweeny, C., Effects of cannabinoids and female exposure on the pituitary-testicular axis in mice: Possible involvement of prostaglandin, Biol. Reprod. 24:315-322 (1981).
6. Dalterio, S., Bartke, A., Roberson, C., Watson, D., and Burstein, S., Direct and pituitary mediated effects of delta-9-tetrahydrocannabinol on the testis, Pharmacol. Biochem. Behav. 8:673-678 (1978).
7. Desoize, B., Leger, C., Banchereau, J., and Nahas, G. G., Inhibitory effects ofdiazepam and other psychotropic drugs on blastogenesis of cultured T lymphocytes, Fed. Proc. 37:739 (1978).

8. Dixit, V. P., Sharma, V. N., and Lohiya, N. K., The effects of chronically administered cannabis extract on the testicular function of mice, Eur. J. Pharmacol. 26:111-114 (1974).
9. Dixit, V.P., and Lohiya, N.K., Effects of cannabis extract in the response of accessory sex organs of adult male mice to testosterone, Indian J. Physiol. Pharmacol. 19:98-100 (1975).
10. Dravland, E., and Meizel, S., Stimulation of hamster sperm capacitation and acrosomal reaction in vitro by glucose and lactate and inhibition by the glycolytic inhibitor alpha-chlorohydrin, Gamete Res. 4:515-523 (1981).
11. Free, J. M., Carbohydrate metabolism in the testis, in "The Testis", Vol. III (A. D. Johnson, W. R. Gomes, and N. L. Vandemark, eds.), pp. 125-192. Academic Press, New York and London, 1970.
12. Fujimoto, G. I., Kostellow, A. B., Rosenbaum, R., Morrill, G. A., and Block, E., Effects of Cannabinoids on reproductive organs in the female Fischer rat, in "Marihuana: Biological Effects" (G. G. Nahas and W. D. M. Paton, eds.), pp. 441-447. Pergamon Press, Oxford, 1979.
13. Harclerode, J., Nyquist, S. E., Nazar, B., and Lowe, D., Effects of cannabis on sex hormones and testicular enzymes of the rodents, in "Marihuana: Biological Effects" (G. G. Nahas and W. D. M. Paton, eds.), pp. 395-405. Pergamon Press, Oxford, 1979.
14. Hembree, W. C., Zeidenberg, P., and Nahas, G. G., Marijuana's effects on human gonadal function, in "Marihuana: Chemistry, Biochemistry and Cellular Effects" (G. G. Nahas, ed.), pp. 521-532. Springer-Verlag, New York, 1976.
15. Huang, H. F. S., Nahas, G. G., and Hembree, W. C., Effects of marijuana inhalation on spermatogenesis ofthe rat, in "Marihuana: Biological Effects" (G. G. Nahas and W. D. M. Paton, eds.), pp. 419-427. Pergamon Press, Oxford, 1979.
16. Husain, S., and Paradise, R. R., Effect of halothane on CO_2 production from glucose, fructose, and pyruvate in rat cerebral cortical slices, J. Neurochem. 21:1161-1166 (1973).
17. Husain, S., and Lame, M., Rat testicular tissue glucose metabolism in the presence of delta-9-tetrahydrocannabinol, Proc. West. Pharmacol. Soc. 22:355-358 (1979).
18. Jakubovic, A., McGeer, E. G., and McGeer, P. L., Biochemical alterations induced by cannabinoids in the leydig cells of the rat testis <u>in vitro</u>: Effects on testosterone and protein synthesis, in "Marihuana: Biological

Effects" (G. G. Nahas and W. D. M. Paton, eds.), pp. 251-264. Pergamon Press, Oxford, 1979.

19. Jakubovic, A., and McGeer, P. L., Biochemical changes in rat testicular cells _in vitro_ produced by cannabinoid and alcohol: Metabolism and incorporation of labeled glucose, amino acids, and nucleic acid precursors, Toxicol. Appl. Pharmacol. 41:473-486 (1977).

20. Jones, R. T., in "Marihuana Research Findings 1976" (R. C. Peterson, eds.), pp. 128-178. National Institute on Drug Abuse Res. Monogr. No. 14, U. S. Govt. Printing Office, Washington, D. C. 1977.

21. Kolodny, R. C., Masters, W. H., Kolodner, R. M., and Toro, G., Depression of plasma testosterone levels after chronic intensive marijuana use, N. Engl. J. Med. 290:872-874 (1974).

22. Kolodny, R. C., Lessin, P., Toro, G., Masters, W. H., and Cohen S., Depression of plasma testosterone with acute marijuana administration, in "The Pharmacology of Marihuana" (M. C. Braude and S. Szara, eds.), pp. 217-225. Raven Press, New York, 1976.

23. Lang, G., and Michal, G., D-glucose-6-phosphate and d-fructose-6-phosphate, in "Methods of Enzymatic Analysis" Vol. 3, (H. U., Bergmeyer, ed.), pp. 1238-1242. Verlag Chemie Weinheim, Academic Press, Inc., New York and London, 1974.

24. Mann, T., and Parsons, U., Effect of testicular hormone on the formation of seminal fructose, Nature, Lond. 160:294 (1947).

25. Michal, G., and Beutler, H. O., D-fructose-1,6-diphosphate, dihydroxyacetone phosphate and d-glyceraldehyde-3-phosphate, in "Methods of Enzymatic Analysis", Vol. 3 (H. U. Bergmeyer, ed.), pp. 1314-1319. Verlag Chemie Weinheim, Academic Press Inc., New York and London, 1974.

26. Perez, L. E., Smith, C. G., and Asch, R. H., Delta-9-tetrahydrocannabinol inhibits fructose utilization and motility in human, rhesus monkey, and rabbit sperm in vitro, Fertil. Steril. 35:703-705 (1981).

27. Peterson, R. M., and Freund, M., Glycolysis by washed suspensions of human spermatozoa, Biol. Reprod. 13:552-556 (1975).

28. Poddar, M. K., and Ghosh, J. J., Neuronal membrane as the site of action of delta-9-tetrahydrocannabinol, in "Pharmacology of Marihuana" (M.C. Braude and S. Szara, eds.), pp. 157-173. Raven Press, New York, 1976.

29. Rawitch, A. B., and Rohrer, R., Delta-9-tetrahydrocannabinol uptake by adipose tissue: Preferential accumulation in gonadal fat organs, Gen. Pharmacol. 10:525-529 (1979).

30. Schwartz, S., Harclerode, J., and Nyquist, S. E., Effects of delta-9-tetrahydrocannabinol administration on marker

proteins of rat testicular cells, Life Sci. 22:7-14 (1978).

31. Shahar, A., Bino, T., Kalay, D., and Hamonnai, T. Z., Effects of delta-9-tetrahydrocannabinol (THC) on the kinetic morphology of spermatozoa, in "The Functional Anatomy of the Spermatozoan" (V. A. Afzelius, ed.), p. 189. Pergamon Press, New York, 1975.

32. Smith, C. C., Besch, N. F., and Asch, R. H., Effects of marijuana on the reproductive system, in "Advances in Sex Hormone Research" (J. A. Thomas and R. L. Singhal, eds.), pp. 273-294. Urban and Schwarzenberg, Baltimore, 1980.

33. Symons, A. M., Teale, J. D., and Marks, V., Effects of delta-9-tetrahydrocannabinol on the hypothalamic-pituitary gonadal system in maturing male rat, J. Endrocrinol. 68:43P-44P (1976).

34. Tamblyn, T., and First, N., Caffeine-stimulated ATP-reactivated motility in a detergent-treated bovine sperm model, Arch. Biochem. Biophys. 181:208-215 (1977).

35. Toro-Goyco, E., Rodriguez, M. B., and Preston, A. M., On the action of delta-9-tetrahydrocannabinol as an inhibitor of sodium and potassium-dependent adenosine triphosphatase, Mol. Pharmacol. 14:130-137 (1978).

36. Zimmerman, A. M., Zimmerman, S., and Raj, A. Y., Effects of cannabinoids on spermatogenesis in mice, in "Marihuana: Biological Effects" (G. G. Nahas and W. D. M. Paton, eds.), pp. 407-418. Pergamon Press, Oxford, 1979.

TOLERANCE TO THE REPRODUCTIVE EFFECTS OF DELTA-9-TETRAHYDROCANNABINOL: COMPARISON OF THE ACUTE, SHORT-TERM, AND CHRONIC DRUG EFFECTS ON MENSTRUAL CYCLE HORMONES

Carol Grace Smith, Ramona G. Almirez
Pamela M. Scher, Riccardo H. Asch

Department of Pharmacology
Uniformed Services University of the Health Sciences
Bethesda, Maryland
and
Department of Obstetrics and Gynecology
University of Texas Health Science Center
San Antonio, Texas

I. INTRODUCTION

The reproductive effects of marijuana and delta-9-tetrahydrocannabinol (THC) have received much attention from the scientific community for the past several years. Early clinical reports indicated that chronic marijuana use may be associated with decreased hormone levels and infertility. Later studies failed to confirm these findings. Studies in laboratory animals clearly demonstrate that THC has pronounced effects on reproductive hormones and on ovulation and spermatogenesis, and have provided much information on how these effects are produced. These studies have not, however, provided much insight into the apparent discrepancy in the pronounced drug effects reported in laboratory animal studies and the less impressive effects of absence of disruptive effects reported in clinical studies. Since much of our knowledge of human reproductive physiology has been obtained from studies in laboratory animals, it is difficult to ascribe these differences to species variations. It is more likely that the discrepancies in laboratory animal studies and the clinical studies are based on differences in experimental designs and

ISBN 0-12-044620-0

failure to consider the role of the development of drug tolerance in the conclusions of these studies.

The sexually mature rhesus monkey is one of the best experimental animal models for extrapolating to the human reproductive system. The female commonly has a 28-day menstrual cycle that is controlled by negative and positive feedback mechanisms between gonadal steroids and pituitary gonadotropins similar to those found in the human menstrual cycle. Specific amount of marijuana can be administered to these animals and reproductive parameters can be examined directly. The purpose of this review is to summarize the effects of acute, short-term (less than 30 days), and chronic treatment with THC on the primate menstrual cycle. Particular emphasis will be place on the studies that examine the development of tolerance to the reproductive effects of THC.

II. RESULTS

A. Acute Effects of THC on Menstrual Cycle Hormones

It is now well established that THC decreases the circulating levels of FSH and LH in various species (1-4) including primates of both sexes (5). This inhibition in ovariectomized rhesus monkeys ranges from 50 to 80% of basal levels and lasts for up to 24 hours after a single dose (dose dependent). This inhibitory effect can be reversed by the administration of the hypothalamic gonadotropin releasing hormone (GnRH) indicating a hypothalamic site of action for the THC (6,7).

Acute administration of THC also causes a decrease in the circulating levels of prolactin for up to 180 minutes in both male and female rhesus monkeys (8) and in other species (9). This effect on prolactin again indicates a hypothalamic site of action for THC.

The acute effects of THC on menstrual cycle hormones have been studied in the rhesus monkey using both _in vivo_ and _in vitro_ techniques (10). In the _in vivo_ studies, THC (2.5 mg/kg) or vehicle (3% Tween 80 in saline) was administered by an intramuscular injection to rhesus monkeys on day 20, 21 or 22 of the menstrual cycle. Progesterone levels were measured at 6 hour intervals for the first 24 hours after treatment. THC caused a significant decrease in progesterone levels during this 24 hour period. This decease was reversed by the administration of human chorionic gonadotropin (HCG) at 6 hours after THC administration (Figure 1). This stimulatory effect on HCG could be observed as early as 30 minutes after injection, and normal progesterone levels were observed from 180 minutes to 48 hours after the HCG injection. These

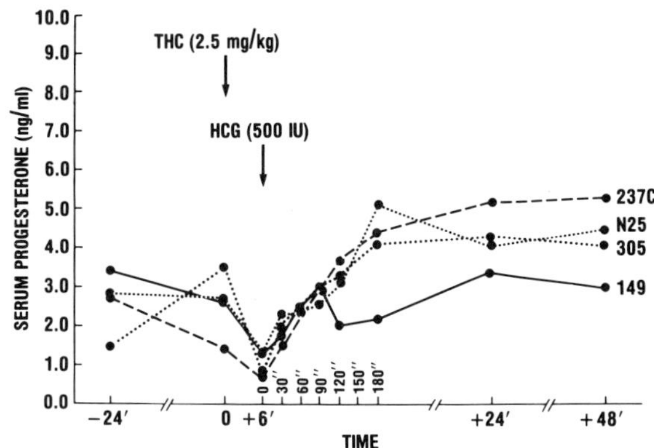

FIGURE 1. The effect of THC (2.5 mg/kg) on progesterone levels during the luteal phase in rhesus monkeys and the reversal of the effect of THC by injection of HCG six hours after the drug injection (cf. ref. 10).

results indicate that the acute effect of THC on progesterone levels is mediated by an indirect effect on pituitary gonadotropins rather than direct effects on the ovarian synthesis and secretion of progesterone.

This conclusion is supported by _in vitro_ studies of basal progesterone production by dispersed cells from the rhesus monkey corpus luteum. The corpora lutea were surgically removed from the ovaries six to eight days after ovulation. These dispersed cells will continue to produce progesterone for several hours without adding gonadotropin to the medium. THC or marijuana extract was added to the cell suspension to a final concentration of up to 50 mcM. Figure 2 shows an example of the production or progesterone by these cells. Neither THC nor marijuana extract had any effect on progesterone production at any concentration up to 50 mcM (limit of drug solubility). However, a number of other _in vitro_ studies with cannabinoids have shown that these drugs disrupt gonadal steroidogenesis, protein and nucleic acid synthesis, glucose utilization, prostaglandin synthesis, and cyclic AMP concentrations in various species including mice, rats and pigs and in various tissues including Leydig cells, granulosa cells and luteal cells (11-15). Clearly, the weight of evidence points to a pronounced _in vitro_ effect of THC on gonadal function.

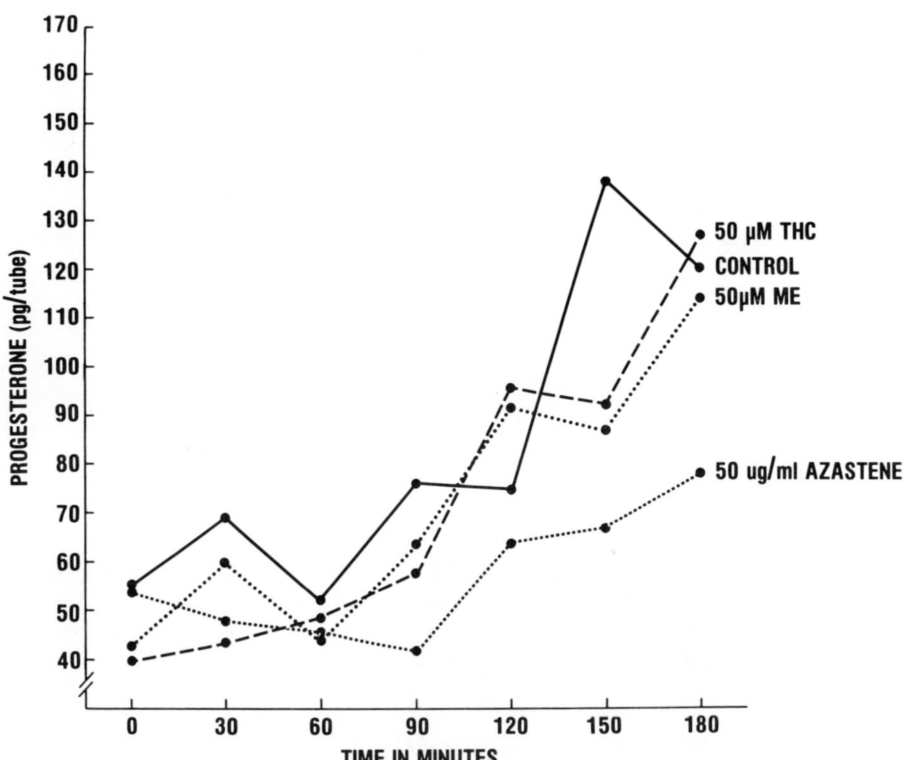

FIGURE 2. Progesterone production by dispersed luteal cells. Neither THC nor marijuana extract showed any effect on progesterone production at concentrations of up to 50 mcM (limit of drug solubility) when compared to control incubations (cf. ref. 10). Azastene (a competitive inhibitor of 3-beta-hydroxysteroid dehydrogenase) was used as a positive control in these studies.

This generates a conflict between the <u>in vivo</u> studies that show no direct effect on gonadal steroid production with these <u>in vitro</u> results; therefore, special attention to the details of the <u>in vitro</u> methods is warranted. All of the cannabinoids studied in these <u>in vitro</u> systems are poorly water soluble. If the solubility of the compound is exceeded, the actual tissue level may be greater than the concentration added to the medium. Unlike the studies with dispersed luteal cells from rhesus monkeys, most of the other <u>in vitro</u> systems use tissues that require the addition of a gonadotropin to the incubation medium to stimulate steroid production. The integrity of the <u>in vitro</u> environment and the function of the polypeptide hormones added to the incubations may be compromised in the presence of these drugs. Until adequate information is available on the actual levels of these drugs in the media and in the tissues and on the chemical identity of the drugs throughout the incubation period, the conclusions drawn from all in vitro studies will remain tentative.

B. Short-term Effects of THC on Menstrual Cycle Hormones

The effects of short-term administration of THC on the menstrual cycle in the rhesus monkey has been studied in our laboratories. One such study examined the effect of THC administration on follicular development and ovulation (16). The rhesus monkeys used in these studies had normal menstrual cycles. The first day of menses was designated as day 1 of the cycle, and ovulation normally occurs on about day 15 (average day 15 +/- 1 day S. D.). In order to determine whether THC administration would affect ovulation in these monkeys, THC (2.5 mg/kg) or vehicle (3% Tween 80 in saline) was injected daily from day 1 to day 18 of the cycle. Blood was drawn daily from day 8 to day 18 of the cycle and then every other day until the occurrence of menses. The hormones that were measured included total estrogens, LH, and progesterone. Serial laparoscopies were done twice weekly to observe follicular maturation, ovulation, and corpus luteum formation. None of the five THC-treated monkeys exhibited estrogen rises of LH surges, and none of the THC-treated monkeys ovulated before the next menses. A typical response is shown in Figure 3. The period of disruption that followed the short-term THC treatment ranged from 55 to 145 days. After this period, normal hormone levels and ovulation were observed in all monkeys. This study shows that the inhibitory effect of THC on gonadotropin secretion is sufficient to disrupt ovulation and that the subsequent disruption of themenstrual cycle may last as long as several months. When exogenous gonadotropins were administered to monkeys treated with THC during the first 18 days of the cycle, ovulation was restored and normal luteal function followed (Figure 4). The successful induction of ovulation and normal luteal function inthis study using exogenous gonadotropins in the presence of antiovulatory doses of THC clearly supports the hypothesis of a central action of the drug rather than an action directly at the gonad. These results are consistent with studies from other laboratories that show that THC treatment causes an inhibition of ovulation in rats (7) and rabbits (3) by a reversible inhibition of gonadotropin secretion.

Similar results were obtained in studies in which THC was administered to rhesus monkeys during the luteal phase of

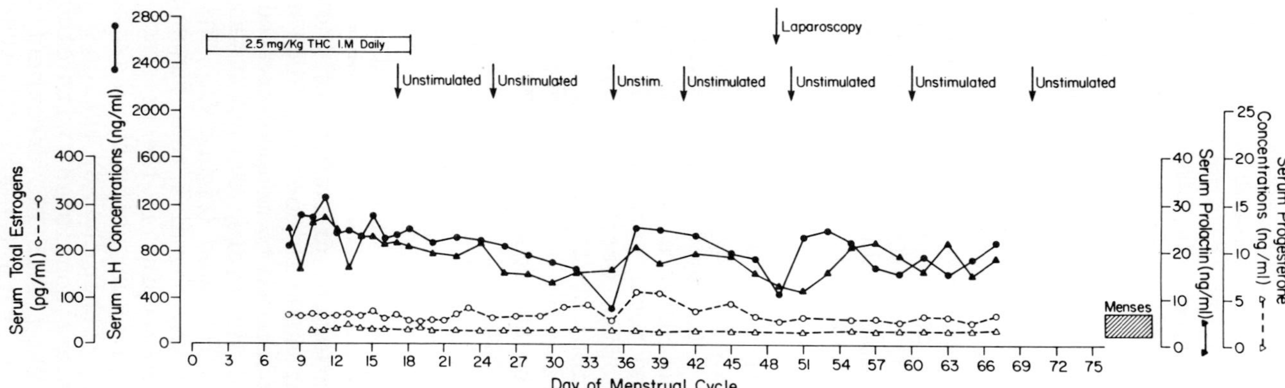

FIGURE 3. The effect of short-term treatment with THC during the follicular phase of the menstural cycle. This figure shows a typical response of a female monkey to daily treatment with THC (2.5 mg/kg I.M. daily) from day 1 to day 18 of the menstural cycle. Drug treatment caused a disruption of the normal cyclic pattern of hormones and an inhibition of ovulation (cf. ref. 16). The effect was observed for several months following discontinuation of drug treatment.

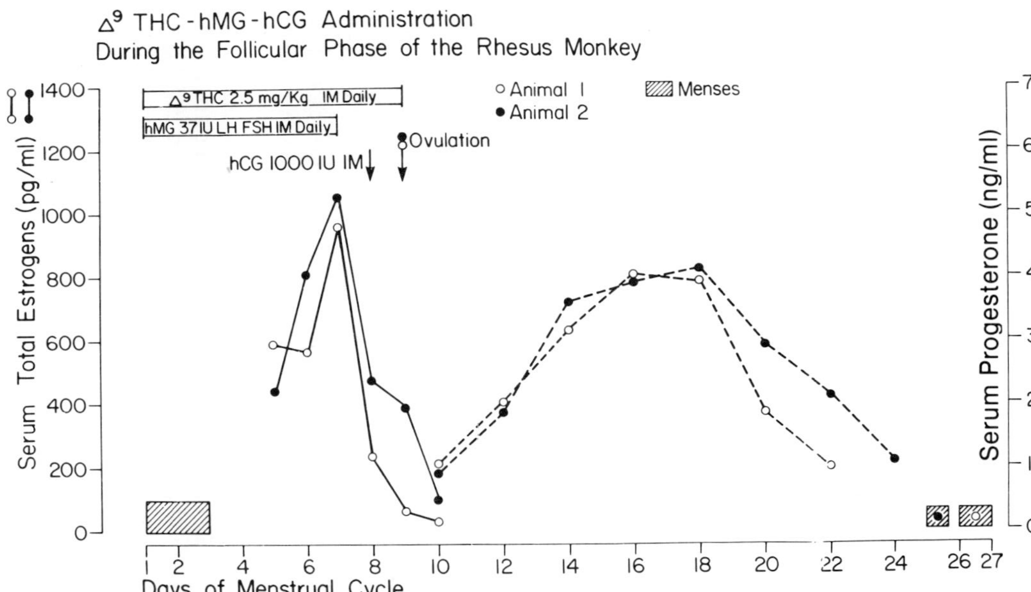

FIGURE 4. Induction of ovulation by the administration of exogenous gonadotropins during short-term treatment with antiovulatory doses of THC in two rhesus monkeys. These monkeys were given hMG (human menopausal gonadotropin) to induce ovarian follicular maturation and hCG (human chorionic gonadotropin) to induce ovulation. The figure shows the original estrogen rise associated with follicular growth and the normal progesterone use during the luteal phase in both THC-treated monkeys.

normal ovulatory cycles (17). The daily administration of THC (2.5 mg/kg) had no effect on serum progesterone levels or on the length of the luteal phase. A typical response is shown in Figure 5. Again, the post-treatment period was marked by an absence of normal levels of estrogens, gonadotropins, and progesterone. The prolactin levels recorded during the post-treatment period were 4 to 5 times greater than prolactin levels in normal ovulatory cycles. A separate study was done in which increasing doses of HCG were administered from Day 6 to Day 10 after ovulation (Day 6, 30 I.U.; Day 7, 60 I.U.; Day 8, 90 I.U.; Day 9, 180 I.U.; Day 30, 360 I.U.). This treatment with HCG during the luteal phase in control animals resulted in augmentation of the progesterone levels to 4-5 times greater than those of control cycles. The daily injections of THC (2.5 mg/kg) had no effect on the HCG-induced progesterone rise when compared to either vehicle treatment or control responses. These results show that THC has no direct effect on luteal function during normal cycles. Further, THC has no direct effect on corpus luteum function stimulatedby HCG administration. The lack of an effect of THC on HCG-stimulated corpus luteum function is particularlyimportant, since this experimental condition mimics progesterone secretion in early pregnancy.

C. Chronic Effects of THC on the Primate Menstrual Cycle

Drug tolerance can be defined as a decrease in pharmacologic response that results from prior exposure to the drug. This phenomenon has been reported with repeated administration of THC in man and laboratory animals to the behavioral and cardiac effects of THC administration. Tolerance can develop by several mechanisms including metabolic tolerance or an increased metabolic clearance of the drug from the body. Cellular or adaptive tolerance occurs when the organ system through homeostatic mechanisms loses its sensitivity to the drug's actions. Either of these mechanisms could be involved in the development of tolerance to the reproductive effects of THC. The chronic studies described here were designed to study the effects of chronic THC on the primate menstrual cycle and to examine the mechanisms involved in the development of tolerance. The study was designed to continue drug treatment for at least one year or until tolerance developed and normal cycles were restored.

Five female rhesus monkeys with normal menstrual cycles were used in this study. Ovulation was detected by monitoring plasma estrogen, LH and progesterone levels and by laparoscopic examination. Daily vaginal swabbings were utilized to detect the onset of vaginal bleeding and duration of menses.

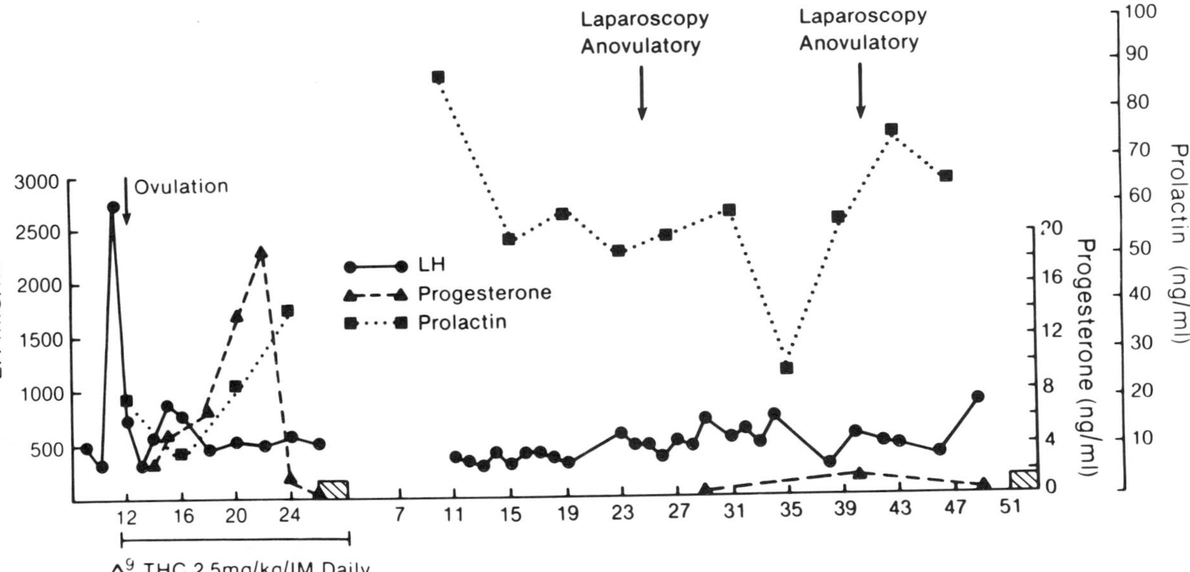

FIGURE 5. The effect of short-term treatment with THC during the luteal phase of the mensural cycle. This figure shows a typical response of a female rhesus monkey to daily treatment with THC from the day of ovulation until the occurrence of menses (hatched bars). Normal progesterone levels were observed during the drug treatment and the luteal phase was of normal length. These monkeys do not ovulate following the luteal phase treatment with THC. This post-treatment period was marked by an absence of normal estrogens, gonadotropins, and progesterone. Prolactin levels were 4 to 5 times greater than those observed in normal ovulatory cycles (cf. ref. 17).

Each monkey was followed for one control cycle and one vehicle treatment cycle before the THC treatment began. On day 1 of the third cycle the monkeys began receiving thrice weekly injections of 2.5 mg/kg THC or 1.25 mg/kg THC. The injections were given on a M-W-F schedule (at noon), and blood sampled on each treatment day immediately before injection.

THC was obtained from the National Institute on Drug Abuse in solution in absolute ethanol. The ethanol was evaporated under a constant stream of nitrogen gas, and the residue was homogenized in Emulphor (polyethoxylated vegetable oil and ethanol) in saline. The drug or vehicle was administered by an intramuscular injection. The blood level of THC obtained with the 2.5 mg/kg dose of THC given 3 times per week in monkeys is equivalent to moderate to heavy use of marijuana (5-6 joints per day; three times per week). Blood levels of THC were measured by RIA where adequate serum was available after hormone measurements (19). The maximum blood level of THC was an average of 300 ng/ml at 60 minutes after injection. The blood level had decreased to an average of 20 ng/ml by 12 hours, and this trough level was maintained until the next dose at 48 hours. These parameters did not change significantly throughout the studies.

All monkeys exhibited normal hormone levels and ovulation during the control and vehicle cycles. Cycle lengths were within normal limits for the colony. After the drug injections began, none of the monkeys ovulated or showed normal hormone levels. The duration of the drug effects (days until next normal menstruation) are shown on Table I. After the tolerance to the drug effects developed, normal cycles were reestablished. Ovulation was again detected laparoscopy and normal hormone levels were observed.

Vehicle administration produced no significant change in prolactin levels. The comparisons shown in Figure 6 were made between pre-treatment prolactin values from control and vehicle cycles (sample size ca. 24 values/monkey); treatment prolactin values during the period of disruption (sample size ca. 48 values/ monkey); and prolactin values during the two cycles after tolerance (sample size 24 values per monkey). There appears to be some decrease in the average prolactin levels during the period of disruption produced by the chronic drug treatment for the three monkeys treated with the 2.5 mg/kg dose of THC (19C; 103C; 237C). Whether this is due to direct drug effects or is secondary to disrupted menstrual cycles cannot be determined. It is clear, however, that the previously observed elevations in prolactin levels following discontinuation of short-term drug treatment are not observed with chronic drug treatment. Some recovery in the average prolactin level was observed after tolerance developed and normal menstrual cycles were restored in these three monkeys.

TABLE I. The Effect of Chronic Treatment with Delta-9-Tetrahydrocannabinol on the Menstural Cycle in Rhesus Monkeys (see Footnote, opposite page)

	CONTROL CYCLE		VEHICLE CYCLE		CHRONIC THC TREATMENT			
					DISRUPTED CYCLES		TOLERANCE	
ANIMAL NO. (THC mg/kg)	DURATION *	OVARIAN** ACTIVITY	DURATION	OVARIAN ACTIVITY	DURATION	OVARIAN ACTIVITY	DURATION	OVARIAN ACTIVITY
19C (2.5mg/kg)	30	Ov-CL	31	Ov-CL	135	NR	30	Ov-CL
103C (2.5mg/kg)	30	Ov-CL	28	Ov-CL	110	NR	29	OV-CL
237C (2.5mg/kg)	30	Ov-CL	34	Ov-CL	103	NR	35	Ov-CL
149A (1.25mg/kg)	25	Ov-CL	28	Ov-CL	100	NR	30	Ov-CL
922C (1.25mg/kg)	25	Ov-CL	22	Ov-CL	70	NR	29	Ov-CL

* Number of days from first day of menses until next normal mense for each cycle or period of time.

**Ovulation (Ov) and corpus luteum (CL) formation or no ovarian activity (NR) as verified by hormone levels and laparoscopy.

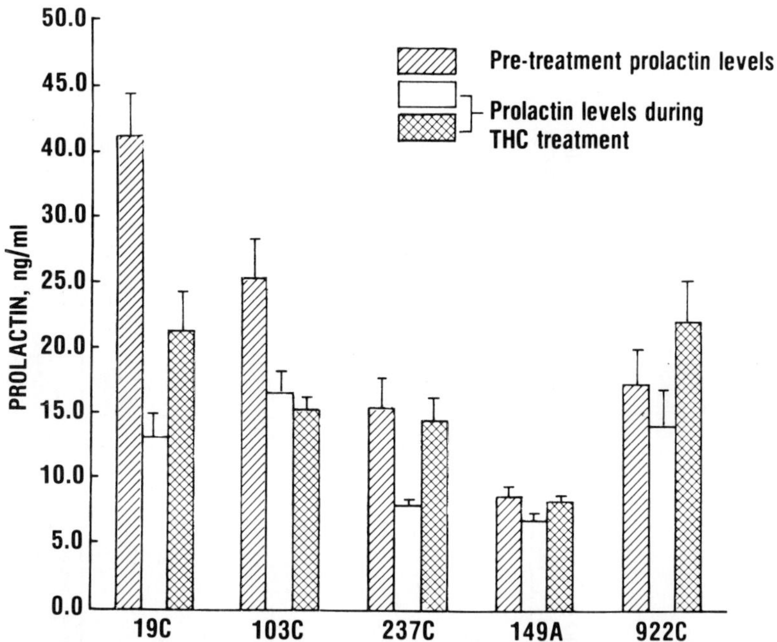

FIGURE 6. Prolactin levels during pretreatment and drug treatment periods for 5 rhesus monkeys treated thrice weekly with 2.5 mg/kg of THC (19C, 103C, 237C) or 1.25 mg/kg of THC (149C and 922C). Hormone measurements were made on blood samples obtained each day before the drug or vehicle was administered. Each bar represents the average (mean +/- SEM) for prolactin levels for each monkey for approximately 24 samples during the anovulatory (open bars) and normal cycles (cross-hatched bars) during chronic drug treatment. These sample numbers are approximations because the cycle durations varied among the monkeys.

TABLE I. (Footnote) In these studies, monkeys were followed for at least one control and one vehicle treatment cycle (hormone levels, laparoscopy, and dates of menses). On the first day of the third cycle, THC injections began, with each monkey receiving an injection on M-W-F of each week. Hormone levels and ovulation were disrupted for the period of time shown for each monkey. Normal cycles were restored with continued THC treatment showing the development of tolerance to THC.

III. DISCUSSION

This chronic study demonstrates the disruptive effects of chronic THC administration on the primate menstrual cycle. Since both gonadotropins and sex steroids are at basal levels during the period of disruption, it is likely that there is a direct suppression of hypothalamic/pituitary activity. This study also demonstrates that with chronic drug treatment tolerance develops to the inhibitory effect of THC and normal cycles are reestablished.

The mechanism for the tolerance to the effect of THC is not known. Tolerance develops to other pharmacologic effects of THC including euphoria and tachycardia. Behavioral tolerance has been reported in rhesus monkeys and was observed in the present study. Preliminary data from this study and complete pharmacokinetic studies in man and laboratory animals indicate that increased drug metabolism or clearance is not a major factor in the development of tolerance (19). It is likely that the tolerance that develops to the reproductive effects of THC is due to adaption of neural mechanisms in the hypothalamus rather than to increased metabolism of the drug.

The results of the present study are consistent with the one clinical study of young women who regularly used marijuana (20). These women experienced changes in menstrual cycles associated with decreased prolactin levels. However, the development of tolerance and return to apparently normal menstrual cycles may mean that normally fertile young women who use marijuana regularly may not notice much change in their menstrual cycles. Drug effects may be more obvious during adolescence, in young women who have some other menstrual irregularities, or if pregnancy occurs. The present studies also demonstrate that the development of tolerance must be considered as a variable in reproductive studies in young men and women who use marijuana and may help to explain some of the conflicting data in human and laboratory animal studies.

REFERENCES

1. Marks, B. H., delta-1-tetrahydrocannabinol and luteinizing hormone secretion, Prog. Brain Res. 39:331 (1973).
2. Dalterio, S., Bartke, A., Roberson, C., Watson, D., and Burstein, S., Direct and pituitary-mediated effects of THC and cannabinol on the testis, Pharmacol. Biochem. Behav. 8:673 (1978).
3. Besch, N. R., Smith, C. G., Besch, P. K., and Kaufman, R. H., The effect of marijuana (delta-9-tetrahydrocannabi-

nol) on the secretion of luteinizing hormone in the ovariectomized rhesus monkey, Amer. J. Obstet, Gynecol. 128:635 (1977).

4. Asch, R. H., Fernandez, E. O., Smith, C. G., and Pauerstein, C. J., Precoital single doses of delta-9-tetrahydrocannabinol blockovulation in therabbit, Fertil. Steril. 31:331 (1979).
5. Smith, C. G., Besch, N. F., and Asch, R. H., Effects of marihuana on the reproductive system, in "Advances in Sex Hormone Research", (J. A. Thomas and R. Singhal, eds.), p. 273. Urban and Schwartzenberg, Baltimore, MD, 1980.
6. Smith, C. G., Besch, N. F., Smith, R. G., and Besch, P. K., Effect of tetrahydrocannabinol on the hypothalamic-pituitary axis in the ovariectomized rhesus monkey, Fertil. Steril. 31:331 (1979).
7. Nir, I., Ayalon, D., Tsafriri, A., Cordova, T., and Lindner, H. R., Suppression of the cyclic surge of luteinizing hormone secretion and of ovulation in the rat by delta-1-tetrahydrocannabinol, Nature 243:470 (1973).
8. Asch, R. H., Smith, C. G., Siler-Knodr, T. M., and Pauerstein, C. J., Acute decreases in serum prolactin concentrations caused by delta-9-tetrahydrocannabinol in nonhuman primates, Fertil. Steril. 32:571 (1979).
9. Kramer, J., and Ben-David, M., Prolactin suppression by (-)-delta-9-tetrahydrocannabinol (THC): involvement of serotonergic and dopaminergic pathways, Endocrinol. 102: 452 (1978).
10. Almirez, R. G., Smith, C. G., and Asch, R. H. The effects of marijuana extract and delta-9-tetrahydrocannabinol on luteal function in the rhesus monkey, Fertil. Steril. 38:000 (1982).
11. Ayalon, D., Nir, I., Cordova, T., Bauminger, S., Puder, M., Naor, Z., Kashi, R., Zor, U., Harell, A., and Lindner H. R., Acute effect of delta-1-tetrahydrocannabinol on the hypothalamo-pituitary-ovarian axis in the rat, Neuroendocrinol. 23:31 (1977).
12. Burstein, S., Hunter, S., and Shoupe, T. S., Cannabinoid inhibition of rat luteal cell progesterone synthesis, Res. Commun. Chem. Pathol. Pharmacol. 24:413 (1979).
13. Dalterio, S., Bartke, A., and Burstein, S., Cannabinoids inhibit testosterone secretion by mouse testes in vitro, Science 196:1472 (1976).
14. Reich, R., Laufer, N., Lewysohn, O, Cordova, T., Ayalon, D., and Tsafriri, A., (1982) In vitro effects of cannabinoids on follicular function in the rat, Biol. Reprod. 27:223 (1982).
15. Jakubovic, A., and McGreer, P. L., In vitro inhibition of protein and nucleic acid synthesis in rat testicular tissue by cannabinoids, in "Marijuana: Chemistry, Biochemis-

try, and Cellular Effects", (G. G. Nahas, W. D. M. Paton, and J. Idanpaan-Heikkila, eds.), p. 223. Springer-Verlag, New York, 1976.

16. Asch, R. H., Smith, C. G., Siler-Knodr, T. M., and Pauerstein, C. J., Effects of delta-9-tetrahydrocannabinol during the follicular phase of the rhesus monkey (macaca mulatta), J. Clin. Endocrinol. Metab. 52:50 (1981).
17. Asch, R. H., Smith, C. G., Siler-Knodr, T. M., and Pauerstein, C. J. Effects of delta-9-tetrahydrocannabinol administration on gonadal steroidogenic activity in vivo, Fertil. Steril. 32:576 (1979).
18. Lemberger, L., and Rubin, A., Cannabis: Role of metabolism in the development of tolerance, Drug Metab. Rev. 8(1):59 (1978).
19. Cook, C. E., Seltzman, H. H., Schindler, V. H., Tallent, C. R., and Chin, M. M., The analysis of cannabinoids in biological fluids, in "Cannabinoid Assays in Body Fluids" (R. L. Hawks, ed.). NIDA Research Monograph, No. 42, U.S. Government Printing Office, Washington, D. C., 1982.
20. Bauman, J. E., Marijuana and the female reproductive system. Testimony before the Subcommittee on Criminal Justice of the Committee on the Judiciary, U. S. Senate, in "Health Consequences of Marijuana Use", p. 85. U.S. Government Printing Office, Washington, D. C., 1980.

INHIBITION OF SUCKLING-INDUCED PROLACTIN SECRETION BY DELTA-9-TETRAHYDROCANNABINOL*

Lee Tyrey
Claude L. Hughes, Jr.

Department of Obstetrics and Gynecology
Duke University Medical Center
Durham, North Carolina

I. INTRODUCTION

Increased postnatal mortality during the first few days of life occurs among the offspring of rats and mice treated during pregnancy or the early postpartum period with delta-9-tetrahydrocannabinol (THC) (1,2). That starvation might be casually related to this poor survival was suggested to Borgen et al. (1) by their observation that milk was not always visible in the stomachs of these pups, in spite of the fact that they were known to have attempted suckling. Considerable support for this idea was gained from cross-fostering experiments in which the offspring of THC-treated dams were transferred to surrogate untreated mothers immediately after birth. In this circumstance, survival of the THC-exposed prodgeny was returned to normal (1), while unexposed pups cross-fostered to the treated mothers did poorly (1,3). The clear implication of these findings is that if starvation is the cause of early postnatal mortality, it must result from maternal, presumable lactational, defects, rather than from some treatment-associated deficiency in the pups themselves.

The initiation and maintenance of normal lactation in the rodent, as in other mammals, is heavily dependent upon the appropriate hormonal environment in which prolactin (PRL) plays a primary and essential role (4). In view of earlier

*Supported by NIDA grant DA-02006.

ISBN 0-12-044620-0

observations that serum PRL concentrations are decreased by THC treatment under a variety of circumstances (5-8), it is possible that PRL secretion, and hence lactation, is compromised by perinatal treatment of mothers with THC. In particular, the surge in PRL secretion induced by each suckling episode, necessary for the continuation of adequate lactation, may be sensitive to the inhibitory effect of THC. The current study was designed to determine if that is the case.

II. MATERIALS AND METHODS

Young adult female rats of the Charles River Crl:CD(SD)BR strain were housed in air-conditioned animal quarters illuminated by fluorescent lighting 14 hrs each day (0500 - 1900 h). Purina Laboratory Chow and water were provided ad libitum.

Vaginal smears were obtained 5-6 days per week by saline lavage and individuals exhibiting proestrous smears were placed overnight with males of the same strain. Mating was confirmed by the presence of a vaginal plug or sperm in the vaginal smear the next morning. Animals later identified as pregnant by palpation or the appearance of red blood cells in the vaginal smears were housed individually and checked each morning to establish the day of parturition. Animals were used in experiments 9 to 15 days postpartum, at which time the number of pups per litter ranged from 7 to 16. The average litter size was 12.4 +/- 2.3 (S.D.).

On the evening before an experiment, all but 2 pups were separated from their mother in order to assure vigorous suckling during the experiment on the next day. The 2 pups remaining with the mother overnight avoided complete deprivation of the suckling stimulus. When necessary, small litters were supplemented with pups of similar age from other litters. The next morning, dams were anesthesized with urethane (1.1 gm/kg BW) and indwelling atrial cannulae for later drug administration and blood withdrawal were inserted via an external jugular vein. Cannulae were filled with heparinized saline (10 U/ml) to maintain patency. After an interval of at least 3 hr, 10 pups, which had been separated from their mother overnight, were returned and allowed to suckle continuously for 2 or 2.5 hrs, depending upon the experiment.

THC in ethanol solution was provided by the National Institute on Drug Abuse. Immediately before use, the ethanol was evaporated at 45-50°C under a continuous stream of nitrogen. The resulting residue was emulsified at a concentration of 1 mg/ml in a vehicle consisting of 10% propylene glycol and 1% Tween-80 in 0.9% saline. THC was administered by iv injection in doses of 0.5 mg/kg BW, a treatment which was highly effective in suppressing PRL secretion in earlier experiments (7). Control animals were treated with an equivalent volume of the vehicle alone.

Two experiments were performed. In the first, mothers were injected with THC or vehicle immediately before return of the pups and the onset of suckling. Blood samples (0.3 ml) were drawn just prior to treatment in order to determine baseline PRL concentrations, and then every 30 min during 2 hrs of suckling and a 1 hr post-suckling period. After each sample, a volume of heparinized saline equivalent to one-half of the sample volume was injected in order to minimize plasma volume loss. In the second experiment, the overall procedure was as in the first, but the injection of THC or vehicle was delayed until after suckling had proceeded for 90 min. After treatment, suckling was allowed to continue for an additional 60 min before the pups were removed.

Blood samples were allowed to clot at room temperature for approximately 1 hr, and then were centrifuged in a Beckman Microfuge B (Beckman Instruments, Palo Alto, CA) for subsequent PRL radioimmunoassay. Serum PRL concentrations were determined by the use of radioimmunoassay materials and methods provided by the NIADDK. Aliquots of 5-25 mcl were assayed in duplicate and the mean result expressed in terms of the NIADDK rat-prolactin RP-1 reference. The within- and among-assay coefficients of variation for 10 mcl aliquots of arat-serum pool containing 105 +/- 10 ng PRL/ml were 2.1% and 13.7%, respectively.

Statistical comparisons were made by analysis of variance with planned single degree of freedom contrasts as appropriate.

III. RESULTS

Serum PRL concentrations in samples obtained before, during, and after suckling from rats treated with THC (0.5 mg/kg BW) or vehicle just prior to an episode of suckling are summarized in Fig. 1A. PRL in the serum of vehicle-treated dams increased from a baseline concentration of 14 +/- 6 (S.E.M.) ng/ml to a high of 215 +/- 47 ng/ml after 120 min of continuous suckling ($p < 0.001$). After removal of the pups at 120 min, the mean serum PRL concentration fell to 74 +/- 25 ng/ml during the ensuing hour ($p < 0.01$). In distinct contrast, the mean serum PRL concentration in dams treated with THC before suckling did not increase significantly, and the concentration of 53 +/- 25 ng/ml reached by the end of the suckling period remained significantly below that attained in the vehicle-treated group ($p < 0.01$). While the mean data for the THC-treated animals as plotted in panel A of Fig. 1 suggest a gradually rising trend in the concentration of serum PRL during suckling, which continues even after removal of the pups, that appearance is not representative of the majority of individuals. The rising trend was imparted to the group data by one animal which displayed what appeared to be a delayed, but otherwise full, PRL response to the suckling stimulus. When that one animal was removed from the group and the data replotted as in Fig. 1B, a better illustration of the more typical response emerges.

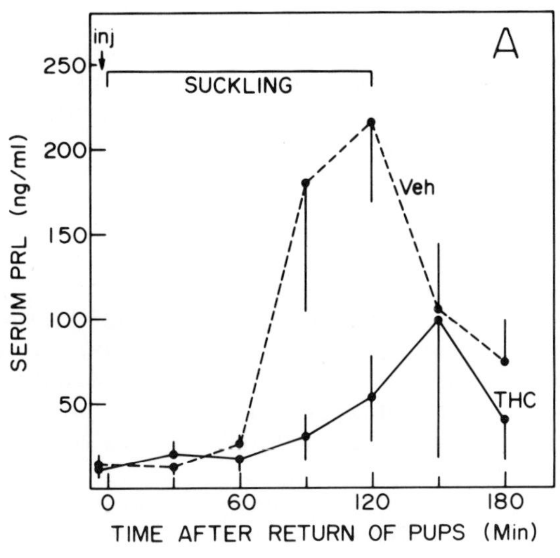

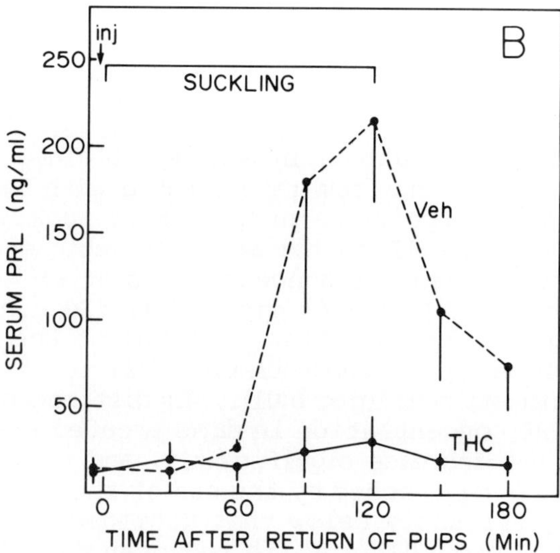

In view of the inhibited PRL response observed following THC administration prior to suckling, it was of interest to determine the effect of THC on the PRL surge that had already become established. Thus, in a second experiment, pups were returned to their mothers after blood samples were drawn for baseline PRL determinations and allowed to suckle continuously for 90 min before injection of the THC or vehicle. After injection, suckling was allowed to continue for an additional 60 min before removal of the pups. The mean serum concentration of PRL in these animals increased from a baseline of 6 +/- 1 ng/ml to 138 +/- 34 ng/ml in response to 90 min of suckling ($p < 0.001$) (Fig. 2). The injection of vehicle alone at that time into half of the animals of this group had no apparent effect. Serum PRL concentrations remained elevated ($p < 0.001$), declining only after removal of the pups an hour later ($p < 0.01$). In the animals treated with THC, on the other hand, the mean serum PRL concentration declined following injection such that by the end of the suckling period it was less than 50% of that registered in the vehicle-treated animals (84 +/-23 vs. 184 +/- 63 ng/ml; $p < 0.05$).

DISCUSSION

The results of the current study unequivocally demonstrate that the PRL surge induced in the lactating rat by the suck-

FIGURE 1. The inhibition of suckling-induced PRL secretion by THC treatment prior to suckling. Serum PRL concentrations (mean +/- S. E. M.) are plotted against time after the return of the pups. (A) Pups were returned at zero-time and allowed to suckle for 120 min before removal. THC (---) or vehicle (---) was injected iv before the onset of suckling as indicated by the vertical arrow. Serum PRL in vehicle-treated mothers (n = 6) increased from a baseline of 14 +/- 6 ng/ml to 215 +/- 47 ng/ml after 120 min of suckling ($p < 0.001$). After removal of the pups, serum PRL fell to 74 +/- 25 ng/ml within 1 hr ($p < 0.01$). In contrast, serum PRL in THC-treated mothers (n = 5) did not increase significantly with suckling, and the level of 53 +/- 25 ng/ml reached at the end of the suckling period remained well below that in the vehicle-treated group ($p < 0.01$). The apparent rising trend of serum PRL in THC animals during and after suckling was imparted to the group data by the inclusion of one animal displaying a delayed, rather than blocked, PRL surge. (B) The data of panel A replotted with omission of the one animal displaying a delayed PRL surge after THC treatment.

ling stimulus is inhibited by THC treatment. A single iv injection of THC in the relatively low dose of 0.5 mg/kg BW just prior to the onset of an episode of suckling prevented the induction of a suckling-induced PRL surge in four of the five animals so treated. In the remaining animal, the surge was delayed, but not prevented, presumably reflecting individual variation in sensitivity to the suppressive action of THC. Similar individual variation in the duration of THC-induced LH suppression has been noted in earlier studies (9,10).

The delay of THC administration until after the suckling-induced PRL surge was already well underway did not prevent expression of its suppressive action. THC injected after 90 min of suckling curtailed PRL secretion and its serum concentration declined even though suckling continued for an additional 60 min. Serum PRL in the vehicle-treated dams, on the other hand, did not fall until the pups were removed from the mother.

The mechanism by which THC inhibits PRL secretion in response to suckling is unknown. However, since THC does not act at the level of the pituitary in the inhibition of other modes of PRL secretion (7), there is little incentive to believe that it might do so in the case of suckling. Nonetheless, that point awaits direct demonstration. Thus, until there is evidence to the contrary, the most reasonable interpretation of the current data suggests that THC action at a site within the nervous system. The results would indicate, therefore, that THC exposure might prevent, or disrupt, conveyance of neural activity which is initiated by suckling and normally culminates in a surge of PRL secretion from the pituitary. Whether this interference might be exerted at the peripheral or central level is, of course, an open question. However, since THC administration also inhibits basal PRL secretion (7) and PRL surges initiated by cervical stimulation (8), it is tempting to speculate that the inhibitory effect of THC on PRL secretion reflects an action at a site along the final common pathway of the PRL neuroendocrine regulatory system. If this is the case, it is unlikely that that site resides in the medial basal hypothalamus (11).

It is worth pointing out that the current study was greatly facilitated, indeed made possible, through the use of urethane anesthesia. Our initial attempts to study the effect of THC on PRL secretion during suckling were frustrated, as were the studies of Bromley et al. (12), by the disruption of nursing behavior caused by THC. The iv administration of THC (0.5 mg/kg BW) to a nursing dam immediately initiated maternal activity which precluded further suckling. Bromley et al. (12) dealt with this problem by removal of the pups from the mother at the time of THC administration. This resulted in a fall in serum PRL in both control and THC groups, but the

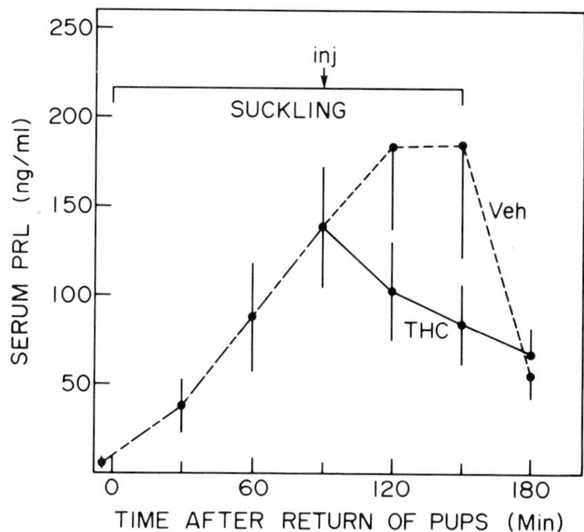

FIGURE 2. The inhibition of suckling-induced PRL secretion by THC treatment during suckling. Serum PRL concentrations (mean +/- S. E. M.) are plotted against time after the return of pups. Pups were returned to mothers (n = 28) at zero-time and allowed to suckle for 150 min before removal. After 90 min of suckling (vertical arrow), half of the mothers were injected with THC (---) and half with vehicle (---). Prior to treatment, serum PRL increased from a baseline of 6 +/- 1 ng/ml to 138 +/- 34 ng/ml in response to suckling ($p < 0.001$). After treatment, PRL remained elevated in the vehicle group ($p < 0.001$), but decreased in the THC group such that by the end of the suckling period the serum PRL concentration was less than 50% of that in vehicle-treated animals (84 +/- 23 vs. 184 +/- 63 ng/ml; $p < 0.05$). Serum PRL in the vehicle-treated group declined only after removal of the pups ($p < 0.01$).

somewhat more rapid decline of serum PRL in the THC animals was interpreted as indicative of an inhibition of suckling-induced PRL secretion. This conclusion was tenuous, however, since the differences in PRL concentrations were not great, and neither the continued secretion of PRL in control animals after removal of the pups nor an unaltered PRL clearance in THC animals were documented. In our study, we chose to circumvent the disruption of nursing behavior by the use of urethane anesthesia. Under the conditions employed, urethane provides prolonged anesthesia, but allows the neuroendocrine reflex response to suckling to remain operational (13). The clear and direct demonstration of THC inhibition of suckling-induced PRL secretion was thus possible.

In that the administration of THC inhibits PRL secretion, including that induced by suckling, it seems likely that the inadequate lactation and early postpartum pup mortality noted by others (1-3) results, in part, if not entirely, from maternal neuroendocrine effects of perinatal THC treatment of the mother. It is important to recognize that this likelihood underscores the need for pup fostering to untreated mothers in experiments where interest is focused on the effects of *in utero* exposure to THC on the offspring, at least when rodents are used as experimental subjects. Whether a similar inhibition of suckling-induced PRL secretion, and hence lactation, exists in the primate is unknown and needs to be investigated. Since basal PRL secretion in the primate is sensitive to THC suppression (14), one might predict that suckling-induced PRL secretion in the primate, as that in the rat, will prove sensitive to the suppressive effects of THC exposure.

ACKNOWLEDGMENTS

The expert technical assistance of Cynthia Thomas and Marylou Everett is gratefully acknowledged. The authors thank the National Institute of Arthritis, Diabetes, Digestive and Kidney Diseases for the materials for prolactin radioimmunoassay, and the National Institute on Drug Abuse for the gift of THC.

REFERENCES

1. Borgen, L. A., Davis, W. M., and Pace, H. B., Effects of synthetic delta-9-tetrahydrocannabinol on pregnancy and offspring in the rat. Toxicol. Appl. Pharmacol. 20:480-486 (1971).
2. Hatoum, N. S., Davis, W. M., Elsohly, M. A., and Turner, C. E., Perinatal exposure to cannabichromene and delta-9-tetrahydrocannabinol: separate and combined effects on viability of pups and on male reproductive system at maturity, Toxicol. Lett. 8:141-146 (1981).
3. Abel, E. L., Day, N., Dintcheff, B. A., and Ernst, C. A. S., Inhibition of postnatal maternal performance in rats treated with marijuana extract during pregnancy, Bull. Psychonom. Soc. 14:353-354 (1979).
4. Tindal, J. S., Neuroendocrine control of lactation, in "Lactation", vol. IV (B. L. Larson, ed.), pp. 67-114.

Academic Press, New York, 1978.

5. Kramer, J., and Ben-David, M., Suppression of prolactin secretion by acute administration of delta-9-THC in rats, Proc. Soc. Exp. Biol. Med. 147:482-484 (1974).
6. Ayalon, D., Nir, I., Cordova, T., Bauminger, S., Puder, M., Naor, Z., Kashi, R., Zor, U., Harell, A., and Lindner, H. R., Acute effect of delta-9-tetrahydrocannabinol on the hypothalamo-pituitary-ovarian axis in the rat, Neuroendocrinol. 23:31-42 (1977).
7. Hughes, C. L., Jr., Everett, J. W., and Tyrey, L., Delta-9-tetrahydrocannabinol suppression of prolactin secretion in the rat: lack of direct pituitary effect, Endocrinol. 109:876-880 (1981).
8. Hughes, C. L., Jr., and Tyrey, L., Effects of (-)-trans-delta-9-tetrahydrocannabinol on serum prolactin in the pseudopregnant rat, Endocr. Res. Commun. 9:25-36 (1982).
9. Tyrey, L., Delta-9-Tetrahydrocannabinol suppression of episodic luteinizing hormone secretion in the ovariectomized rat, Endocrinol. 102:1808-1814 (1978).
10. Tyrey, L., Delta-9-Tetrahydrocannabinol: a potent inhibitor of episodic luteinizing hormone secretion, J. Pharmacol. Exper. Therap. 213:306-308 (1980).
11. Hughes, C. L., Jr., Everett, J. W., and Tyrey, L., Effects of delta-9-tetrahydrocannabinol on serum prolactin in female rats bearing CNS lesions: implications for site(s) of drug action, this volume.
12. Bromley, B. L., Rabii, J., Gordon, J. H., and Zimmerman, E., Delta-9-tetrahydrocannabinol inhibition of suckling-induced prolactin release in the lactating rat, Endocr. Res. Commun. 5:271-278 (1978).
13. Burnet, F. R., and Wakerley, J. B., Plasma concentrations of prolactin and thyrotrophin during suckling in urethane-anaesthetized rats, J. Endocrinol. 70:429-437 (1976).
14. Asch, R. H., Smith, C. G., Siler-Knodr, T. M., and Pauerstein, C. J., Acute decreases in serum prolactin concentrations caused by delta-9-tetrahydrocannabinol in nonhuman primates, Fertil. Steril. 32:571-575 (1979).

EFFECTS OF DELTA-9-TETRAHYDROCANNABINOL ON SERUM PROLACTIN IN FEMALE RATS BEARING CNS LESIONS: IMPLICATIONS FOR SITE OF DRUG ACTION

Claude L. Hughes, Jr.[1]
John W. Everett
Lee Tyrey[2]

Departments of Obstetrics and Gynecology and Anatomy
Duke University Medical Center
Durham, North Carolina

I. INTRODUCTION

Delta-9-tetrahydrocannabinol (THC), the primary psychoactive constituent of marijuana (1), acutely suppresses serum prolactin (PRL) concentrations in male (2,3) and ovariectomized (4) or proestrous (5) female rats. The PRL-suppressive effect of THC appears to depend upon a central nervous system (CNS) site of action, since THC failed to alter serum PRL in hypophysectomized pituitary-autografted rats (4), block the TRH-induced PRL rise in rhesus monkeys (6), or reduce PRL secretion from rat pituitary glands incubated *in vitro* (4). To investigate possible CNS sites of THC action, we administered THC to young adult female rats that had been previously subjected to hypothalamic or limbic system lesions.

II. MATERIALS AND METHODS

Two to four month-old female rats of the Charles River Crl:CD(SD) BR strain (180-260 g BW) were maintained in air-conditioned quarters with 14 hours of light daily (0500 h-

[1]Supported in part by NIH training grant GM-07046.
[2]Supported by NIDA grant DA-02006.

ISBN 0-12-044620-0

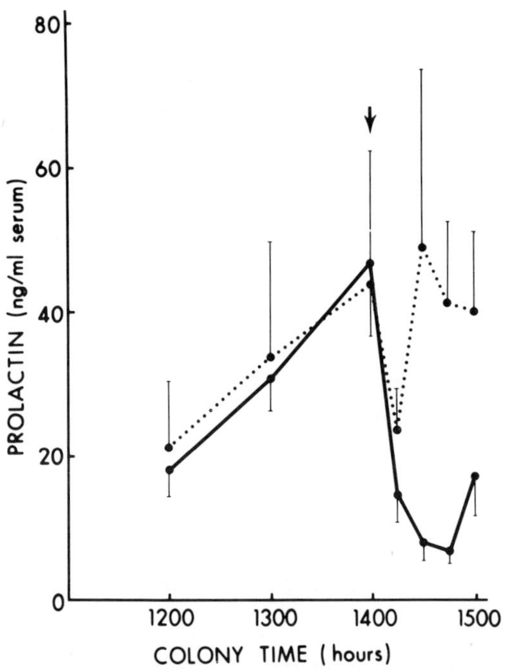

FIGURE 1. Serum PRL concentrations (mean +/- SE) on diestrus-1 in sham-operated rats. Vehicle alone (n = 5; .....) or 0.5 mg THC/kg BW (n = 4:_____) was injected iv at 1400 h. Within the THC group, PRL levels at 1415 h, 1430 h and 1445 h were significantly reduced ($p < 0.05$) relative to the level at 1400 h. Post-treatment PRL levels in the THC group were significantly lower than both the pre-treatment levels within the THC group ($p < 0.05$) and the post-treatment levels in the control group ($p < 0.01$). Administration of vehicle was without effect ($p < 0.05$).

1900 h) and with Purina Laboratory Chow and water available *ad libitum*. Daily vaginal smears were recorded and only rats demonstrating at least two consecutive 4- or 5-day estrous cycles immediately before use were selected for lesioning.

CNS lesions were placed in animals under ether anesthesia with the aid of a small animal stereotaxic apparatus (David Kopf Instruments, Tujunga, CA). In order to control for possible nonspecific effects of surgery, control animals were subjected to sham operations performed with a slender scalpel blade (number 11) oriented in a frontal plane. The blade was lowered bilaterally 1.9 mm from the midline to a point 3.5 mm above and 6.7 mm anterior to ear bar zero (EBZ). Animals were

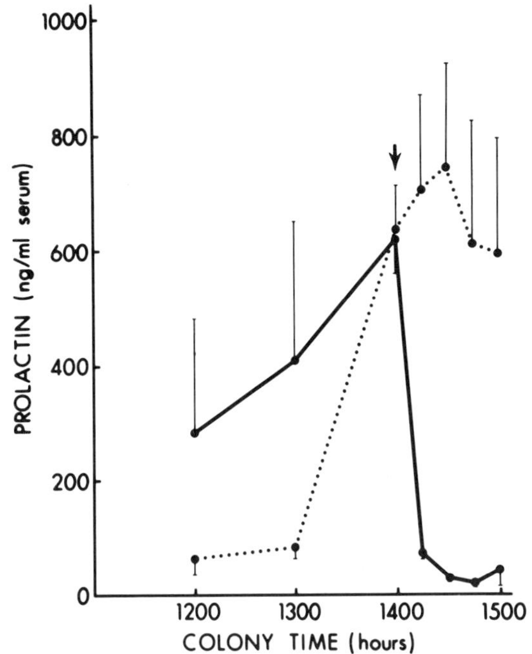

FIGURE 2. Serum PRL concentrations (mean +/- SE) on proestrus in sham-operated rats. Vehicle alone (n = 5; .....) or 0.5 mg THC/kg BW (n = 4; _____) was injected iv at 1400 h. Post-treatment PRL levels in the THC group were significantly lower than pre-treatment levels within the THC group ($p < 0.01$) and post-treatment levels in the vehicle group ($p < 0.01$). Administration of vehicle was without effect ($p < 0.05$).

used 23 to 59 days after sham-operation.

Complete hypothalamic deafferentations (CHD) were performed with a spring-loaded, bayonet-shaped knife which had a vertical blade of 1.9 mm and a 1.3 mm radius of swing. With the head of the animal mounted in the stereotaxic apparatus with the incisor bar adjusted to a point 5 mm below the horizontal plane passing through the earbars, the blade tip was oriented rostrally at a position 7.7 mm anterior to EBZ, and the knife was lowered in the midline to the base of the skull. The blade was rotated counterclockwise through a full 360°, and then through an additional 90° to insure a complete cut rostrally. The blade was then returned to the starting position and the knife was withdrawn. The placement of the cut was designed to put its most rostral extension just caudal to

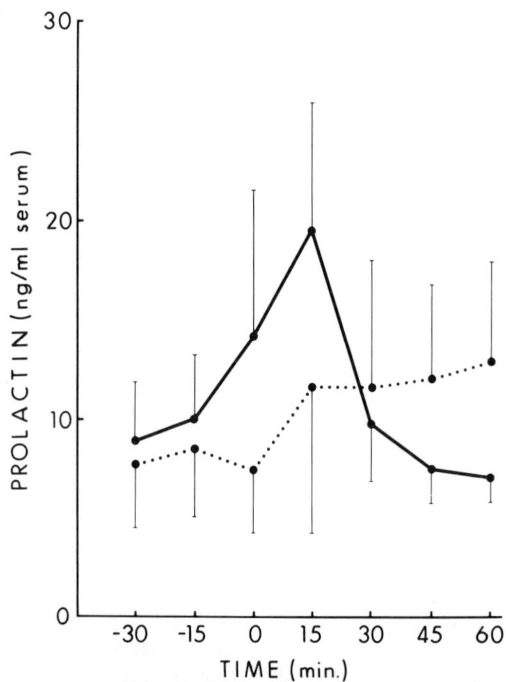

FIGURE 3. (A) Serum PRL concentrations (mean +/- SE) in CHD rats. Vehicle alone (n = 2; .....) or 0.5 mg THC/kg BW (n = 6; _____) was injected iv at t = 0 min. Statistical comparisons revealed no significant differences between pre- and post-treatment levels within or between groups at any sampling interval ($p < 0.05$). (B) A parasagittal sketch of the approximate location of lesions in CHD rats.

the suprachiasmatic nuclei. Animals were used 31 to 37 days later.

Frontal cuts at the level of the suprachiasmatic nuclei (frontal suprachiasmatic cuts; FSC) were produced with two different knifes. Cuts confined to the frontal plane were produced with a spring-loaded 4 mm straight-edged knife. With the incisor bar fixed 4 mm below the earbars, the blade was oriented in a frontal plane 6.4 anterior to EBZ. Centered over the midline, the blade was lowered through the brain to the base of the skull, and immediately withdrawn. Frontal cuts with arcing posterolateral extensions were produced with the same bayonet-shaped knife used for CHD. With the head oriented as for the straight frontal cuts, the blade tip was positioned rostrally 8.1 mm anterior to EBZ and lowered in the midline to the base of the skull. A sweeping frontal cut was produced by rotating the blade 90° counterclockwise, and then

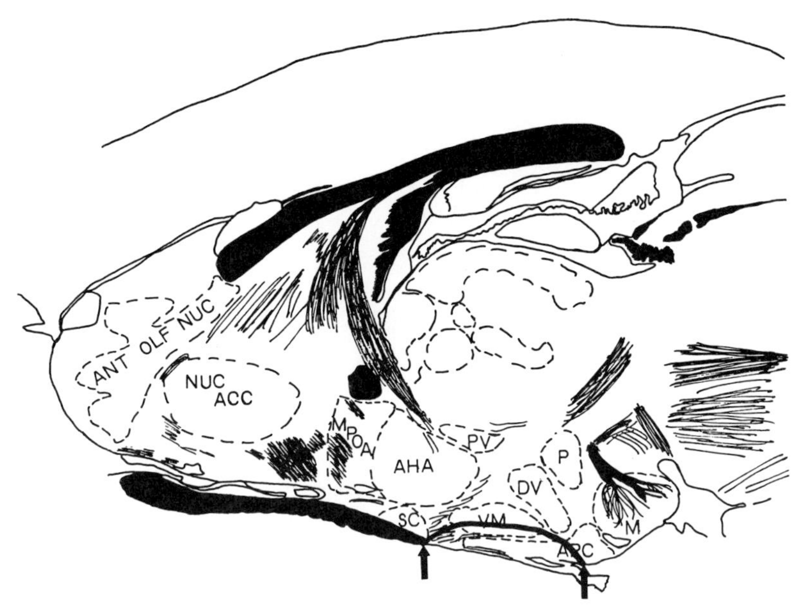

back through 180° to the opposite side. The blade was then returned to the starting point and withdrawn. Animals were used 22 to 56 days after lesioning.

Cuts just rostral to the suprachiasmatic nuclei (presuprachiasmatic cuts; PSC) were produced with the same bayonet-shaped knife used for CHD. The head of the rat was mounted in the stereotaxic apparatus with the incisor bar 5 mm below the earbars. With the tip of the knife oriented rostrally, the knife was lowered to the base of the skull in the midline 9.5 mm rostral to EBZ. The knife was rotated 90° counterclockwise, then 180° clockwise, before it was returned to the starting point and withdrawn. These rats exhibited a reduction in food and water intake over the first 5 to 15 days post-operatively. Consequently, they were fed by gavage until food and water intake improved. Each rat was given 1.5 to 2.0 ml of a soy protein formula ("Isomil", Ross Laboratories, Columbus, Ohio) 3 or 4 times daily during this recovery interval. Animals were used 21 to 48 days after lesioning.

Lateral cortico-hypothalamic tract sections (LCHTS) were performed with a semi-cylindrical knife. The knife radius was 2.5 mm and a notch of 1.0 mm width and 4.0 mm height was located at the midpoint of the curved knife edge. With the incisor bar 3 mm below EBZ, the knife was positioned, concavity posterior, such that its posterior edges were located 7.9 mm anterior to EBZ and then lowered in the midline to the base

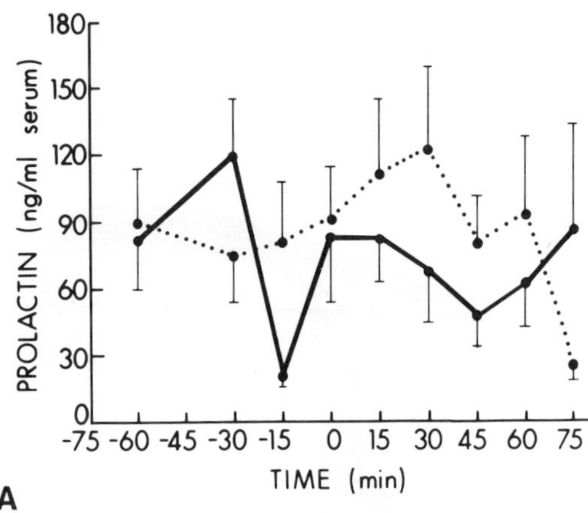

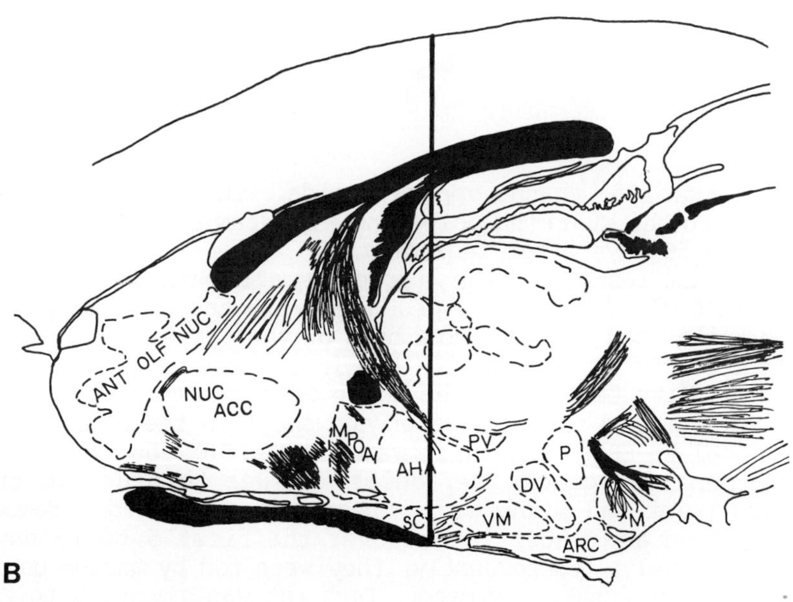

FIGURE 4. (A) Serum PRL concentrations (mean +/- SE) in FSC rats. Vehicle alone (n = 12; .....) or 0.5 mg THC/kg BW (n = 12; ______) was injected iv at t = 0 min. There were no significant differences between pre- and post-treatment levels within or between groups ($p < 0.050$). (B) A parasagittal sketch of the approximate location of frontal cuts produced with the straight edged knife. (C) A parasagittal sketch of the approximate location of frontal cuts produced with the bayonet-shaped knife.

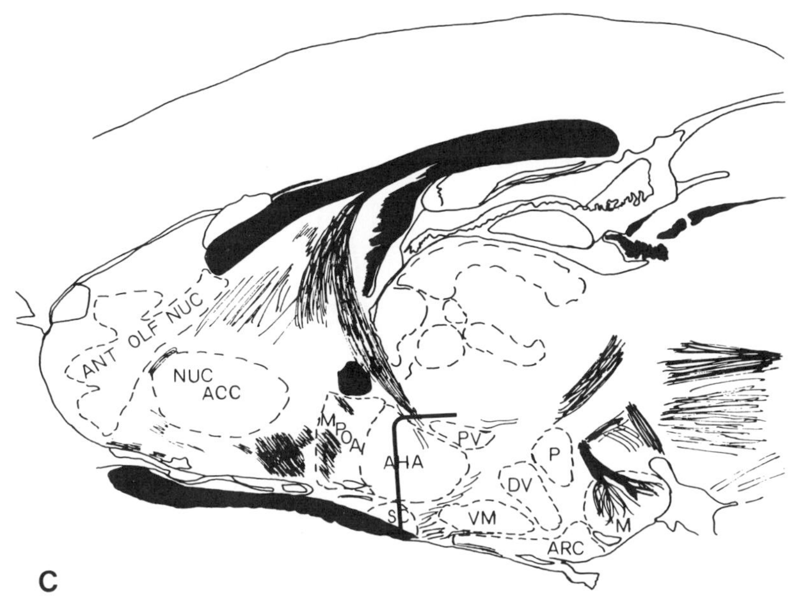

of the skull. The central notch in the blade allowed preservation of the anterior cerebral arteries. Animals were used 18 to 34 days later.

Amgdalofugal projections to caudal septal and rostral preoptic areas, identifiable as the diagonal band of Broca, were sectioned (DBBS) with a 2.2 mm straight-edged knife. With the incisor bar fixed 4 mm below EBZ, the blade was oriented in the sagittal plane 1.3 mm to either side of the midline and lowered bilaterally to the base of the skull. The caudal edge of the knife was located 8.6 mm anterior to EBZ. Animals were used 22 to 31 days later.

Stria terminalis sections (STS) were performed bilaterally with a 4 mm straight-edged knife oriented in the frontal plane 6.2 mm anterior to EBZ. With the incisor bar 4 mm below EBZ, the blade was centered 3.0 mm to either side of the midline and lowered to a point 2.0 mm above EBZ. Animals were used 28 to 33 days later.

Dorsal longitudinal fascilculus sections (DLFS) were performed with a 2.2 mm straight-edged knife. With the incisor bar 4 mm below EBZ and the blade oriented in the frontal plane 3.4 mm anterior to EBZ and centered over the midline, the knife was lowered to a point 1.5 mm above EBZ. Animals were used 23 to 56 days later.

An ethanol solution of THC of greater than 95% purity was provided by the National Institute on Drug Abuse. Prior to use, the alcohol was evaporated under nitrogen at 45-50°C and

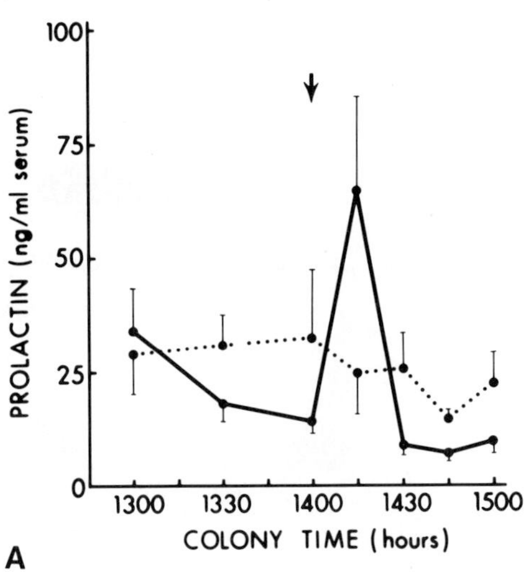

FIGURE 5. (A) Serum PRL concentrations (mean +/- SE) in PSC rats. Vehicle alone (n = 8; .....) or 0.5 mg THC/kg BW (n = 9; _____) was injected iv at 1400 h. PRL levels within the vehicle group did not differ significantly ($p < 0.05$) over the sampling interval. Within THC group, the PRL level at 1415 h was significantly increased ($p < 0.05$) relative to that at 1400 h, while those from 1430 h through 1500 h did notdiffer significantly ($p < 0.05$) from the pre-treatment level. PRL in the THC group at 1415 h was elevated ($p < 0.01$) above that in the vehicle group, but no between group differences were detected at other times. (B) Sketch of the approximate location of lesions in PSC rats.

the residue was emulsified in a vehicle consisting of 10% propylene glycol and 1% Tween-80 in 0.9% saline. The appropriate THC dose was always administered in a volume of0.5 ml/kg BW, with several animals receiving vehicle alone.

The intravenous (iv) administration of THC or vehicle and serial sampling of blood were carried out in unrestrained, fully alert rats by means of intra-atrial cannulae. Cannulae were filled with heparinized saline (10 U/ml) and implanted under ether anesthesia 2-3 hours prior to drawing the initial blood sample. Seven blood samples (0.4 ml each) were typically drawn every 15 min with 0.2 ml replacement with heparinized saline to minimize plasma volume changes and to maintain cannula patency. Blood samples were allowed to clot at room temperature for approximately one hour and then were centrifuged at 1500 x g for 15 min at 4°C. Sera were aspirated and stored at -20°C for later radioimmunoassay.

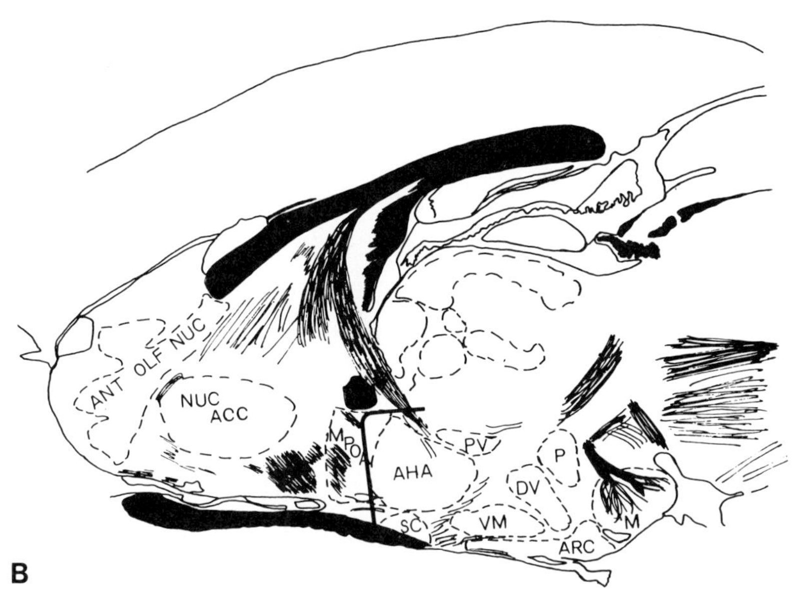

B

Upon completion of the experiment, rats were perfused through the ventral aorta with 0.9% saline and then with 10% formalin in saline. Brains were later removed and embedded in paraffin. Serial sections (18 microns) were cut and stained with Luxol fast blue and neutral red for microscopic examination to determine the location and extent of all lesions. Sketches of selected sections were prepared by direct projection.

Serum PRL concentrations were determined by a double antibody radioimmunoassay utilizing materials provided by the NIADDK. Aliquots of sera (100 mcl or less) were assayedin duplicate and the mean result expressed in terms of the NIADDK rat PRL reference RRP-1. Within and among assay coefficients of variation for the measurement of PRL in aliquots of a rat serum pool containing 15.0 ng PRL.ml were 4.5% and 10.1%, respectively. The assay sensitivity was 0.6 ng PRL/ml serum, and no value fell below that level in these studies.

Serum PRL levels were subjected to one-way analysis of variance with partitioning of the sums of squares for planned between group comparisons, compared by the Student's _t_-test or paired _t_-test, as appropriate.

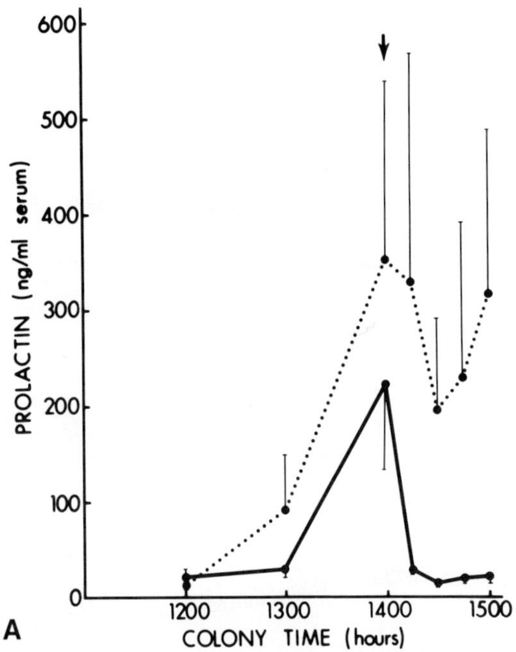

FIGURE 6. (A) Serum PRL concentrations (mean +/- SE) on proestrus in LCHTS rats. Vehicle alone (n = 4; .....) or 0.5 mg THC/kg BW (n = 4; ______) was injected iv at 1400 h. Post-treatment PRL levels in the THC group were significantly reduced from 1415 through 1500 h relative to that at 1400 h ($p < 0.05$). Post-treatment PRL levels in the THC group were also significantly lower than those in the vehicle group ($p < 0.01$). Vehicle administration did not alter serum PRL levels ($p < 0.05$). Both groups show the expected proestrus PRL rise prior to treatment. (B) Sketch of the approximate rostrocaudal extent of lesions in LCHTS rats.

III. RESULTS

A. Sham-Operated Rats

Rats subjected to sham-operation suffered limited CNS damage in a region approximately 1 mm in width which extended vertically through the dorsal cortex to reach approximately 1 mm into the underlying corpus striatum. These rats had regular 4- or 5-day estrous cycles post-operatively and were treated with 0.5 mg THC/kg BW or vehicle at 1400 h on the day of either diestrus-1 or proestrus. As shown, in Fig. 1, mean serum PRL in diestrus rats ranged from approximately 20 to 50

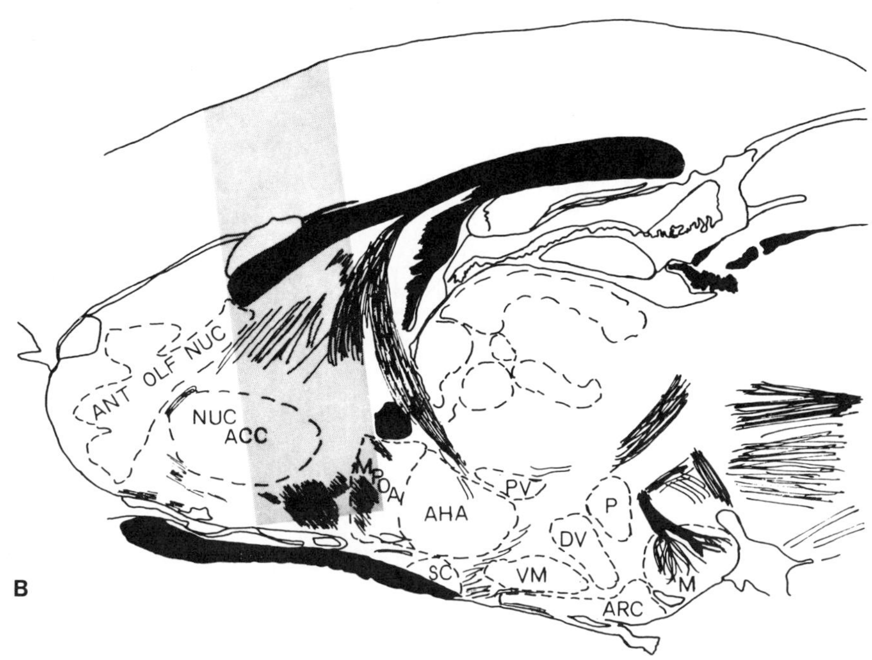

ng/ml prior to treatment. After treatment with THC, PRL was decreased within 15 min and remained suppressed 45 min after injection, relative to either post-treatment levels in the vehicle group ($p < 0.01$) or to the immediate pre-treatment level within the THC group ($p < 0.05$). Vehicle injection was without effect.

Mean serum PRL concentrations in proestrus rats averaged approximately 600 ng/ml at the time of THC or vehicle injection at 1400 h (Fig. 2). PRL levels in the vehicle-treated group remained in the range of 600 to 800 ng/ml in samples drawn during the hour following treatment, while over the same interval serum PRL in the THC-treated rats was suppressed to below 100 ng/ml ($p < 0.05$).

B. Complete Hypothalamic Deafferentation

CHD rats showing predominantly leukocytic vaginal smears following deafferentation were treated with either vehicle alone or 0.5 mg THC/kg BW. Mean serum PRL in these animals ranged from 5 to 20 ng/ml throughout the sampling interval (Fig. 3A) and neither vehicle nor THC injection altered serum PRL levels. An apparent small increase in serum PRL in the THC group 15 min following injection was not statistically

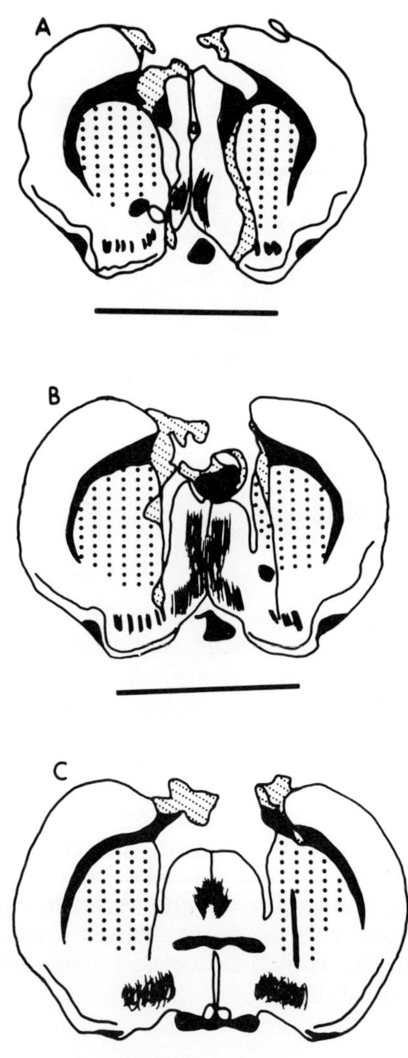

FIGURE 7. Projection sketches of frontal sections of a representative brain from a LCHTS rat at the (A) mid-nucleus accumbens level, (B) caudal nucleus accumbens level and (C) rostral preoptic area level. The fine stippling indicates the region of gliosis and the bar beneath each section provides a 4 mm reference scale. The coarse stippling indicates the extent of the corpus striatum at the several levels.

significant ($p < 0.05$). The location and extent of the CHD lesions are shown in Fig. 3B, with the surviving mediobasal "island" of tissue approximately delineated by the arcing line which extends from the caudal edge of the suprachiasmatic nuclei to a point just caudal to the separation of the infundibular stem from the basal hypothalamus. The surviving isolated brain region thus included predominantly the arcuate nucleus and the lower portions of the ventromedial nuclei.

C. Frontal Suprachiasmatic Cuts

FSC rats showing predominantly cornified vaginal smears were treated with vehicle or 0.5 mg THC/kg BW. Mean serum PRL levels varied widely and ranged from 20 to 123 ng/ml serum during the sampling interval (Fig. 4A). PRL concentrations in individual animals in both vehicle and THC groups showed wide variation from sample to sample with no apparent correlation with experimental manipulations. Neither vehicle nor THC produced statistically detectable alterations in serum PRL during the post-treatment interval. Fig. 4B illustrates the approximate location of the cut produced with the straight edged knife (4 rats group), and Fig. 4C that for the bayonet-shaped knife (8 rats group). FSC by either technique interrupted connections between the mediobasal hypothalamus and rostral structures at a mid-to-caudal level of the suprachiasmatic nuclei. There were no differences in the response to treatment between these two subgroups.

D. Presuprachiasmatic Cuts

PSC rats showed variations in postsurgical vaginal smear patterns, but did not show regular cyclicity. Smears were predominantly cornified with occasional leukocytic types. PSC rats were treated on a day showing a leukocytic smear which was immediately preceded by one or more days of cornified smears. Vehicle alone did not alter serum PRL (Fig. 5A), but THC treatment (0.5 mg/kg BW) at 1400 h increased the mean PRL concentration 15 min later ($p < 0.05$) to a level which was significantly greater than the concurrent level in the vehicle group ($p < 0.01$). Subsequent PRL levels in the THC group did not differ from the pretreatment level within that group or from post-treatment levels in the vehicle group. The location and extent of the PSC lesions are illustrated in Fig. 5B. These lesions consisted of an arcing cut from a level just anterior to the anterior hypothalamic area andsuprachiasmatic nuclei to a more caudal and lateral level at approximately the caudal edge of the suprachiasmatic nuclei.

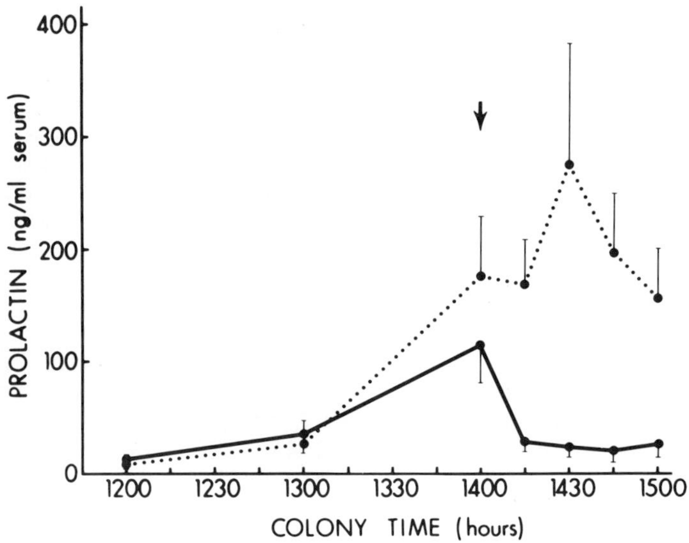

FIGURE 8. (A) Serum PRL concentrations (mean +/- SE) on proestrus in DBBS rats. Vehicle alone (n = 7; .....) or 0.5 mg THC/kg BW (n = 8;______) was injected iv at 1400 h. Post-treatment PRL levels in the THC group were significantly lower than both the 1400 h level in the THC group ($p < 0.05$) and the post-treatment levels in the vehicle group ($p < 0.01$). Vehicle administration did not alter serum PRL levels ($p < 0.05$). (B) Sketch of the approximate rostrocaudal extent of lesions in DBBS rats.

E. Lateral Corticohypothalamic Tract Sections

LCHTS rats had regular 4- or 5-day estrous cycles, and vehicle alone or 0.5 mg THC/kg BW was injected at 1400 h on a day of proestrus. Although vehicle administration did not significantly alter serum PRL (Fig. 6A), THC administration markedly suppressed PRL concentrations at all post-treatment times sampled, both with respect to the 1400 h level in the THC group, ($p < 0.05$) and the post-treatment levels in the vehicle group ($p < 0.01$). Both groups showed the expected proestrus rise in serum PRL prior to treatment. Figs. 6B and 7 illustrate the approximate location and extent of lesions in LCHTS rats. These lesions were bilateral arcs which extended from the mid-region of the nucleus accumbens caudally and laterally to a level immediately anterior to the transverse portion of the anterior commissure. The most ventral portions of the diagonal band of Broca were preserved in these animals.

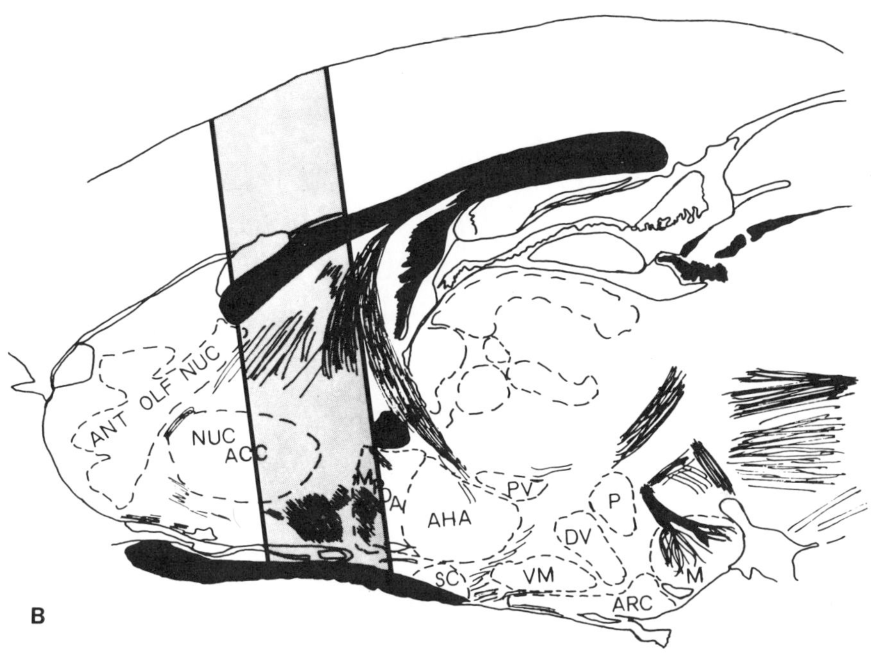

F. Diagonal Band of Broca Sections

DBBS rats showed regular 4- or 5-day estrous cycles and were treated on a day of proestrus by the injection of either vehicle or 0.5 mg THC/kg BW at 1400 h. While the vehicle alone did not alter serum PRL concentrations (Fig.8A), THC significantly suppressed serum PRL levels relative to both the 1400 h level in the THC group ($p < 0.05$) and the post-treatment PRL levels in the vehicle group ($p < 0.01$). Both groups show the proestrus PRL rise. Figs.8B and 9 illustrate the approximate location and extent of lesions in DBBS rats. These lesions have a rostrocaudal extent which approximates those in the LCHTS rats. In the DBBS rats, however, the linear bilateral lesions extended completely to the base of the brain and thus transected ventral connections between the amygdalae and the more medial portions of the septal and preoptic areas.

G. Stria Terminalis Sections

STS rats showed regular 4- or 5-day estrous cycles and were injected with vehicle or 0.5 mg THC/kg BW at 1400 h on a

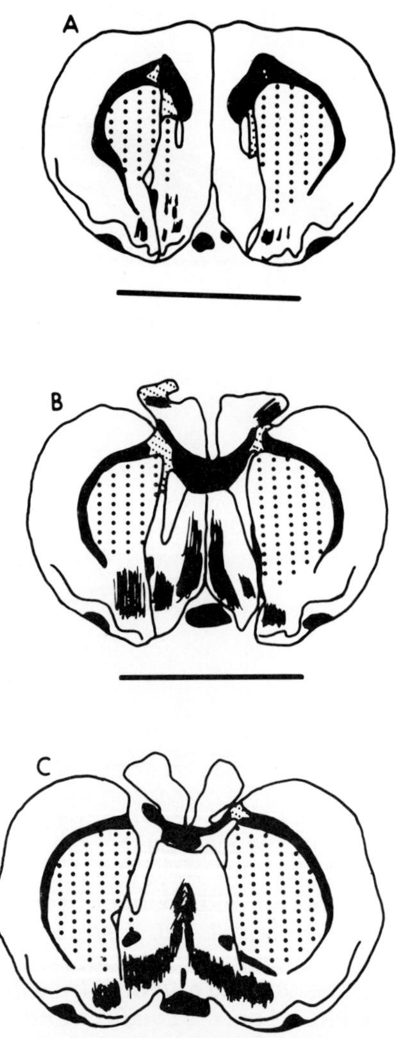

FIGURE 9. Projection sketches of frontal sections of a representative brain from a DBBS rat at the (A) mid-nucleus accumbens level, (B) caudal nucleus accumbens level and (C) rostral preoptic area level. The fine stippling indicates the region of gliosis and the bar beneath each section provides a 4 mm reference scale. The coarse stippling indicates the extent of the corpus striatum at the several levels.

day of proestrus. While vehicle alone did not alter serum PRL (Fig. 10A), post-treatment PRL levels in the THC group were significantly lower than both the THC group pretreatment level ($p < 0.01$) and the post-treatment levels in the vehicle group ($p < 0.01$). Figs. 10B and 10C illustrate the approximate location and extent of lesions in STS rats. These bilateral lesions severed the stria terminalis and destroyed a portion of the nearby corpus striatum.

H. Dorsal Longitudinal Fasciculus Sections

DLFS rats showed regular 4- or 5-days estrous cycles and were treated with either vehicle alone or 0.5 mg THC/kg BW at 1400 h on a day of proestrus. Although vehicle was without significant effect (Fig. 11A), serum PRL was suppressed at all post-treatment times in the THC group relative to both the THC group pretreatment level at 1400 h ($p < 0.05$) and the post-treatment PRL levels in the vehicle group ($p > 0.01$). Figs. 11B and 11C illustrate the approximate location and extent of lesions in the DLFS rats. These lesions damaged the periventricular region and adjacent midline brain tissue at the level of the posterior commissure and the caudal portion of the mamillary complex. The midline periventricular connections between the hypothalamus and the midbrain were thus disrupted, but the more ventrolateral connections by way of the medial forebrain bundle and associated fiber systems remained intact.

IV. DISCUSSION

Since the current evidence indicates that the site of THC action in the suppression of PRL is within the CNS (4,6), we studied the effects of THC on serum PRL in rats previously subjected to hypothalamic or limbic system lesions in order to more precisely define potential CNS loci of THC action. Experiments with sham-operated rats demonstrated a PRL suppression following THC treatment which was similar to that previously reported for male (2) and ovariectomized female rats, with suppression detectable within 15 min and persistence for at least 1 h after a dose of 0.5 mg THC/kg BW. These results suggested that the stress of stereotaxic CNS surgery would not in itself compromise the expression of THC action on PRL secretion.

Because the mediobasal hypothalamus (MBH) is widely accepted as the major brain region involved in the regulation of PRL release from the anterior pituitary, the lack of effect of THC on PRL secretion in rats previously subjected to CHD provides important information. These data suggest that THC does not suppress PRL secretion by action at a site within the

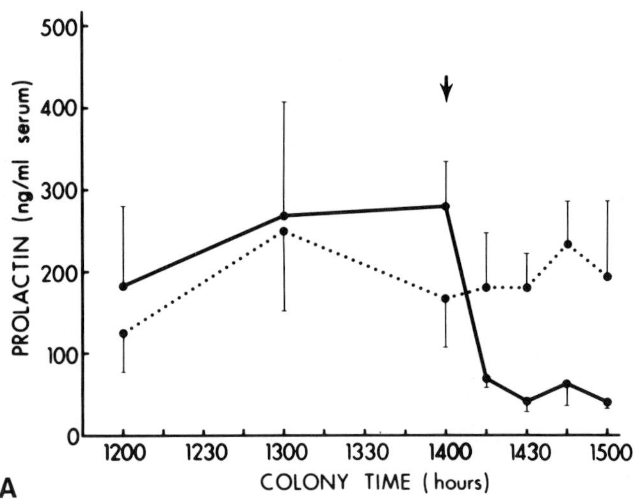

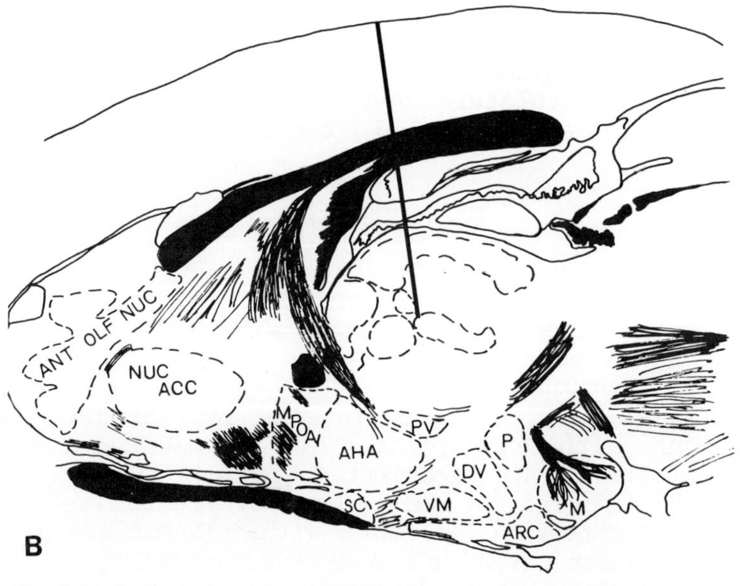

MBH, and therefore, presumably not by action on those elements most directly involved in PRL regulation. While it is possible that the low pretreatment PRL levels in CHD animals many have compromised our ability to detect a decrease in serum PRL which may have resulted from THC action within the MBH, the observations with the FSC animals provide some reassurance against this point. The ineffectiveness of THC in FSC rats, in which pretreatment PRL was not low, implies that the sup-

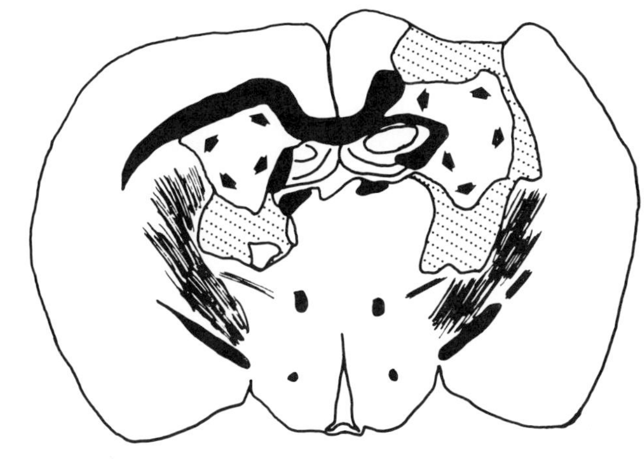

FIGURE 10. (A) Serum PRL concentrations (mean +/- SE) on proestrus in STS rats. Vehicle alone (n = 5; .....) or 0.5 mg THC/kg BW (n = 5; _____) was injected iv at 1400 h. Post-treatment PRL levels in the THC groups were significantly lower than both pretreatment levels within the THC group ($p < 0.01$) and post-treatment levels in the vehicle group ($p < 0.01$). Vehicle administration did not alter serum PRL levels ($p < 0.05$). (B) Sketch of the approximate location of lesions in STS rats. (C) Projection sketch of a frontal section of a representative brain from a STS rat at the level of the arcuate nucleus and median eminence. The stippling indicates the region of gliosis, the arrow indicate tissue-free spaces and the bar beneath the section provides a 4 mm reference scale.

pression of PRL by THC depends either upon the anterior hypothalamic region destroyed by these lesions, or upon the rostral connections which pass through this region into the MBH.

The fact that THC failed to suppress PRL levels in animals having FSC lesions produced with two different knife types which caused different local damage, and also failed to suppress serum PRL in PSC rats in which the lesions were located more rostrally near the junction of the medial preoptic and anterior hypothalamic areas, argues rather strongly in favor of the disruption of some critical fiber pathway. The remarkable brief rise in serum PRL in PSC rats remain unexplained, but may represent the unmasking of a THC-sensitive PRL-stimulatory mechanism; however further exploration of the possibility is necessary.

THC action at a site outside of the MBH with communication of its PRL suppressive effects over rostral afferent pathways into the MBH would be the interpretation most consistent with

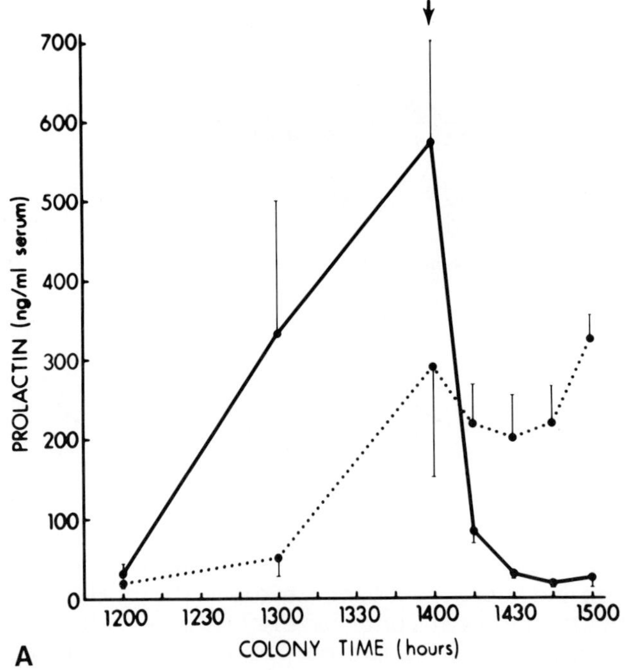
700
600
500
400
300
200
100
0
PROLACTIN (ng/ml serum)
1200
1230
1300
1330
1400
1430
1500
COLONY TIME (hours)
A

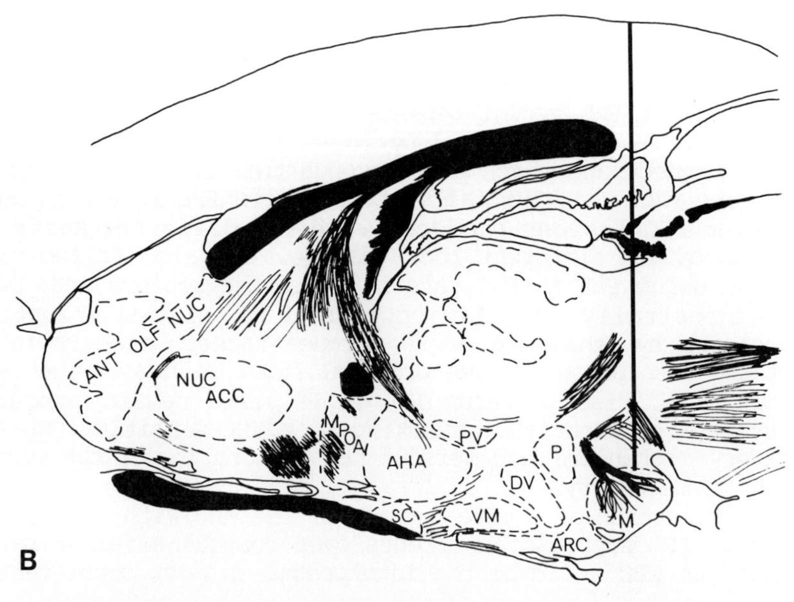
ANT OLF NUC
NUC ACC
MPOA
AHA
PV
P
DV
SC
VM
M
ARC
B

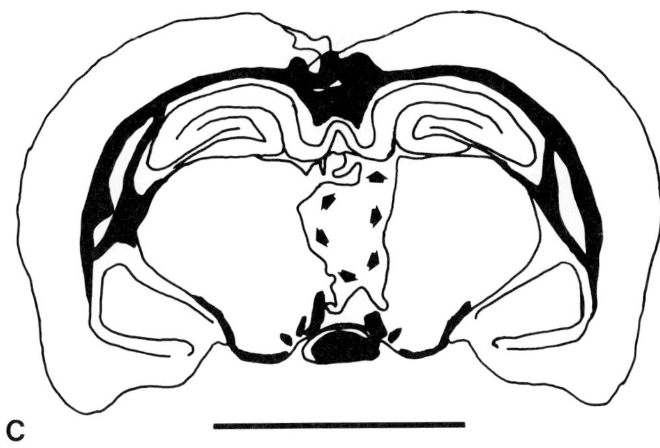

FIGURE 11. (A) Serum PRL concentrations (mean +/- SE) on proestrus in DLFS rats. Vehicle alone (n = 6; .....) or 0.5 mg THC/kg BW (n = 7; _____) was injected iv at 1400 h. PRL levels were significantly decreased at all post-treatment times in the THC group relative to that at 1400 h ($p < 0.05$). Post-treatment PRL levels in the THC group were also significantly lower than those in the vehicle group ($p <0.01$). Vehicle administration did not alter serum PRL levels ($p < 0.05$). (B) Sketch of the approximate location of lesions in DLFS rats. (C) Projection sketch of a frontal section of a representative brain from a DLFS rat at the level of the caudal portion of the mamillary nuclei. The bar beneath the section provides a 4 mm reference scale. The arrows indicate the margins of the lesion, a midline tissue-free space.

the data obtained from CHD and frontal cut animals. However, no indication is provided by these data as to whether the pertinent structures for THC action reside within the immediately rostral preoptic area or at other more distant sites. While earlier workers (7) found little regional localization of ^{3}H-THC within the rat brain after intraperitoneal injection of the labeled compound, Yashpal and Henry (8) more recently reported that after intravenous administration ^{3}H-THC was localized to the amygdala, striatum, cerebellum, and periaqueductal grey, but, notably, not to a hypothalamus or mesencephalic reticular formation, Thus an extra-hypothalamic site remote from the MBH for THC action appears quite tenable, and therefore, the effects of THC on serum PRL were determined in rats previously subjected to destruction of several extra-hypothalamic pathways believed to be functionally pertinent to the control of PRL secretion.

Septal lesions which interrupted the presumptive PRL-regulatory pathway from the orbitofrontal neocortex to the preoptic area by way of the lateral corticohypothalamic tract (9) failed to prevent the suppression of PRL after THC administration. In addition, although amygdaloid lesions can influence PRL secretion (10), lesioning of the ventral projections from the amygdala to the medial preoptic via the diagonal band of Broca, or sectioning of the dorsal stria terminalis pathway failed to prevent THC suppression of PRL secretion. Finally, midline lesions of the periventricular structures at the diencephalic-mesencephalic junction which included the dorsal longitudinal fasciculus interrupted the ascending PRL-regulatory pathway described by Tindal and Knaggs (9), but did not alter the suppressive effect of THC. These data suggest that the THC-induced suppression of serum PRL does not depend upon a site of action within the orbitofrontal neocortex or amygdala, and that if THC acts at a site in the midbrain, the essential rostral projections to the hypothalamus do not pass via fiber systems which are midline at the level of the diencephalic-mesencephalic junction.

In summary, the current data suggests that THC acts at a site or sites outside of the MBH to suppress PRL secretion in the rat, but that suppression does not appear to dependon hypothalamic projections from the orbitofrontal neocortex, amygdala, and a midbrain periventricular areas which have been implicated in the control of PRL secretion. Other extra-hypothalamic sites of potential importance in the preoptic, septal, hippocampal, mesencephalic and dorsal thalamic regions remain to be evaluated as to their possible role in the mediation of the PRL-suppressive action of THC.

ACKNOWLEDGMENTS

The data reported herein were submited by C.L.H. in partial fulfillment of the requirements for the degree of Doctor of Philosophy at Duke University. The authors thank the National Institute of Arthritis, Diabetes and Digestive and Kidney Disease for the gift of materials used in the prolactin radioimmunoassay, and the National Institute on Drug Abuse for the gift of THC.

REFERENCES

1. Mechoulam, R., Marijuana Chemistry, Science 168:1159 (1970).
2. Kramer, J., and Ben-David, M., Suppression of prolactin secretion by acute administration of delta-9-THC in rats,

Proc. Soc. Exper. Biol. Med. 147:482 (1974).
3. Kramer, J., and Ben-David, M., Prolactin suppression by (-)-delta-9-tetrahydrocannabinol (THC): involvement of serotonergic and dopaminergic pathways, Endocrinol. 103:452 (1978).
4. Hughes, C. L., Everett, J. W., and Tyrey, L., Delta-9-Tetrahydrocannabinol suppression of prolactin secretion in the rat: lack of direct pituitary effect, Endocrinol. 109:876 (1981).
5. Ayalon, D., Nir, I., Cordova, T., Bauminger, S., Puder, M., Naor, Z., Kashi, R., Zor, U., Harell, A., and Lindner, H. R., Acute effects of delta-1-tetrahydrocannabinol on the hypothalamo-pituitary-ovarian axis in the rat, Neuroendocrinol. 23:31 (1977).
6. Asch, R. H., Smith, C. G., Siler-Kohdr, T. M., and Pauerstein, C. J., Acute decreases in serum prolactin concentrations caused by delta-9-tetrahydrocannabinol in nonhuman primates, Fert. Steril. 32:571 (1979).
7. Layman, J. M., and Milton, A. S., Distribution of tritium labelled delta-1-tetrahydrocannabinol in the rat brain following intraperitoneal administration, Brit. J. Pharmacol. 42:308 (1971).
8. Yashpal, K., and Henry, J. L., Delta-9-tetrahydrocannabinol: central distribution after intravenous administration in the awake rat, Fed. Proc. 38:1402 (ABS) (1979).
9. Tindal. J. S., and Knaggs, G. S., Pathways in the forebrain of the rat concerned with the release of prolactin, Brain Res. 119:211 (1977).
10. Peters, J. A., and Gala, R. R., The effect of corticomedial amygdaloid lesions on prolactin secretion in male and female rats, Endocrinol. 106:1665 (1980).

Section V NEUROPHARMACOLOGIC ASPECTS

PHARMACOLOGICAL ACTIVITY OF DELTA-9-THC METABOLITES AND ANALOGS OF CBD, DELTA-8-THC AND DELTA-9-THC*

Billy R. Martin
Louis S. Harris
William L. Dewey

Department of Pharmacology
Medical College of Virginia
Virginia Commonwealth University
Richmond, Virginia

I. INTRODUCTION

The first systematic study of the structure-activity relationships of cannabinoids was carried out by Adams (1). Since these early investigations in the 1940's, publications from several laboratories (2-5), including our own (6-10), have appeared which describe some of the structural requirements for cannabinoid activity. By and large, the emphasis has been placed on establishing which structural modifications alter behavioral activity rather than the other pharmacological properties of the cannabinoids. One aspect has been the structural changes caused by metabolism, specifically with regard to whether or not metabolic processes activate or inactivate the naturally occurring cannabinoids (11). There is now evidence that shows that delta-9-tetrahydrocannabinol (THC) can exert behavioral effects itself without conversion to 11-hydroxy-delta-9-THC (6) or to other active metabolites (12-13). Of course, it has been confirmed that metabolites are pharmacologically active, but to what extent they contribute to the behavioral actions of THC has not been established (3,4,14-16). A second consideration of the structural requirements for cannabinoid activity (as reviewed by Razdan, this volume) is the implication that behavioral effects are

*Supported in part by NIDA grants DA-00490 and DA-00574.

ISBN 0-12-044620-0

mediated through a receptor mechanism (17). However, the search for cannabinoid receptors has been hampered by the lack of an antagonist.

The current interest in cannabinoids as potential therapeutic agents has cast a new direction on studies of structure-activity relationships. With the possibility that cannabinoids may eventually be useful in the treatment of a variety of diseases and/or their symptomatology (18,19), there is a need to develop cannabinoids that are more specific in their effects. In contrast to the early studies in which the interest was on increasing behavioral activity of cannabinoids through structural modifications, there is now a need in many cases to decrease the CNS effects and increase the therapeutic effectiveness of the cannabinoids.

We report here the pharmacological activity of a large number of newly synthesized metabolites and analogs of the cannabinoids in an effort to further characterize the structural requirements for behavioral activity as well as to attempt to separate other pharmacological effects from the behavioral effects. These compounds were evaluated for their ability to alter spontaneous activity and body temperature in mice, to block convulsions in mice and to produce static ataxia in dogs.

II. METHODS

A. Synthesis of Cannabinoids

3'-Hydroxy- and (+/-)-3',11-dihydroxy-delta-9-THC were synthesized as described previously (16). The synthesis of the remaining analogs will be described elsewhere. All drugs were prepared for pharmacological testing by dissolving 100 mg in 1 ml of a 1:1 mixture of emulphor (GAF Corp., Linden, NJ) and ethanol with the aid of a sonicator. Appropriate dilutions were made with the addition of emulphor:ethanol:saline (1:1:18).

B. Spontaneous Activity and Body Temperature in Mice

In order to conserve a limited supply of drug, rectal temperature and spontaneous activity were recorded in the same animal. Male ICR mice (22-30 g) were housed in the laboratory for 24 hr before treatment. The ambient temperature of the laboratory, which varied from 21 to 24° from day to day, was recorded at the beginning and end of each experiment. Rectal temperature was determined by a thermistor probe (inserted 25 mm) and a telethermometer (Yellow Springs Instrument Co., Yellow Springs, Ohio) just prior to vehicle or drug administration. Following the initial temperature determinations, mice were injected i.v. with either vehicle or drug (0.1 ml/10 g body weight) and immediately placed individually in photocell activity chambers. After the animals were placed in the chambers, interruptions of the photocell beams were recorded for ten minutes. The results were expressed as percent of control and the ED50's and their confidence limits were determined by the method of Litchfield and Wilcoxon (20). The mice were removed from the activity chambers and rectal temperature measured immediately and at 10 min intervals up to 60 min after drug administration. At least six mice were tested at each dose.

C. Overt Behavior in Dogs

The ability of cannabinoids to produce static ataxia (an effect unique to psychoactive cannabinoids) and other characteristic behavioral effects described by Walton et al. (21) was examined in mongrel dogs of either sex (8-12 kg). Prior to drug administration, the animals were observed for their degree of spontaneous activity, gait, tail-tuck, etc. The animals were then injected i.v. with the drug or vehicle (1 ml per 5 kg body weight) and observed for the occurrence of the signs described in Table I and rated according to the scale. Most of the signs were present for any given score. The animals were rated at 5 min intervals by three observers who were unaware of the drug treatment. The maximum scores (which usually occurred at 30 min) were averaged for each dog. A typical test session consisted of five animals that received either vehicle, 0.2 mg/kg of THC, or one of three other cannabinoid treatments.

D. Anticonvulsant Activity

For anticonvulsant activity against electroshock, mice were treated with vehicle or test drug i.v. 10 min prior to an electrical stimulus (60 Hz, 400 V) administered through ear clips. The number of animals exhibiting the maximal seizure (hind-limb extension) and the number of deaths were recorded for each group (10 mice per group). For protection against pentylenetetrazol-induced seizures, the mice were pretreated with the vehicle or test drug either 10 min (i.v.) or 30 min (i.p.) before i.p. administraton of 75 mg/kg of metrazol (Knoll Pharmaceutical Company, Whippany, N. J.). The number of animals exhibiting clonic and tonic convulsions and the

TABLE I. Quantification of Cannabinoid Behavioral Effects in Dogs

Score	CNS Depression[a]	Static Ataxia[b]	Prancing	Hyperreflexia[c]	Tail-Tucked
0					
1	+	3-5 min	-	-	-
2	+	2-3 min	+/-	+/-	+/-
3	+	1-2 min	+	+	+
4	++	< 1 min	+	++	+
5	++	30 sec	+	++	+
6	+++	Prostrate	N/A	++	+

[a] +slight decrease in spontaneous activity, ++moderate depression, +++severe depression and cannot be aroused.

[b] Animal sways forward and backward and/or side to side after standing in one position for the indicated time.

[c] Exaggerated reflex to an object thrust at their face. -absent, +slight, ++severe.

number of deaths per group were recorded. The results from both tests were expressed as percent of vehicle-treated mice.

II. RESULTS AND DISCUSSION

A. Metabolites of THC

There has been considerable interest in the side-chain hydroxylated metabolites of delta-8- and delta-9-THC since it has been demonstrated that they are formed in a number of species (5,22,23), including humans (24). The cannabinoids may be hydroxylated only in the side chain or di- and trihydroxylated in the side chain and at positions 11 and/or 8. The monohydroxylated metabolites (side chain) in the delta-8-THC series have been shown to exhibit cannabinoid activity (5,25) but those in the delta-9-THC series have not been investigated. 3'-Hydroxy-delta-9-THC was synthesized and tested for cannabinoid activity. The results in Table II show that this metabolite has a pharmacological profile similar to that of delta-9-THC. The major difference between the two is 3'-OH-delta-9-THC is almost 3 times more potent that delta-9-THC in all three tests. These results are consistent with those reported for the delta-8-THC series (5,15). To our knowledge, the metabolites hydroxylated both in the side chain and at position 11 have not been tested for cannabinoid activity. Indeed, they might be expected to have little activity based upon the relative inactivity of compounds such as 8,11-diOH-delta-9-THC. Therefore, (±)-3',11-diOH-delta-9-THC was synthesized and tested for cannabinoid activity (Table II). The dihydroxylated metabolite had cannabinoid activity in all three tests but was approximately three times less potent that delta-9-THC. Hydroxylation at either position 3' or 11 enhances THC activity 3 or 4 (Table VII) fold, respectively, but hydroxylation at both positions decreases activity. This attenuation in potency may well be due to the increased polarity with a resultant diminuation in brain penetrability.

Clearly, these two metabolites have the potential of contributing to the behavioral pharmacology of THC. The biodisposition studies of cannabinoids carried out thus far have not revealed large quantitites of metabolites in brain so that it would appear that these metabolites play a relatively minor role in the expression of cannabinoid activity. Few, if any, studies have been conducted with the sole intention of measuring 3'-OH- and 3',11-diOH-delta-9-THC in brain during periods of delta-9-THC induced behavioral activity, thereby making it difficult to assess their true contributions. However, our

TABLE II. Pharmacological Activity of Delta-9-THC and Metabolites

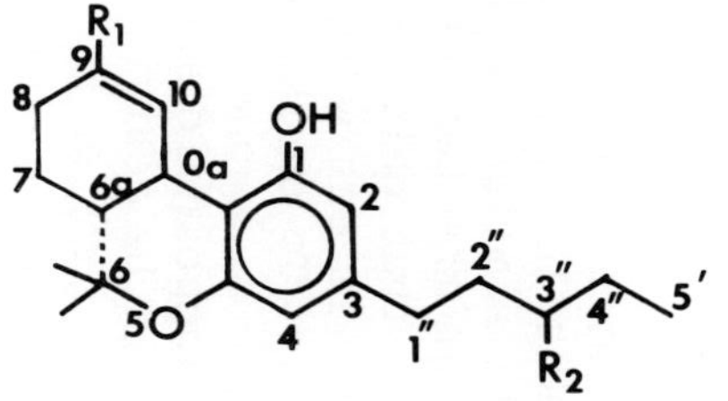

COMPOUND	NAME	R_1	R_2	SPONTANEOUS ACTIVITY[A]	HYPOTHERMIA DOSE	HYPOTHERMIA Δ^0 C	STATIC ATAXIA DOSE	STATIC ATAXIA SCORE	(N)
	Δ^9-THC	CH_3	H	3.2 (1.7 - 6.2)	2.5	3.4	0.1	1	(3)
					5.0	4.4	0.2	3	(4)
					7.5	4.6	0.4	4	(2)
					10.0	5.0			
1	3'-OH-Δ^9-THC	H	OH	0.8 (0.4 - 1.5)	0.1	1.2	0.05	1	(2)
					0.3	2.1	0.1	2	(2)
					1.0	3.6	0.2	5	(2)
					3.0	4.9			
					10.0	8.4			
2	3',11-DiOH-Δ^9-THC	OH	OH	8.7 (3.6 - 20.8)	3.0	1.3	0.2	1	(1)
					6.0	1.1	0.5	3	(2)
					10.0	3.9			
					30.0	5.2			

[A] ED_{50} (C.L.) mg/kg

data suggest that if they do contribute in a significant way, it would be to the overall pharmacological effect rather than to a specific THC action.

B. Oxepine Derivatives of THC

It has generally been assumed that the intact benzopyran system is necessary for behavioral activity because the opening of the pyran ring (to form CBD, for example) leads to complete loss of behavioral activity. In order to investigate the importance of the B ring (Table III) further, two novel analogs of THC were prepared in which the pyran was expanded to a seven-membered ring with an exo-cyclic methylene rather than gem di-methyls (Table III). These two alterations in the pyran ring essentially elimated cannabinoid activity in all three tests as demonstrated by compound 3. It may be that expansion of the pyran ring results in sufficient realignment of the two remaining rings to cause loss of activity. Interestingly, when the pentyl side chain of 3 was replaced with a 1,2-dimethylheptyl side chain (4), effects on spontaneous activity and body temperature were restored almost completely but the compound was at least 5 times less active that THC in the dog static ataxia test. This separation in the composite effects of THC is difficult to attribute to any one of the three structural changes that were made. However, it is well known that branching the side chain enhances cannabinoid activity as first shown by Adams (1). It may be that the structural requirements for altering spontaneous activity and hypothermic effects are less strict than those for the dog static ataxia test which may account for the fact that the dimethylheptyl side chain enhances activity in mice more readily than in the static ataxia test in dogs.

C. Substitution at the 11 Position

The discovery that the 11-hydroxy metabolite of THC exhibited potent cannabinoid activity (25) served to demonstrate the importance of the 11 position. Several structural modifications of this position have been reported previously. Removal of the 11 position for THC does not abolish behavioral activity, but merely reduces it 50-60% (6). On the other hand, when the double bond is delta-9,11 rather than delta-9,10, the behavioral activity is reduced dramatically (26). The addition of a methyl (6) or methoxy (9) group to position 11 also reduces, but does not eliminate, behavioral activity. A series of delta-8-THC analogs were recently synthesized in which aromatic and aliphatic hydrocarbon groups were substi-

TABLE III. Pharmacological Activity of Delta-9-THC Analogs

COMPOUND	STRUCTURE	SPONTANEOUS ACTIVITY[A]	HYPOTHERMIA DOSE	HYPOTHERMIA Δ°C	STATIC ATAXIA DOSE	STATIC ATAXIA SCORE (N)
Δ^9-THC	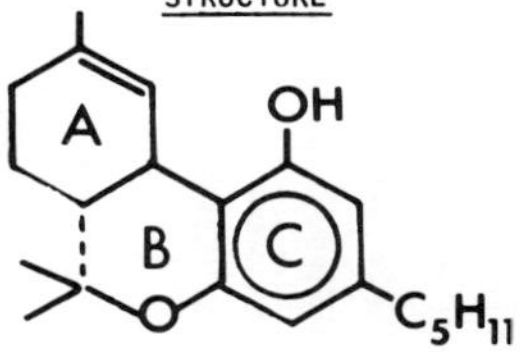	3.2 (1.7 - 6.2)	2.5	3.4	0.1	1 (3)
			5.0	4.4	0.2	3 (4)
			7.5	4.6	0.4	4 (2)
			10.0	5.0		
3	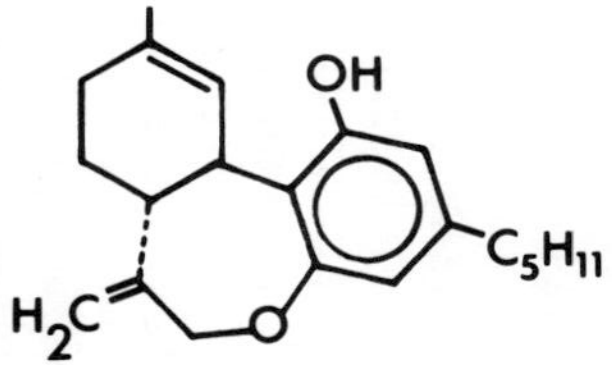	41% at 100 mg/kg	30	0	2.0	0 (2)
			100	0	5.0	0 (1)
4	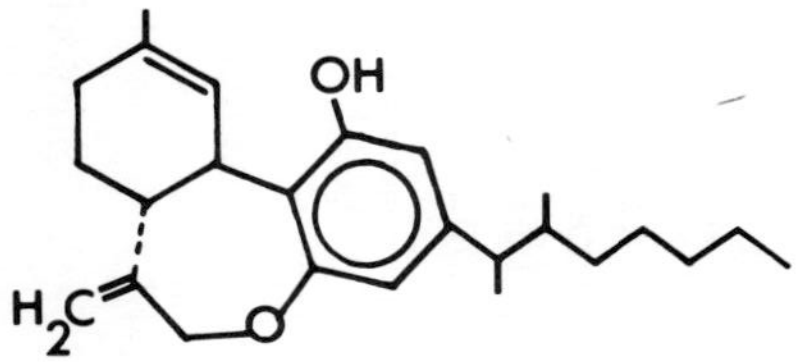	4.2 (1.5 - 11)	5	0.3	0.5	0 (3)
			10	4.5		
			30	5.3		

[A] ED_{50} (C.L.) mg/kg

tuted for the 11 methyl. The effect of these analogs on spontaneous activity and body temperature of mice is depicted in Table IV. All of these compounds were 4-5 times less effective than delta-8-THC in producing hypoactivity with the exception of the phenyl derivative (5) which was almost 10 times less potent. The hypothermic effect was also reduced in all of these compounds, with the exception of the butyl derivative (8). The two exceptions provided by the phenyl and butyl substitutions are probably anomalies rather than unique structural requirements for specific cannabinoid actions. From these data, it appears that optimum activity occurs when a methyl group is at position 9.

TABLE IV. Pharmacological Activity of Delta-8-THC Analogs

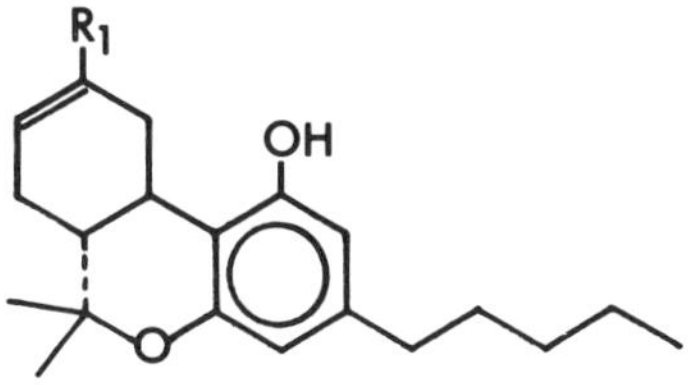

COMPOUND	NAME	R_1	SPONTANEOUS ACTIVITY[A]	HYPOTHERMIA[B] DOSE	Δ°C
	Δ^8-THC	CH_3	7.1 (4.5-11.2)	5 10 20	0.2 0.7 2.7
5	9-nor-9-Phenyl-Δ^8-THC	C_6H_5-	67 (44-102)	30 100	1.3 1.9
6	9-nor-9-Benzyl-Δ^8-THC	$C_6H_5CH_2$-	32 (10-101)	30 60	0.7 1.2
7	9-nor-9-Isopropyl-Δ^8-THC	$(CH_3)_2CH$-	26 (11-60)	30 100	0.4 0.9
8	9-nor-9-(n)Butyl-Δ^8-THC	$(CH_3)(CH_2)_3$-	32 (17-61)	30 60	4.3 5.0
9	9-nor-9-(1-Hydroxy)-propyl-Δ^8-THC	$CH_3CH_2C(OH)H$-	39 (24-61)	30 60	0 0.9
10	11-N-Methyl-Δ^8-THC	CH_3NCH_2-	11 (6-20)	5 10 20	0 0 0.4

[A] ED50 (C.L.) mg/kg

[B] Dose in mg/kg

D. Substitutions on the C-ring

Alterations in the substituents on the C ring have generally resulted in a marked reduction in behavioral activity. Edery et al. (2) found that addition of methyl, ethyl, carbomethoxy or acetyl groups at positions 2 or 4 attenuated behavioral effects in rhesus monkeys. Also, we have shown that interposing the phenolic hydroxyl with the pentyl side chain eliminated behavioral activity but did not alter the cardiovascular effects (8). An analog of delta-8-THC in which a hydroxyl group was added at position 2 was recently synthesized by Razdan (synthesis to be published elsewhere) and the structure is shown in Table V. 2-Hydroxy-delta-8-THC (12) was almost as active as delta-8-THC in producing hypoactivity but was inactive in decreasing body temperature. In contrast, 11 (the O-methyl derivative of 12) was less effective in producing both hypoactivity and hypothermia. It will be interesting to see if 2-OH-delta-8-THC produces static ataxia in dogs. Hydroxylation at the 2 position may well attenuate cannabinoid behavioral activity without altering its general CNS depres-

TABLE V. Pharmacological Activity of Delta-8-THC Analogs

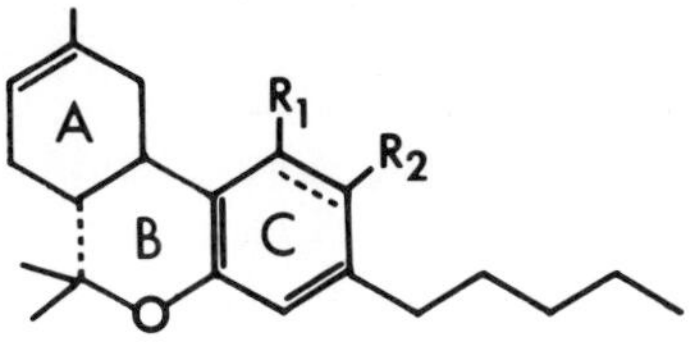

COMPOUND	NAME	R_1	R_2	SPONTANEOUS ACTIVITY[A]	HYPOTHERMIA[B] DOSE	Δ°C
	Δ^8-THC	OH	H	7.1 (4.5-11.2)	5	0.2
					10	0.7
					20	2.7
11	2-OH-O-METHYL-Δ^8-THC	OCH_3	OH	40 (10-163)	30	0.4
					100	2.4
12	2-OH-Δ^8-THC	OH	OH	10 (3-33)	3	0.4
					10	0.5
					30	0.2
13	Δ^8-THC-1,2-BISQUINONE	=O	=O	12 (5-32)	3	0.4
					10	0.7
					20	1.9
					30	2.2

sant properties. The delta-8-THC-1,2-bisquinone (13) was also synthesized and tested for activity. Suprisingly, the bisquinone was only slightly less potent that delta-8-THC in its effects on spontaneous activity and hypothermia. Edery et al. (2) have reported that delta-8-THC-1,4-bisquinone was at least 100 times less active that delta-8-THC in producing behavioral effects in monkeys. It may be that the 1,2-bisquinone will also be devoid of behavioral effects in the dog.

E. Analogs of CBD

The anticonvulsant activity of CBD has been studied extensively and antiseizure activity has been observed, albeit somewhat weak, in a variety of tests (see Karler and Turkanis ref. 27, for additional discussion). Recently, Razdan synthesized a gamma-aminobutyric acid (GABA) derivative of CBD (14, Table VI) in an effort to increase the anticonvulsant activity of CBD (the synthesis will be described elsewhere). In addition, an N-ethylamine derivative (15, Table VI) was also prepared. These analogs were compared to CBD for their ability to alter spontaneous activity, body temperature and produce lethality as well as anticonvulsant activity. The results in Table VI show that CBD is capable of producing hypoactivity and hypothermia at high doses, although it is considerably less potent than delta-9-THC. The addition of a GABA functional group increased the effect on spontaneous activity slightly and body temperature to a somewhat greater degree. The striking difference between CBD and the GABA analog was the greater lethality of the latter. In addition, GABA, a known amino acid inhibitory neurotransmitter, waspractically devoid of any effects in doses up to 400 mg/kg when given i.v. It may be that the analog serves as a vehicle for allowing GABA to penetrate brain much in the same way that chlorination of GABA (to form bacloflen) increases its brain penetrability (28). One might also expect the GABA analog to effect motor coordination, which it did not do in doses up to 30 mg/kg as measured in the inverted-screen test as described previously (29).

When an N-ethylamine group was added at position 10 (15), the effect on spontaneous activity was enhanced 10 fold (compared to CBD) and was nearly equivalent to that produced by THC. In addition, the lethality was much greater than that of CBD. A dose of 6 mg/kg (i.v.) produced 88% lethality within 5 min of the injection. A reliable LD50 could not be determined due to a very steep dose-response curve.

The anticonvulsant activity of compounds 14 and 15 were compared to that of CBD in mice treated with either electroshock or pentylenetetrazol. CBD at doses of 65 mg/kg i.v.

TABLE VI. Pharmacological Activity of Cannabidiol (CBD) Analogs[a]

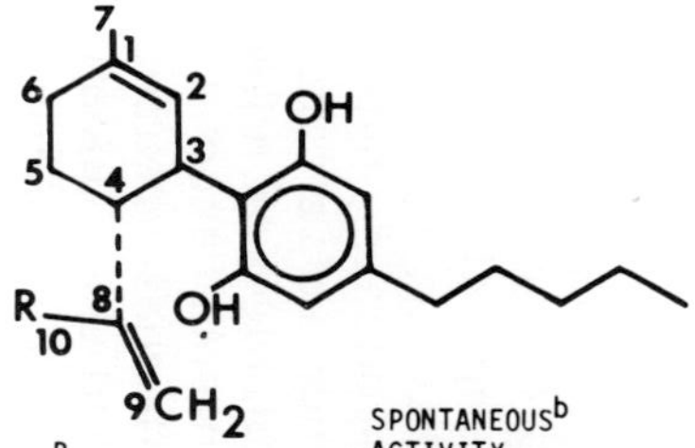

COMPOUND	NAME	R	SPONTANEOUS[b] ACTIVITY	HYPOTHERMIA[c] DOSE	Δ^0 C	LETHALITY[d]
	CBD	CH_3-	40 (25 -65)	50 75 100	0.5 2.2 2.6	> 100
14	10-(3-Aminobutyryl-amido)-CBD	$NH_2(CH_2)_3CONHCH_2$-	30 (23 - 38)	25 30 35	1.3 2.0 2.1	41 (37 - 47)
15	10-(N-Ethylamino)-CBD	$CH_3CH_2NHCH_2$-	4 (1.4 - 11.6)	2.5 5.0	0 1.2	<6.0
	Gamma-Aminobutyric acid	---	f	400	1.4	ND[e]

[a]Monoterpenoid numbering system due to lack of a pyran ring in CBD.

[b]ED_{50} (C.L.) mg/kg

[c]Dose of mg/kg

[d]LD_{50} (C.L.) mg/kg

[e]Not determined

[f]13% effect at 400 mg/kg

completely blocked tonic seizures and death induced by electroshock. Compounds 14 and 15 were inactive at doses up to 25 and 5 mg/kg, respectively. In the pentylenetetrazol-treated mice, CBD (45 mg/kg, i.v.) did not block clonic seizures but did block tonic seizures (72% of vehicle-treated animals) and lethality (38%). Compound 14 produced a 31 and 21% blockade of tonic seizures and lethality, respectively, at a dose of 25 mg/kg, i.v. Higher doses could not be given due to its lethality. Compound 15 was without effect on either pentylenetetrazol-induced tonic seizures or lethality at a dose of 5 mg/kg, the highest dose permissible without producing death. Compound 15 was also given i.p. at a dose of 25 mg/kg 30 min prior to penylenetetrazol and it only produced a 24% blockade of pentylenetetrazol-induced tonic seizures and did not prevent deaths. The addition of an N-ethyl or a GABA functional group does not appear to impart greater anticonvulsant activity to CBD.

F. Evaluation of Miscellaneous THC and Cannabinol (CBN) Derivatives in the Dog Static Ataxia Test

The behavioral activity of a variety of analogs is presented in Table VII. Methylation of the phenolic hydroxyl group (16) of THC reduced behavioral activity almost 25 fold, whereas methylation of 11-hydroxy-delta-8-THC produced a compound (19) that was about three fold less potent than delta-8-THC. These reductions in activity are consistent with the data presented in Table V in which methylation of the phenolic hydroxyl in 2-OH-delta-8-THC attenuated its effect on spontaneous activity almost 4-fold.

In our earlier discussion of the oxepine derivatives with the exo methylene unit (3), we stressed that possible realignment of the molecule due to expansion of the pyran ring might have resulted in the loss of activity. It may also be that replacement of the gem dimethyls with a methylene unit reduces activity. Loev et al. (30) have shown that a ketone at position 6 reduces cannabinoid activity. When an hydroxyl group was substituted for one of the gem dimethyls, behavioral activity was not altered. Replacement of the dimethyl groups with a carbonyl to form analog 23 resulted in loss of activity. This abolition of activity could have been due to any one of the structural changes in compound 23. However, compound 22 differs from 23 only in that it has the 6,6-dimethyls rather than the ketone and it exhibits weak cannabinoid activity. Therefore, these results, taken together, suggest that both gem dimethyls are not necessary for behavioral activity but certain structural modifications at position 6 can result inaltered behavioral activity. The position of the double

TABLE VII. Evaluation of Other Cannabinoids in the Dog Static Ataxia Test At Least Three Doses of Each Compound was Tested, Usually with Two or More Dogs/Dose

COMPOUND	NAME	STRUCTURE	ACTIVITY RELATIVE TO Δ^9-THC	COMMENTS
	Δ^9-THC		1.0	
	Δ^8-THC		0.4	
16	O-Methyl-Δ^9-THC	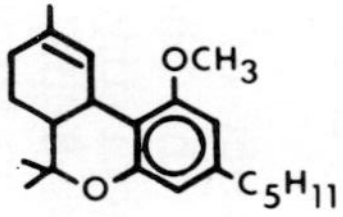	0.04	
17	6-nor-6β-OH-Δ^9-THC	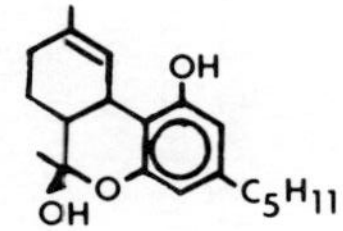	1.0	
18	11-OH-Δ^9-THC	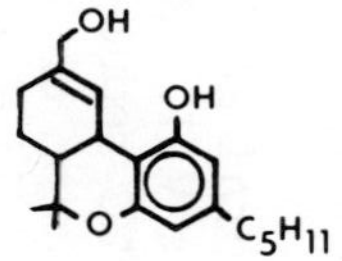	4.0	a
19	11-Methoxy-Δ^8-THC	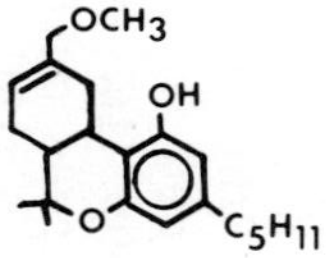	0.1	[a]0.3 compared to Δ^8-THC

COMPOUND	NAME	STRUCTURE	ACTIVITY RELATIVE TO Δ^9-THC	COMMENTS
20	(±)-11-OH-Δ^{6a-10a}-THC	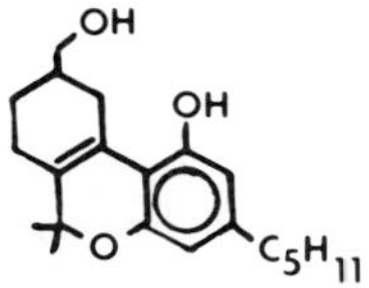	< 1.0	Difficult to assess due to rapid onset of effects and short duration.
21	9-<u>nor</u>-9β-OH-Δ^{10}-THC	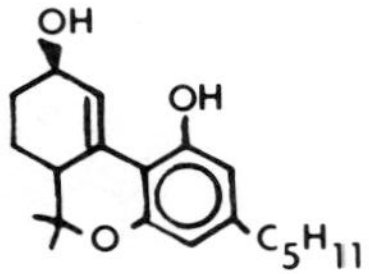	0.4	b
22	9-<u>nor</u>-9-OH-Δ^{10}-THC	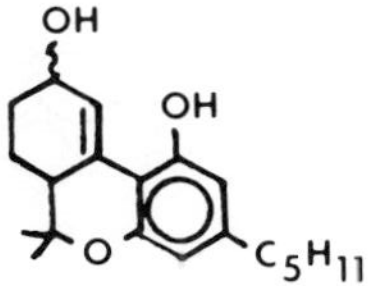	0.2	
23	6,6,9-tri-<u>nor</u>-6-oxo-9-OH-Δ^{10}-THC	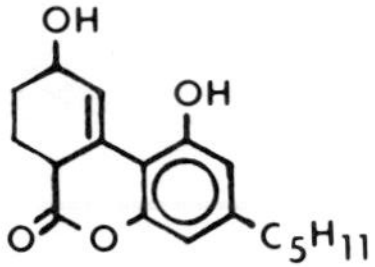		Causes marked sedation at 2.0 mg/kg, otherwise not cannabinoid.

TABLE VII. (Continued)

COMPOUND	NAME	STRUCTURE	ACTIVITY RELATIVE TO Δ^9-THC	COMMENTS
	CBN		∼ 0.2	Severe CNS depression after 5.0 mgkg
24	9-*nor*-CBN	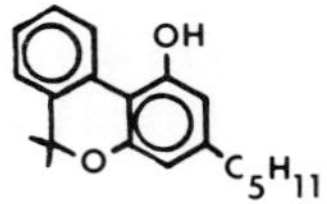 OH, C_5H_{11}	0.2	
25	9-nor-9-OH-CBN	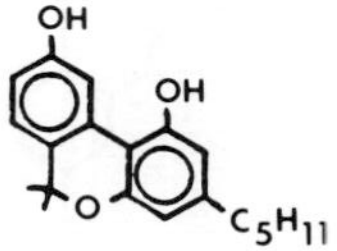 OH, OH, C_5H_{11}		[b]Not cannabinoid severe CNS depression after 10 mg/kg
26	11-OH-CBN	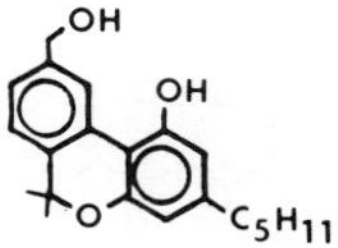 OH, OH, C_5H_{11}	∼ 0.5	Somewhat variable response. All of the typical cannabinc signs were seen after 1.0 mg/kg before the animal became prostrate.
27		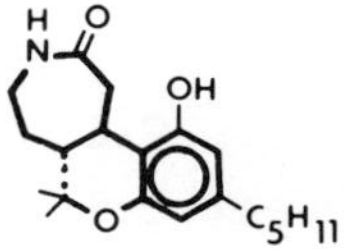 H, N, O, OH, C_5H_{11}	0.5	
28		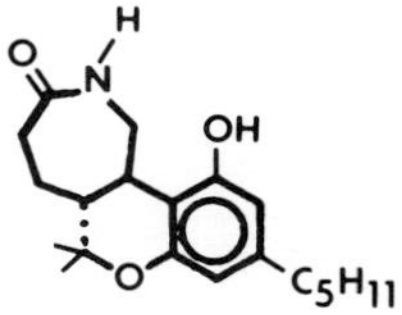 H, N, O, OH, C_5H_{11}		Not cannabinoid up to 8 mg/kg

COMPOUND	NAME	STRUCTURE	ACTIVITY RELATIVE TO Δ^9-THC	COMMENTS
29		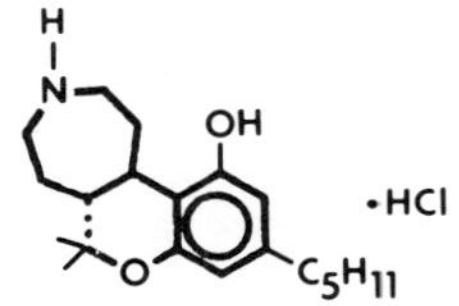 ·HCl		Marked CNS depression at 8 mg/kg, few other cannabinoid signs
30		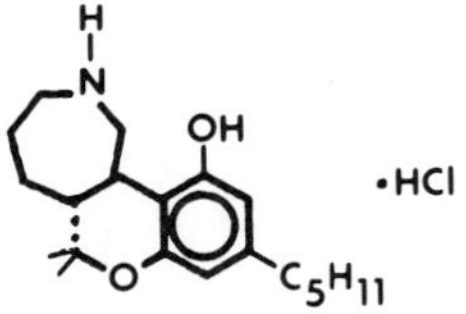 ·HCl		Marked CNS depression at 8 mg/kg, few other cannabinoid signs
31		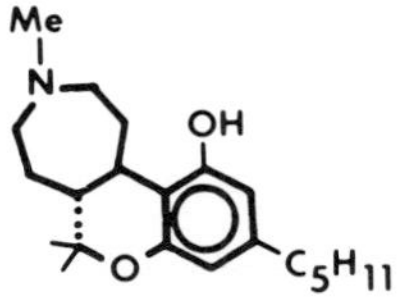	0.1	
32		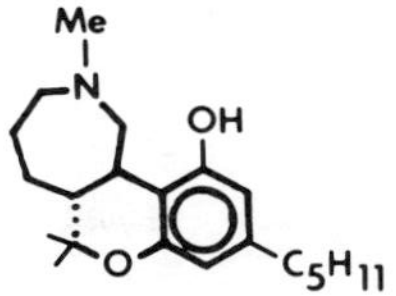		Slight CNS depression at 8 mg/kg, few other signs

[a] Reported previously by Wilson-*et al.* (9)

[b] Reported previously by Wilson *et al.* (33)

bond in delta-9-THC appears to be of considerable importance since delta-6a,10a-THC is less active than delta-9-THC (2,30). The activity of (+/-)-11-OH-delta-6a,10a-THC (20) was somewhat less than that of delta-9-THC but at least 4 times less than that of 11-OH-delta-9-THC (18). Behavioral activity was also decreased when the double bond was in position 10 as shown in 21 and 22. Analog 23 was inactive but several important changes were made in this structure.

There has also been some interest in CBN since it has been shown to possess weak cannabinoid effects in humans (31). Removal of the 11-methyl (24) did not diminish CBN's behavioral activity (Table VII). Actually, its potency is somewhat comparable to that of 11-nor-delta-9-THC (6). When thell-methyl position was replaced with a hydroxyl group (25), cannabinoid behavioral activity was eliminated completely. This is a contradistinction toll-nor-9-beta-OH-hexahydrocannabinol, which is much more active than THC (7). As in THC, 11-hydroxylation of CBN (26) results in increased behavioral activity (Table VII). 11-Hydroxy-CBN, a known metabolite of CBN (32), is approximately one-half as active as delta-9-THC.

The last group of compounds, synthesized by Drs. Rice and Iorio of the National Institutes of Health, are benzopyranoazepines, which for the most part are considerably less active that THC. The most active of these derivatives was azepine-10-one (27), which had approximately half the activity of THC. The azepine-9-one (28) and the two unsubstituted azepines (29 and 30) were completely devoid of cannabinoid effects in the dog static ataxia test, with the exception of CNS depression at high doses. The N-methyl azepine derivatives (31 and 32) exhibited little, if any, effects in this test.

III. SUMMARY

The results presented herein demonstrate several structural changes that either attenuate or enhance cannabinoid potency. The 3'-hydroxy metabolite was more potent than THC, whereas dihyroxylation at positions 3' and 11 diminished, but did not eliminate, activity. In addition, 11-hydroxylation of CBN increased cannabinoid behavioral potency almost two and one-half times.

Alterations in the A ring and its substituents also produced dramatic changes in cannabinoid potency. Substitution of bulky hydrocarbon groups at position 9 reduced effects on spontaneous activity and body temperature, in general. The addition of an N-methyl substituent at position 11 did not alter spontaneous activity. Also, changes in the position of the double bond greatly reduced behavioral potency. When the

A ring was changed to a heterocyclic 7-membered ring (benzopyranoazepine), cannabinoid effects were attenuated.

Changes in the pyran (B) ring all served to reduce cannabinoid activity in one way or another. Expansion of the pyran ring to an oxepine, replacement of the gem dimethyl groups with a ketone or methylene resulted in diminution of cannabinoid effects.

Several changes were made in the phenolic ring (C), such as methylation of the phenolic hydorxyl (reduces activity), addition of an hydroxyl group at position 2 (no loss in producing hypoactivity), and formation of a 1,2-bisquinone (no loss in producing hypoactivity).

Selected structural modifications appeared to alter some of the cannabinoid effects more than others. Compounds with increased ability to produce hypoactivity relative to hypothermia included the oxepine with the DMHP side chain (4), 11-N-methylamino-delta-8-THC (10), 2-OH-delta-8-THC (12), and 10-(N-ethylamino)-CBD (15). There was only one compound tested that had a greater effect on body temperature relative to its effects on spontaneous activity and that was11-nor-9-butyl-delta-8-THC (8). It appears that compounds that are potent in producing both hypoactivity and hypothermia are likely to produce behavioral effects as measured in the dog static ataxia test. Compounds that only diminish spontaneous activity in mice at high doses probably lack cannabinoid behavioral effects, CBD being a prime example. Also, several compounds (Table VII) produced marked sedation in dogs, yet no other signs were present. These data do show that it is possible to get some separation of cannabinoid effects. Certainly the general depressant properties were retained in some of the analogs when the other cannabinoid behavioral effects were lost.

ACKNOWLEDGMENTS

The authors acknowledge the technical assistance of Ramona Winkler. Delta-9-, 11-hydroxy-delta-9-, delta-8-THC, CBD and CBN were provided by NIDA. Compounds 1-15 were synthesized by Dr. Raj Razdan and his colleagues at the SISA Institute for Research, Cambridge, MA. Compound 16 was synthesized by Dr. I. M. Uwaydah while he was in this department. Compounds 17, 19-26 were prepared by Drs. R.S. Wilson and E. L. May. Finally, compounds 27-32 were synthesized by Drs. K. Rice and M. A. Iorio at the National Institutes of Health.

REFERENCES

1. Adams, R., Marihuana, Harvey Lect. 37:168-197 (1942).
2. Edery, H., Grunfeld, Y., Ben-Zvi, Z., and Mechoulam, R., Structural requirements for cannabinoid activity, Ann. N. Y. Acad. Sci. 191:40-50 (1971).
3. Mechoulam, R., and Edery, H., Structure-activity relationships in the cannabinoid series, in "Marihuana, Chemistry, Pharmacology, Metabolism and Clinical Effects" (R. Mechoulam, ed.), pp. 101-136. Academic Press, New York, 1973.
4. Hollister, L. E., Structure-activity relationships in man of cannabis constituents and homologs and metabolites of delta-9-tetrahydrocannabinol, Pharmacol. 11:3-11 (1974).
5. Agurell, S., Binder, M., Fonseka, K., Lindgren, J.-E., Leander, K., Martin, B. R., Nilsson, I. M., Nordqvist, M., Ohlsson, A., and Widman, M., Cannabinoids: metabolites hydroxylated in the pentyl side chain, in "Marihuana, Chemistry, Biochemistry and Cellular Effects" (G. G. Nahas, ed.), pp. 141. Springer-Verlag, New York, 1976.
6. Martin, B. R., Dewey, W. L., Harris, L. S., Beckner, J., Wilson, R. S., and May, E. L., Marihuana-like activity of new synthetic tetrahydrocannabinols, Pharmacol. Biochem. Behav. 3:849-853 (1975).
7. Wilson, R. S., May, E. L., Martin, B. R., and Dewey, W. L., 9-Nor-9-hydroxyhexahydrocannabinols, Synthesis, some behavioral and analgesic properties and comparisons with the tetrahydrocannabinols, J. Med. Chem. 19:1165-1167 (1976).
8. Adams, M. D., Earnhardt, J. T., Martin, B. R., Harris, L. S., Dewey, W. L., and Razdan, R. K., A cannabinoid with cardiovascular activity but no overt behavioral effects, Experientia 33: 1204-1205 (1977).
9. Wilson, R. S., Martin, B. R., and Dewey, W. L., Some 11-substituted tetrahydrocannabinols, Synthesis and comparison with the potent cannabinoid metabolites, the 11-hydroxytetrahydrocannabinols, J. Med. Chem. 22: 879-882 (1979).
10. Martin, B. R., Balster, R. L., Razdan, R. K., Harris, L. S., and Dewey, W. L., Behavioral comparisons of the stereoisomers of tetrahydrocannabinols, Life Sci. 29:565-574 (1981).
11. Mechoulam, R., Marihuana Chemistry, Science 168:1159-1166 (1970).
12. Martin, B. R., Agurell, S., Krieglstein, J., and Rieger, H., Perfusion of the isolated rat brain with ^{14}C-delta-1-tetrahydrocannabinol, Biochem. Pharmacol. 26:2307-2309 (1977).

13. Carney, J. M., Balster, R. L., Martin, B. R., and Harris, L. S., Effects of systemic and intraventricular administration of cannabinoids on schedule-controlled responding in the squirrel monkey, J. Pharmacol. Exp. Ther. 210:399-404 (1979).
14. Perez-Reyes, M., Timmons, M. C., Lipton, M. A., Davis, K. H., and Wall, M. E., Intravenous injection in man of delta-9-tetrahydrocannabinol and 11-OH-delta-9-tetrahydrocannabinol, Science 177:633-635 (1972).
15. Ohlsson, A., Widman, M., Carlsson, Ryman, T., and Strid, C., Plasma and brain levels of delta-6-THC and seven monooxygenated metabolites correlated to the cataleptic effect in the mouse, Acta Pharmacol. Toxicol. 47:308-317 (1980).
16. Handrick, G. R., Duffley, R. P., Lambert, G., Murphy, J. G., Dalzell, H. C., Howes, J. F., Razdan, R. K., Martin, B. R., Harris L. S., and Dewey, W. L., 3'-Hydroxy- and (+/-)-3',11-dihydroxy-delta-9-tetrahydrocannabinol (THC); biologically active metabolites of delta-9-THC, J. Med. Chem. (in press).
17. Harris, L. S., Carchman, R. A., and Martin B. R., Evidence for the existence of specific cannabinoid binding sites, Life Sci. 22:1131-1138 (1978).
18. Cohen, S., and Stillman, R. C. (eds.), "The Therapeutic Potential of Marihuana." Plenum, New York and London, 1976.
19. Harris, L. S., Dewey, W. L., and Razdan, R. K., Cannabis, its chemistry, pharmacology and toxicology, in "Handbook of Experimental Pharmacology", volume 45 (W. R. Martin, ed.), pp. 371-429. Springer-Verlag, Berlin, Heidelberg, New York, 1977.
20. Litchfield, L. T., and Wilcoxon, F. A., A simplified method of evaluating dose effect experiments, J. Pharmacol. Exp. Ther. 96:99-113 (1949).
21. Walton, R. P., Martin, L. F., and Keller, J. H., The relative activity of various purified products obtained from American grown hashish, J. Pharmacol. Exp. Ther. 62:239-251 (1938).
22. Wall, M. E., and Brine, D. R., Identification of cannabinoids and metabolites in biological materials by combined gas-liquid chromatography-mass spectrometry, in "Marihuana: Chemistry, Biochemistry, and Cellular Effects" (G. G. Nahas, ed.), pp. 51-62. Springer-Verlag, New York, Heidelberg, Berlin, 1976.
23. Harvey, D. J., Martin B. R., and Paton, W. D. M., Compartive <u>in vivo</u> metabolism of delta-1-tetrahydrocannabinol (THC), cannabidiol (CBD) and cannabinol (CBN) by several species, in "Recent Developments in Mass Spectrometry in

Biochemistry and Medicine" (A. Frigerio, ed.), pp. 161-184. Plenum, New York and London, 1978.

24. Halldin, M. M., Widman, M., v.Bahr, C., Lindgren, J.-E., and Martin, B. R., Identification of in vitro metabolites of delta-1-tetrahydrocannabinol formed by human livers, Drug. Met. Disp. (in press).
25. Christensen, H. D., Freudenthal, R. I., Gidley, J. T., Rosenfeld, R., Boegli, G., Testino, L., Brine, D. R., Pitt, C. G., and Wall, M. E., Activity of delta-8- and delta-9-tetrahydrocannabinol and related compounds in the mouse, Science 172:165-167 (1971).
26. Binder, M., Edery, H., and Porath, G., Delta-7-tetrahydrocannabinol, a non-psychotropic cannabinoid: structure-activity considerations in the cannabinoid series, in "Marihuana: Biological Effects" (G. G. Nahas and W. D. M. Paton, eds.), pp. 71-80. Pergamon Press, New York, 1979.
27. Karler, R., and Turkanis, S. A., Cannabis and epilepsy, in "Marihuana: Biological Effects" (G. G. Nahas and W. D. M.Paton, eds.), pp. 619-641. Pergamon Press, New York, 1978.
28. Faigle, J. W., and Keberle, H., The metabolism and pharmacokinetics of Lioresal, in "Spacticity - A Topical Survey" (W. Bukmayer, ed.), pp. 94-100. Han Huber Publications, Vienna, 1972.
29. Martin, B. R., Vincek, W. C., and Balster, R. L., Studies on the disposition of phencyclidine in mice, Drug Metab. Disp. 8:49-54 (1980).
30. Loev, B., Bender, P. E., Dowalo, F., Macko, E., and Fowler, P. J., Cannabinoids, Structure-activity studies related to 1,2-dimethylheptyl derivations, J. Med. Chem. 16:1200-1206 (1973).
31. Perez-Reyes, M., Timmons, M. C., Davis, K. H., and Wall, M. E., A comparison of the pharmacological activity in man of intravenously administered delta-9-tetrahydrocannabinol, cannabinol, and cannabidiol, Experientia 29: 1368-1369 (1973).
32. Widman, M., Dahmen, K., Leander, K., and Petersson, K., In vitro metabolism of cannabinol in rat and rabbit livers, Synthesis of 2"-, 3"-, and 5"-hydroxy-cannabinol, Acta, Pharm. Suec. 12:385 (1975).
33. Wilson, R. S., May, E. L., and Dewey, W. L., Some 9-hydroxycannabinoid-like compounds, Synthesis and evaluation of analgesic and behavioral properties, J. Med. Chem. 22:886-888 (1979).

THE DISCRIMINATIVE STIMULUS PROPERTIES OF DELTA-9-TETRAHYDROCANNABINOL: GENERALIZATION TO SOME METABOLITES AND CONGENERS[1]

Robert D. Ford[2]
Robert L. Balster
William L. Dewey
John A. Rosecrans
Louis S. Harris

Department of Pharmacology
Medical College of Virginia
Virginia Commonwealth University
Richmond, Virginia

I. INTRODUCTION

Animals can be readily trained to choose which of two response levers to press for reinforcement dependent upon whether they received a drug or vehicle injection. Such drug discriminations have become important in behavioral pharmacology because they can be used to classify drugs. Animals tested with drugs similar to the training drug respond as if they had received the training drug and respond primarily on the lever which was correct after drug injections, i.e., they generalize the stimulus properties of the training drug to the test drug. Animals tested with drugs dissimilar from the training drug respond either on the lever which was correct after vehicle injections during training or distribute their responses on both levers. Generally speaking, drug clas-

[1]Supported in part by NIDA grant DA-00490. Send reprint requests to L. S. Harris.
[2]Postdoctoral Fellow supported by NIDA training grant DA-07027. Present address: Department of Phaarmacology, University of Maryland Dental School, Baltimore, Maryland.

ISBN 0-12-044620-0

sifications using this procedure result in grouping together drugs with similar pharmacological properties which produce similar subjective effects in intoxicated humans (1).

Delta-9-tetrahydrocannabinol (THC) has been used as a training drug in about 15 drug discrimination studies in a variety of species. It functions effectively and generalization tests with other drugs provide evidence for the specificity of the procedure. A number of investigators have proposed the use of a THC-vehicle discriminations in animals as a test for drugs with marijuana-like intoxicating effects in humans (2-5). In this paper we report more extensively on the results of our testing of various synthetic cannabinoids and THC metabolites in rats trained to discriminate THC from vehicle in a two-bar operant task. Prelimnary conclusions were included in earlier reports (5,6).

II. METHODS

A. Subjects

Fifteen male Holtzman rats with no previous experimental history which weighed between 311 and 391 g when given free access to food and water were used. They were deprived of food until they reached 80 percent of their free-feeding weights, and subsequently maintained at this weight by adjusted feedings after each experimental session. Except for an hour each day consumed by injections and the experimental session, rats were housed individually with free access to water.

B. Apparatus

Training and testing of rats was carried out in standard operant chambers equipped with two response bars. A bar press with a force of approximately 15 g constituted a response. Centered in the wall between the two bars was an opening through which a 0.1 ml mixture of sweetened condensed milk and tap water (1:2) could be made accessible by means of an electrically operated dipper. Each chamber was illuminated by a six-watt bulb and placed in a ventilated enclosure for light and sound attenuation. Solid state programming equipment and electromechanical counters were used to control the experimental contingencies and record data.

C. Procedure

Thirty minutes prior to their first introduction to the experimental chamber, eight rats were injected with 3.0 mg/kg of THC, while the additional seven rats were injected with vehicle. Subsequently, daily injections were administered on a double alternation regimen, so that two consecutive injections of THC alternated wth two consecutive injections of vehicle. Training to bar-press was completed in the first four consecutive sessions, during which each response on one bar resulted in milk presentation, while responding on the other bar had no programmed consequence. The correct bar was determined by whether the prior injection was THC or vehicle. For eight rats the left bar was correct after THC and the right bar correct after the vehicle. The converse was true for the remaining rats. These bar-injection pairings remained fixed for each rat throughout the study. After the initial training, session length was set at 30 minutes and rats were placed on a fixed ratio-10 (FR-10) schedule of reinforcement, where 10 responses on the correct bar resulted in milk presentation. Responses on both bars were recorded.

D. Types of Sessions

Starting with Session 5, there were three types of sessions used in the study and they are designated training, check (C), and test (T) sessions. All sessions had in common that they began 30 minutes after an i.p. injection and responses on both bars were recorded. Training sessions were of two kinds since they followed the injection of either THC or vehicle and lasted 30 minutes, throughout which the reinforcer was presented on a FR-10 schedule for responding on the appropriate bar. Check sessions (C) also followed injections of either 3.0 mg/kg THC or vehicle, but for the first 2.5 minutes of the session the reinforcer was not presented. The initial 2.5 minutes of a check session provided a measure of stimulus control of responding by THC or vehicle, and the session was completed with 27.5 minutes of FR-10 reinforcemet on the appropriate bar. A test session (T) folllowed the injection of THC doses other than 3.0 mg/kg or doses of novel cannabinoids. A test session lasted only 2.5 minutes during which no reinforcement was given, and this provided a measure of stimulus generalization to 3.0 mg/kg THC and vehicle injection.

E. Order of Sessions

The basic order of session types was a double alternation

of daily THC and vehicle (V) training sessions (THC, THC, V, V, THC, THC, etc.). This order was altered starting with session 30 when a check session (C) occurred every 3rd session (THC, THC, C, V, THC, C, etc.). Whether a check session was preceded by a 3.0 mg/kg THC or vehicle injection was determined by the double alternation sequence. In determining a THC dose-response curve, a test session occurred every 3rd session in the place of a check session. During the period when doses of novel cannabinoids were tested, a check session occurred every 3rd session and a test session every 6th session.

F. Drug Procedure

The 15 rats were divided into two groups that were distinguished by the novel cannabinoids tested in each. The number of animals tested was largely determined by the amount of drug available. The order of drugs tested and number of animals used for Group I were: delta-9-THC (N = 7); 11-OH-delta-9-THC (N = 7); 8alpha-OH-delta-9-THC (N = 2); 8beta-OH-delta-9-THC (N = 3); 8alpha,11-diOH-delta-9-THC (N = 3); 8beta,11-diOH-delta-9-THC (N = 2); 11-nor-9beta-OH-HHC (N = 7); delta-9-THC (N = 6); 11-OH-delta-8-THC (N = 6). The order of drugs tested and number of animals used for Group II were: 11-nor-9alpha-OH-HHC (N = 8); 11-nor-delta-8-THC (N = 7); cannabidiol (N = 4); abnormal cannabidiol (N = 4); delta-9-THC (N = 8); 11-OH-delta-8-THC (N = 8).

The structure of the metabolites tested are presented in Figure 1, while the structures of the synthetic and other natural products are shown in Figure 2. In pure and suspension form, the cannabinoids were stored in the dark at about 4°C until used. The suspending agent used for the cannabinoids were emulphor (EL 620), which was prepared as described (7,8). On each day of administration, stock suspensions were diluted with saline so that the volume injected was 1 ml/kg, except in cases where a dose larger than 30.0 mg/kg was given. To administer the 60.0 mg/kg dose of 11-nor-delta-8-THC and the 100.0 mg/kg doses of cannabidiol and abnormal cannabidiol volumes of 2.0 ml/kg and 3.3 ml/kg, respectively, were used. Vehicle control injections during training were 1 ml/kg of saline solution containing emulphor and ethanol, to correspond with the amount of emulphor and ethanol in the 3.0 mg/kg THC training dose. In testing for generalization to THC, the vehicle injection for a particular test drug consisted of a saline solution which corresponded in volume and in emulphor and ethanol concentration to that in the dose of drug tested.

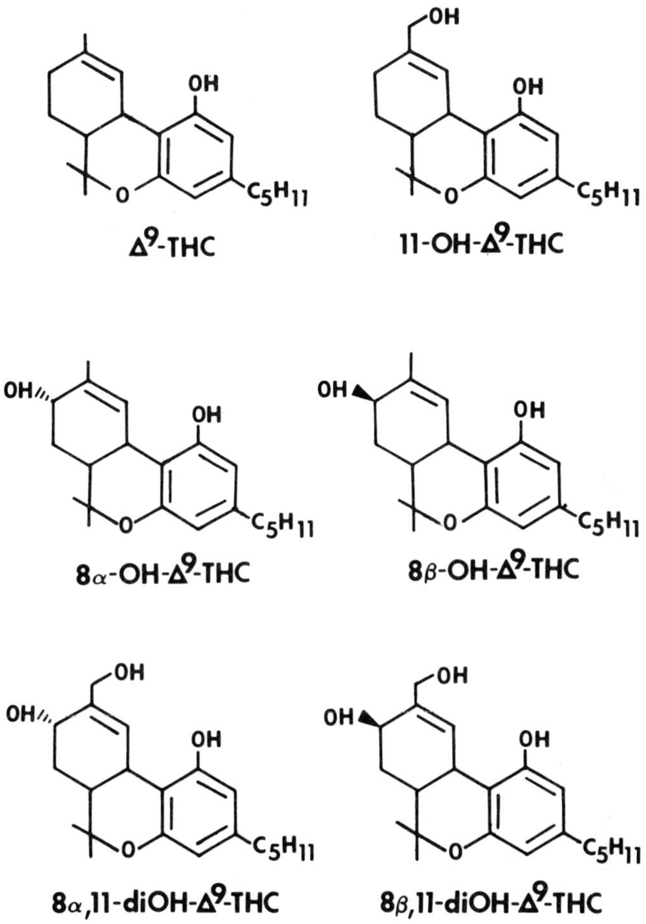

FIGURE 1. Structures of THC and its metabolites.

G. Measurement of Drug Effects

The results to be reported are based upon the number of responses on each of the two bars during the 2.5 min. extinction periods which constituted test sessions or initiated check sessions. Responding during extinction periods gives a measure of stimulus generalization to vehicle and the 3.0 mg/kg THC training dose. Drug effects are characterized throughout this paper as the mean response rate during extinction periods and the percent THC bar-responses. The results of test sessions were compared for statistical significance to the most proximate vehicle check session using a two-tailed, paired *t*-test.

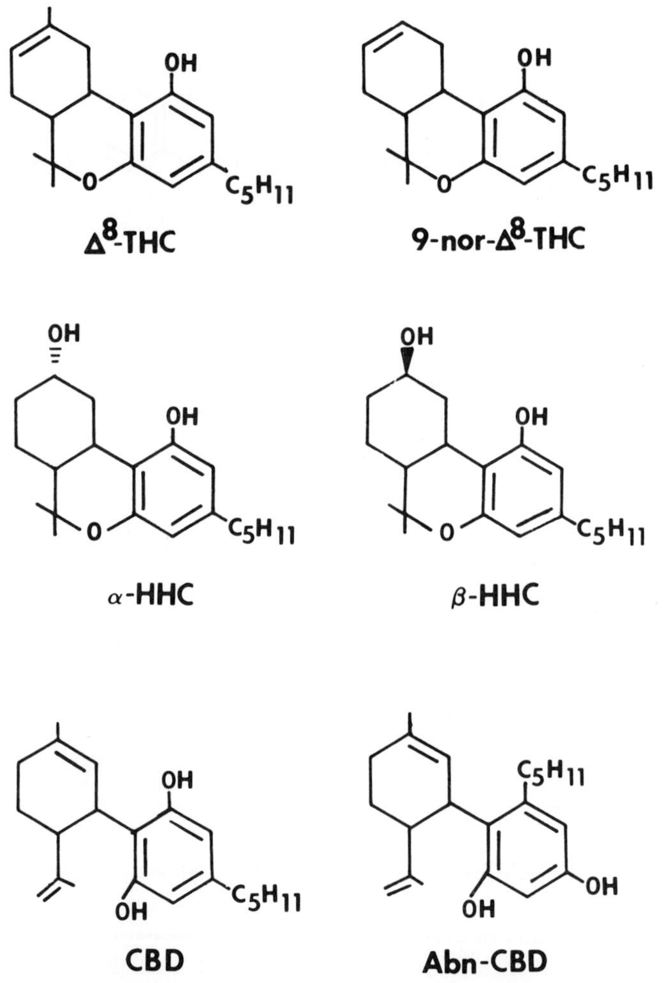

Δ^8-THC 9-nor-Δ^8-THC

α-HHC β-HHC

CBD Abn-CBD

FIGURE 2. Stuctures of delta-8-THC and the congeners tested.

III. RESULTS

A. THC as a Discriminative Stimulus

Figure 3 shows the effects produced by various doses of THC as percent THC bar responses and response rates. When tested in 7 rats at the beginning of the study (open circles), the largest dose of 4.0 mg/kg produced the highest proportion of THC bar responses, while the smallest dose of 0.3 mg/kg

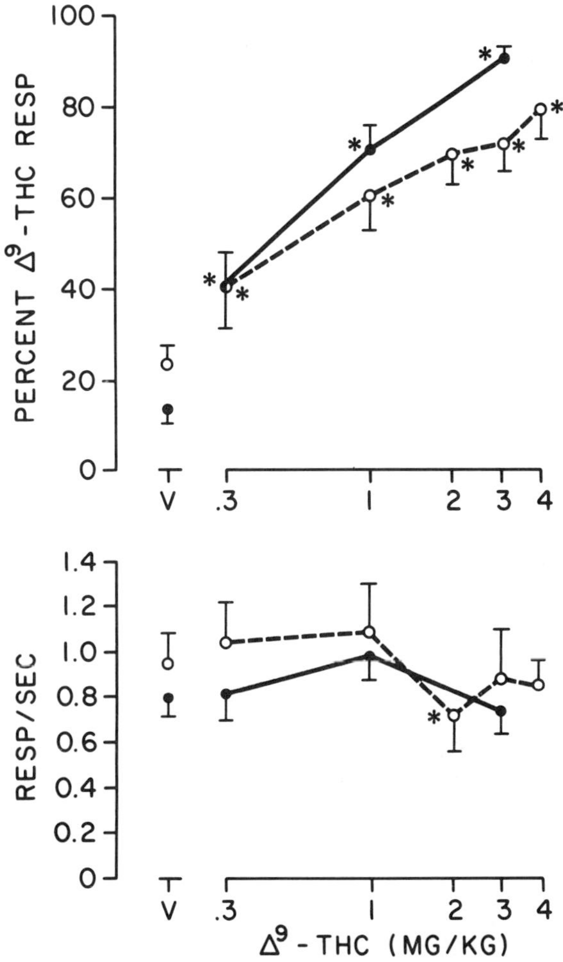

FIGURE 3. Effects of THC on percent THC-bar responses and response rate. Abscissas: dose, log scale. Ordinates: percent THC responses and response rate during 2.5 minute extinction periods. Open circles, first determination (N = 7); closed circles, second determination (N = 14). The points at V are the mean of vehicle injections. Each point represents the mean of one observation in each rat. The vertical lines show one standard error above and below the mean. (*$p < 0.05$ compared to vehicle)

resulted in the highest proportion of responses on the vehicle bar. Similar results were obtained when a THC dose-response curve was determined in 14 rats near the end of the study and following the testing of other cannabinoids (closed circles). These two dose-response curves, together with the results from check sessions throughout the study, indicate that THC functioned in a dose-related manner as a discriminative stimulus, and that stimulus control of responding by 3.0 mg/kg THC and vehicle injections remained relatively stable during the testing of a number of THC metabolites and congeners.

The effects on mean response rates produced by THC doses is shown in the bottom plot of Figure 3. Thoughout the study there was a higher variability associated with response rates than that obtained for percent THC bar responses. As shown, there was a small but significant ($p < 0.05$) decrease in mean response rate produced by 2.0 mg/kg THC when tested at the beginning of the study in these seven rats. This small decrease in mean response rate may be due to the level of training of this group, where behavioral tolerance had not yet completely developed to the disruptive effects of THC. This explanation is further suggested since significant changes from vehicle values were not produced by other THC doses in this determination nor when the THC dose response curve was redetermined in all 14 remaining rats near the end of the study.

B. Generalization of 11-OH-delta-9-THC to THC

Results of test doses of 11-OH-delta-9-THC on percent THC bar responses and mean response rates are shown in Figure 4. The two points on the left of each plot show the result of check sessions where the 3.0 mg/kg training dose of THC produced 88 percent and vehicle 22 percent of total responses on the THC bar, while response rates did not differ. Test doses of 11-OH-delta-9-THC were generalized to THC as a function of dose. 11-OH-delta-9-THC at a dose of 0.1 mg/kg resulted in 34 percent of the total responses being on the THC bar, while 0.3 and 1.0 mg/kg produced 73 and 97 percent, respectively. Mean response rate, on the other hand, decreased as a function of dose. While the 3.0 mg/kg dose of THC did not alter the mean response rate, it was markedly decreased by 1.0 mg/kg of the 11-hydroxy metabolite. Thus, at 1/3 the THC training dose, the 11-hydroxy metabolite produced THC-like discriminative stimulus effects and markedly decreasd the mean response rate.

C. Generalization of 11-OH-delta-8-THC to THC

The effects of 11-OH-delta-8-THC, also indicated in Fig.

4, are much like those of 11-OH-delta-9-THC in both potency of stimulus effects and concomitant response rate decreasing effects. Both metabolites are about three times as potent as THC in producing similar stimulus effects. In addition, at equi-

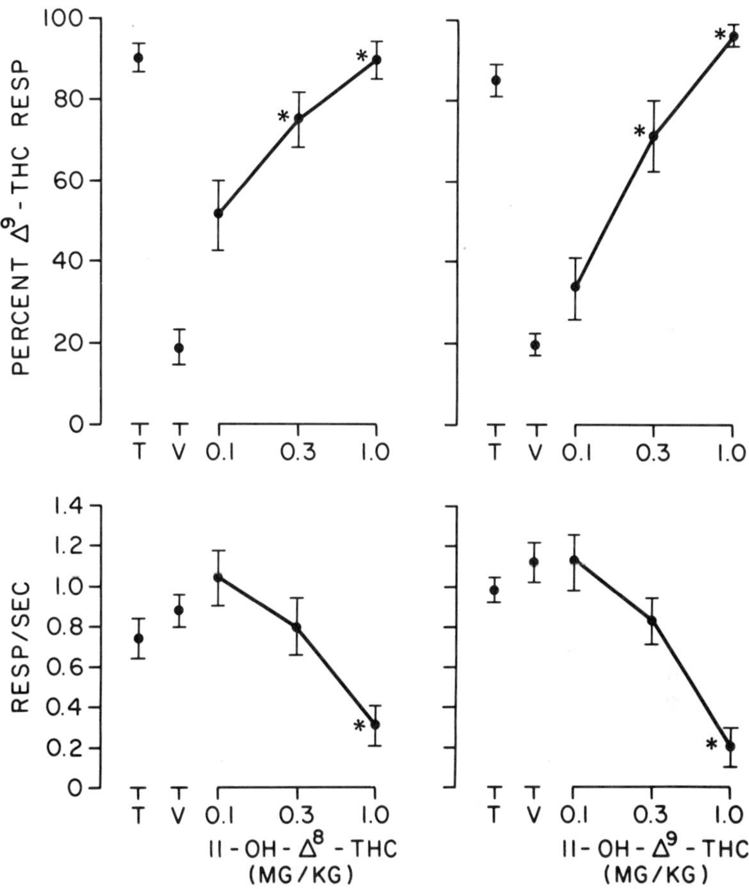

FIGURE 4. Effects of 11-OH-delta-9- and delta-8-THC on the percent of THC responses and response rate. Abscissas: dose, log scale. Ordinates: percent THC responses and response rate during 2.5 minute extinction periods. The points at the left of the four plots are the result of THC and vehicle check sessions and represent the mean of two observations in 7 rats for 11-OH-delta-9-THC and the mean of two observations in 14 rats for 11-OH-delta-8-THC. Each point at doses of 11-OH-delta-9-THC and 11-OH-delta-8-THC represents the mean of one observation in 7 and 14 rats, respectively. The vertical lines show one stan-dard error above and below the mean. (*$p < 0.05$ compared to vehicle)

potent doses for producing discriminative stimulus effects, the 11-hydroxy metabolites have a response rate decreasing component which the parent THC largely lacks.

D. Generalization of 11-nor-delta-8-THC to THC

Figure 5 shows the effects produced by graded doses of 11-nor-delta-8-THC. As indicated in the top plot of percent THC bar responses, a 10.0 mg/kg dose produced vehicle-like effects. At a dose of 60.0 mg/kg, 11-nor-delta-8-THC generalized to THC. Thus, 11-nor-delta-8-THC was about 1/20 as

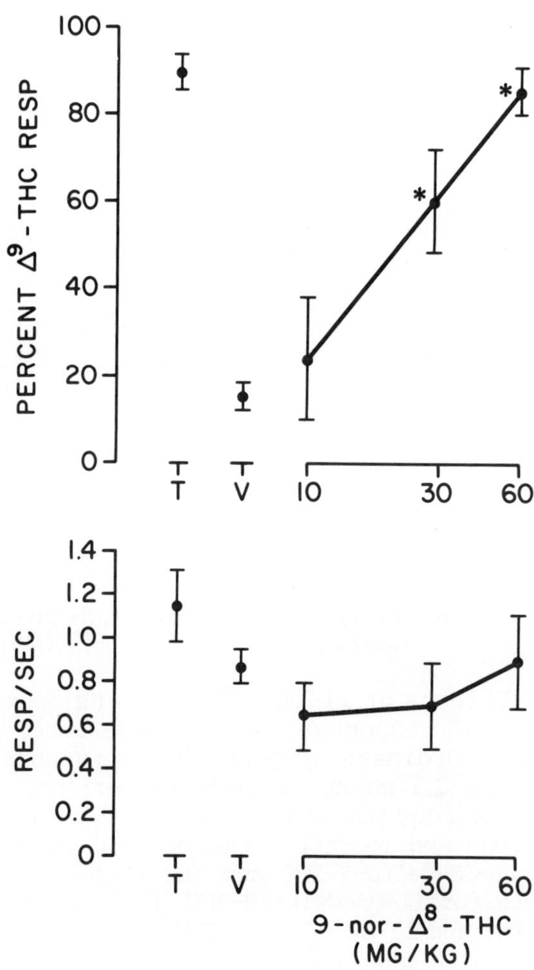

potent as THC. As shown in the bottom plot of Figure 5, mean response rates after 11-nor-delta-8-THC were not significantly different from vehicle values.

E. Generalization of 11-nor-9beta-OH-HHC (9beta-HHC) to THC

As shown in Figure 6, 9beta-HHC generalized to THC as a function of dose and in a manner very similar to the 11-hydroxy metabolites. 9beta-HHC produced THC-like stimulus effects at 1/3 the dose of THC. Also like 11-OH-delta-9-THC, 1.0 mg/kg 9beta-HHC markedly decreased mean response rate.

F. Effects of 11-nor-9alpha-OH-HHC (9alpha-HHC)

Fig. 6 shows that 9alpha-HHC had no effect on mean response rate over a 10-fold range of doses and at a dose 10 times that of 9beta-HHC, which markedly decreased responding. However, 9alpha-HHC produced a distribution of responding different from vehicle and 3.0 mg/kg THC. Over this 10-fold dose range, 9alpha-HHC resulted in responses being more evenly distributed on the two response bars.

G. Effects of 8alpha-OH-delta-9-THC; 8beta-OH-delta-9-THC; 8alpha,11-diOH-delta-9-THC; and 8beta,11-diOH-deta-9-THC

We used all the drug available to us and tested high doses of these metabolites in a selected small number of animals which had the most stable performances. The results are shown in Table I. None of the metabolites were significantly different from vehicle. There was no indication that 8alpha-OH-delta-9-THC and the dihydroxy metabolites producted THC-like effects at doses 4 to 10 times the THC training dose. The results with 8beta-OH-delta-9-THC were only mildly suggestive

FIGURE 5. Effects of 11-nor-delta-8-THC on the percent of THC responses and response rate. Abscissas: dose, log scale. Ordinates: percent THC responses and response rate during 2.5 minute extinction periods. The points at the left of the two plots are the result of THC and vehicle check sessions and represent the mean of two observations in 7 rats. Each point at doses of 11-nor-delta-8-THC represents the mean of one observation in 7 rats (14 sessions). The vertical lines show one standard error above and below the mean. (*$p < 0.05$ compared to vehicle)

of THC activity, and this was not significantly different from vehicle effects.

H. Lack of Generalization of THC to Cannabidiol and Abnormal Cannabidiol

As indicated in Table I, neither the plant constituent cannabidiol nor its synthetic analog abnormal cannabidiol were generalized to THC at doses of 30.0 and 100.0 mg/kg.

IV. DISCUSSION

THC functioned well as a discriminative stimulus for lever-choice behavior in rats. This has been observed in many other studies with rats (2-5,9-10) and pigeons (12,13). A training dose of about 3.0 mg/kg THC has been consistently successful for drug discrimination in rats. At this dose we obtained excellent stimulus control, greater than 80% correct bar responding, during check sessions. This dose of THC had specificity for discriminative stimulus effects since no differences were seen between overall response rates on THC and vehicle sessions. Rats trained under these conditions can be

TABLE I. Results of Generalization Tests with Secondary Delta-9-THC Metabolites, Cannabidiol and Abnormal Cannabidiol

Drug	Dose (mg/kg)	N	Percent of THC Responses	
			Mean	S.E.M.
8alpha-OH-delta-9-THC	15	2	28.0	14.4
	30	2	26.9	5.9
8beta-OH-delta-9-THC	3	3	20.4	6.8
	15	3	29.8	9.9
	30	3	50.8	11.9
8alpha-11-diOH-delta-9-THC	12	3	21.0	7.8
8beta-11-diOH-delta-9-THC	12	2	6.1	3.3
Cannabidiol (CBD)	30	4	6.8	4.4
	100	4	19.1	9.4
Abnormal CBD	30	4	15.9	14.7
	100	4	13.0	9.0

repeated tested with other drugs to determine if the stimulus control exerted by THC will be genralized to them.

Of the drugs we tested for generalization to the THC cue, only the 11-hydroxy (11-OH) metabolites of both delta-9- and delta-8-THC and the synthetic cannabinoids 11-nor-delta-8-THC and 11-nor-9beta-OH-HHC resulted in levels of THC bar responding comparable to that obtained with THC itself. The 11-OH

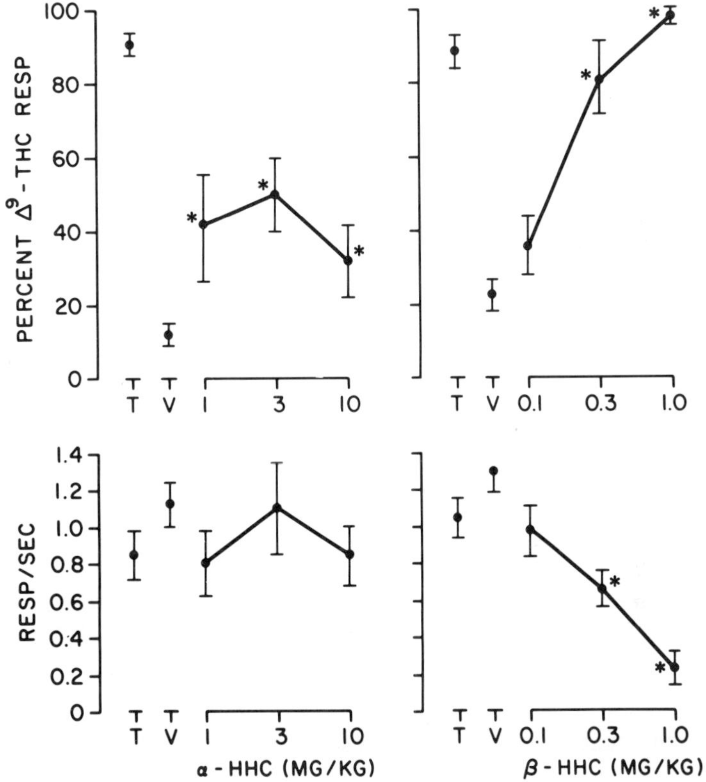

FIGURE 6. Effects of 11-nor-9beta-OH-hexahydrocannabinol (9beta-HHC) and 9alpha-HHC on the percent of THC responses and response rate. Abscissas: dose, log scale. Ordi-nates: percent THC responses and response rate during 2.5 minute extinction periods. The points at the left of the two plots are the result of THC vehicle check sessions and represent the mean of two observations in 7 rats for 9b-HHC (14 sessions) and in 8 rats for 9alpha-HHC (16 sessions). Each point at doses of 9beta-HHC and 9alpha-HHC represents the mean of one observation in 7 and 8 rats, respectively. The vertical lines show one standard error above and below the mean (*$p < 0.05$ compared to vehicle)

metabolites of delta-9- and delta-8-THC have been reported by others as well to be generalized to THC in rats (3,4,13) and pigeons (13). The greater potency of the metabolites over THC was also seen in these other studies. These compounds produce marijuana-like subjective effects in humans (14,15) and are more potent than THC in humans as well. Other drugs that produce marijuana-like effects in humans and that are generalized to THC in animal studies include hashish extract, delta-8-THC and nabilone (2,4).

There was an interesting difference between the results with THC and with both 11-OH metabolites in our study suggesting that their effects, although similar, may not be equivalent. Unlike THC, where greater than 80% drug bar responding could readily be produced by doses that had no effects on overall response rates, both 11-OH-delta-9- and -delta-8-THC only produced complete generalization at doses that markedly suppressed responding. These compounds way be less specific for marijuana-like subjective effects with a greater propensity for behavioral disruption at intoxicating doses.

The two synthetic cannabinoids, 9beta-HHC and 11-nor-delta-8-THC, which were generalized to THC by rats, have not been evaluated for marijuana-like effects in humans, however, we would predict effects similar to THC. Generalization to THC by 9beta-HHC in rats has also been reported by Weissman (4), and this compound as well as 11-nor-delta-8-THC shares many pharmacological properties with THC in animal tests (16,17). The fact that both these compounds cannot be 11-hydroxylated but yet retain THC-like effects suggests that 11-OH metabolites of THC are not solely responsible for the effects of THC. This is consistent with our finding that THC produces behavioral effects when injected directly into the brains of monkeys at a time when no metabolic conversion has occurred (18). The 9alpha-isomer of HHC was not generalized to THC demonstrating the importance of the orientation of the 9-substituent relative to the plane of the cyclohexane ring for hexahydrocannabinols.

We tested both alpha and beta isomers of the 8-OH and 8,11-diOH metabolites of THC for THC-like discriminative stimulus effects. We were limited by the availability of only small supplies of these compounds. None of them were completely generalized to THC. The monohydroxy metabolites were tested up to 30 mg/kg, 30 times the lowest dose of THC that resulted in appreciable THC bar responding. Jarbe and McMillan also tested both of these compounds at comparable doses in pigeons for generalization to THC and also found no activity (13). Both the alpha and beta 8,11-diOH metabolites were also without THC-like effects at 12 mg/kg in our study and at 10 mg/kg in the study using pigeons (13). However, Jarbe and McMillan were able to test higher doses of the 8beta,11-diOH compound (40 mg/kg) and found evidence for generalization to THC. Thus, the lack of THC-like effects of the 8-OH and 8,11-diOH metabolites of THC may be more quantitative than qualitative. Nonetheless, their relative lack of potency compared to THC (at least 30 fold), combined with their relatively low levels in brain after THC or marijuana administration, suggests that they contribute little if anything to the acute CNS effects of marijuana.

Cannabidiol and abnormal cannabidiol were not generalized to THC at doses up to 100 mg/kg. Similar results for cannabidiol have been reported by others (4,12,19). Cannabidiol also lacks marijuana-like effects in humans (20).

We believe that these results point again to the utility of a drug discrimination based on THC in animals as a sensitive and specific method for demonstrating THC-like behavioral effects of drugs. It also appears to predict well drugs that will produce marijuana intoxication in humans. Cannabinoids such as delta-8-THC, 11-OH-delta-9-THC, 11-OH-delta-8-THC, and nabilone, which produce these effects, are generalized to THC in animal studies. Cannabinoids such as cannabidiol and the 8-OH and 8,11-diOH metabolites of THC, which are essentially inactive in humans, are not generalized to THC in animal studies. Tests in humans of potent cannabinoids such as 9beta-HHC and SP-111 (13), which are generalized to THC by rats, would help confirm the predictive value of this procedure. It is also important to point out that drugs from other classes, including other hallucinogens, such as LSD, mescaline, and phencyclidine, are not generalized to THC nor is THC generalized to them (see reviews 3-5). Thus, this method has greater specificity.

ACKNOWLEDGMENTS

The authors gratefully acknowledge the supply of drugs from Dr. Robert Willette at the National Institute on Drug Abuse, Drs. Raymond Wilson and Everette May at the National Institutes of Health, and Dr. Raj Razdan at the Sheehan Institute For Research.

REFERENCES

1. Barry, H., III., Classification of drugs according to their discriminable effects in rats, Fed. Proc. 33:1814-1824 (1974).

2. Jarbe, T. U. C., and Henriksson, B. G., Discriminative response control produced with hashish, tetrahydrocannabinols (delta-8- and delta-9-THC), and other drugs, Psychopharmacologia 40:1-16 (1974).
3. Krimmer, E. C., and Barry, H., III., Discriminable stimulus properties of drugs, in "Discriminative Stimulus Properties of Drugs" (H. Lal, ed.), pp. 121-135. Plenum Publishing Co., New York, 1977.
4. Weissman, A., Generalization of the discriminative stimulus properties of delta-9-tetrahydrocannabinol to cannabinoids with therapeutic potential, in "Stimulus Properties of Drugs: Ten Years of Progress" (F. C. Colpaert and J. A. Rosencrans, eds.), pp. 99-122. Elsevier/North-Holland Biomedical Press, Amsterdam, 1978.
5. Balster, R. L., and Ford, R. D., The discriminative stimulus properties of cannabinoids: A review, in "Drug Discrimination and State Dependent Learnings", (B. T. Ho, D. W. Richards, III, and D. L. Chute, eds.), pp. 131-147. Academic Press, New York, 1978.
6. Ford, R. D., and Balster, R. L., The discriminative stimulus properties of delta-9-tetrahydrocannabinol: Generalization to some metabolites and derivatives, Fed. Proc. 34:743 (1975).
7. Craddock, J. C., Davignon, J. P., Litterst, C. L., and Guarino, A. M., An intravenous formulation of delta-9-tetrahydrocannabinol using a nonionic surfactant, J. Pharm. Pharmacol. 25:345 (1973).
8. Carney, J. M., Uwaydah, I. M., and Balster, R. L., Evaluation of a suspension system for intravenous self-administration studies of water-insoluble compounds in the rhesus monkey, Pharmacol. Biochem. Behav. 7:357-364 (1977).
9. Jarbe, T. U. C., Johansson, J. O., and Hendriksson, B. G., Characteristics of tetrahydrocannabinol (THC)-produced discrimination in rats, Psychopharmacol. 48:181-187 (1976).
10. Bueno, O. F. A., Carlini, E. A., Finkelfarb, E., and Suzuki, J., delta-9-Tetrahydrocannabinol, ethanol, and amphetamine as discriminative stimuli-generalization tests with other drugs, Psychopharmacologia 46:235-243 (1976).
11. Jarbe, T. U. C., Johanssen, J. O., and Hendriksson, B. G., delta-9-Tetrahydrocannabinol and pentobarbital as discriminative cues in the mongolian gerbil (Meriones unguiculatus), Pharmacol. Biochem. Behav. 3:403-410 (1975).
12. Jarbe, T. U. C., Hendriksson, B. G., and Ohlin, G. C., delta-9-THC as a discriminative cue in pigeons: Effects of delta-8-THC, CBD, and CBN, Arch. int. Pharmacodyn. et Therap. 228:68-72 (1977).

13. Jarbe, T. U. C., and McMillan, D. E., delta-9-THC as a discriminative stimulus in rats and pigeons: Generalization to THC metabolites and SP-111, Psychopharmacol. 71:281-289 (1980).
14. Hollister, L. E., Structure-activity relationships in man of cannabis constituents, and homologs and metabolites of delta-9-tetrahydrocannabinol, Pharmacology 11:3-11 (1974).
15. Lemberger, L., Marty, R., Rodda, B., Forney, R., and Rowe, H., Comparative pharmacology of deta-9-tetrahydrocannabinol and its metabolite, 11-OH-delta-9-tetrahydrocannabinol, J. Clin. Invest. 52:2411-2417 (1973).
16. Wilson, R. S., May, E. L., Martin, B. R., and Dewey, W. L., 9-nor-delta-9-hydroxyhexahydrocannabinols: Synthesis, some behavioral and analgesic properties, an comparison with tetrahydrocannabinols, J. Med. Chem. 19:1165-1167 (1976).
17. Martin, W. R., Dewey, W. L., Harris, L. S., Beckner, J., Wilson, R. S., and May, E. L., Marihuana-like activity of new synthetic tetrahydrocannabinols, Pharmacol. Biochem. Behav. 3:849-853 (1975).
18. Carney, J. M., Balster, R. L., Martin, B. R., and Harris, L. S., Effects of systemic and intraventricular administration of cannabinoids on schedule-controlled responding in the squirrel monkey, J. Pharmacol. Exper. Therap. 210:399-404).
19. Zuardi, A. W., Finkelfarb, E., Bueno, O. F. A., Musty, R. E., and Karniol, I. G., Characteristics of the stimulus produced by the mixture of cannabidiol with delta-9-tetrahydrocannabinol, Arch. int. Pharmacodyn. et Therap. 249:137-146 (1981).
20. Perez-Reyes, M., Timmons, M. C., David, K. H., and Wall, E. M., A comparison of the pharmacological activity in man of intravenously administered delta-9-tetrahydrocannabinol, cannabinol and cannabidiol, Experientia 29:1308-1309 (1973).

ENHANCED REACTIVITY AND DECREASED FOOD INTAKE IN MICE TREATED CHRONICALLY WITH DELTA-9-TETRAHYDROCANNABINOL

William Semple
Richard E. Musty

Department of Psychology
University of Vermont
Burlington, Vermont

I. INTRODUCTION

Consummatory behavior in humans (1,2) and animals (3) may be increased shortly after administration of low doses of delta-9-tetrahydrocannabinol (THC), however, higher doses, especially when administered chronically, typically result in decreases in daily total food consumption in rats, the most popular subject for animal studies of this type (4-8).

There are several lines of evidence that connect THC with enhanced emotionality and reactivity. One of the principal indices of emotionality in animals is defecation (9). Chronic THC injections [2.5 mg/kg, 45 minutes before open field (O.F.) trials] block the decrease in open field defecation normally seen over trials in rats with initially high levels of O.F. defecation, and result in a several-fold increase in O.F. defecation over trials in rats with an initially low level of O.F. defecation (10). Sjoden et al. also found increased open field defecation following THC administration (11). THC treatment also produces vocalization during handling in rats (12,13) and hypersensitivity to tactile and auditory stimuli in mice (14). These signs of increased reactivity disappeared by 3-12 hours after THC administration.

In human subjects given chronic high doses of THC orally (70 mg/kg daily and above) several times daily, irritability is not noted during intoxication, but becomes noticeable by 12 hours after cessation of drug treatment, as measured by the Irritability Scale of the Nurses' Observation Scale for

The Cannabinoids: Chemical, Pharmacologic, and Therapeutic Aspects

ISBN 0-12-044620-0

Inpatient Observation (15). An earlier study, by Williams, et al., reported that prisoners given 17 joints of marijuana daily for 39 days felt "jittery" when the drug was discontinued, but the doctors and nurses involved did not observe any signs of an abstinence syndrome (16). A lack of classical opiate-type withdrawal symptoms was likewise noted by Allentuck and Bowman, who did, however, note that "the after-math of marijuana intoxication resembles an alcoholic "hangover" (17).

In animals, hyperexcitability upon withdrawal of THC, as measured by changes in electroshock thresholds, provides some support for the notion of a withdrawal hypersensitivity following chronic THC administration (18). The demonstration of increased defecation following THC treatment and of a withdrawal syndrome including increased defecation and urination following chronic administration of very high doses of THC (70 mg/kg/day) (19), further demonstrates that cessation of THC treatment can result in withdrawal signs.

In the present study, the measure of reactivity used was the mouse's immediate behavioral reaction to the daily I.P. injection procedure. This reaction could consist of vocalization, defecation, urination, or a combination of these behaviors. Since the measure was taken 24 hours after the previous THC or vehicle injection, a type of "hangover reactivity" was measured, which is operationally similar to Carlini's 24 hours post-injection measures of operant rope-climbing behavior, which demonstrated a defecit, relative to controls, that attenuated over a period of 7 daily injections (20).

The use of this measure permits assessment of reactivity at a time, 24 hours post-injection, which had not been previously observed on a continuous daily basis, so novel information on THC and reactivity was gained.

II. METHODS

A. Subjects

Eighty-one random bred female albino CD-1 mice from Canadian Breeding Laboratories served as subjects. The mice were approximately ten weeks old at the start of the study, and were housed individually. Treatment groups were matched on food intake. Subjects were maintained on a 10L/14D light cycle, with light onset at 8 A. M.

B. Apparatus

Subjects were housed in clear plastic cages 17.5 cm wide by 27.5 cm long by 12.0 cm deep, with mesh covers on top, and wood shavings on the floor. A wooden block 4.5 cm by 9.5 cm by 95 cm was placed inside each cage for gnawing activity, since food was liquid.

The liquid diet consisted of a mixture of 25% Carnation Slender Chocolate Diet Drink and 75% Enfamil Concentrated Infant Formula (undiluted). The diet was mixed daily and placed in graduated drinking tubes constructed from 30 ml plastic syringes and metal drinking spouts. The amount of food left from the previous day's 25 ml supply was recorded for each animal daily at 2 P. M. prior to cleaning and refilling the drinking tubes.

THC was prepared in 0.09% saline and 0.5% Tween 80 solution. All injections were given with a 1 ml plastic disposable syringe fitted with a 25 gauge stainless steel needle. All injections occurred between 11 A. M. and noon, and drug solution concentrations were such that a 30 g mouse received a 0.1 ml volume for proper dosage, and volume was adjusted according to each mouse's weight. All drug and control solutions were refrigerated except during daily injections.

C. Procedure

The mice were allowed a five day period to become familiar with the liquid diet, then intake data for a subsequent 13 day Baseline Food Intake Period (Days 1-13 of the study) were used to form 9 groups of 9 mice each, matched on food intake.

The nine groups were designated and treated as follows:

1. 0.5THC: injection habituated and given 0.5 mg/kg/day THC during the drug treatment phase;
2. 1THC: injection habituated, 1.0 mg/kg/day THC;
3. 4THC: injection habituated, 4.0 mg/kg/day THC;
4. 10THC: injection habituated, 10.0 mg/kg/day THC;
5. SAL: injection habituated, saline control group;
6. TW80: injection habituated, Tween 80 and saline (vehicle) control group;
7. NSAL: non-injection habituated, saline control group;
8. N1THC: non-injection habituated, 1.0 mg/kg/day THC;
9. NIC: non-injection habituated, non-injected control group.

The nine-day injection habituation phase of the experiment took place on Days 15 through 23, and consisted of a single daily I.P. injection of 0.1 ml of a .09% saline solution at 11 A. M. for each injection habituated animal.

The Injection Habituation Period was followed by a 16 day period (Days 24-39) of daily I.P. drug or control injections for mice in all groups except NIC. A 14 Dryout Period (no injections) followed on Days 40-53.

Over the last three days of the Injection Habituation Period and throughout the Drug Injection Period, as well as during a three day injection reactivity retest on Days 54 through 56 following the Dryout Period, each incident of vocalization, defecation or urination (VDU) was noted for each subject as it was injected. The number of subjects in each group exhibiting a reaction (VDU) on any day were summed over three day blocks and analyzed by X^2 test.

Figure 1 summarized the experimental schedule.

III. RESULTS

A. Food Intake

Average food intake in each phase for mice in each group is summarized in Figure 2. As can be seen, the two higher dose drug groups (4THC and 10THC) showed a greater decrease in food intake from the Injection Habituation Period to the Drug Injection Period than low dose (1THC and 0.5THC) and SAL and TW80 groups (which continued to receive appropriate control injections throughout the drug injection period.) In addition, food intake of the 10THC group remained depressed for most of the Dryout Period.

While no differences between groups were evident during the Injection Habituation Period ($F_{(8,72)} = 1$, $P < 0.25$), a nine group repeated measures ANOVA revealed a significant effect of groups ($F_{(8,72)} = 2.19$, $P < 0.05$) over the 17 day Drug Injection Period (Days 24 through 40). Further two group ANOVAS of Drug Period food intake indicated that this effect

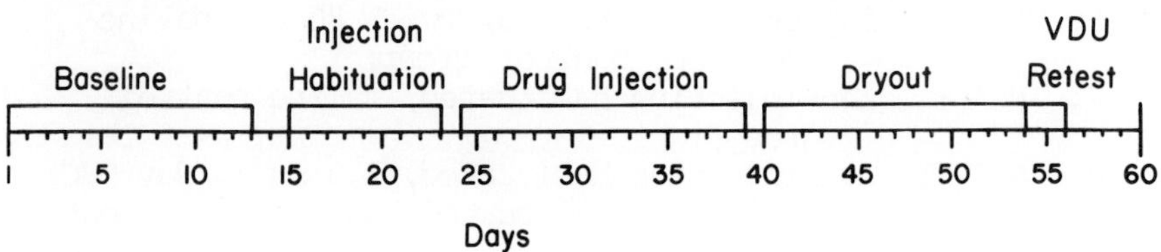

FIGURE 1. Experiment schedule.

of groups was largely due to the difference between the three highest drug dosage groups (1THC, 4THC, and 10THC) and the control and low dose drug (0.5THC) groups; the TW80 (vehicle), NIC and NSAL control groups all showed uniformly higher levels of food intake than did the groups receiving the three highest dose levels of THC.

B. Behavioral Reactivity

As can be seen in Figure 3, high doses of THC (4 and 10 mg/kg/day) resulted in an increased reactivity over the Drug Injection Period, relative to controls.

Since the total number of subjects reacting (80 and 69, respectively) over the Injection Period in the two high dose drug groups (4THC and 10THC) did not differ greatly and showed little difference in time course of the response, their data was combined for graphic presentation and Chi^2 analysis. Data for the two lower dose THC groups (1THC and 0.5THC) and for the two injection habituated control groups (SAL and TW80) were likewise combined across pairs of groups and three day periods for similar reasons: similarity of treatments and scores, and the need to reduce variance across days.

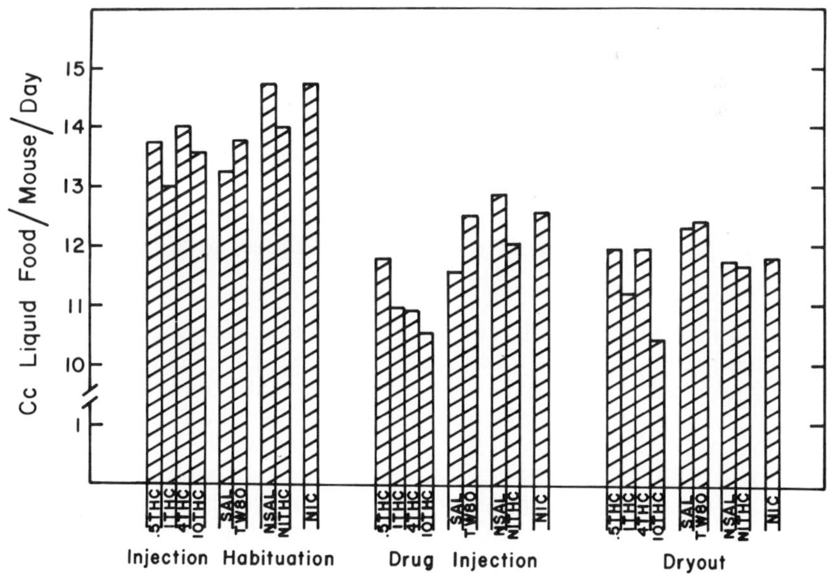

FIGURE 2. Average food intake during injection habituation, drug injection, and dryout periods

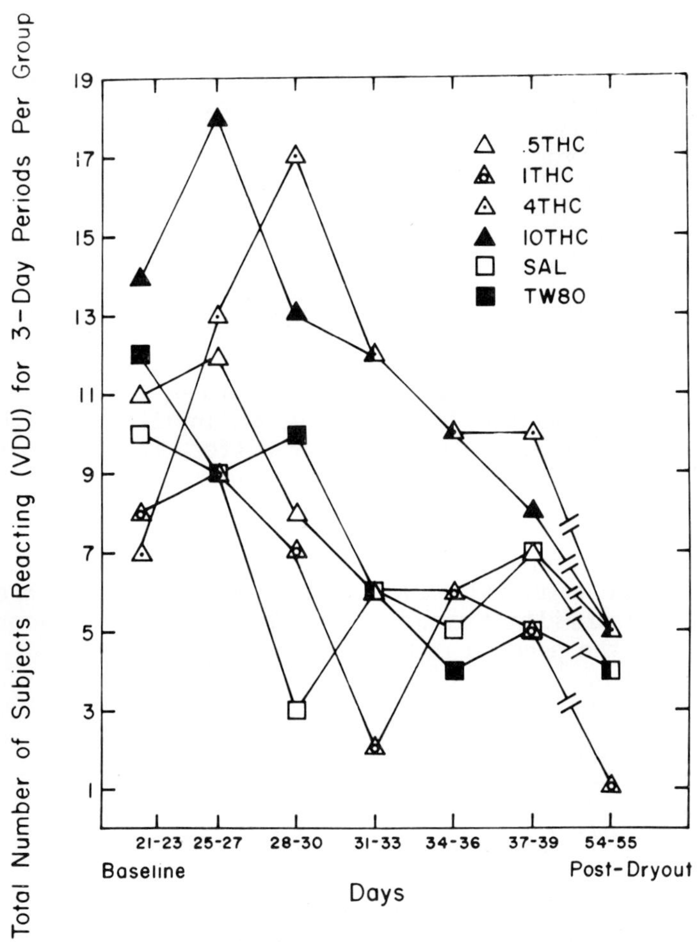

FIGURE 3. Total number of subjects reacting over 3-day blocks in each group of injection-habituated mice.

As can be seen in Figure 4, all three pairs of injection-habituated groups are approximately equal for Baseline Days 21 to 23 (the last three days of injection habituation), ($Chi^2 = 0.36$, $P < 0.1$), with between 19 and 22 Ss reacting in each combined pair of groups. Following initiation of drug injections, the 4THC and 10THC groups show an increase of about 50% in reactivity to injection so that over one half of the subjects responded expressively to the injection.

The difference between these three pairs of groups was significant at the 0.05 level ($X^2 = 7.2$, 2 dF) for Days 25 through 27, and was significant at the 0.002 level ($Chi^2 = 13.8$, 2 dF) for Days 28 through 30.

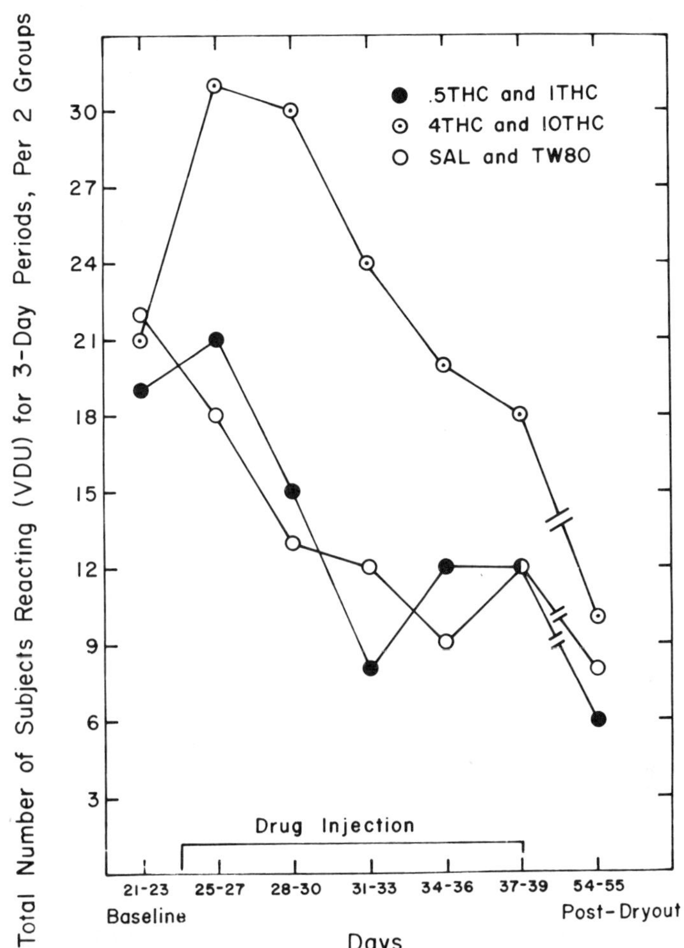

FIGURE 4. Total number of mice reacting to injections over 3-day blocks in paired groups.

As illustrated in Table I, the increased reactivity to injection seen in the 4THC and 10THC groups was due to increased vocalization at both dose levels and increased frequency of defecation as well by mice in the 10THC group, which defecated twice as often as mice in the 0.5THC, 1THC, SAL and TW80 groups.

Thus the higher rate of responding in the high dose THC groups lasted for about a week, following which a sharp decline occurred which almost exactly followed the slope of decline seen about a week earlier in control and low dose THC groups. During this decline, the high dose THC subjects were still more reactive than control or low dose subjects. The 4 THC and 10THC groups reached the low, habituated level of reactivity seen in the low dose and control groups aboutnine days after these latter groups reached it.

Vocalization was uniformly the most frequent response to injection, accounting for 46 to 72 percent of the reactions to injection seen in a group over the Injection Period. Defecation accounted for 25 to 41 percent of reactions, and urination for 0 to 18 percent of reactions to injections.

Thus the two higher doses of THC resulted in a significant increase in the number of mice reacting to the injection procedure by vocalizing, defecating, or urinating. This increase in reactivity occurred after only one injection for 10THC mice and after three daily injections for 4THC mice, and lasted for a total of seven and five days, respectively. Both groups experienced equal delays in the course of habituation of the VDU reaction.

IV. DISCUSSION

The results of the present experiment with mice confirm previous findings across a range of other species of anorexic effects of chronic moderate doses of THC (21), and also demonstrate that dose levels of 4.0 and 10.0 mg/kg/day are associated with a short-term (24 hour post-injection) withdrawal or "hangover" hypersensitivity to a noxious stimulus (the I.P. injection procedure) in the mouse.

THC induced anorexia in mice is essentially similar to that seen in studies using rats. The lack of tolerance over 16 days to suppression of food intake in mice receiving 4.0 and 10.0 mg/kg/day of THC parallels a lack of tolerance over nine (6) and 19 days (5) of administration of 2.5 mg/kg/day in rats, and the lack of tolerance to food intake supression over 15 days of 4.0 mg/kg/day THC found by Drewnowski and Grinker (7).

The increase in reactivity to injection, which 4.0 and 10.0 mg/kg daily of THC produced 24 hours post-injection, is unusual in the literature: changes in reactivity to stimulation such as vocalization in response to pressing have typically been looked for and noted sooner after injection than in the present study. Paton described a 3 hour time course for 9-THC-induced vocalization (in response to mild tactile stimuli such as gentle handling) in the rat, vocalizationbeing interpreted as a sign of distress rather than pain (22). Holtzman, Lovell, Jaffe and Freeman found a hypersensitivity

TABLE I. Frequency of Vocalization, Defecation, and Urination in Each Group

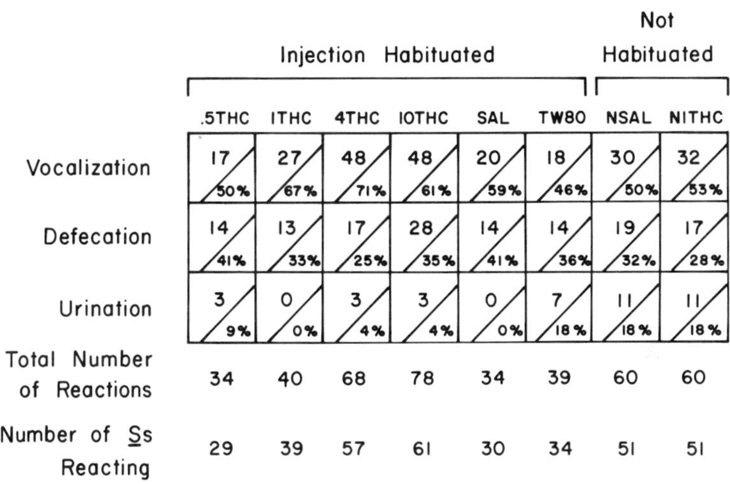

	Injection Habituated						Not Habituated	
	.5THC	1THC	4THC	10THC	SAL	TW80	NSAL	N1THC
Vocalization	17 / 50%	27 / 67%	48 / 71%	48 / 61%	20 / 59%	18 / 46%	30 / 50%	32 / 53%
Defecation	14 / 41%	13 / 33%	17 / 25%	28 / 35%	14 / 41%	14 / 36%	19 / 32%	17 / 28%
Urination	3 / 9%	0 / 0%	3 / 4%	3 / 4%	0 / 0%	7 / 18%	11 / 18%	11 / 18%
Total Number of Reactions	34	40	68	78	34	39	60	60
Number of Ss Reacting	29	39	57	61	30	34	51	51

to tactile and auditory stimuli in THC treated mice, the hypersensitivity disappearing by 3 to 4 hours post-injection (14). Rosenkrantz and Braude administered daily THC inhalations to rats using a smoking machine, and found that spontaneous vocalization developed overa period of 4 to 5 days (similar to the gradual development of the vocalization response in the present experiment for mice receiving 4.0 mg/kg/day, where enhanced vocalization were evident 24 hours after the first THC injection), and that normal behavior returned at 6 hours post-injection (22). Carlini and Kramer found that rats vocalized in response to being touched after injection with 30 to 50 mg/kg of marijuana extract, and described return to normal behavior by 12 to 15 hours post-injection (13).

The present study illustrates the rapid development over one to three days (depending on dose) of a THC induced 24 hour "hangover by hypersensitivity" to stimulation, which is similar to the hyperexcitability to stimuli found soon after THC administration by Lowe (24), Carlini and Kramer (13), and Holtzman et al. (14).

The results of this study indicate that THC can enhance reactivity to mildly stressful stimuli 24 hours after drug administration.

Recent studies demonstrate that physiological (heart rate) and behavioral reactivity to stress is increased during marijuana intoxication in humans, (25-27).

Together, these finding raise the possibility that reactivity to stress or performance demands may be altered in humans as much as a day after marijuana administration. This hypothesis is currently being tested in our laboratory.

REFERENCES

1. Abel, E. L., Marijuana, anagrams, memory, & appetite, Nature, 231:260 (1971).
2. Hollister, L. E., Hunger and appetite after single doses of marijuana, alcohol, and dextroamphetamine, Clin. Pharmacol. Therap. 12:44-49 (1971).
3. Brown, J. E., Kassouny, M., and Cross, J. K., Kinetic studies of food intake and sucrose solution preference by rats treated with low doses of delta-9-tetrahydrocannabinol, Behav. Biol. 20:104-110 (1977).
4. Fernandes, M., Rating, D., and Kluwe, S., The influence of subchronic tetrahydrocannabinol - cannabis treatment on food- and water-intake, body weight and body temperature of rats, Acta Pharmacol. Toxicol. Suppl. 29:89 (1971).
5. Sjoden, P., Jarbe, T. U., and Henriksson, B. G., Influence of tetrahydrocannabinols (delta-8-THC and delta-9-"THC) on body weight, food, and water intake in rats, Pharmacol Biochem. Behav. 1:395-399 (1973).
6. Sofia, R. D., and Barry, H., Acute and chronic effects of delta-9-tetrahydrocannabinol on food intake by rats, Psychopharmacologia 39:213-222 (1974).
7. Drewnowski, A., and Grinker, A., Food and water intake, meal patterns and activity of obese and lean Zucker rats following chronic and acute treatment with delta-9-tetrahydrocannabinol, Pharmacol. Biochem. Behav. 9:619-630 (1978).
8. Miczek, K. A., Chronic delta-9-tetrahydrocannabinol in rats: Effect on social interactions, mouse killing, motor activity, consummatory behavior, and body temperature, Psycholpharmacol. 60:137-146 (1979).
9. Walsh, R. M., and Cummins, R. A., The open-field test: A critical review, Psychol. Bull. 83:482-504 (1976).
10. Masur, J., Martz, R. M. W., and Carlini, E. A., Effects of acute and chronic administration of Cannabis sativa and (-)-delta-9-tetrahydrocannabinol on the behavior of rats in an open-field arena, Psychopharmacol. 19:388-397 (1971).

11. Sjoden, P., Jarbe, T. U. C., and Henriksson, B. G., Effects of long-term administration and withdrawal of tetrahydrocannabinols (delta-8-THC and delta-9-THC) on open-field behavior in rats, Pharmacol. Biochem. Behav. 1:243-249 (1973).
12. Henriksson, B. G. and Jarbe, T., Cannabis-induced vocalization in the rat, Pharm. Pharmacol. 23:457-458 (1971).
13. Carlini, E. A., and Kramer, C., Effects of cannabis sativa (marijuana) on maze performance of the rat, Psychopharmacol. 7:175-181 (1965).
14. Holtzman, D., Lovell, R. A., Jaffe, J. H., and Friedman, D. X., Delta-9-tetrahydrocannabinol: Neurochemical and behavioral effects in the mouse, Science 163:1464-1467 (1969).
15. Jones, R. T., and Benowitz, N., The 30-day trip: Clinical studies of cannabis tolerance and dependence, in "Pharmacology of Marijuana", Vol. 2, (M. C. Braude and S. Szara, eds.), pp. 627-642. Raven Press, New York, 1976.
16. Williams, E. G., Himmelsbach, C. K., Wikler, A., Rubel, D. C., and Lloyd, B. J., Studies on marijuana and parahexyl compound, Public Health Reports 61:(29):1059-1083 (1946).
17. Allentuck, S., and Bowman, K. M., The psychiatric aspects of marijuana intoxication, Amer. Psych. 99:248-251 (1942).
18. Karler, R., and Turkanis, S. A., Hyperexcitability upon withdrawal from marijuana, Fed. Proc. 34(3):782 (1975).
19. Kaymakcalan, S., Ayhan, I. H., and Tulunay, F. C., Naloxone-reduced or postwithdrawal abstinence signs in delta-9-tetrahydrocannabinol-tolerant rats, Psychopharmacol. 55:243-249 (1977).
20. Carlini, E. A., Tolerance to chronic administration of cannabis sativa (marijuana) in rats, Pharmacol. 1:135-142 (1968).
21. Abel, E. L., Cannabis: Effects on hunger and thirst, Behav. Biol. 15:255-281 (1975).
22. Paton, W. D. M., Pharmacology of Marijuana, Ann. Rev. Pharmacol. 15:191-220 (1975).
23. Rosenkrantz, H., and Braude, M. C., Acute, subacute, and 23-day chronic marijuana inhalation toxicities in the rat, Toxicol. Pharmacol. 28:428-441 (1974).
24. Lowe, S., Studies on the pharmacology and acute toxicity of compounds with marijuana activity, J. Pharmacol. Exp. Ther. 88:154-161 (1946).
25. Klonoff, H., Marijuana & Driving in real-life situations, Science 186:317 (1974).
26. Naliboff, B., Rickles, W., Cohen, M., and Naimark, R., Interaction of marijuana and induced stress: Forearm

blood flow, heart rate, and skin conductance, Psychophysiol. 13(6):517-522 (1976).

27. Phil, R., Spiers, P., and Shae, D., The disruption of marijuana intoxication, Psychopharmacol. 52:227-230 (1977).

EFFECTS OF CANNABINOIDS ON NEUROTRANSMITTER RECEPTORS IN THE BRAIN*

Alan S. Bloom

Department of Pharmacology and Toxicology
Medical College of Wisconsin
Milwaukee, Wisconsin

I. INTRODUCTION

Although it was first reported over 15 years ago that cannabinoids can affect biogenic amine neurotransmitters (1), the role of these transmitters in the many actions of marijuana is still not well understood. Furthermore, it is evident from reviewing past literature (for review, see 2) that there is not total agreement as to what the effects of various cannabinoids are on dopaminergic, noradrenergic and serotonergic containing neurons. Delta-9-tetrahydrocannabinol (THC) and other behaviorally-active cannabinoids increase the synthesis and turnover of dopamine and norepinephrine in rat and mouse brain while producing little or no change in endogenous levels of catecholamines (3,4). This indicates that THC can increase the utilization of the catecholamine neurotransmitters. The observed increase in synthesis was not a side effect of drug-induced hypothermia (5). Moreover, THC increases the synthesis of dopamine and norepinephrine in a synaptosomal preparation suggesting that cannabinoids can have a direct action on neuronal elements (6).

THC and other cannabinoids can also effect other functional aspects of catecholaminergic neurotransmisson. THC alters the active uptake of biogenic amine neurotransmitters and their precursors into synaptosomes (6-9) and also transmitter release from synaptosomes. In addition, THC can alter the activity of enzymes involved in the synthesis and degrada-

---

*Supported by NIDA grant DA-00124.

ISBN 0-12-044620-0

tion of the catecholamines. Chronic treatment with THC has been reported to increase the activity of tyrosine in rat brain (10). THC has also been reported both to increase (11) or inhibit (12) monoamine oxidase. THC also inhibits the activity of Na^{+}-K^{+}-ATPase which is involved in the active re-uptake of the monoamine neurotransmitters (8,13).

In contrast to the large number of reports on the effects of cannabinoids on other aspects of dopaminergic and noradrenergic systems, there has been only one published report of cannabinoid effects on receptors for these transmitters. In these studies (14), we observed that THC _in vitro_ increased the binding of the beta-adrenergic antagonist, ^{3}H-dihydroalprenolol (DHA) to beta-adrenergic receptors in the mouse cerebral cortex. This effect was also produced by 11-OH-delta-9-THC but not by cannabidiol (CBD). The chronic _in vivo_ administrationof THC caused a decrease in the density (B_{max}) of DHA binding sites with no change in their apparent affinity (K_d) for DHA.

In further studies on the interactions of cannabinoids with the beta-receptor (see Hillard and Bloom; this volume) we found that THC affected the binding beta-antagonists but had little effect on beta-agonists. The question was then asked: are these changes specific to the beta-adrenergic receptor or can THC affect other membrane-bound neurotransmitter receptors in the same manner. As part of our attempt to answer that question, we have examined in some detail the effects of cannabinoids on dopamine receptors in the mouse corpus striatum.

There are many studies demonstrating the existence of more than one type or form of receptor for dopamine in the brain (see review by Seeman, 15). Therefore, two different ligands were used in the present study. It is fairly well accepted that there is a binding site that has nanomolar affinity for neuroleptics such as haloperidol and micromolar affinity for dopamine and other agonists. This is often referred to as the D_2 site. Binding to this site was determined using ^{3}H-spiperone, a neuroleptic of the butyrophenone class. Conversely, there are dopamine binding sites that bind dopamine and other agonists with low nanomolar affinity and neuroleptics with high nanomolar or micromolar affinity. Seeman refers to these as D_3 sites (15). Binding to this type of site was examined using the ligand ^{3}H-ADTN (2-amino-6,7-dihydroxy-1,2,3,4-tetrahydronaphthalene), as agonist.

II. METHODS

A. Materials

Male ICR outbred, Swiss, albino mice were purchased from ARS/Sprague-Dawley (Madison, WI) and housed grouped with *ad libitum* access to food and water. Cannabinoids were provided by the National Institute on Drug Abuse. Butaclamol was a gift of Ayerst Research Laboratories. ^{3}H-Spiperone and ^{3}H-ADTN were purchased from New England Nuclear Corp. All other chemicals were obtained from standard commercial sources.

In all studies mice were housed in a temperature and humidity controlled room with a 12 hour light-dark cycle. Mice were sacrificed by decapitation and the brains removed. Corpus striata were dissected from the brains by using the method described by Glowinski and Iverson (16) modified for the mouse brain. Washed membranes were prepared from striatal tissue using the methods described below. Protein concentration was determined using a modification of the dye binding method of Bradford (17) from Bio-Rad Laboratories.

B. Measurement of 3H-Spiperone Binding

The binding of spiperone to membranes from mouse corpus striatum was measured using a modification of the methods described by Quik and Iversen (18). Tissue was homogenized in 50 vol cold Tris HCl buffer (50 mM, pH 7.7) using a glass and Teflon homogenizer. The homogenate was centrifuged at 40,000 x g for 10 min and the supernatant discarded. The pellet was resuspended in 50 vol of cold Tris buffer and again centrifuged at 40,000 x g for 10 min. The resultant pellet was resuspended in 100 vol of 50 mM (pH 7.7) Tris buffer containing 120 mM NaCl, 5 mM KCl, 2 mM $CaCl_2$, 1 mM $MgCl_2$, 10 mM pargyline and 0.1% ascorbic acid. A 2 ml incubation volume was used and contained about 0.5 mg of membrane protein. Samples were pre-incubated with the appropriate cannabinoid or its Emulphor-ethanol vehicle (19) for 5 min at 37°C. The emulphor vehicle was found to be without significant effect on ^{3}H-spiperone binding over the concentration range used. Incubations were started by the addition of the ^{3}H-spiperone (25-800 pM) and terminated after 10 min by filtration through GF/B glass fiber filters. The filters were then washed twice with 5 ml of the incubation buffer and the bound radioactivity determined. Samples were also incubated with 0.1mcM (+)-butaclamol. Specific binding of ^{3}H-spiroperidol was defined as total binding minus binding in the presence of 0.10 mcM (+)-butaclamol.

C. Measurement of 3H-ADTN Binding

The binding of ^{3}H-ADTN to mouse striatal membranes was determined using a modification of the method described by Creese and Snyder (20). Membranes were prepared as described above, except the final resuspension was in 50 mM Tris (pH 7.1) buffer containing in a 1 ml incubation volume, 1 mM $MnCl_2$ and 0.1% ascorbic acid. Specific binding of ^{3}H-ADTN was determined by subtracting binding in the presence of 4 mcM dopamine from binding in the absence of excess dopamine. Cannabinoids were suspended using a polyvinylpyrrolidone (PVP) vehicle (21) since an emulphor vehicle significantly decreased binding.

D. Data Analysis

All experiments were repeated three or four times. Overall analysis of results was performed using analysis of variance. Treatment comparisons to control group values were performed by using Dunnett's modification of the t-test or the students test (22). K_d and B_{max} values were determined by either the method of Scatchard (23) or directly from the binding data by non-linear regression (24). IC50 values were determined from logit plots of binding competition data and K_i values were estimated by the method of Cheng and Prusoff (25).

III. RESULTS

The effects of several concentrations of THC on the specific binding of ^{3}H-spiperone were examined first. The results of this study are shown in Fig. 1. It can be seen that THC produced a concentration related inhibition of spiperone binding. Significant inhibition ($p < 0.05$) was produced by the 10 and 30mcM concentrations. The 30 mcM concentrationreduced binding to 60% of the vehicle control level. 11-OH-delta-9-THC, an active THC metabolite, and cannabidiol (CBD), a cannabinoid without the psychoactive properties of THC, also decreased spiperone binding. Significant ($p < 0.05$) inhibition of binding was produced by 30 mcM concentrations ofeach cannabinoid (Fig. 2). All three cannabinoids decreased specific spiperone binding to the same degree.

In order to further investigate the interaction of THC with spiperone binding, the effects of THC on the equilibrium binding properties were then examined. In this study, spiperone concentrations between 25 and 800 pM were used. Spiperone binding in the presence of emulphor vehicle was saturable (Fig. 3 - inset) and appeared to bind to one class of sites

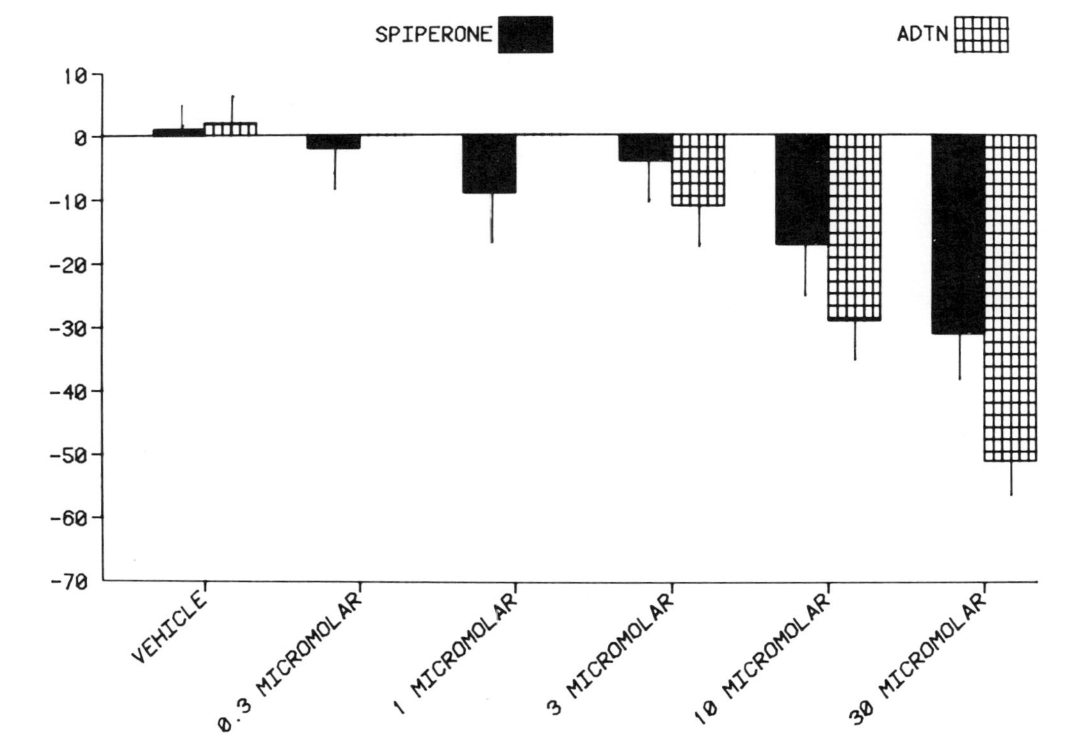

FIGURE 1. Effects of THC on the specific binding of ^{3}H-spiperone and ^{3}H-ADTN to membranes from mouse corpus striatum. Values are expressed as percent change from non-drug control samples and are the mean +/- S.E.M. of 4 to 6 experiments. ^{3}H-spiperone content was 0.3 nM. Binding in control samples was 99.4 +/- 7.4 fmol/mg of protein for spiperone and 75.6 +/- 8.5 fmol/mg of protein for ADTN.

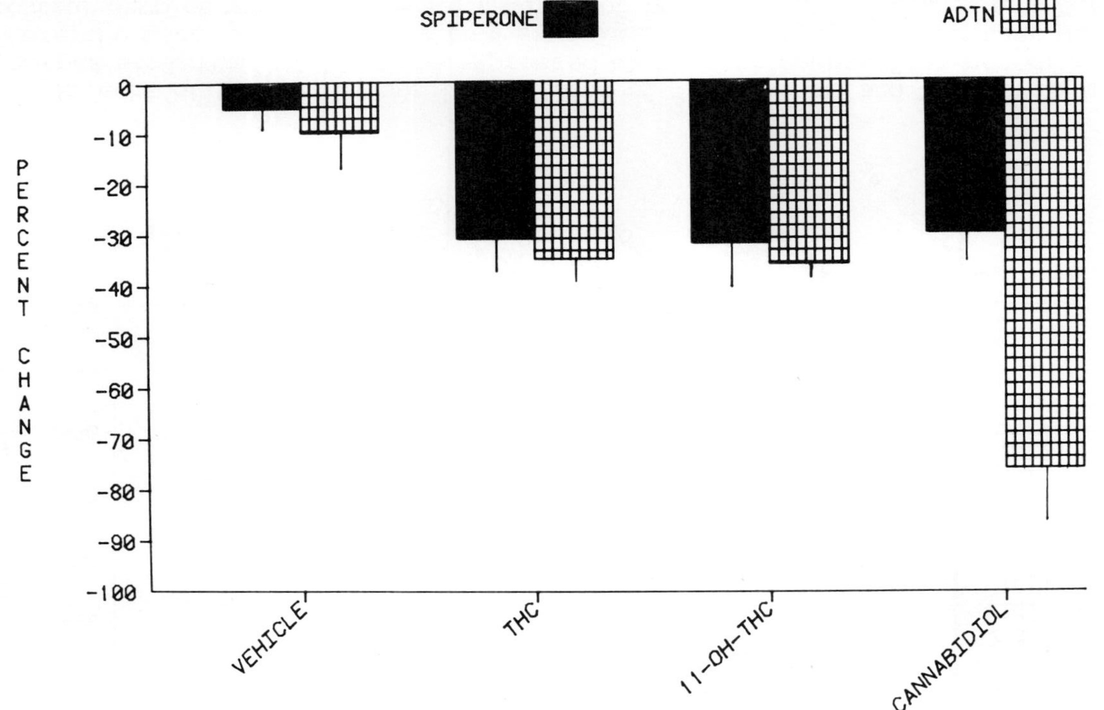

FIGURE 2. Effects of cannabinoids on the specific binding of ^{3}H-spiperone and ^{3}H-ADTN to membranes from mouse corpus striatum. Values are expressed as percent change from non-drug control samples and are the mean +/- S.E.M. of 3 or 4 experiments. Drug concentration was 30 mcM for all cannabinoids. Ligand concentrations were the same as in Fig. 1.

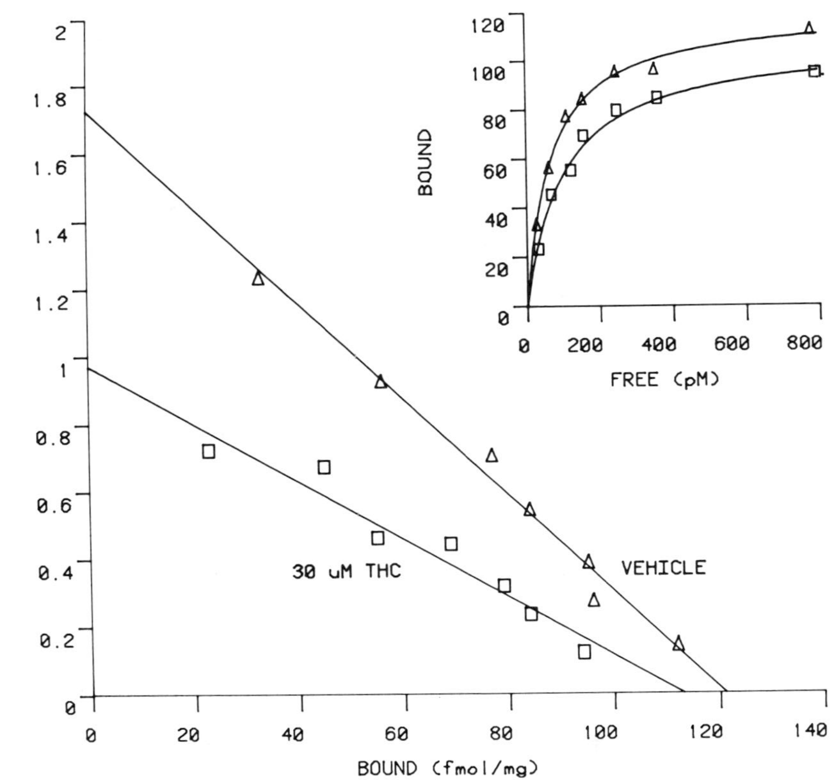

FIGURE 3. Effect of 30 mcM THC on the equilibrium binding properties of ^{3}H-spiperone. Values plotted are the mean of 3 or 4 experiments. Spiperone concentrations were between 50 and 800 pM.

with a K_d of 70 mcM and a B_{max} of 132 pmol/mg of protein. The 30mcM concentration of THC altered the equilibrium binding properties of spiperone. The K_d was increased to 114 pM. This was a statistically significant ($p < 0.05$) 70% decrease in receptor affinity. The Scatchard plot remained linear in the presence of THC. There was also a slight but not statistically significant decrease in the B_{max} parameter. The K_d increase is dependent upon the concentration since a 20 mcM concentration of THC (data not shown) produced an increase of 36% as opposed to a 70% change with the 30 mcM concentration.

Equilibrium binding parameters were also determined in the presence of 30 mcM CBD. The results of this study are shown in Table I. There was a significant increase (260%) in the K_d produced by CBD. There was a slight decrease in the B_{max} that did not reach statistical significance.

The effects of THC and CBD on the binding of dopaminergic agonists and antagonists to spiperone binding sites was then examined. This was accomplished by generating competition curves using dopamine, apomorphine, haloperidol and (+)-butaclamol in the presence of the above mentioned cannabinoids or their vehicle. The effects of a 30 mcM concentration ofTHC are shown in Table II. In vehicle-treated preparations, agonists demonstrated IC_{50} values in the high nanomolar or low micromolar range and antagonists had low nanomolar IC_{50}s. This indicated that spiperone was binding to a site with D_2 (15) properties. IC_{50} values for both dopamine and apomorphine were significantly reduced by the 30 mcM concentration of THC. With K_i values were calculated taking into account the change in spiperone K_d produced by THC, agonist affinities for the D_2 site were enhanced 2 fold by THC.

IC_{50} values for haloperidol and butaclamol were not significantly changed by THC. Therefore, K_i values for the antagonists were increased, thus, their affinities for the D_2 site decreased, as was the case for spiperone when measuredby direct binding.

TABLE I. Effects of Cannabidiol on the Binding Characteristics of ^{3}H-Spiperone

	Kd pM[a]	B_{max} fmol/mg protein[a]
Vehicle	59 (9)	120 (20)
CBD	154 (13)[b]	100 (11)

[a]Mean (+/- S.E.M.) of 3 to 4 experiments.
[b]$p < 0.05$ when compared to vehicle group.

The effect of CBD on agonist and antagonist binding is shown in Table III. Neither agonist nor antagonist IC_{50} values were significantly affected by a 30 mcM concentration of CBD. Therefore, K_i values for both agonists and antagonists were increased by CBD.

TABLE II. Effects of 30 mcM THC on the Displacement of ^{3}H-Spiperone Binding

	IC_{50}[a]		K_i[a]	
	Vehicle	THC	Vehicle	THC
Agonists:				
Dopamine (mcM)	13.5 (1.5)	4.9 (1.1)[b]	2.5	1.3
Apomorphine (nM)	224 (10)	64 (6)[b]	42.4	17.6
Antagonists:				
Haloperidol (nM)	9.2 (0.5)	8.8 (1.3)	1.7	2.4
(+)-Butaclamol (nM)	1.1 (0.1)	1.1 (0.1)	0.21	0.30

[a]Mean (+/- S.E.M). of 3 to 4 experiments.
[b]$p < 0.05$ compared to vehicle group.

TABLE III. Effects of 30 mcM-CBD on the Displacement of ^{3}-H-Spiperone Binding

	IC_{50}[a]		K_i[a]	
	Vehicle	THC	Vehicle	THC
Agonists:				
Dopamine (mcM)	10.1 (0.8)	8.8 (1.3)	1.6	3.4
Apomorphine (nM)	213 (73)	189 (13)	33.7	64.0
Antagonists:				
Haloperidol (nM)	9.9 (1.1)	10.1 (1.7)	1.6	3.4
(+)-Butaclamol (nM)	1.4 (0.2)	1.6 (0.3)	0.22	0.54

[a]Mean (+/- S.E.M.) of 3 to 4 experiments.

The effects of cannabinoids on the binding of ^{3}H-ADTBN, a dopaminergic agonist were also examined. In these studies PVP was used as the cannabinoid vehicle since emulphor significantly decreased the binding of ^{3}H-ADTN. The specific binding of ^{3}H-ADTN was inhibited by THC in a concentration related manner (Fig. 1). Significant ($p < 0.05$) decreases in binding were caused by the 3, 10 and 30 mcM concentrations. ADTN binding was also decreased by 30 mcM concentrations of 11-OH-delta-9-THC and CBD (Fig. 2). CBD was significantly ($p < 0.05$) more effective than the other cannabinoids. Binding was reduced by 73% with the 30 mcM concentration of CBD.

The effects of THC and CBD on the equilibrium binding properties of ^{3}H-ADTN are shown in Table IV. Unlike their effects on spiperone binding, neither cannabinoid significantly changed the K_d when compared to vehicle controls. However, there were significant decreases in the B_{max} produced by both THC and CBD. B_{max} values were decreased 50% by 20 mcM THC and 65% by 20 mcM CBD. K_d and B_{max} values could not be accurately obtained in the presence of 30 mcM CBD because ofthe large decrease in binding.

IV. DISCUSSION

The results of these studies demonstrate interactions between cannabinoids and dopamine receptors that are complex in their nature. The cannabinoids tested have different effects on D_2 and D_3 type receptors. Furthermore, THC and CBD differentially affected binding to the D_2 receptors. Lastly, the effects of the cannabinoids on binding to dopamine recep-

TABLE IV. Effects of THC and CBD on the Binding Characteristics of ^{3}H-ADTN

Drug	Concentration mcM	K_d (nM)[a] Vehicle	K_d (nM)[a] Drug	B_{max} (fmol/mg-protein)[a] Vehicle	B_{max} (fmol/mg-protein)[a] Drug
THC	20	2.3 (0.4)	2.1 (0.6)	66 (6)	33 (6)[b]
	30	1.9 (0.3)	1.7 (0.1)	71 (18)	25 (8)[b]
CBD	20	2.0 (0.3)	1.5 (0.2)	81 (17)	28 (17)[b]

[a]Mean (+/- S.E.M.) of 3 to 4 experiments.
[b]$p < 0.05$ when compared to vehicle group.

tors were quite different than their effects on binding to beta-adrenergic receptors in the mouse brain (14; Hillard and Bloom, this volume).

THC, 11-OH-delta-9-THC and CBD all inhibited the specific binding of ^{3}H-spiperone to membranes from mouse corpus striatum. Analysis of the binding data indicated that the decrease in binding resulted from a decrease in the apparent affinity (an increase in K_d) of the receptor for ^{3}H-spiperone. The increase in K_d produced by the 30 mcM concentration ofCBD (260%) was greater than the change produced by the same concentrationof THC (70%). The specific binding of the dopaminergic agonist ^{3}H-ADTN was also decreased by all three of the cannabinoids used in these studies. Again, CBD was more effective than THC. However, the decrease in binding appeared to be the result of a decrease in the B_{max} (the theoretical number of binding sites) rather than a change in K_d as was the case for spiperone. Thus it appears that cannabinoids interact differently with D_2 and D_3 receptors. This is not surprising since it appears that D_2 and D_3 sites are separate and distinct molecular entities. The binding of agonist and antagonist ligands differ in their sensitivity to guanyl nucleotides (26) and lesions, and in their sub-cellular and cellular localization (15).

THC, although it decreased the binding of dopaminergic antagonists, appeared to increase the affinity of agonists at ^{3}H-spiperone binding sites. Agonist IC_{50} and K_i values for spiperone binding were reduced by 30 mcM THC. CBD did not produce this effect on agonist binding. It reduced the affinity of both agonists and antagonists. Previous studies indicate that there are differences in the binding of agonists and antagonists to ^{3}H-spiperone binding sites. For example, GTP reduces the agonist inhibition of ^{3}H-spiperidol binding itself. Furthermore, the enhancement of agonist binding argues against the probability that the increased spiperone dissociation constant is the result of competitive antagonism by THC at D_2 binding sites. Rather it seems that THC is altering the properties of the receptor site rendering it less favorable to antagonists and more favorable to agonists. Changes such as this could be the result of changes in the membrane environment that the receptor resides in. The concept that the cell membrane is a primary site of action for THC is supported by the work of Gill and Lawrence (27) who found that THC increased the fluidization and disordering of liposomes, and Bach et al. (28) who demonstrated similar effects using synthetic membranes. Gill and Lawrence reported that this effect was specific for those cannabinoids having marijuana-like behavioral activity since cannabinol and cannabidiol produced effects opposite to those of THC, while 11-OH-delta-9-THC was more active than THC. In other studies THC has been shown to alter the activity of several membrane associated enzymes such as NADH-oxidase (29,30), acetylcholinesterase (31) and various ATPases (8,13). Similarly, cannabinoids can decrease the high affinity uptake of several neurotransmitters into synaptosomes (7,32). These studies indicate that the interaction of THC with membranes may result in changes in the functional compounds such as enzymes. Thus similar changes in other protein compounds such as receptors are also possible.

The importance of the changes observed in these studies to the psychoactive actions of THC is not clear. Since ^{3}H-spiperone and ^{3}H-ADTN binding are inhibited by both THC and CBD, it seems unlikely that this action is of great significance to psychoactivity. On the other hand, the selective enhancement of agonist binding to D_2 sites by THC but not CBD may be of more significance. The significance of this observation is due more to the differences in the effects of THC and CBD on a membrane bound entity rather than the fact that the entity is a dopamine receptor. Similarly, we have observed that THC but not CBD can enhance binding of antagonist to beta-adrenergic receptors in mouse brain (14). The relative role of any of these receptor systems in the effect of the cannabinoids is as yet unknown.

In summary, the studies described here indicate that THC and other cannabinoids can alter the binding of ligands to several different membrane bound neurotransmitter receptors. Furthermore the effects described are selective for both the cannabinoid and the receptor. Different cannabinoids can affect the same receptor differently; and different receptors can be affected differently by the same cannabinoid. Lastly, since THC is highly associated with synaptic membranes after its _in vivo_ administration (33) and can alter membrane physical properties such as fluidity, it is possible that the effects on receptors are due to cannabinoid induced changes in the membrane environment that neurotransmitter receptors reside in. Thus it is possible that membranes can serve as a selective recognition site for the different cannabinoids.

ACKNOWLEDGMENTS

The authors thanks Jan Greathouse and Therese Dieringer for their fine technical assistance.

REFERENCES

1. Holtzman, D., Lovell, R. A., Jaffe, J. H., and Freedman, D. X., l-delta-9-tetrahydrocannabinol: Neurochemical and behavioral effects in the mouse, Science 163:1464-1467 (1969).
2. Harris, L. S., Dewey, W. L., and Razdan, R. K., Cannabis: Its chemistry, pharmacology, and toxicology, in "Handbook of Experimental Pharmacology" (W. R. Martin, ed.), pp. 372-429. Springer-Verlag, Berlin, 1976.
3. Maitre, L., Baumann, P. A., and Delini-Stula, A., Neurochemical tolerance to cannabinols, in "Cannabis and its Derivatives" (W.D.M. Paton and J. Crown, eds.), Pharmacology and Experimental Psychology, Oxford University Press, London, 1972.
4. Bloom, A. S., Johnson, K. M., and Dewey, W. L., The effects of cannabinoids on body temperature and brain catecholamine synthesis, Res. Comm. Chem. Path. Pharm. 20:51-57 (1978).
5. Bloom, A. S., and Kiernan, C. J., Interaction of ambient temperature with the effects of delta-9-tetrahydrocannabinol on brain catecholamine synthesis and plasma corticosterone levels, Psychopharmacology 67:215-219 (1980).
6. Bloom, A. S., Effect of delta-9-tetrahydrocannabinol on the synthesis of dopamine and norepinephrine in mouse brain synaptosomes, J. Pharmacol. Exp. Ther. 221:97-103 (1982).
7. Banerjee, S. P., Snyder, S. H., and Mechoulam, R., Cannabinoids: Influence on neurotransmitter uptake in rat brain synaptosomes, J. Pharmacol. Exp. Ther. 194:74-81 (1975).
8. Hershkowitz, M., Goldman, R., and Raz, A., Effect of cannabinoids on neurotransmitter uptake, ATPase activity and morphology of mouse brain synaptosomes, Biochem. Pharmacol. 26:1327-1331 (1977).
9. Johnson, K. M., and Dewey, W. L., Effects of delta-9-THC on the synaptosomal uptake of ^{3}H-tryptophan and ^{3}H-choline, Pharmacology 17:83-87 (1978).
10. Ho, B., T., Taylor, D., and Englert, L. F., The effect of repeated administration of (-)-delta-9-tetrahydrocannabinol on the biosynthesis of brain amines, Res. Comm. Path. Pharmacol. 5:851-954 (1973).
11. Banerjee, A., Poddar, M. K., Sara, S., and Ghosh, J., Effect of delta-9-tetrahydrocannabinol on monoamine oxidase activity of rat tissue <u>in vivo</u>, Biochem. Pharmacol. 24:1435-1436 (1975a).
12. Schurr, A., and Livne, A., Differential inhibition of mitochondrial monoamine oxidase from brain by hashish

components, Biochem. Pharmacol. 25:1201-1203 (1976).

13. Bloom, A. S., Haavik, C. O., and Strehlow, D., Effects of delta-9-tetrahydrocannabinol on ATPases in mouse brain subcellular fractions, Life Sci. 23:1399-1404 (1978).

14. Hillard, C. J., and Bloom, A. S., Delta-9-tetrahydrocannabinol-induced changes in beta-adrenergic receptor binding in mouse cerebral cortex, Brain Research 235:370-377 (1982).

15. Seeman, P., Brain dopamine receptors, Pharmacol. Reviews 32:229-312 (1980).

16. Glowinski, J., and Iversen, L. L., Regional studies of catecholamines in the rat brain. I. The disposition of (^{3}H)-norepinephrine,(^{3}H)-dopamine and (^{3}H)-dopa in various regions of the brain, J. Neurochem. 13:655-669 (1966).

17. Bradford, M. M., A rapid and sensitive method for the quantitation of microgram quantities of protein utilizing the principle of protein-dye binding, Anal. Biochem. 72:248-254 (1976).

18. Quik, M., and Iversen, L. L., Regional study of ^{3}H-spiperone binding and dopamine-sensitive adenylate cyclase in rat brain, Eur. J. Pharmacol. 56:323-330 (1979).

19. Cradock, J. C., Davignon, J. P., Litterst, G. L., and Guarino, A. M., An intravenous formulation of delta-9-tetrahydrocannabinol using anon-toxic surfactant, J. Pharm. Pharmacol. 24:345 (1973).

20. Creese, I., and Snyder, S. H., Dopamine receptor binding of ^{3}H-ADTN (2-amino-6,7-dihydroxy-1,2,3,4-tetrahydronaphthalene) regulated by guanyl nucleotides, Eur. J. Pharmacol. 50:459-461 (1978).

21. Fenimore, D. C., and Loy, P. R., Injectable dispersion of delta-9-tetrahydrocannabinol in saline using polyvinylpyrrolidone. J. Pharm. Pharmacol. 23:310 (1971).

22. Winer, B., "Statistical Principles in Experimental Design." McGraw-Hill Book Company, New York, 1972.

23. Scatchard, G., The attractions of proteins for small molecules and ions, Ann. N. Y. Acad. Sci. 51:660-672 (1948-49).

24. Graybill, F. A., "Introduction to matrices with applications in statistics." Wadsworth Publishing Company, Belmont, CA, 1969.

25. Cheng, Y. C., and Prusoff, W. H., Relationship between the inhibition constant and the concentration of inhibitor which causes 50 percent inhibition (I_{50}) of an enzymatic reaction, Biochem. Pharmacol. 22:3099-3108 (1973).

26. Creese, I., Usdin, T. B., and Snyder, S. H., Dopamine receptor binding regulated by guanine nucleotides, Mol. Pharmacol. 50:459-461 (1978).

27. Gill, E. W., and Lawrence, D. K., The physiochemical mode of action of tetrahydrocannabinol on cell membrane, in "The Pharmacology of Marihuana" (M. C. Braude and S. Szara, eds.) pp. 147-155. Raven Press, New York, 1976.
28. Bach, D., Raz, A., and Goldman, R., The interaction of hashish compounds with planar lipid bilary membranes (BLM), Biochem. Pharmacol. 25:1241-1244 (1976).
29. Bartova, A., and Birmingham, M. K., Effect of tetrahydrocannabinol and deoxycorticosterone on brain and adrenal NADH-oxidase activity, Fed. Proc. 31:481 (1972).
30. Bartova, A., and Birmingham, M. K., Effect of delta-9-tetrahydrocannabinol on mitochondrial NADH-oxidase activity, J. Biol. Chem. 251:5002-5006 (1976).
31. Laurent, B., and Roy, P. E., Alteration of membrane integrity by delta-9-tetrahydrocannabinol, Int. J. Clin. Pharm. 12:261-266 (1975).
32. Johnson, K. M., Ho, B. T., and Dewey, W. L., Effects of delta-9-tetrahydrocannabinol on neurotransmitter accumulation and release mechanisms of rat forebrain synaptosomes, Life Science 19:347-356 (1976).
33. Dewey, W. L., Martin, B. R., Beckner, J. S., and Harris, L. S., A comparison of the subcellular distribution of cannabinoids in the brains of tolerant and nontolerant dogs, rats, mice after injecting radiolabeled delta-9-tetrahydrocannabinol, in "Marihuana: Chemistry, Biochemistry and Cellular Effects" (G. G. Nahas, ed.), pp. 349-365. Springer-Verlag, New York, 1976.
34. Seeman, P., Chau-Wong, M., and Moyyen, S., The membrane binding to morphine, diphenylhydantoin, and tetrahydrocannabinol, Can. J. Physiol. Pharmacol. 50:1193-1200 (1972).

FURTHER STUDIES OF THE INTERACTION OF DELTA-9-TETRAHYDROCANNABINOL WITH THE BETA-ADRENERGIC RECEPTOR*

Cecilia J. Hillard
Alan S. Bloom

Department of Pharmacology and Toxicology
Medical College of Wisconsin
Milwaukee, Wisconsin

I. INTRODUCTION

The ability of delta-9-tetrahydrocannabinol (THC) to influence the structure and function of biological membranes is well documented. The partition coefficient of THC into crude brain synaptosomal membranes is on the order of 12,000, indicating that THC has an extremely high affinity for the membrane (1). Lawrence and Gill demonstrated that THC dissolved in and increased the fluidity of spin-labeled liposomes, which are synthetic phospholipid bilayers (2). Furthermore, they found that the less potent (+)-stereoisomer of THC produced a smaller change and that cannabidiol and cannabinol, cannabinoids devoid of THC-like psychoactivity, decreased membrane fluidity.

THC can exert a wide range of effects on membrane associated systems as well. For example, THC has been shown to affect neurotransmitter uptake systems (3,4), membrane bound enzyme systems (5-7) and glucose efflux (8). These findings suggest that a mechanism of THC action could be a primary alteration in the physical properties of the phospholipid bilayer of the membrane (e.g., increased fluidity) which secondarily effects the functioning of membrane associated macromolecules.

*Supported by NIDA grant DA-00124.

ISBN 0-12-044620-0

To further investigate this hypothesis, we have begun to study the effects of THC on the beta-adrenergic receptor in membranes from mouse cerebral cortex. Our initial studies demonstrated that the psychoactive cannabinoids THC and 11-OH-delta-9-THC, when administered _in vitro_, biphasically increased the binding of the beta-adrenergic ligand ^{3}H-dihydroalprenolol (^{3}H-DHA) to mouse cerebral cortical membranes (9). We found that cannabidiol, a cannabinoid devoid of THC-like psychoactive properties, did not affect ^{3}H-DHA binding. Results within this limited range of cannabinoids suggestthat the increase in ^{3}H-DHA binding is specific for the psychoactive cannabinoids. These results provide another example of THC-induced changes in a membrane-bound entity.

We now report further studies of the interaction of _in vitro_ THC and cerebral cortical beta-adrenergic receptors. We have extended the analysis of the effect of THC on ^{3}H-DHA binding and have investigated the effects of THC on agonist binding as well. These results allow further insight into the mechanism of THC-induced alterations in the beta-adrenergic receptor system.

II. MATERIALS AND METHODS

Delta-9-Tetrahydrocannabinol (generously supplied by NIDA) was administered using an Emulphor (GAF, New York, NY)-ethanol-buffer vehicle in 0.5:0.5:9 proportion (10). Sotalol hydrochloride was a gift from Ayerst Laboratories (New York, NY). All other drugs were obtained from the usual commercial sources.

The beta-adrenergic binding assay was carried out using a modification of the method of Alexander et al. (11). Male ICR outbred mice (ARS, Madison, WI) weighing 20-30 g were used in all studies. After sacrifice, cerebral cortices were removed, pooled and homogenized in 10 volumes of cold 0.25 M sucrose buffer containing 5 mM Tris-HCl (pH 7.4) and 1 mM $MgCl_2$. The homogenate was centrifuged at 800 x g for 20 min; the resulting supernatant was recentrifuged at 14,000 x g for 14 min. The final pellet was resuspended in cold 75 mM Tris HCl (pH 7.4) buffer containing 25 mM $MgCl_2$ to yield a final protein concentration of approximately 0.5 mg/ml. The total incubation volume was 1.0 ml; 10 mcM dl-propranolol was added to half the incubates to account for nonspecific binding. After preincubation of tissue with drugs at 37°C, ^{3}H-DHA (30-60 Ci/mmol, Amersham, Arlington Heights, IL) was added and the incubation was continued for 15 min. Bound and free ^{3}H-DHA were separated using filtration under reduced pressure through

Whatman GF/B glass fiber filters. Specific binding was calculated by subtracting the amount of ^{3}H-DHA bound in the presence of dl-propranolol (non-specific binding) from the amount of ^{3}H-DHA bound in the absence of dl-propranolol. The protein content of each homogenate was estimated using the Bio-rad (Bio-Rad Laboratories, Richmond, CA) dye-binding method of Bradford (12).

Binding data were analyzed using standard methods. The dissociation constant K_D, and binding site density, B_{max}, were estimated from the plot of ^{3}H-DHA bound versus ^{3}H-DHA bound/^{3}H-DHA free using the method of Scatchard (13). The K_D is equal to the negative reciprocal of the slope and B_{max} is equal to the x-intercept; slope and intercept were estimated using linear regression. In competition studies, the IC_{50} values (concentration of cold ligand that reduced ^{3}H-DHA bound by 50%) and 95% confidence intervals were obtained from plots of log concentration of unlabeled ligand versus % ^{3}H-DHA bound using linear regression. Pseudo Hill plots, i.e., log ligand concentration versus log (% ^{3}H-DHA bound/100-% ^{3}H-DHA bound), were also constructed for each ligand. The pseudo Hill coefficient, or slope, was estimated using linear regression.

III. RESULTS

The effect of 10 mcM THC on ^{3}H-DHA binding to the beta-adrenergic receptor of mouse cerebral cortical membranesis shown in Figure 1. In previous studies, we found that the maximum increase in ^{3}H-DHA binding occurred at 10 mcM THC (9). The saturation curves of ^{3}H-DHA binding in the presence of 10 mcM THC or equivalent vehicle show an increase in ^{3}H-DHA binding at all ^{3}H-DHA concentrations with THC treatment. Scatchard analysis of the data is also shown in Figure 1. In the presence of vehicle, the Scatchard plot is linear with a derived K_D (dissociation constant) of 1.86 nM and a B_{max} (binding site density) of 58.6 fmol/mg protein. However, with 10 mcM THC, the Scatchard plot of ^{3}H-DHA binding is shifted to the right and becomes curvilinear.

A curvilinear Scatchard plot is indicative of multiple classes or forms of ^{3}H-DHA binding sites. In Figure 2, a two binding site model was assumed and estimates of the binding parameters were obtained using a curve stripping technique. The low affinity (high K_D) site was assigned parameters close to those obtained in the presence of vehicle alone; the K_D value is 2.5 nM and B_{max} is 70 fmol/mg protein. The high affinity site that results when the low affinity site is "stripped out" has a K_D of 0.4 nM and a B_{max} of 15 fmol/mg

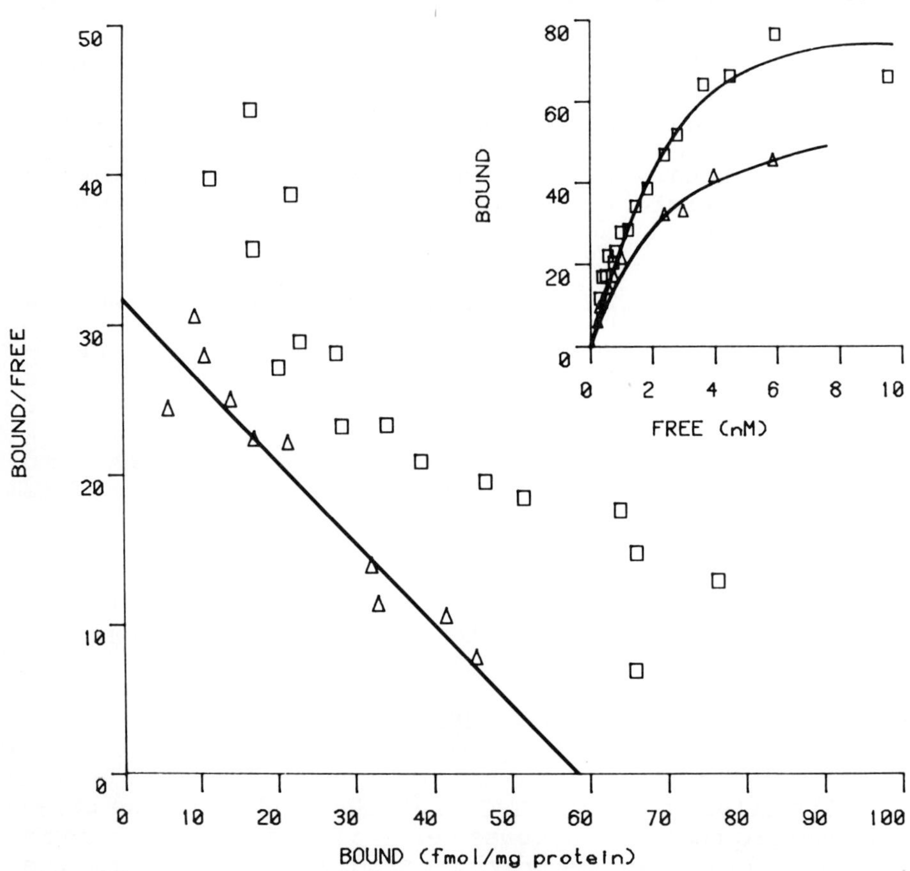

FIGURE 1. Scatchard plots of ^{3}H-DHA binding obtained in the presence of 10 mcM THC (squares) and equivalent vehicle (triangles) are shown. The data points are derived from the saturation curves shown in the inset. The solid line is the best linear fit to vehicle data using linear regression analysis. Inset: Saturation curves of ^{3}H-DHA binding obtained in the presence of 10 mcM THC (squares) and equivalent vehicle (triangles). Each point is the mean of 3-5 experiments.

protein. When these two binding sites are graphically added, the curve shown in Figure 2 is obtained.

Competition studies were carried out in order to determine whether THC produced the same change in binding of both agonists and antagonists to the receptor. In all of the competition studies, ^{3}H-DHA was used at a concentration of 7.0 nM. In Figure 3, the effect of 10 mcM THC on dl-propranolol competition with ^{3}H-DHA is shown. The competition curve is shifted to the left in the presence of THC, corresponding to a change in IC_{50} from 80.4 nM to 36.2 nM (Table I). Pseudo Hill plots

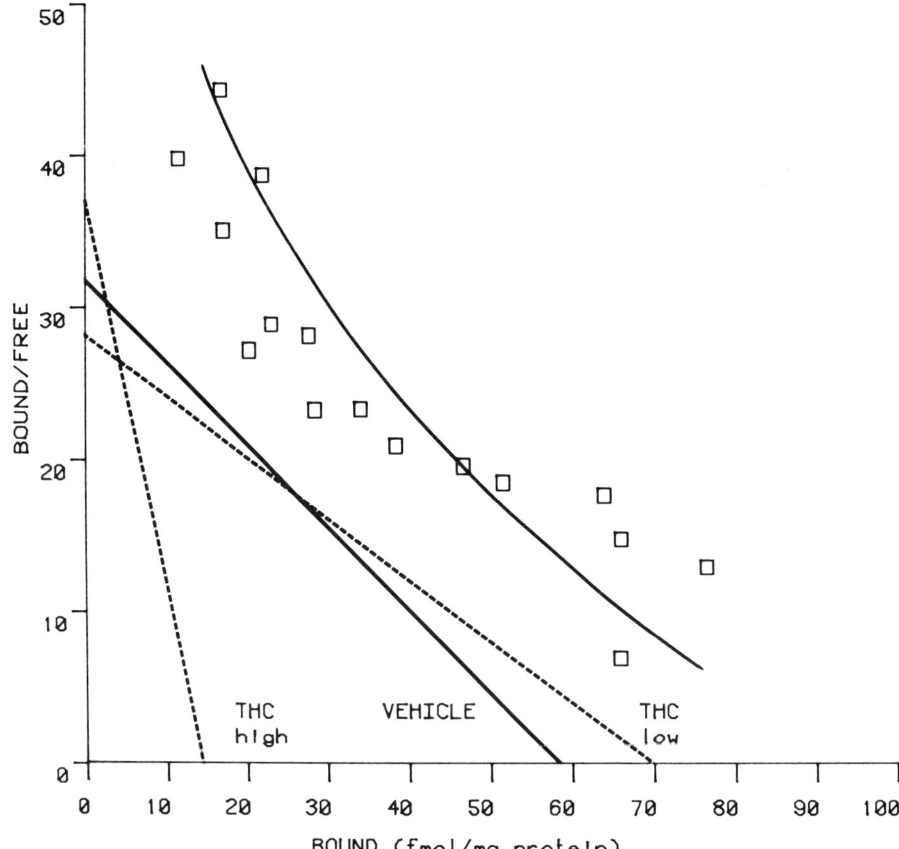

FIGURE 2. Scatchard plot of ^{3}H-DHA binding in the presence of vehicle (solid line) and 10 mcM THC (squares). The high and low affinity sites derived using curve stripping areshown with dashed lines. The Scatchard plot that would be expected from ^{3}H-DHA to these two sites is shown by the curved solid line.

of the competition data are linear in the presence of both 10 mcM delta-9-THC and vehicle (Figure 3). The pseudo Hill coefficient, however, is lower in the presence of THC; 0.73 compared to 1.10 in the presence of vehicle (Table I).

The effect of 10 mcM THC on the competition of the agonist isoproterenol with ^{3}H-DHA is shown in Figure 4. In contrast to its effect on antagonist binding, THC shifts the isoproterenol competition curve to the right. This shift corresponds to a change in IC_{50} from 0.63 mcM to 1.49 mcM with THC treatment (Table I). The pseudo Hill plots are both linear with a slight decrease in pseudo Hill coefficient in the presence of THC.

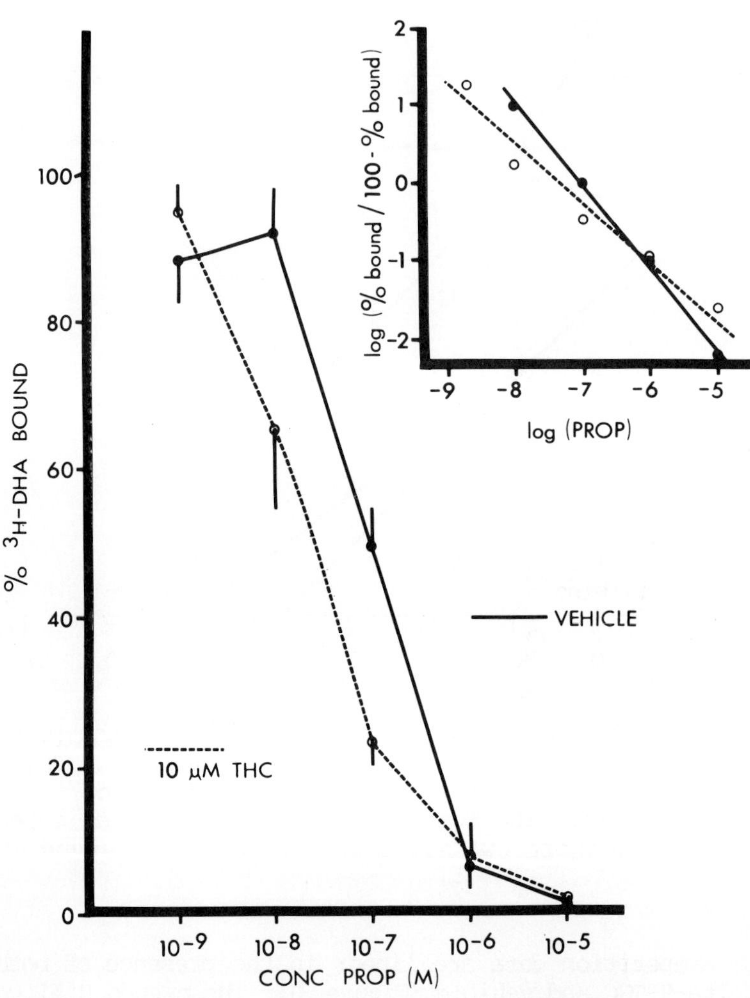

FIGURE 3. The % ^{3}H-DHA bound at various propranolol concentrations in the presence of vehicle (solid circles and line) and 10 mcM THC (open circles and dashed line) are shown. Each point is the mean of 3-5 experiments; vertical lines represent S.E.M. Inset: Pseudo Hill plots of propranolol competition with ^{3}H-DHA in the presence of vehicle and 10 mcM THC (key, as above) are shown. Each point is derived from competition curves shown. Lines are drawn using linear regression analysis.

In Table I are listed the IC_{50} values and pseudo Hill coefficients for propranolol and isoproterenol as well as several other beta-adrenergic receptor ligands. THC reduced the IC_{50} values for all the antagonists investigated. This occurs regardless of the lipid solubility of the antagonist, practolol and sotalol being relatively lipid insoluble ligands (14). The pseudo Hill coefficients of all the antagonists are reduced by THC. Interestingly, the pseudo Hill coefficients for practolol and sotalol are less than one but still decrease in the presence of THC. All of the antagonist pseudo

TABLE II. Effects of THC On Competition of Agonists and Antagonists with ^{3}H-DHA[a]

Competing Ligand	IC50[b]		Pseudo Hill Coefficient[c]	
	Vehicle	10 mcM THC	Vehicle	10 mcM THC
Antagonists:				
Propranolol	80.4 (58.7-110.3)	36.2 (27.8-47.0)	1.10	0.73
Alprenolol	29.4 (18.2-42.6)	8.1 (6.8-9.6)	0.91	0.64
Practolol	21.4 (17.3-26.4)	11.8 (9.9-13.9)	0.76	0.50
Sotalol	1.84 (1.53-2.21)	0.98 (0.93-1.03)	0.54	0.49
Partial Agonist:				
Dichloro-isoproterenol	95.7 (88.3-103.8)	167.0 (141-198)	0.50	0.59
Agonists:				
Isoproterenol	0.63 (0.53-0.75)	1.49 (1.36-1.62)	0.63	0.48
Norepinephrine	7.26 (6.37-8.28)	12.52 (10.2-15.3)	0.47	0.59
Epinephrine	6.17	11.22	0.64	0.49

[a] ^{3}H-DHA concentration was 7.0 nM in all studies.

[b] Units are in nM for antagonists and partial agonist and in mcM for agonists (95% confidence interval).

[c] IC_{50} values and pseudo Hill coefficients were obtained from plots of combined data from 3-5 experiments as outline in the Methods section.

Hill plots were qualitatively similar to that shown for propranolol.

The effects of THC on agonist binding are the opposite of the effects of THC on antagonist binding. The IC_{50} values of all the agonists were increased in the presence of THC. The pseudo Hill coefficients are all less than one in the presence of vehicle and changed slightly and inconsistently in the presence of THC. The partial agonist, dichloroisoproterenol, appears agonist-like, since the IC_{50} is increased and pseudo Hill coefficient is slightly increased in the presence of THC.

IV. DISCUSSION

In these studies we have demonstrated that THC increases the binding of antagonists but not agonists to the beta-adrenergic receptor binding site of cerebral membranes. The increase in antagonist binding is accompanied by a decrease in pseudo Hill coefficient while there is no consistent change in the pseudo Hill coefficients or agonists. The differential effects of THC on agonist and antagonist binding indicate a complex interaction of THC with the beta-adrenergic receptor system.

In a previous report from our laboratory, we demonstrated that THC increased the binding of ^{3}H-DHA to beta-adrenergic receptors (9). In that paper, the slopes of Scatchard plots, constructed from a limited number of ligand concentrations, were steepened in the presence of THC but appeared to remain essentially linear. We concluded that the increase in ^{3}H-DHA binding due to a decrease in K_D (increase in affinity). In the present paper, we have increased the number of ligand concentrations used and still find that THC increases ^{3}H-DHA binding. However, a Scatchard plot of these data is distinctly curvilinear in the presence of THC.

The most likely cause of a nonlinear Scatchard plot is ligand binding to more than one class or form of binding sites, each having a different affinity for the ligand. In Fig. 2, we assumed a two binding site model and solved for the K_D and B_{max} of each site a using graphic curve-stripping method. However, when the two sites are added back together, the resulting curve poorly approximates the actual data. It appears more likely that this Scatchard plot is the result of binding to a range of binding sites with a continuum of K_D values. Therefore, THC changes the character of the ^{3}H-DHA binding sites from a single class of sites to a heterogeneous pool with several, perhaps a continuum of K_D values. This interpretation was also confirmed by our inability to fit this data to a two site model using nonlinear regression techniques.

The effects of THC on the binding of four unlabeled antagonists were assessed using competition studies. The IC_{50} values of all the antagonists are decreased in the presence of THC. The antagonist affinities are apparently increased, although actual K_i values cannot be calculated since an estimate of a single K_D for ^{3}H-DHA in the presence of THC is not easily made.

When agonists are used as the competing ligands, the IC_{50} values are increased in the presence of THC. Since the binding of ^{3}H-DHA itself is increased by THC, it is difficult to determine whether the increase in agonist IC_{50} is due to a real reduction in agonist binding or is a reflection of the increase in ^{3}H-DHA binding with no actual change in agonist binding. In either case, agonist binding is not increased by THC at a concentration which increases antagonist binding.

The slope of pseudo Hill plot of the competing ligand, called the pseudo Hill coefficient, provides an indication of the complexity of the binding process. A pseudo Hill coefficient of less than one will result if the ligand binds to more than one binding site with differing affinities. This reasoning probably explains the low pseudo Hill coefficient for practolol in the presence of vehicle. Practolol has a higher affinity for the beta-1 subtype than for the beta-2 subtype of the beta-adrenergic receptor.

Recent evidence suggests that the low pseudo Hill coefficient observed with agonists results from the formation of a ternary complex between the beta-adrenergic receptor and a guanine nucleotide binding protein (G-protein) within the membrane (15). It is thought that the binding of an agonist to the receptor produces a conformational change in the receptor that allows its association with the G-protein into a ternary complex. Such a conformational change does not occur with antagonist binding. In the absence of GTP, the complex is stable and has a high affinity for the agonist. In the presence of GTP, the ternary complex dissociates and the affinity of the receptor for the agonist decreases. These changes in the receptor are reflected by changes in agonist pseudo Hill coefficients. In the absence of GTP, the majority of agonist binding is to the ternary complex, with high affinity and a low pseudo Hill coefficient. In the presence of GTP, the majority of agonist binding is to the receptor alone having lower affinity and a pseudo Hill coefficient closer to one. Since antagonist binding does not induce the formation of a ternary complex, the pseudo Hill coefficients are approximately one and affinities are the same in the presence and absence of GTP.

The competition studies in these experiments were done in the absence of GTP and agonist pseudo Hill coefficients are less than one in the presence of vehicle. THC treatment appears to have no effect on agonist pseudo Hill coefficient. The pseudo Hill coefficients of the antagonists alprenolol and propranolol are approximately one in the presence of vehicle. Practolol has a low pseudo Hill coefficient for the reason mentioned above. Sotalol, which is reported to be a nonselective antagonist, has a low pseudo Hill coefficient in our study for reasons which are not apparent. In the presence of THC, the pseudo Hill coefficients of the antagonists are all reduced.

The changes in antagonist binding produced by THC, an increase in affinity and decrease in pseudo Hill coefficient, tend to make antagonist binding more agonist-like. It is possible that THC affects the ability of the receptor to discriminate between agonists and antagonists. In the presence of THC, binding of either an agonist or an antagonist has the characteristics of binding to the receptor in a ternary "state". It is possible that THC either promotes the formation of the ternary complex in the absence of any ligand or allows any binding event to result in the change in receptor conformation that is associated with ternary complex formation. To speculate on a mechanism for such a change, it is plausible that THC could act on the membrane to alter the environment of the receptor and G-protein. There is evidence that agents which increase membrane fluidity can affect beta-adrenergic receptor activation (16).

The effects of THC on ^{3}H-DHA binding itself are consistent with this proposal. Binding of ^{3}H-DHA is increased and the Scatchard plot indicates that ^{3}H-DHA binds to more than one form of binding site with THC treatment. It is conceivable that THC could produce a graded change in receptor conformation leading to a spectrum of affinity states. At one end of the spectrum would be the completely unassociated receptor with a low affinity for the ligand and at the other end, the receptor associated with G-protein in a ternary complex having a high affinity for ^{3}H-DHA and other beta-adrenergic ligands.

Although we do not suggest that THC induced changes in binding to beta-adrenergic receptors are a prime cause of the behavioral effect of THC, these data indicate that cannabinoids can have significant effects on the properties of membrane bound entities. These studies offer further support for the hypothesis that the membrane is a primary site of cannabinoid action.

REFERENCES

1. Roth, S. H., and Williams, P. J., The nonspecific membrane binding properties of delta-9-tetrahydrocannabinol and the effects of various solubilizers, J. Pharm. Pharmacol. 31:224-230 (1979).
2. Lawrence, D. K., and Gill, E. W., The effects of delta-1-tetrahydrocannabinol and other cannabinoids on spin-labeled liposomes and their relationship to mechanisms of general anesthesia, Mol. Pharmacol. 11:595-602 (1975).
3. Banerjee, S. P., Snyder, J. H., and Mechoulam, R., Cannabinoids: Influence on neurotransmitter uptake in rat brain synaptosomes, J. Pharmacol. Exp. Ther. 194:74-81 (1975).
4. Johnson, K. M., Ho., B. T., and Dewey, W. L., Effects of delta-9-tetrahydrocannabinol on neurotransmitter accumulation and release mechanisms in rat forebrain synaptosomes, Life Sci. 19:347-356 (1976).
5. Banerjee, A., Podar, M. R., Saha, S., and Ghosh, J. J., Effect of delta-9-tetrahydrocannabinol on monoamine oxidase activity of rat tissues in vivo, Biochem. Pharmacol. 24:1435-1436 (1975).
6. Bloom, A. S., Haavik, C. O., and Strehlow, D., Effects of delta-9-tetrahydrocannabinol onATPases in mouse brain subcellular fractions, Life Sci. 23:1399-1404 (1978).
7. Gawienowski, A. M., Chatterjee, D., Anderson, P. J., Epstein, D. L., and Grant, W. M., Effect of delta-9-tetrahydrocannabinol on monoamine oxidase activity in bovine eye tissues in vitro, Invest. Ophtal. Visual Sci. 22:482-485 (1982).
8. Schurr, A., Sheffer, N., Graziani, Y., and Livine, A., Inhibition of glucose efflux from human erythrocytes by hashish components, Biochem. Pharmacol. 23:2005-2009 (1974).
9. Hillard, C. J., and Bloom, A. S., Delta-9-tetrahydrocannabinol-induced changes in beta-adrenergic receptor binding in mouse cerebral cortex, Brain Res. 235:370-379 (1982).
10. Craddock, J. C., Davignon, J. P., Litterst, G. L., and Guarino, A. M., An intravenous formulation of delta-9-tetrahydrocannabinol using a nonionic surfactant, J. Pharm. Pharmacol. 25:345-349 (1973).
11. Alexander, R. W., Davis, J. N., and Lefkowitz, R. J., Direct identification and characterization of beta-adrenergic receptors in rat brain, Nature 258:437-439 (1975).
12. Bradford, M. M., A rapid and sensitive method for the quantitation of microgram quantities of protein utilizing the principle of protein-dye binding, Anal. Biochem.

72:248-252 (1976).
13. Scatchard, G., The attractions of proteins for small molecules and ions, Ann. N. Y. Acad. Sci. 51:660-672 (1949).
14. Cruikshank, J. M., The clinical importance of cardioselectivity and lipophilicity in beta blockers, Amer. Heart J. 100:160-178 (1980).
15. Molinoff, P. B., and Minneman, K. P., Biochemical and functional aspects of the interactions of agonists and antagonists with beta-adrenergic receptors, in "Psychopharmacology and Biochemistry of Neurotransmitter Receptors" (Yamamura, Olsen and Usdin, eds.), pp. 171-182. Elsevier North Holland, Inc., New York, 1980.
16. Levitzki, A., The beta-adrenergic receptor and its mode of coupling to adenylate cyclase, Crit. Rev. Biochem. 10:81-112 (1981).

MONOAMINE OXIDASE AND CANNABIS: SPECIES, TISSUE, AND DRUG SELECTIVITY

Avital Schurr
Benjamin M. Rigor

Department of Anesthesiology
University of Louisville School of Medicine
Louisville, Kentucky

I. INTRODUCTION

The interaction of cannabis components with monoamine oxidase (EC 1.4.3.4. amine: O_2 oxidoreductase, MAO) has been studied for several reasons. First, MAO plays a key role in the metabolism of monoamines in brain tissue (1). Secondly, interaction of cannabinoids with biological membranes is a paramount feature of their effect (2-8). Finally, since MAO can be isolated from both brain and liver tissues using similar means, it would be possible to discern tissue selectivity with respect to the drug effect.

Monoamine oxidase is believed to be an enzyme with multiple activities. Whether or not these activities are a result of the existence of multiple forms of the enzyme is still under debate (9-12). Nevertheless, the effect of inhibitors on these activities is a major component of this debate. The ability of different MAO inhibitors to exert selective inhibition usually depends on the substrate specificity (13, 14). Moreover, MAO preparations from different species (human, pig, beef, rat) tissues (brain, liver, kidney) give rise to differences in substrate specificity and inhibitor selectivity (11). Hence, the involvement of MAO with the psychoactivity of cannabis, or with any other of its effects, has to be tested using more than one source of the enzyme and more than one substrate.

Four different sources for MAO were used in the present study; human brain and liver and procine brain and liver. A variety of substrates was used to follow the two distinct

The Cannabinoids: Chemical, Pharmacologic, and Therapeutic Aspects

ISBN 0-12-044620-0

activities of MAO. Type A activity is believed to be responsible for the deamination of 5-hydroxytryptamine (5-HT, serotonin). Type B activity deaminates 2-phenylethylamine (PEA) and benzylamine (BA). Since MAO is a lipoprotein containing some 20 moles of phospholipids per mole of protein (1), we examined the hypothesis that these phospholipids may function as the site of interaction with the lipophylic cannabinoids.

Various cannabinoids including delta-9-tetrahydrocannabinol (THC) and cannabidiol (CBD) and a crude extract of cannabis were used and compared in this study.

II. METHODS

A. Preparation of Mitochondria

Mitochondria were prepared according to Tipton (15) with the exception that the mitochondria (protein concentration of 10 mg/ml) were stored frozen in sucrose 0.25 M, pH 7.6.

B. Solubilization of Monoamine Oxidase

The mitochondrial preparation (stored frozen overnight) was allowed to thaw at room temperature, and the suspension was then sonicated in a sonifier 100 W at an amplitude of 8 microns peak to peak, for 15 min. The sonicate was then centrifuged at 100,000 g for 120 min. Temperature was kept under 4°C through all the treatments. The supernatant (soluble MAO) was decanted and used for the assay of enzyme activity.

C. Assay of MAO Activity

Either spectrophotometric (16) or radiochemical (17) determination of the deamination products of the different substrates was used.

D. Effects of Cannabinoids

Aliquots of ethanolic stock solutions of cannabis extract and the various cannabinoids were mixed with the assay buffer before adding the MAO preparation. Ethanol was included in the control tubes at the same final concentration (0.33% v/v). Following a preincubation period of 30 min at 37°C, the enzymatic reaction was initiated by adding the substrate.

E. Chloroformic Extraction of Soluble MAO Preparation

To a given volume of soluble MAO preparation, THC or CBD were added to a final concentration of about 30-60 mcg per mg protein. In the controls ethanol replaced THC or CBD. After an incubation of 30 min at room temperature, the mixture was extracted with 3 volumes of cold chloroform by vigorous mixing for 5 min. Following centrifugation at 10,000 g for 20 min the upper aqueous layer was collected, a stream of N_2 was passed over it to assure the removal of chloroform, and then the preparation was assayed for enzyme activity. The extraction procedure must take place no later than 24 hr after the sonication step.

F. Preparation of Liposomes

Liposomes were prepared according to Alhanaty and Livne (7) in KPi buffer, 50 mM, pH 7.4 using various phospholipids.

G. Cannabis Extract

Cannabis (hashish) was extracted twice with petroleum ether (1 g in a total of 100 ml). The extract included about 25% of the hashish solid materials. Stock solutions were prepared in ethanol.

H. Fractionation and Isolation of Cannabinoids from Cannabis Extract

Silca gel (GF) preparative thin layer chromatography (TLC) plates were used with toluene: chloroform: methanol (100: 10:1, by volume) as a solvent system. The R_f values of the different fractions were determined by using UV light. To assure that cannabinoids were actually detected, the following procedure was used: Fractions were scraped from the preparative TLC plate and were re-extracted from the silica gel with chloroform: methanol (10: 1, by volume). Samples of these re-extracted fractions were applied to a silca gel (GF) analyticalTLC plate, and developed with the same solvent system as above. After drying, the plate was sprayed with ethanolic solution of Black K Salt (1 mg/ml) (18). Purple spots, if apparent on the TLC plate, indicate the presence of cannabinoids.

I. Data Presented

Each of the experiments was repeated at least four times in duplicate, yielding identical patterns. Duplicates agreed within 5% experimental error, and representative experiments are shown.

III. RESULTS

A. Effects of Cannabinoids and Hashish Extract on Pig Brain MAO

MAO activity of pig brain mitochondria was inhibited by THC and hashish (cannabis) extract. Fig. 1 shows that the inhibition was dependent on preincubation with the cannabinoids. In contrast, CBD was ineffective even after one hour

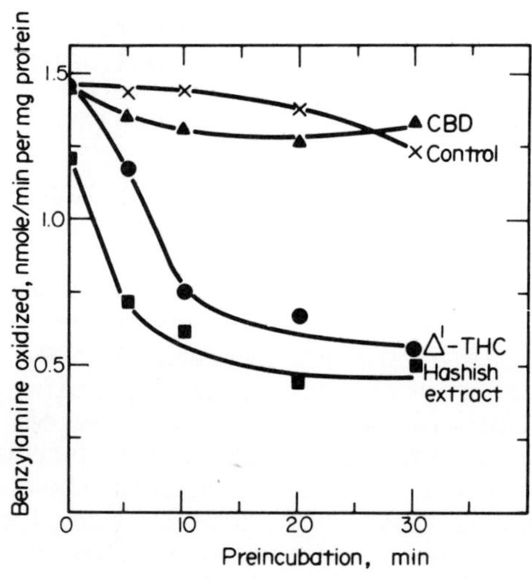

FIGURE 1. The inhibition of pig brain MAO activity by THC and hashish extract as affected by preincubation with the cannabinoids. Aliquots of the mitochondrial suspension (1 mg protein in 3 ml KPi buffer, pH 7.4) were incubated at 37°C with one of the following drugs (in mcg/mg protein): THC, 94; CBD, 94; hashish extract, 19.

of incubation with the mitochondrial preparation. The extent of inhibition of pig brain MAO by THC or by the cannabis extract was dose-dependent (Fig. 2), the extract being about ten times more potent than THC.

Unlike THC and the Extract, CBD was essentially ineffective at a wide concentration range (Fig. 2). If administered concomitantly, CBD is known to interfere with the effects of THC in man (19) and in experimental animals (20). CBD is able to counteract in vitro the inhibitory effect of THC on MAO of pig brain mitochondria (Fig. 3). CBD also partially diminishes the inhibitory effect of the extract. If CBD is added at the onset of the reaction, following the preincubation period, it no longer interferes with the inhibitory effect of THC. When CBD is added during the pretreatment with the THC the interference is proportional to the duration of the concomitant incubation.

When other MAO substrates were used, the activity of pig brain mitochondrial MAO was inhibited also by THC and hashish extract (Fig. 4). Again, CBD, was found to be ineffective. Different degrees of inhibition with THC were found for the

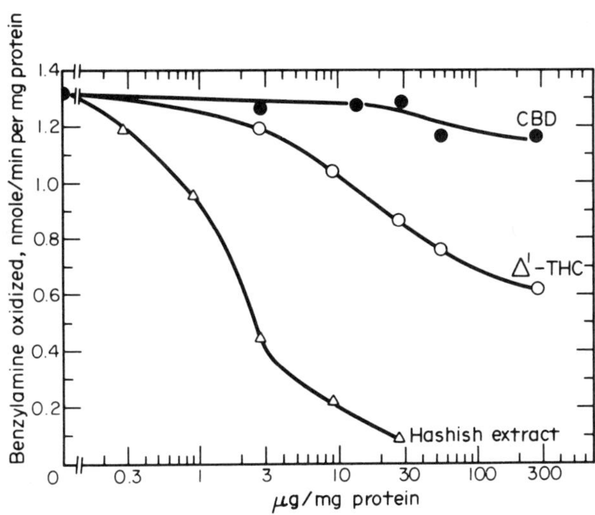

FIGURE 2. Effect of THC, CBD and hashish extract of pig brain MAO activity. Preincubation time: 30 min.

different substrates, ranging from 80% inhibition when dopamine was the substrate to about 25% when tryptamine was used. The extract was inhibitory at a much lower dose and its effect varied as well according to the substrate tested. Phenylcyclopropylamine (SKF-385), a known competitive MAO inhibitor, was used for comparison at a final concentration of 3.3 mcM.

Study of the kinetic parameters of the enzyme activity in the presence of THC and increasing concentrations of the different substrates, revealed that the inhibition produced was of noncompetitive type, independent of the substrate used (Fig. 5). This phenomenon suggests that the cannabinoids are not interacting directly with the active site of MAO but rather with a different moiety of the enzyme or the membrane in which it is embedded. If the interaction of THC with MAO takes place through a membranal component, separation of the enzyme from the membrane by means of solubilization should abolish the inhibitory effect of the cannabinoid. If, on the other hand, THC affects MAO activity directly or through a phospholipid moiety of the enzyme itself, then the cannabinoid must also affect the soluble enzyme, although no membrane or membranal particles are present. To solubilize the enzyme,

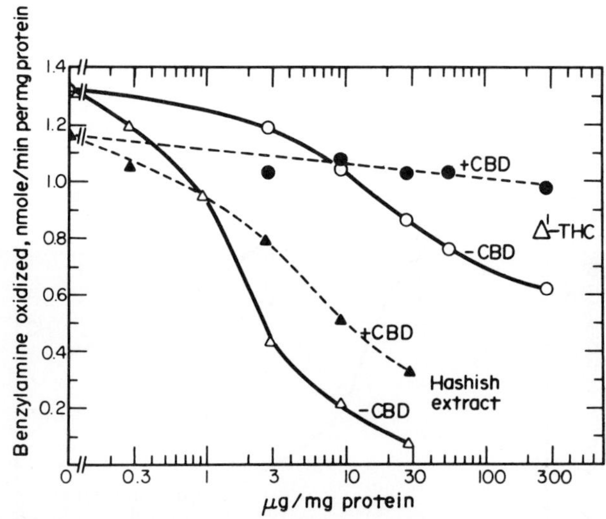

FIGURE 3. Inhibitory effect of THC and hashish extract interfered with by CBD. Preincubation time: 30 min. Where indicated, CBD (135 mcg/mg protein) was added along with the inhibitor.

the technique of Tipton (15) was adopted, mainly because it avoids the use of detergents, which are very difficult to remove after the solubilization. The soluble enzyme thus obtained was found to be inhibited by THC (Table I,Trmnt. I).

Based on this finding it was assumed that the probable lipophylic component through which the cannabinoids interact with the enzyme, is part of, or bound to, the enzyme itself. MAO phospholipids are likely to serve this function and therefore attempts were made to extract the phospholipids from the enzyme. Table I summarizes the various treatments carried out for this purpose. The extraction alone, irrespective of the solvent used (Trmnts. II, III) did not abolish the inhibitory effect of THC.

It has been shown by Sklenovsky et al. that THC causes an increased disruption of firm complexes of phospholipids from

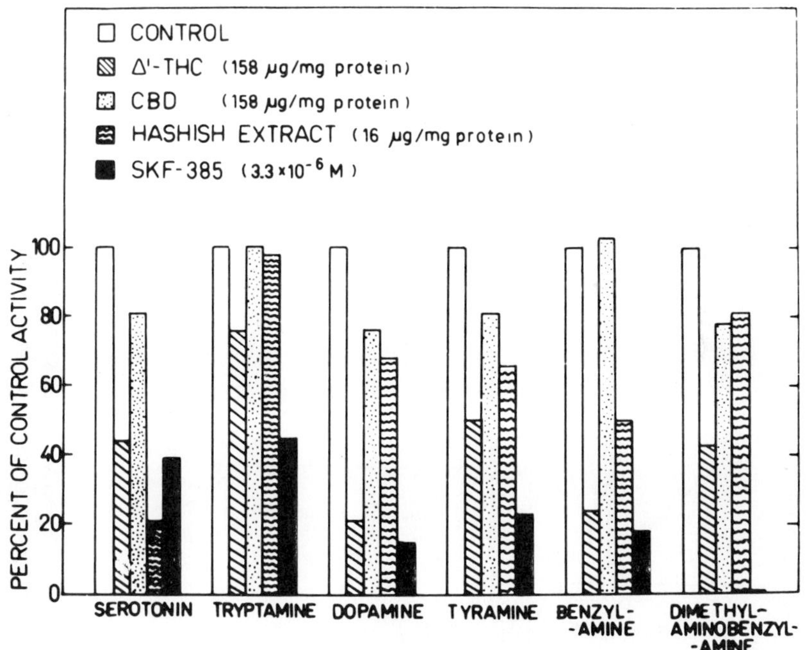

FIGURE 4. The effects of THC, CBD, hashish extract and SKF-385 on pig brain MAO activity in the presence of 1 mM of various substrates (except tryptamine, which was present at 5 mM). The drugs were preincubated with the enzyme preparation for 30 min before adding the substrate. The enzyme activity in the presence of each substrate and in the absence of any inhibitor is 100% of control activity.

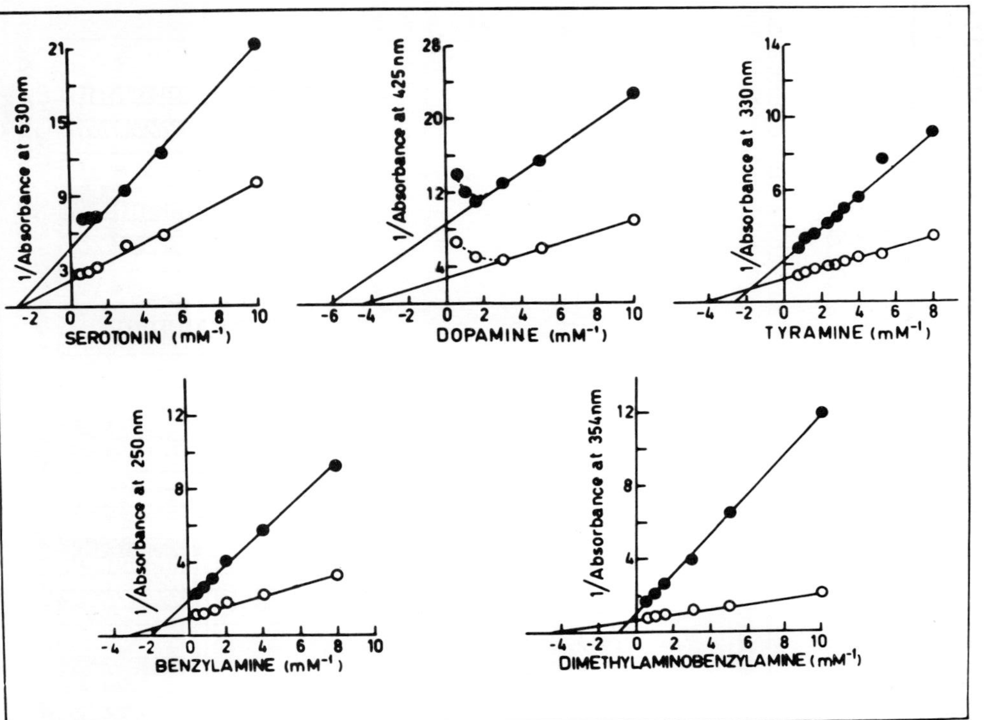

FIGURE 5. Lineweaver-Burk plots of MAO activity with various substrates in the presence (●) or absence (O) of 158 mcg THC per mg protein. Preincubation time: 30 min. Enzyme source: pig brain.

TABLE I. The Effects of Delta-1-THC and CBD on Pig Brain MAO Activity in Soluble Preparation Before and After Various Organic Extraction Procedures

Treatment		MAO activity[a]		
		Control	THC[b]	CBD
I	None	1.00	35	88
II	2-Butanone extraction[c]	0.76	32	82
III	Chloroformic extraction	0.75	36	86
IV	Chloroformic extraction in the presence of THC	0.75	81	169
V	Chloroformic extraction in the presence of CBD	0.73	100	155

[a]MAO activity in the control: nmoles benzylamine oxidized/min/mg protein. In the presence of the cannabinoids: percent (%) of the control.

[b]The cannabinoid dosage: 50 mcg/mg protein.

[c]The extraction was done according to ref. 26.

brain tissue and thus increases the extractability of these substances (21). Following Treatment IV (Table I), when soluble MAO was preincubated with THC (see methods) and then extracted with chloroform, the inhibitory effect of the cannabinoid was indeed drastically reduced. Since CBD is capable of competing with THC, probably for the same site on the MAO molecule, it might cause the "labilization" of the phospholipid complexes similarly to THC. Treatment V in Table I clearly indicates that this is the case. To determine whether the cannabinoids incubated with the enzyme were extracted into the chloroform phase, tritiated THC and CBD were used in this procedure. The results show that no more than 3% of the cannabinoids remained within the aqueous (enzyme) phase after the chloroformic extraction. Thus a resolution obtained between the MAO and the extractable factor, which is responsible for the enzyme sensitivity to THC. This enabled us to examine the capacity of various phospholipids to restore the sensitivity of MAO to this cannabinoid by adding them, one by one, as liposomes, to the extracted enzyme. As can be seen from Fig. 6, phosphatidylcholine (PPC) reconstituted the inhibitory effect of THC on pig brain mitochondrial MAO activity. Moreover, PPC increased the MAO activity to the level of the untreated (soluble) enzyme and even higher. These effects of PPC were found to be concentration-dependent (Fig. 7). The optimal concentration was 1.1 mg/mg protein, while lower and higher concentrations were less effective. Other phospholipids examined were much less effective (Fig. 6).

B. Effects of Cannabinoids and Hashish Extract on Pig Liver MAO

MAO activity of pig liver mitochondria is not affected by either THC, CBD or hashish extract (given at doses of 94, 94 and 19 mcg/mg protein, respectively). The lack of effect was independent of the substrate used.

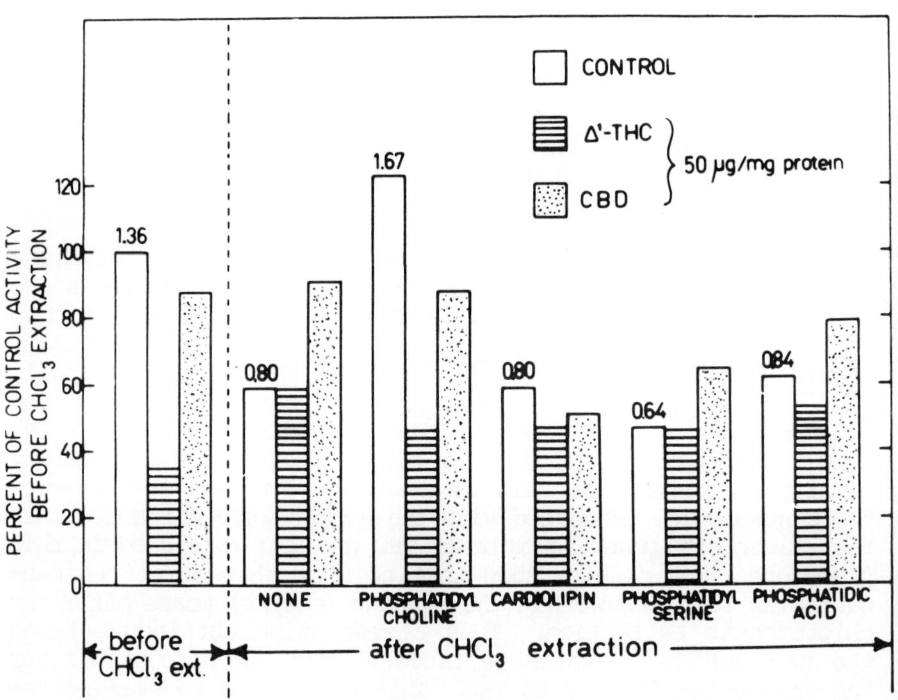

FIGURE 6. The sensitivity of soluble MAO to THC and CBD before and after chloroformic extraction (Treatment V in Table I) and in the presence of 1 mg of various phospholipids per mg of protein added after the extraction. The numbers at the heads of the columns are specific activity of pig brain MAO expressed as nmoles benzylamine oxidized/min/mg protein.

C. Effects of Cannabinoids and Hashish Extract on Human Brain MAO

Unlike pig brain MAO, the human enzyme displayed insensitivity to THC (Figs. 8 and 9, open triangles). The ineffectiveness of this cannabinoid was independent of the substrate used. The cannabis extract on the other hand, inhibited the activity of human brain MAO almost to the same degree it did pig brain MAO. However, the inhibition of the human enzyme by hashish extract was found to be substrate-dependent. Phenylethylamine (PEA) deamination (type B activity) was inhibited to a higher degree than the deamination of 5-hydroxytryptamine (5-HT, type A activity), (Figs. 8 and 9, open circles).

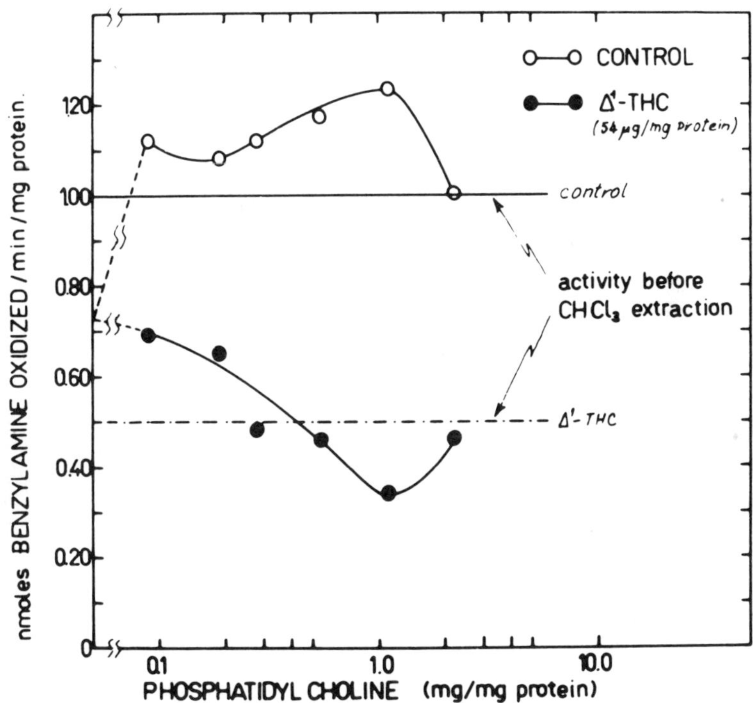

FIGURE 7. The effect of added quantities of phosphatidylcholine on the activity of soluble pig brain MAO, extracted according to Treatment V in Table I, and its sensitivity to THC. Preincubation time: 30 min.

D. Effects of Cannabinoids and Hashish Extract on Human Liver MAO

THC was innocuous in inhibiting the human liver MAO as it was with the brain enzyme (Figs. 8 and 9, closed triangles). However, the liver MAO displayed high sensitivity to hashish extract, higher than that of the brain enzyme (Figs. 8 and 9, closed circles). This is in contrast to pig liver MAO that was found to be insensitive to cannabinoids.

The potency of the cannabis extract in inhibiting human and pig brain MAO and human liver MAO prompted us to try to isolate the responsible component(s). Shown in Fig. 10 are the R_f values and the abilities of cannabis extract (CE), THC, CBD, and 11 different fractions of cannabinoids isolated from CE, to inhibit human liver MAO activity. When screening tests like the one shown in Fig. 10 were conducted, liver mitochondria and benzylamine (BA) were used for the following reasons: a) Human liver MAO was found to be more sensitive to CE than the brain enzyme. b) The type B activity of the enzyme (deamination of BA or PEA) exhibited higher sensitivity to CE than the type A activity (deamination of 5-HT). c) The

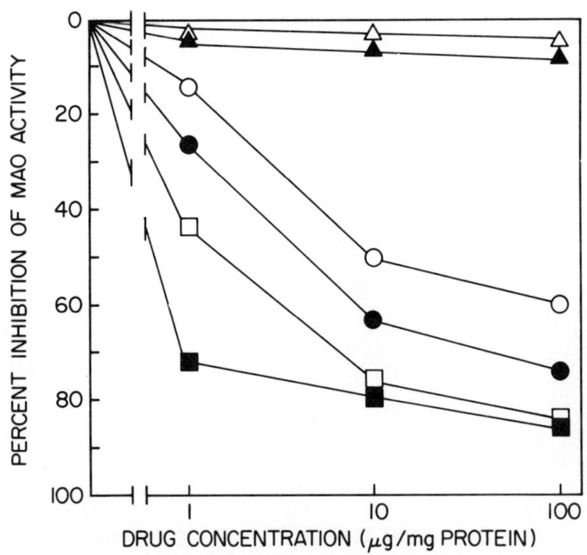

FIGURE 8. Inhibition of human brain (open symbols) and liver (closed symbols) MAO activity by cannabis extract (circles), fraction F_4 (squares), and THC (triangles), using 10 mcM PEA as a substrate.

assay of the enzyme activity with BA is a spectrophotometric one, easier and faster to perform than the radiochemical assay, yet sensitive enough for first screening purposes. Each fraction shown in Fig. 10 including CE, THC and CBD, was tested for its inhibitory effect on MAO at a concentration of 100 mcg/mg protein. As can be seen, fractions F_4, F_5, and F_6 were the most potent as MAO inhibitors. In our study we focused on fraction F_4 only. Upon spraying the TLC plate with Black K Salt solution, this fraction appeared as two purple spots, indicating the presence of two cannabinoids with R_f values of 0.67 and 0.71. These two spots were seen also under UV light and so were all the other cannabinoids. The Black K Salt spraying and the UV light produced identical cannabinoid maps.

The effect of fraction F_4 on both human brain and liver MAO was found to be dose-dependent (Figs. 8 and 9, Squares). Like CE, F_4 was more effective in inhibiting the deamination of PEA (Fig. 8) than the deamination of 5-HT (Fig. 9). Again, like CE, fraction F_4 was found to be more potent against human liver MAO than against the brain enzyme. Moreover, F_4 displayed higher potency than CE in inhibiting MAO activity with

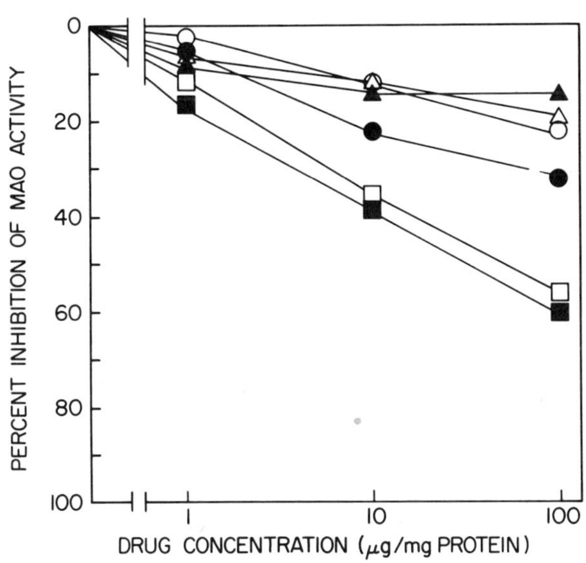

FIGURE 9. Inhibition of human brain (open symbols) and liver (closed symbols) MAO activity by cannabis extract (circles), fraction F_4 (squares), and THC (triangles), using 500 mcg 5-HT as a substrate.

either tissue or substrate; 1 mcg/mg protein of F_4 produced the same degree of inhibition as 10 mcg/mg protein of CE.

IV. DISCUSSION

Biogenic amines have been implicated in the expression of the psychoactivity of cannabis (22-25). Increased levels of biogenic amines and catecholamines were found in experimental animals in vivo after administration of cannabis extract and THC, the psychoactive component of cannabis. Several mechanism may account for these elevated levels: a) Changes in the uptake rates of these compounds into their sites of action, b) changes in their turnover rate, c) changes in their biosynthesis or rate of biotransformation.

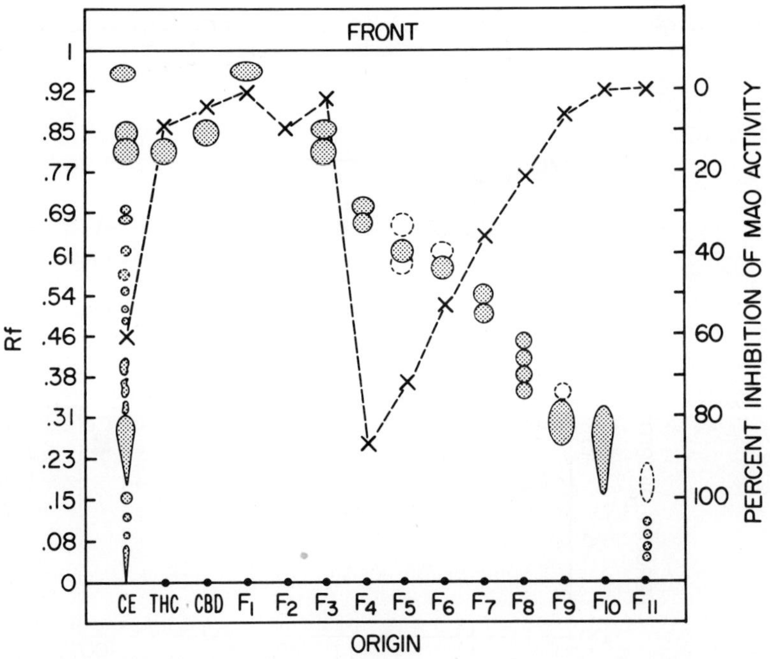

FIGURE 10. TLC fractionation of cannabis extract with toluene:chloroform:methanol (100:10:1, by volume), the R_f values of the different fractions, and the degree of human liver MAO inhibition (X) produced by each fraction (see text for details).

Monoamine oxidase (MAO), an enzyme embedded in the outer mitochondrial membrane, has an important role in the metabolism of endogenous monoamines in the brain (1) and as such may be considered as a possible site for the action of cannabis. The fact that MAO is a lipoprotein makes it even more favorable as a candidate for interaction with the lipophylic cannabinoids. Since we began the study by examining the effects of THC and CBD on pig brain MAO, we were very encouraged to find the pronounced effect of the former on the enzyme activity and the lack of effect of the latter. On the other hand the potency of hashish extract as an MAO inhibitor could not be explained by its content of THC alone (ca. 10%), and one has to assume either a synergistic effect of THC and other cannabinoids or the presence of a much more potent component than THC within this extract. Nevertheless, the tissue selectivity that was displayed by the cannabinoids, inhibiting pig brain MAO without affecting the activity of the liver enzyme, prompted us to continue and investigate the nature of the interaction between the cannabinoids and MAO. The noncompetitive type of inhibition exerted by THC on MAO activity led to the assumption that the interaction of the cannabinoid with the enzyme is not taking place at the active site of MAO. Rather it occurs with a lipophylic moiety of the enzyme or its membranal microenvironment. Solubilizing the enzyme by extracting it from the mitochondrial membrane did not abolish the inhibitory effect of THC. This result indicates that the component, which THC is interacting with, is tightly bound to MAO. We attempted to extract such a component with organic solvents like 2-butanone or chloroform, without success (Table I, Trtmnts. II and III). However, using the chloroform extraction procedure in the presence of THC (Table I, treatment IV), we abolished the inhibitory effect of this cannabinoid. Furthermore, CBD, could also be used instead of THC in the chloroformic extraction to obviated the effect of the latter. CBD has no effect on pig brain MAO, but counteracts the effect of THC on the enzyme (Fig. 3). Using radiolabeled THC and CBD, we showed that 97% of these cannabinoids were extracted into the chloroformic phase (Table I, Trtmnts. IV and V). Postulating that the factor thus extracted is a phospholipid, liposomes were prepared from different phospholipids and were incubated with the extracted enzyme to examine their ability to restore the sensitivity of pig brain MAO to THC. Of the four phospholipids tested, PPC was the only one to reconstitute the inhibitory effect of THC. Moreover, it seems that the ability of this phospholipid is dose related. This phenomenon suggests that the interaction between MAO, PPC and THC is stoichiometric. An optimum concentration of 1.1 mg PPC per 1.0 mg protein was found maximum enzyme activity and inhibition by THC.

A schematic model which outlines our proposal for the mode of action of THC in inhibiting pig brain MAO activity is shown in Fig. 11. The dotted squares in this scheme represents the polypeptide chain of MAO, the open circles are phospholipids and the triangle "S" is the substrate. When CBD or THC are added, they interact with the phospholipids which are bound to the enzyme by this interaction (B_2). When soluble MAO (A) is treated with chloroform, to give form D, the phospholipids are not extractable unless the enzyme is preincubated with either CBD or THC. The extracted enzyme (C) is not inhibited by THC. Phospholipids like PPC, could reassociate with the extracted MAO to reconstitute the complex which is sensitive to THC.

One might conclude from these results that MAO is involved in the psychoactivity of THC. Since the enzyme is inhibited by this cannabinoid and not by CBD, such inhibition would result in elevated levels of monoamines. Thus in turn could lead to the known psychotomimetic signs produced by cannabis. However, when the effect of THC was tested on human brain MAO,

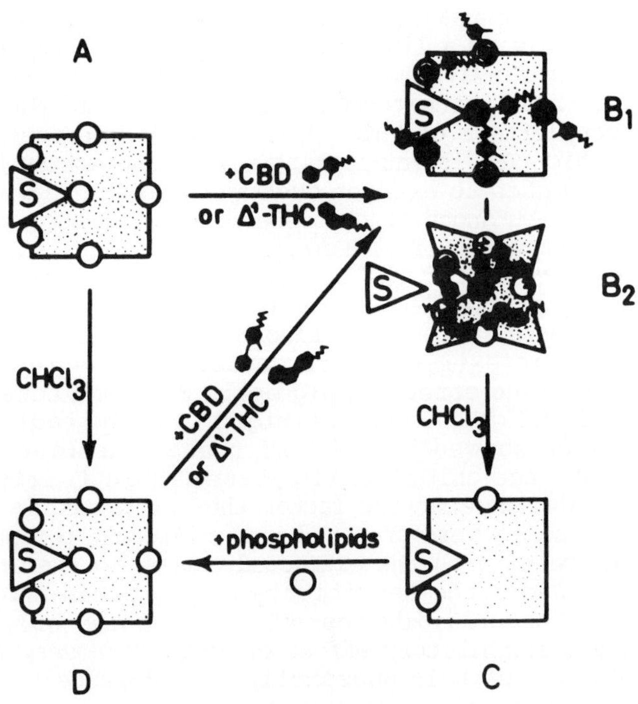

FIGURE 11. Mechanism of inhibition of pig brain MAO activity by THC (see text for details).

none was found. Species selectivity, like tissue selectivity, indicates the existence of differences among different MAO preparation which could lead to different sensitivities to THC. This is especially true if one assumes the presence of different phospholipid moieties with which the cannabinoids are interacting.

However, this is not the case with the cannabis extract which inhibits both pig and human brain MAO, and also liver MAO. Moreover, this extract is ten times more active than THC. Does that mean that the component, or components, in cannabis which is responsible for MAO inhibition, is more specific than THC? Since THC content in the extract cannot account for the strong inhibition of the enzyme activity, the only other explanation is a synergism between THC and other cannabinoids within the extract. The fractionation results (Fig. 10) demonstrate clearly that other cannabinoids, not THC, are responsible for the inhibition of MAO activity produced by cannabis extract. The potential of these components as MAO inhibitors is much greater than that of THC and their specific activity is increasing with the increase in their purity.

Though the differential effect of THC and CBD on pig brain MAO activity alone cannot explain the psychoactivity of the former, the lack of its effect on the human brain enzyme excludes such explanation completely. Nevertheless, the present study emphasizes the importance of species and tissue selectivity in the different effects exerted by THC and other cannabinoids. Moreover, drug selectivity toward different cannabinoids by in vitro preparations is a phenomenon of which we should be aware.

Inasmuch as this study is concerned, the enigma of the psychoactivity of THC is yet to be solved. However, the potential of cannabis as a source of possible therapeutic agents is clear. Fraction F_4 is, undoubtedly, only one of many which contain cannabinoids with even greater selectivity and specificity than THC.

REFERENCES

1. Nagatsu, J., in "Biochemistry of Catecholamines", Vol. 131. University Park Press, Tokyo, 1973.
2. Chari-Bitron, A., Life Sci. 10:1273 (1971).
3. Chari-Bitron, A., and Bino T., Biochem. Pharmacol. 20:473 (1971).
4. Mahonney, J. M., and Harris, R. A., Biochem Pharmacol. 21:1217 (1972).
5. Raz, A., Schurr, A., and Livne, A., Biochem. Biophys. Acta 274:269 (1972).

6. Raz, A., Schurr, A., Livne, A., and Goldman, R., Biochem. Pharmacol. 22:3129 (1973).
7. Alhanaty, E., and Livne, A., Biochem Biophys. Acta. 339:146 (1974).
8. Schurr, A., Sheffer, N., Graziani, Y., and Livne, A., Biochem. Pharmacol. 23:2005 (1974).
9. Houslay, M. D., Tipton, K. F., and Youdim, M. B. H., Life Sci. 19:467 (1976).
10. Jain, M., Life Sci. 20:97 (1978).
11. Fowler, C. J., Callingham, B. A., Mantle, T. J., and Tipton, K. F., Biochem. Pharmacol. 27:97 (1978).
12. Schurr, A., Life Sci. 30:1059 (1982).
13. Johnston, J. P., Biochem. Pharmacol. 17:1285 (1968).
14. Knoll, J., and Magyar, K., Adv. Biochem. Psychopharmacol. 5:339 (1972).
15. Tipton, K. F., Eur. J. Biochem. 4:103 (1968).
16. Schurr, A., Porath, O., Krup, M., and Livne, A., Biochem. Pharmacol. 27:2513 (1978).
17. Schurr, A., Ho, B. T., and Schoolar, J. C., J. Pharm. Pharmacol. 33:165 (1981).
18. de Faubert Maunder, M. J., Bull. Narc. 26:19 (1974).
19. Karniol, I. G., Shirakawa, I., Kasinsky, N., Pfeferman, A., and Carlini, E. A., Eur. J. Pharmacol. 28:172 (1974).
20. Borgenn, A. L., and Davis, W. M., Res. Commun. Chem. Path. Pharmacol. 1:663 (1974).
21. Sklenovsky, A., Navratil, J., Hrbek, J., and Skrabal, J., Act. Nerv. Sup., Praha 17:67 (1975).
22. Bose, B. C., Saifi, A. Q., and Bhagwat, A. W., Archs. Int. Pharmacodyn. Ther. 147:291 (1964).
23. Holzmann, D., Lovell, R. A. , Jaffe, J. H., and Freedman, D. X., Science 163:1464 (1969).
24. Ho, B. T., Taylor, D., Fritchie, G. E., Englert, L. F., McIssac, W. M., Brain Res. 38:163 (1972).
25. Paton, W. D. M., Ann. Rev. Pharmacol. 15:191 (1975).
26. Olivecrona, T., and Oreland, L., Biochemistry, 10:332 (1971).

ELECTROPHYSIOLOGICAL EFFECTS OF THC ON CORTICAL SENSORY EVOKED ACTIVITY*

D. M. Wilkison

Department of Pharmacology and Toxicology
Medical College of Wisconsin
Milwaukee, Wisconsin

I. INTRODUCTION

A large body of information has been assembled which describes the effects of marijuana and its psychoactive components, the tetrahydrocannabinols. The investigations of the mechanism of action by which these compounds alter central nervous system function has proceeded in two complimentary directions, the neurochemical actions and the electrophysiological actions of cannabinoids. Studies on the electrophysiological actions of delta-9-tetrahydrocannabinol (THC) have produced information which suggest THC has actions in virtually every region of the CNS, cortex, limbic structures, hypothalamus, and spinal cord. The numerous effects of THC at these sites, both excitation and inhibition, have made generalized conclusions as to the neuronal actions of the cannabinoids elusive.

Since many of the effects of THC reported in man are related to changes in visual, auditory, and tactile perception (1,2), we are studying the effects of the cannabinoids on central sensory processing. Sensory perception is influenced by many factors beyond any specific sensory system. Subtle drug effects on perception may be the result of alterations in the integration of all sensory information. This could occur in central sensory area that receive multiple sensory information, i.e., areas outside classical sensory afferent pathways that respond to sensory stimulation in a nonspecific hetero-

---

*Supported in part by NIDA grants DA-01754 and DA-00124.

ISBN 0-12-044620-0

topic manner. Cortical sites that have such nonmodality specific representation have been described in cats (3-6). These areas receive afferent sensory information from thalamic nuclei, which also exhibit multisensory activity through pathways that are, in part, parallel to the primary sensory pathways, and many neurons in these areas individually respond to more than one sensory modality (7). A systematic exploration of the electrophysiological effects of the cannabinoids on sensory-evoked activity provides necessary information on the site of action of THC and the processes of sensory perception that are affected by THC in particular and, more generally, by the wide class of compounds that alter sensory function.

Other investigators have studied the effects of THC on sensory-evoked and electrically-evoked activity in sensory areas of the CNS. Low doses of THC generally increased cortico-cortical evoked responses whereas high doses of THC were found to be depressant. Auditory-evoked potentials also were enhanced by THC in the restrained, conscious cat. This was accompanied by an increased latency and broader peak of the evoked potential (8).

Thus, we have compared the effects of THC and a synthetic analog of THC, dimethylheptylpyran (DMHP) on visual and somatosensory evoked potentials in areas which are modality specific and in areas which receive multimodality information.

II. METHODS

Cats of both sexes, 2.5 - 4.5 kg, were anesthetized initially with halothane, and the trachea and femoral vein were cannulated. Cats were then transferred to alpha-chloralose anesthesia, 70 mg/kg, and the halothane discontinued. Cannulae were placed in the descending aorta via the femoral artery to monitor blood pressure. Cats were placed in a stereotaxic frame and the cortex was exposed bilaterally. Rats were anesthetized with alpha-chloralose-urethane and the femoral vein cannulated prior to placement in stereotaxic frame.

Subdural cortical, Platinum-ball electrodes were placed on the primary visual cortex (area 18), the primary somatosensory cortex (area 4), and the anterior marginal association cortex. Subcortical recording and stimulating electrodes were placed stereotaxically according to the atlases of Jasper and Ajmone-Marsan (9), and Pellegrino and Cushman (10). Coaxial, insulated electrodes were made from 23 ga. stainless steel tubing and an insulated 0.01 inch stainless steel center element. They were positioned in the dorsal lateral geniculate nucleus (LGN) or ventral posterolateral nucleus of the thalamus (VPL) for recording evoked bioelectric activity. Coaxial electrodes were placed in optic chiasm (OX) for stimulation of the visual system. Parallel stainless steel electrodes with a 1-cm (cat) or 3-mm (rat) pole separation were placed subdermally under the radial nerve for stimulation of the somatosensory system.

All cats were immobilized with a succinylcholine-saline drip, 1 mg/ml, and artificially ventilated to an end-tidal CO_2 level of 2.5-4.0%. Rats were allowed to respire spontaneously. Two to three hours elapsed after completion of surgery prior to the start of the experimental sessions. All recording sites were mapped to locate the site of maximal evoked potentials in response to stimulation of OX (0.05 msec., 0.5-1.0 mA), or radial nerve (0.5 msec., 0.05-1.0 mA), or both. The stimulus rate was once every four seconds (0.25 Hz).

Polygraphic records were made of end tidal CO_2, blood pressure, and bioelectric activity for cat studies. Rectal temperature was monitored and maintained between 36.5-37.5^{o}C. Bioelectric activity was amplified with band-pass filters set at 3 and 3,000 Hz for primary cortical activity, 1.0-3,000 Hz for association cortex activity, and 3-10,000 Hz for deep nuclei activity. Electrical activity was either digitized "on-line" at appropriate rates and/or recorded on FM magnetic tape for subsequent processing.

Stimulus intensities were set as multiples of the threshold intensities required to elicit a primary cortical response for each sensory pathway. Experimental data was derived from responses evoked by stimulation of radial nerve at 1x, 2x, and 4x threshold or by stimulation of OX at 2x, 4x, and 8x threshold. Baseline and vehicle controls were established in each cat prior to drug administration.

At termination of the experiments, electrode sites were lesioned at 2 mA for 10 seconds and the brain perfused _in situ_ with saline followed by 10% formalin saline containing 0.5% sodium ferrocyanide. Electrode sites were documented utilizing techniques described elsewhere (11).

Individual evoked potentials were digitized at appropriate rates (1,000-16,000 samples per second). Mean and standard deviations were calculated for each ensemble of 25 potentials. Latency-corrected mean, standard deviation, and standard error of mean of the latency and amplitude of the significant peaks of each potential were determined in order to characterize the ensemble. Drug effects were determined by the present change in amplitude of the evoked potential. Vehicle control effects were determined by comparing the 30-minute post-vehicle response to the pre-vehicle-baseline response. Responses after drug, 30-120 minutes, were compared to the post-vehicle responses. Thus, negative percent effects represented depression of the evoked potential amplitude and positive effects were facilitation. Significances of drug effect were determined by means of paired T-tests or analysis of variance.

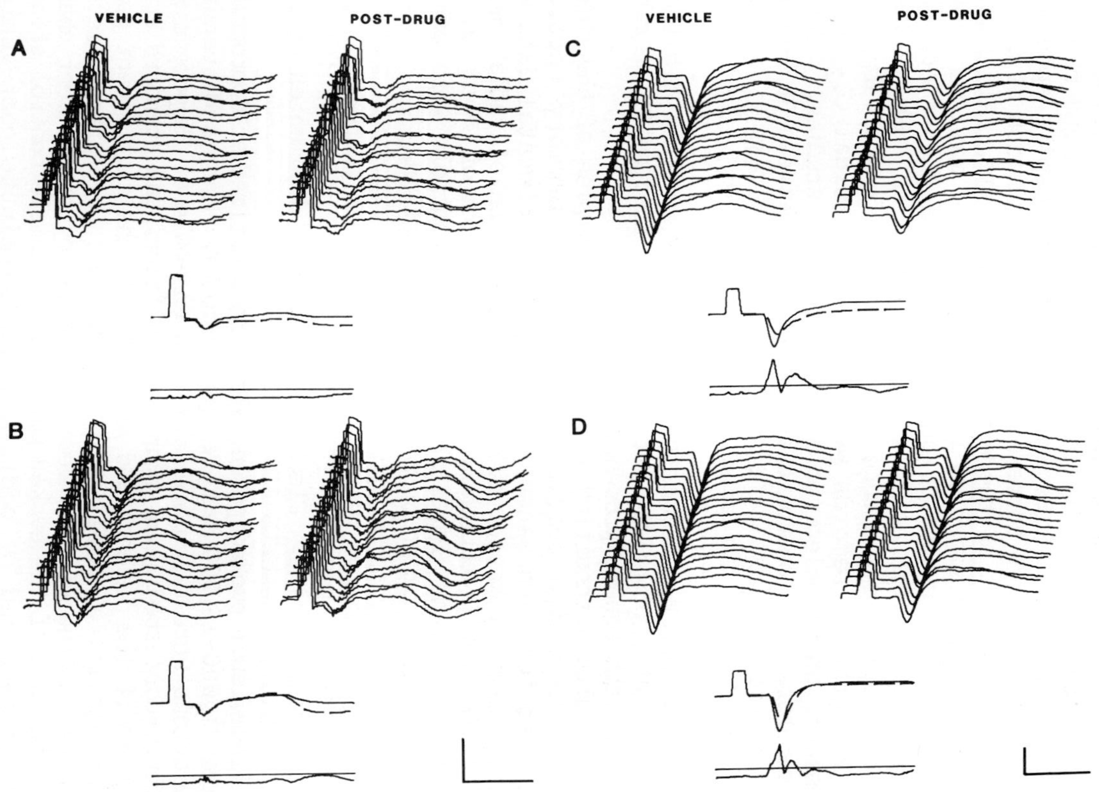
VEHICLE
POST-DRUG
VEHICLE
POST-DRUG
A
C
B
D

THC and DMHP in 95% ethanol were dissolved in equal volumes of emulphor and diluted with water to 5 mg/ml. Vehicle consisted of ethanol substituted for drug.

III. RESULTS

In general, somatic activity was elicited by electrical stimulation of the radial nerve in cats and rats. The afferent somatic evoked activity was recorded from the contralateral primary somatosensory cortex and corresponding ventral posterolateral nucleus of the thalamus (VPL). Additionally in cats, somatosensory evoked activity was recorded from the anterior marginal association (AMA) cortex, a cortical site which receives multisensory information.

The positive wave of the somatosensory-evoked potential (SEP), recorded from the cortex of chloralose-anesthetized cats, was delayed by administration of THC (0.25-4.90 mg/kg) in a dose-dependent manner. Figure 1 illustrates the increase in the latency of the SEP elicited by radial nerve stimulation induced by 2 mg/kg THC. Somatic afferent activity at VPL was not significantly delayed (2 +/- 1.4%) by 2 mg/kg THC in 8 cats, which exhibited a 13 +/- 2% delay in the cortical response. THC depressed the amplitude of the cortical response only at the 4 mg/kg dose when moderate to high stimulation intensities were used. Responses to low, near threshold stimulus intensities were often depressed by THC such that detection and quantification of the response was not possible. These very small SEP to weak somatosensory stimulation were completely obscured in 5 of 12 cats. DMHP produced effects similar to THC but was more potent especially in depressing the amplitude of the cortical SEP. Figure 2 summarizes the dose response relationship for THC and DMHP on the cortical SEP in the cat elicited by electrical stimulation of the peripheral radial nerve.

FIGURE 1. Effects of THC on SEP at VPL and primary cortex. Individual SEP were simultaneously recorded from VPL (A,B) and primary somatosensory cortex (C,D) after vehicle (VEHICLE) and 30 minutes after 2 mg/kg THC (POST-DRUG). Potentials were evoked by two levels of stimulation: low (A,C) and high (B,D). Below each set of SEP are the superimposed averages, vehicle (-) and post-THC (--). Under each pair of averages the statistical T-values are illustrated, t = 7.5. Stimulation immediately followed calibration pulse, 5 msec, -500 mcV, positive voltage downward.

The relative lack of effect of THC on the somatosensory-evoked potential recorded in VPL suggested that the site of action for the cortical effects of THC may be either in the sensory processing and projection of information from VPL or in the integration at area 3 cortex itself. To distinguish between these two possibilities, cats were prepared as before except after the VPL and cortex were mapped the VPL was stimulated and the cortical SEP recorded. Figure 3 illustrates the effect of THC, 2 mg/kg, on the SEP evoked by stimulation of radial nerve or VPL and recorded at one cortical site. Stimulation of VPL evoked a positive wave on the cortex similar to that elicited by electrical stimulation of the radial nerve, albeit, with a shorter latency. THC produced similar effects on the cortical activity evoked from each site. The major effect of THC on cortical SEP as illustrated in Figure 3 was a slowing of the surface positive wave. This was most readily seen as the lengthened duration and increase in the latency of the peak. In five cats the latency of the positive wave was increased 10.8 +/- 1.5% for radial nerve-evoked and 12.1 +/- 2.6% for VPL-evoked responses.

Similar effects were observed in the cat anesthetized with chloralose-urethane and spontaneously respiring. The latency of the cortical potential evoked by electrical stimulationof the contralateral forepaw was increased following administration of THC in 5 rats (10 +/- 3.2%).

The effects of THC on the other sensory pathways were determined to evaluate the specificity of the action on the somatosensory system. In contrast to the effects on cortical SEP the visual evoked response to electrical stimulation of the optic chiasm was not altered by THC. However the auditory evoked potential did exhibit an increased latency after THC.

THC produced effects on sensory-evoked potentials in areas outside the classical sensory afferent pathways. The cortical association areas of the cat, in particular, anterior marginal which exhibits sensory evoked potentials from visual and somatosensory modalities in a heterotopic manner, was depressed by THC. In contrast to the primary sites, however, the visual-evoked activity recorded at the anterior marginal cortex was more depressed than the somatosensory evoked potential by 2 mg/kg THC (42 +/- 5.2% vs 21 +/- 8%) (Figure 4).

IV. DISCUSSION

Several studies on the effects of THC on sensory electrophysiology (8,12-14) in experimental animals and in man (2,15,16) have reported combinations of facilitation and depression and no effect. The absence of a unifying effect of

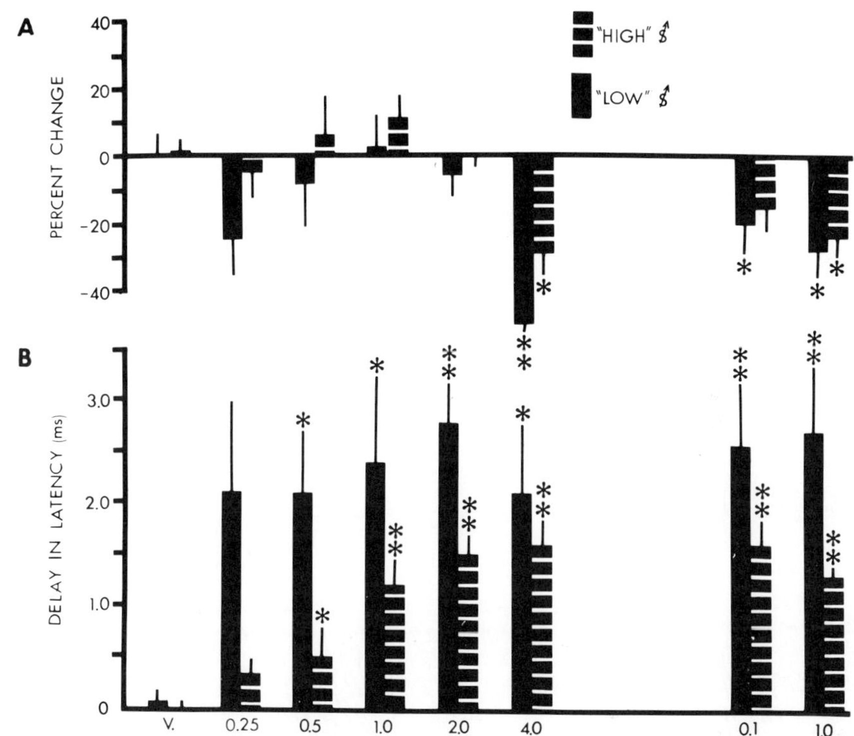

FIGURE 2. Dose-response effects of THC and DMHP. The effects of THC, 0.25-4.0 mg/kg, and DMHP, 0.1-1.0 mg/kg, on the primary SEP are displayed. Effects on amplitude (A) are displayed as percent change in peak amplitude and changes in latency (B) are expressed as the increase in latency. Data for low and high stimulus intensities are presented. (*, $p < 0.05$; **, $p < 0.01$)

THC on sensory activity in the CNS suggests that the actions of THC are dependent on the sensory modality and brain site. Dose, as well, can clearly alter the quality and direction of the effects of THC (17,18). Our present study, investigating three modalities of sensory perception in sensory-specific and convergent areas under the same conditions and often within preparation, supports the argument for specificity of action for THC.

In the chloralose-anesthetized cat the primary visual system appeared least sensitive to THC. The effect on auditory

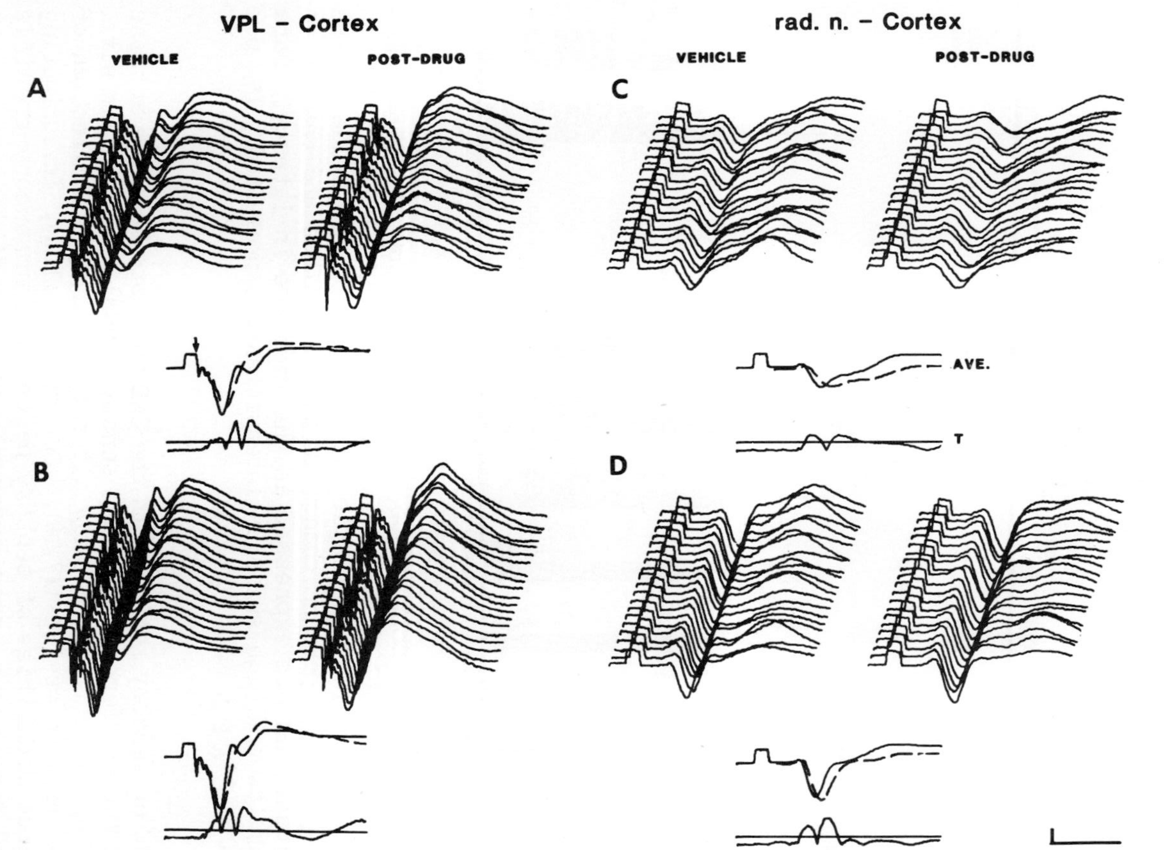

VPL - Cortex
rad. n. - Cortex
VEHICLE
POST-DRUG
VEHICLE
POST-DRUG
A
B
C
D
AVE.
T

sensory potentials were in agreement with those reported by Guha and Pradhan (8) in restrained conscious cats. This similarity and the similarities between the cat and rat experiments in the present study indicates that the effects of THC were not unduely confounded by the alpha-chloralose anesthesia.

The slowing of the cortical SEP without significant alteration in VPL activity suggests THC may act to reduce cortical responsiveness in area 3. The greater effect on activity evoked by low intensity stimulation in comparison to high intensity stimulation suggests that THC increased the threshold for cortical activation or response in the somatosensory pathway. More coherent information, e.g., that evoked by stronger stimuli, may be less affected by THC. This hypothesis would account for the relative little effect on primary visual activity evoked by electrical stimulation of optic chiasm where transmission through LGN may maintain a greater degree of coherence activity than that along the longer multisynaptic somatosensory pathway.

Evoked potentials on the cortical surface are the reflection of slow potentials (EPSP's and IPSP's) in the anisotropic cortical layers (19,20). The positive and negative waves have been attributed to different cell-types in the cortical layers. The positive wave may arise from the afferent connections to the stellate cells (20-22). Towe (23) has identified a population of nonpyramidal cells in the somatosensory cortex of the alpha-chloralose-anesthetized cat which discharge in relationship with the positive wave. It is possible that THC may depress the activity of these stellate cells and/or pyramidal cells which do not extend axons through the pyramids thus slowing the cascade of synaptic events. Whether this action could account for the sensory-specificity or not requires further studies.

FIGURE 3. The effect of THC on primary SEP. Individual SEP were collected 30 minutes after vehicle (VEHICLE) and 30 minutes after 2 mg/kg THC (POST-DRUG). SEP were elicited by: low intensity VPL stimulation (A); high intensity VPL stimulation (B); low intensity radial nerve stimulation (C); and high intensity radial nerve stimulation (D). Below each set of SEP's are the superimposed averages of vehicle (-) and post-THC (--). Under each pair of averages a statistical "t" is displayed illustrating the magnitude of the difference of the average scaled by the pooled standard error, t = 7.5 is indicated. Electrical stimulation immediately follow the calibration pulse, 500 mcV, 5 msec. All responses were derived from the same cortical site. (from ref. 25, with permission.)

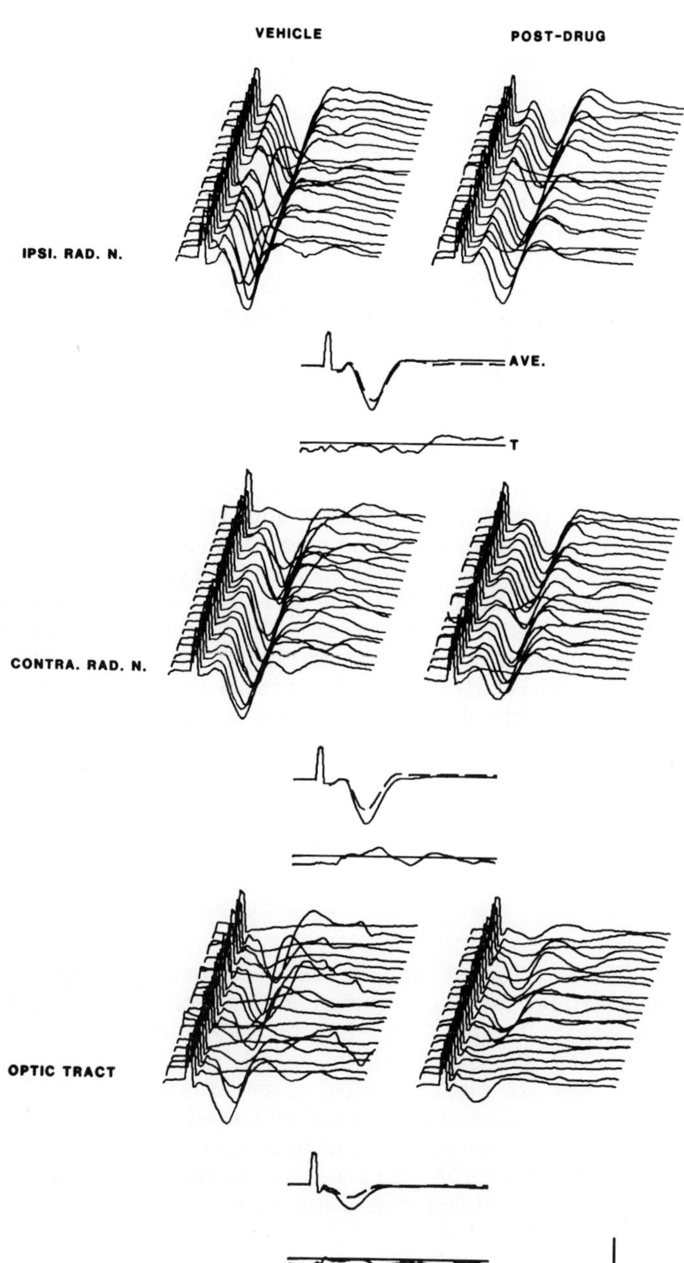
VEHICLE
POST-DRUG
IPSI. RAD. N.
AVE.
T
CONTRA. RAD. N.
OPTIC TRACT

Less functional detail is known about the cortical areas which receive multisensory information. However, multisensory neurons do predominate in these areas (6,24). In contrast to the relatively greater effect on somatosensory specific potentials over visual potentials, in the anterior marginal cortex the visual optic chiasm-evoked activity was depressed to a greater extent than activity evoked by somatosensory, radial nerve, stimulation. THC-induced alterations in activity in anterior marginal cortex may be the result of direct cortical effects or effects on subcortical, integrative thalamic regions that project to the association cortex. Additional data is needed to distinguish between these possibilities. Boyd and coworkers (12,13) reported enhancedcortico-cortical potentials after THC in the squirrel monkey. This finding is of interest because the cortical pathway studied was from primary somatosensory to association multisensory cortex. Although sensory evoked potentials in association cortex do not rely upon the integrity of the primary cortex, the potentials Boyd et al. (12,13) recorded may not be mediated entirely by the cortex. The evidence does suggest a facilatory action of THC in somatosensory elaboration to associative areas. The data presented in this report of a relative depression of visual information arriving at association cortex could be the result of such enhancement in the somatosensory pathways combined with a more generalized depression of sensory integration at either cortical or subcortical sites. A similar depression of association activity was observed after LSD (25) and may be involved in the sensory dissociation produced by drugs which alter sensory perception.

ACKNOWLEDGMENT

We thank M. Savio for his technical assistance.

FIGURE 4. Effects of THC on anterior marginal cortex. Potentials were evoked by stimulation of ipsilateral radial nerve (IPSI.RAD.N); contralateral radial nerve (CONTRA.RAD.N); and optic chiasm (OPTIC TRACT). Display is similar to Figures 1 and 3. All recordings are from a single cortical site. THC consistently depressed optic chiasm-evoked potentials more than radial nerve-evoked activity.

REFERENCES

1. Isbell, H., Gorodetzky, C. W., Jasinski, D., Claussen, U., Spulak, F. V., and Korle, F., Effects of (-)-delta-9-tetrahydrocannabinol in man, Psychopharmacologia 11:184-188 (1967).
2. Hosko, M. J., Kochar, M. S., and Wang, R. I. H., Effects of orally administered delta-9-tetrahydrocannabinol in man, Clin. Pharmacol. Ther. 14:344-352 (1973).
3. Amassian, V. E., Studies on organization of a somesthetic association area, including a single unit analysis, J. Neurophysiol. 17:39-58 (1954).
4. Dubner, R., and Rutledge, L. T., Recording and analysis of converging input upon neurons in cat association cortex, J. Neurophysiol. 27:620-634 (1964).
5. Thompson, R. F., Johnson, R. H., and Hoopes, J. J., Organization of auditory somatic sensory, and visual projection to association fields of cerebral cortex in the cat, J. Neurophysiol. 26:343:364 (1963).
6. Thompson, R. F., Bettinger L. A., Birch, H., and Groves, P. M., Comparison of evoked gross and unit responses in association cortex of wakingcat, Electroencephalogr. Clin. Neurophysiol. 27:146, 151 (1969).
7. Albe-Fessard, D., and Fessard, A., Thalamic integrations and their consequences at the telencephalic level, Prog. Brain Res. 1:115-148 (1963).
8. Guha, D., and Pradhan, S. N., Effects of mescaline, delta-9-tetrahydrocannabinol and pentobarbital on the auditory evoked responses in the cat, Neuropharm. 13:755-762 (1974).
9. Jasper, H. H., and Ajmone-Marsan, C., "A Stereotaxic Atlas of the Diencephalon of the Cat". Ottawa, National Research Council of Canada, 1954.
10. Pellegrino, L. J., and Cushman, A. J., "A Stereotaxic Atlas of the Rat Brain". Appleton-Century-Crofts, New York, 1967.
11. Hosko, M. J., Technique for rapid, permanent documentation of intracerebral electrode sites, Physiol. Behav. 14:367-378 (1975).
12. Boyd, E. S., Boyd, E. H., Muchmore, J. S., and Brown, L. E., Effects of two tetrahydrocannabinols and of pentobarbital on corticocortical evoked responses in the squirrel monkey, J. Pharmacol. Exp. Ther. 176:480-488 (1971).
13. Boyd, E. S., Boyd, E. H., and Brown, L. E., The effects of some drugs on an evoked response sensitive to tetrahydrocannabinols, J. Pharmacol. Exp. Ther. 189:748-758 (1974).

14. Wilkison, D. M., Pontzer, N., and Hosko, M. J., Slowing of cortical somatosensory evoked activity by delta-9-tetrahydrocannabinol and dimethylheptylpyran in alpha-chloralose-anesthetized cats, Neuropharm. 21:705-709 (1982).

15. Rodin, E., Domino, E. F., and Porzak, J. P.: The marijuana-induced "social-high" neurological and electroencphalographic concomitants, J. Amer. Med. Assoc. 213:1300-1302 (1970).

16. Jones, R. T., and Stone, G. C., Psychological studies of marijuana and alcohol in man, Psychopharmacol. (Berl.) 18:108-117 (1970).

17. Turkanis, S. A., Cliu, P., Borys, H. K., and Karler, R., Influence of tetrahydrocannabinol and cannabidiol on photically evoked after-discharge potentials, Psychopharmacol. 56:207-212 (1977).

18. Tramposch, A., Sangdee, C., Franz, D. N., Karler, R., and Turkanis, S. A., Cannabinoid-induced enhancement and depression of cat monosynaptic reflexes, Neuropharm. 20:617-621 (1981).

19. Li, C. L., Cortical intracellular synaptic potentials, J. Cell. Comp. Physiol. 58:153-167 (1961).

20. Creutzfeldt, O. D., Neuronal mechanisms underlying the EEG, in "Basic Mechanisms of the Epilepsies" (H. H. Jasper, A. A. Ward, Jr., and A. Pope, eds.), pp. 397-420. Little, Brown and Co., Boston, 1969.

21. Li, C. L., Cullen, C., and Jasper, H. H., Laminar microelectrode studies of specific somatosensory cortical potentials, J. Neurophysiol. 19:111-130 (1956).

22. Jones, E. G., and Powell, T. P. S., An electron microscopic study of the laminar pattern and mode of termination of the afferent fibre pathways in the somatic sensory cortex of the cat, Phil. Tran. R. Soc. Lond. B 257:45-62 (1970).

23. Towe, A. L., On the nature of the primary evoked response, Exp. Neurol. 15:113-139 (1966).

24. Robertson, R. T., Mayers, K. S., Teyler, T. J., Bettinger, L. A., Birch, H., Davis, J. L., Phillips, D. S., and Thompson, R. F., Unit activity in posterior association cortex of cat, J. Neurophysiol. 38:780-794 (1974).

25. Wilkison, D. M., and Hosko, M. J., Differential effects of lysergic acid diethylamide, methysergide, and cyproheptadine on modality-specific and nonspecific sensory evoked potentials, J. Pharmacol. Exp. Ther., in review (1982).

DELTA-9-TETRAHYDROCANNABINOL: SITE OF ACTION FOR AUTONOMIC EFFECTS*

Michael J. Hosko
William T. Schmeling
Harold F. Hardman

Department of Pharmacology and Toxicology
Medical College of Wisconsin
Milwaukee, Wisconsin

I. INTRODUCTION

Numerous studies have demonstrated that the cannabinoids are potent agents capable of producing a spectrum of pharmacological effects. These actions range from subtle psychoactive effects that almost certainly are mediated at forebrain and diencephalic loci, to autonomic effects that are manifested by alterations in respiration, blood pressure, temperature regulation and heart rate.

Studies from this as well as from other laboratories demonstrate that delta-9-tetrahydrocannabinol (THC), the primary psychoactive component of marijuana, has pronounced ability to induce hypotension and bradycardia in experimental animals. The ability of THC to induce hypotension is not compromised by transection of the neuraxis at the midcollicular level but is abolished by high cervical section. Figures 1 and 2 demonstrate the effects of systemically administered THC on blood pressure and temperature in cats with midcollicular and high cervical transections. The neuraxis was transected under halothane anesthesia. In the case of the midcollicular transections, the forebrain was destroyed by coagulation before discontinuing anesthesia. In the C-1 cord transected animals, a large needle was passed axially along the rostral reticular formation and a coagulating current was

*Supported by NIDA grant DA-00124.

ISBN 0-12-044620-0

applied to destroy the brainstem before discontinuing anesthesia. The animals were maintained on artificial respiration.

Intravenous administration of THC to midcollicular transected animals produced significant decreases in blood pressure (Figure 1) and heart rate when compared to vehicle controls. Within 30 minutes after THC administration, body temperature was significantly depressed when compared to controls (Figure 2). The hypotension and bradycardia elicited by THC administration in these unanesthetized cats with midcollicular transections agree well with previous reports using anesthetized cats with similar transections, and is comparable to the responses obtained in intact anesthetized cats (1). Administration of the second dose (4.0 mg/kg) of THC, produced

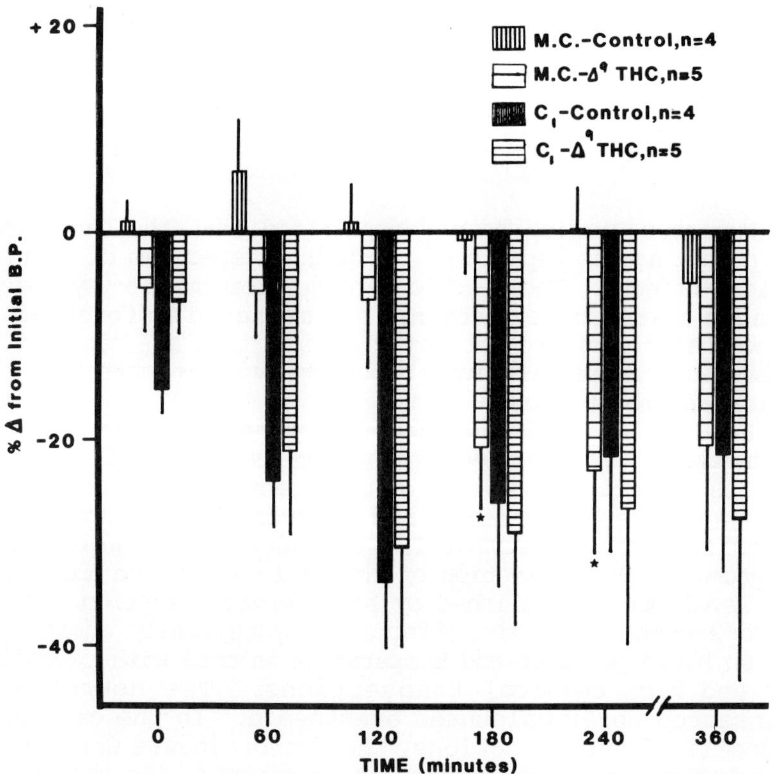

FIGURE 1. Effect of THC on blood pressure in midcollicular (MC) and spinal (C-1) transected cats. Control animals received vehicle in appropriate volume at 60, 120, and 240 minutes. The THC animals received vehicle at 60 minutes, 2 mg/kg THC (i.v.) at 120 minutes and 4 mg/kg THC (i.v.) at 240 minutes.

minimal additional effects. The somatic effects produced by the cannabinoids characteristically exhibit tachphylaxis in experimental animals. Vehicle produced no significant effects on body temperature, heart rate, or blood pressure.

The C-1 transected animals were used to establish the rate of body temperature loss in cats incapable of significant centrally mediated thermoregulation. Figure 2 demonstrates that the rate of temperature loss in C-1 transected animals receiving THC was statistically indistinguishable from C-1 transected animals receiving vehicle alone. These data indicate that in C-1 transected preparations, THC produced few if any peripheral effects that contribute to body temperature loss. The cardiovascular effects of THC were also absent in

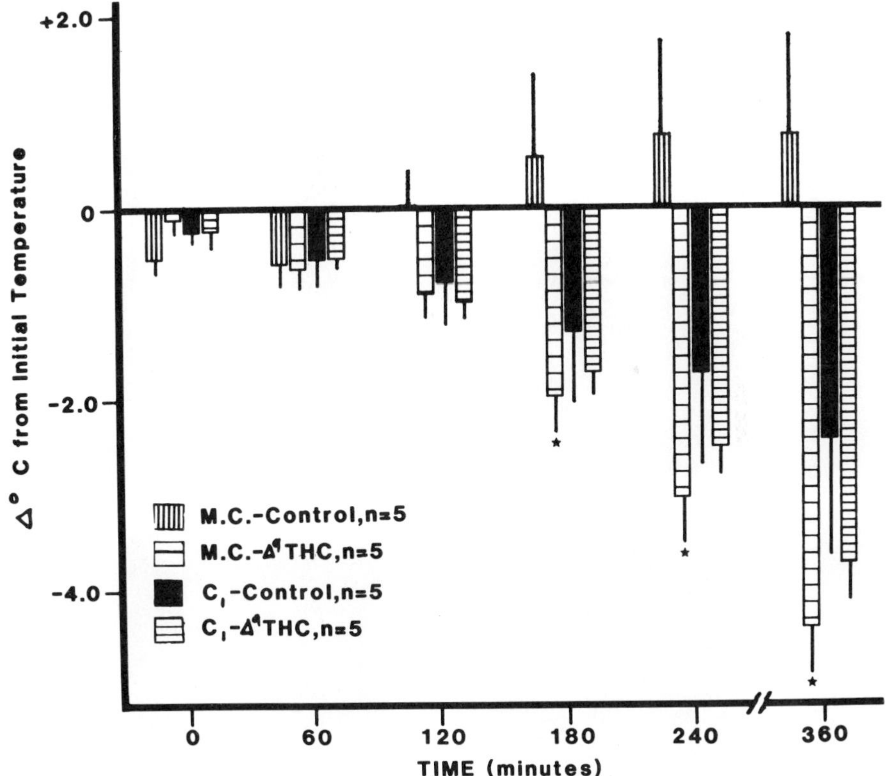

FIGURE 2. Effect of THC on body temperature in midcollicular (MC) and spinal (C-1) transected animals. Control cats received vehicle in appropriate volume at 60, 120 and 240 minutes. The THC animals received vehicle at 60 minutes, 2 mg/kg THC at 120 minutes ad 4 mg/kg THC at 240 minutes.

I.L.C. RESPONSES EVOKED FROM HYPOTHALAMUS

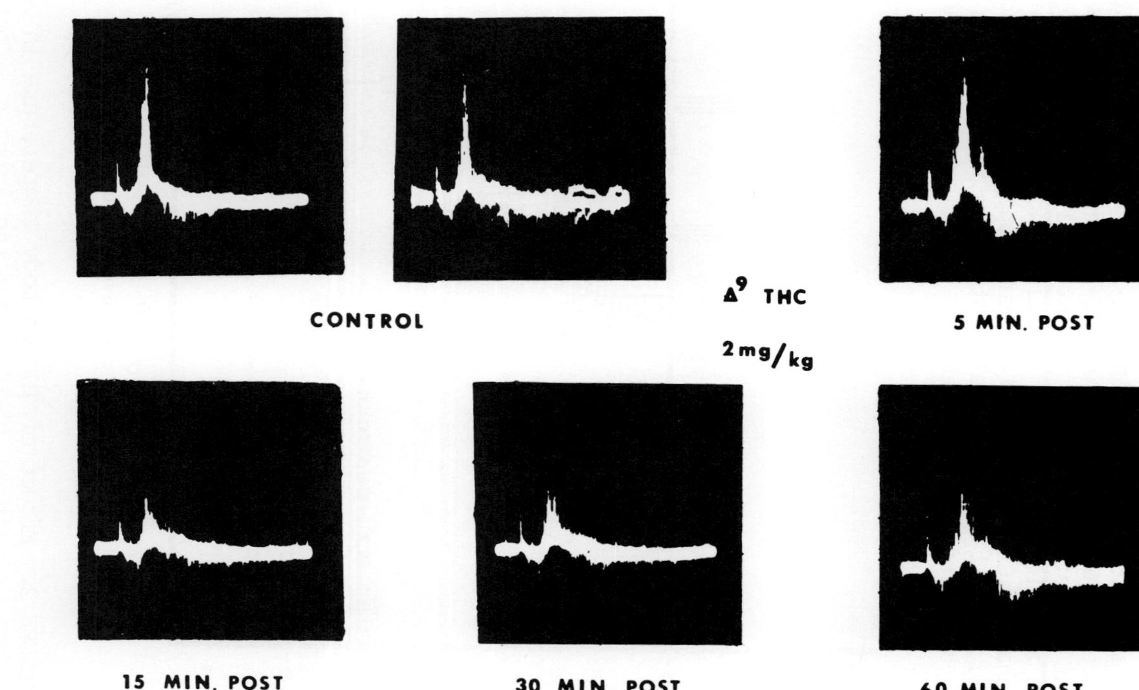

C-1 transected animals (Figure 1). Figure 2 further demonstrates that administration of THC to midcollicular preparations resulted in a rate of body temperature loss that closely approximated the rate seen in C-1 transected (control) animals.

In summary, the hypothermic response to THC, however mediated, was largely absent after low neuraxis transection at C-1, but was essentially unaffected by higher midcollicular transections which spared neuronal pools that subserve the autonomic nervous system. The hypothermic response exhibited by the midcollicular transected animals was essentially the same as that observed in intact animals (2).

In order to test the hypothesis that THC may exert some of its cardiovascular effects by disrupting sympathetic outflow, we have monitored evoked activity in the intermediolateral cell column (ILC) of the thoracic cord before and after THC administration (3). Hypothalamic cardiovascular pressor centers project to the ILC by monosynaptic as well as by polysynaptic pathways via the rhombencephalon.

II. RESULTS AND DISCUSSION

Male and female cats were anesthetized with chloralose-urethane IP. The femoral artery and vein were cannulated for recording BP and for administration of drugs. After appropriate surgical exposures, a coaxial stimulating electrode was positioned in the hypothalamus to elicit pressor responses. A tungsten recording microelectrode was positioned in ILC between T-1 and T-5. The hypothalamic electrode was used to deliver single square wave pulses (0.3 msec, 0.5-3.0 V) at 0.5 Hz. Figure 3 illustrates typical potentials evoked in ILC by stimulation of hypothalamic pressor sites. Each trace represents 10 superimposed responses to stimuli delivered at 2 second intervals. Five minutes after THC administration the evoked activity in the ILC is augmented. The augmented

FIGURE 3. Effects of THC on intermediolateral cell column field potentials evoked by stimulation of a hypothalamic pressor site in the cat. Each trace represents 10 superimposed potentials. Controls were taken 15 to 30 minutes after vehicle was administered. Panel A, 5 minutes after THC (2 mg/kg i.v.) increased amplitude coincided with a transient blood pressure increase. Panels B, C, D = 15, 30 and 60 minutes post THC. Blood pressure was reduced during B and C and was beginning recovery at D.

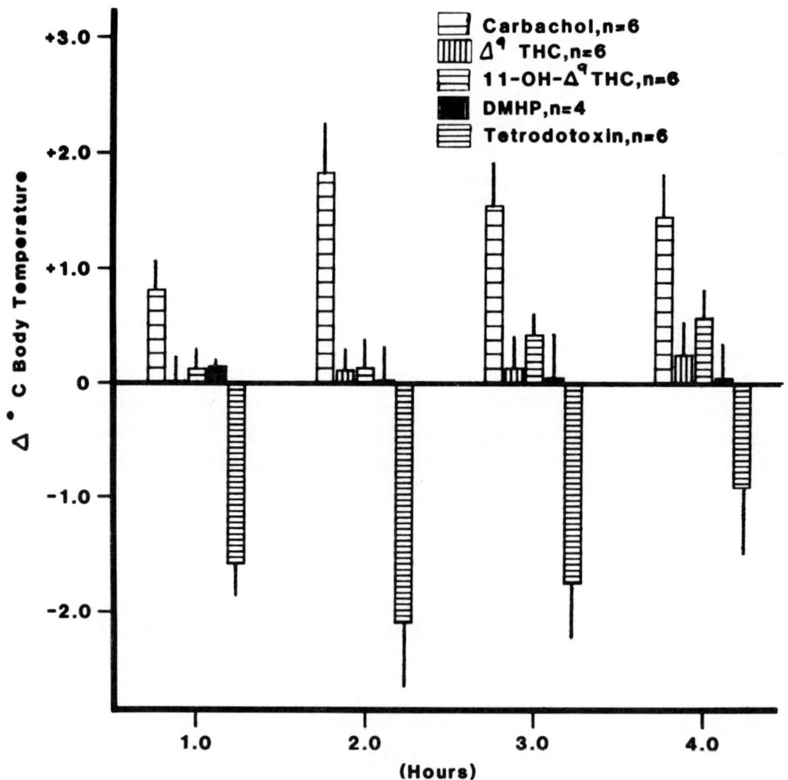

FIGURE 4. Lack of effect of microinjected cannabinoids on telemetered deep body temperature after administration to proven chemosensitive sites of the preoptic hypothalamus in chronic, unrestrained cats. Both carbachol and tetrodotoxin induced significant changes in body temperature. The effects of the cannabinoids were within the temperature variation monitored during a 2 hour vehicle control period. Drugs were administered at four to seven day intervals in a Latin square design. Carbachol, 5.5 mcg; THC, 100 mcg; 11-hydroxy-THC, 100 mcg; dimethylheptylpyran, 100 mcg; tetrodotoxin 75 ng.

response coincided with a slight, transient increase in blood pressure which sometimes occurs after IV THC administration. At 15 through 30 minutes post THC, the evoked responses in ILC are depressed. This time span corresponds to the period of peak blood pressure depression. By 60 minutes the evoked response is returning toward control levels. This coincides with the return of blood pressure toward control levels.

These data suggest that THC alters central processing of cardiovascular afferent input as well as sympathetic outflow to the cardiovascular system.

The cardiovascular response to cannabinoid administration is severely compromised by high spinal section (C-1), but not by transection at midcollicular levels. Attenuation of the pressor response to common carotid occlusion and the depressor response to carotid sinus nerve stimulation has been demonstrated after administration of THC (4). These findings support the conclusion that the primary site responsible for the cardiovascular actions of the cannabinoids is between the mesencephalon and C-1.

In a previous study from this laboratory (5), we demonstrated that in the rat, the preoptic region of the anterior hypothalamus was not the primary site of action for THC hypothermia. Studies in cats with brainstem transections at various levels along the neuraxis indicate that the primary site

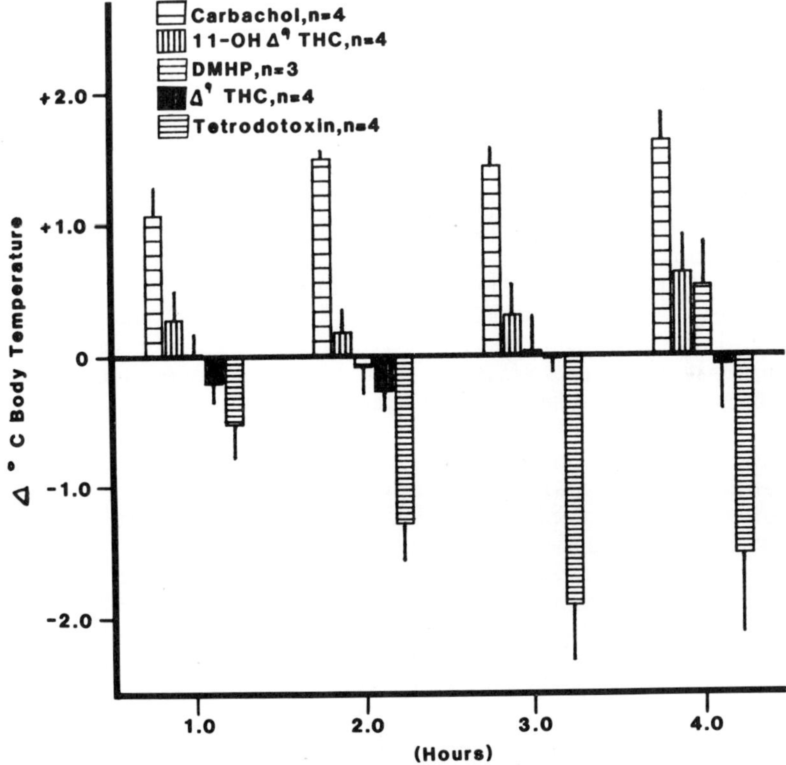

FIGURE 5. Lack of effect of microinjected cannabinoids on telemetered deep body temperature after administration to proven chemosensitive sites in the posterior hypothalamus in chronic, unrestrained cats. See Figure 4 for details.

of action is in the caudal brainstem. To further challenge this hypothesis we applied cannabinoids directly to proven hypothalamic chemosensitive thermoregulatory sites in cats with implanted microinjection guides. In order to allow undisturbed observation of behavioral response to the microinjection, temperature telemetry units were implanted into the peritoneal cavity at the same time the guide tubes were implanted.

Following surgery, the animals received 100,000 units of penicillin for three consecutive days. A minimum of ten days was allowed for recovery.

Each animal received the following drugs: 11-Hydroxy-delta-9-tetrahydrocannabinol (11-OH-THC), 100 mcg (5.0 mcl); delta-9-tetrahydrocannabinol (THC), 100 mcg (8.9 mcl); carbamylcholine (Carbachol), 5.5 mcg (3.0 mcl); tetrodotoxin, 75 ng (1.5 mcl); dimethylheptylpyran (DMHP), 100 mcg (8.0 mcl). The drugs were microinjected into the target sites at five- to seven-day intervals using a Latin square design.

Figures 4 and 5 demonstrate that while carbachol and tetrodotoxin evoked statistically significant alterations in body temperature, intracerebral microinjection of THC, 11-OH-THC or DMHP at doses of 100 mcg produced little or no effect. In order to control for the various vehicles utilized, sterile water, saline and one and two times the normal cannabinoid vehicle concentration (all 8.0 mcl volume) were microinjected into documented chemosensitive sites. No significant alteration in body temperature was observed. To insure that the lack of response to THC microinjection was not due to an insufficient dose, doses of THC as high as 400 mcg (8.0 mcl) were made into proven chemosensitive sites in four cats before the animals were sacrificed. Even at these doses, no significant temperature effects were elicited.

It should be noted that tetrodotoxin and carbachol were included in the cannabinoid microinjection series in a sequence determined by the Latin square design. In every instance, the response elicited by the second dose virtually replicated the thermal and behavioral response elicited by the test dose that established chemosensitivity for the site. This observation indicated that the initial administration of carbachol and tetrodotoxin or, subsequently, the rather large volume (8 mcl) used to administer the cannabinoids did not functionally damage the target site. The differential behavioral effects elicited by the various test agents administered into different sites further suggest that there was minimal, if any, diffusion of the drugs into the ventricles.

At the end of the microinjection sequence, parenteral administration of THC, 11-OH-THC and DMHP (1 or 2 mg/kg) produced hypothermia in every animal, demonstrating that the implanted animals were capable of responding to the test agents. The magnitude of the hypothermic response to parenterally administered agents was consistent with previously published results. The animals were able to respond to external stimuli, however, they made no attempt to conserve body temperature, i.e., there was no evidence of shivering, piloerection or curling or huddling of the body. Deep core temperature recorded 24 hours after intraperitoneal or intravenous injection was always at or near control levels. In general, administration of the cannabinoids by the intravenous route produced a greater hypothermic response than that produced by the intraperitoneal route (6).

We have shown acute lateral intraventricular injection of cannabinoids to induce significant hypothermia in a number of different species. Figure 6 compares the hypothermic action

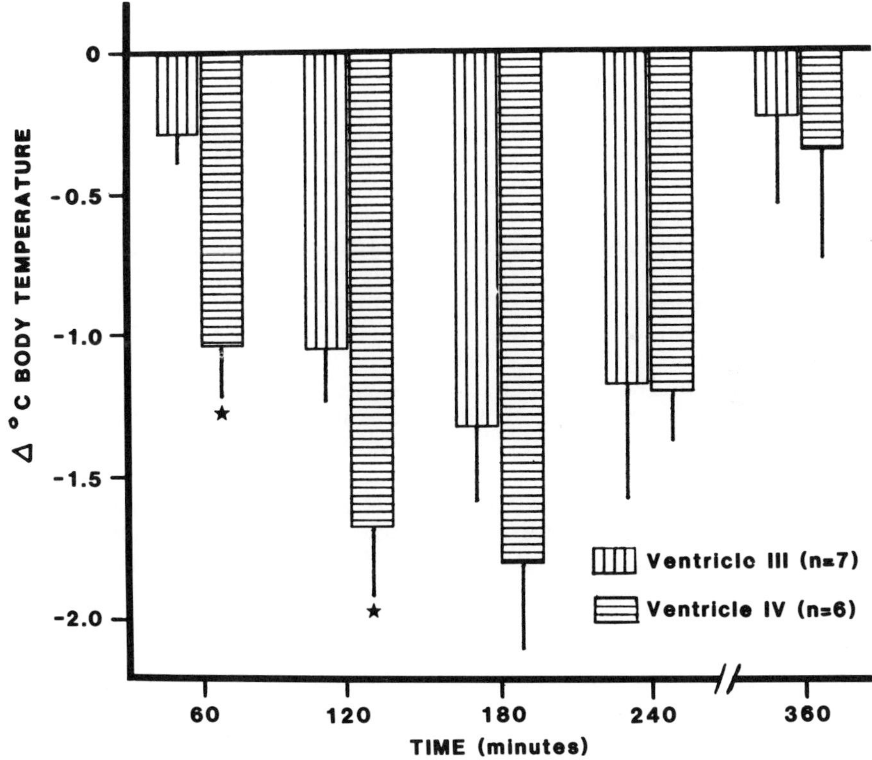

FIGURE 6. Hypothermia induced by THC administered to Ventricle III and IV in chronic unrestrained cats. Temperature was monitored by telemetry. Vehicle produced no significant hypothermia. *Significantly different from Ventricle III administration.

of THC after administration into the third and fourth ventricle in chronically implanted unanesthetized cats. In order to avoid handling the animals, temperature was recorded by telemetry.

Microinjection of 100 mcg THC (in 8.0 mcl) into ventricle III elicited minimal hypothermic effects. Microinjections of 500 mcg of THC (in 40.0 mcl) produced a significant hypothermic response. Onset of temperature depression was slow with little effect during the first hour post-injection. Peak hypothermia, 1.0-2.5^{o}C, was reached 2-4 hours after microinjection. Behavioral manifestations included bilateral nictitating membrane relaxation, mild ataxia, and tremor, slight decrease in response to auditory or tactile stimuli, and some autonomic effects including defecation, urination, and emesis.

Microinjection of THC (500 mcg in 40.0 mcl) into ventricle IV produced significant hypothermic responses. Temperature decrease began within 15 min of administration and reached peak levels at 1.5-3.0^{o}C within 1-2 hours. After injection, cats exhibited bilateral pupillary dilation and nictitating membrane relaxation. Vocalization and urination or defecation was also seen in 3 animals. Vehicle microinjections did not elicit changes in body temperature or behavior.

The hypothermic response to intracisternal administration of THC resulted in a more rapid onset and reached a greater maximum than that produced by ventricle III administration.

Intravenous administration of 500 mcg of THC produced significantly less hypothermia than intracisternal or intraventricular administration. Vehicle produced no significant alteration in body temperature.

Thermosensitive anterior hypothalamic neurons (pre-optic region) have been studied in cats anesthetized with either urethane or chloralose in an attempt to characterize the hypothermic action of THC at the neuronal level. One hundred and seventy-eight single neurons were isolated and subjected to thermal challenge, 66 were found to reproducibly alter firing frequency at a significant level (thermosensitivity, T.S., 0.75). Twenty-one of these units met the criteria for primary thermodetectors, 34 were heat-sensitive interneurons and 11 were cold-sensitive interneurons. Administration of THC (1.0-2.0 mg/kg i.v.) decreased the spontaneous firing and increased the T.S. of the primary thermodetector units. THC also increased the spontaneous firing frequency as well as the T.S. of heat-sensitive interneurons, while decreasing both the T.S. and spontaneous firing of cold-sensitive interneurons. The decreased spontaneous firing of primary thermodetectors could result from altered facilitory or inhibitory influences converging on these cells. The increased thermosensitivity is consistent with the hypothesis that the preoptic region modulates cannabinoid-induced hypothermia (7).

In preliminary studies, a high percentage (70%) of the units we have isolated in the medulla exhibited some thermosensitivity to local thermal challenge. Of the medullary units exhibiting some thermosensitivity, 47% demonstrated thermosensitive convergence to heating and/or cooling of spinal cord and/or preoptic region. The firing rate response to such convergent driving varies from neuron to neuron. Selected, stable thermosensitive units were challenged by systemic administration of small doses (0.5-2.0 mg/kg) of THC. Typically, THC decreases the spontaneous firing rate while the T.S. was differentially altered. Nonthermosensitive neurons (controls), exhibited little or no change in firing patterns after THC. These studies document the presence of thermosensitive neurons in the medulla. Many of these units receive convergent information from other known thermosensitive sites. These preliminary unit studies add support to our contention that the caudal brainstem is the principal site of action for THC induced hypothermia.

In anesthetized cats, THC has a marked depressant effect on spontaneous respiration. Figure 7 illustrates microelectrode recordings from medullary inspiratory neurons in two anesthetized animals. Note that the "inspiratory unit" begins firing immediately before the onset of inspiration and terminates firing prior to the onset of expiration. After i.v. THC administration, frank apneusis is evident in animal RC-15, while a shift toward apneustic respiration is demonstrated by animal RC-20. After THC the inspiratory neurons continue to fire for extended periods with concomitant maintenance of inspiration.

Doses of THC above 2 mg/kg reduce respiration rate by at least 50%. However, most striking, was the production of apneusis. Although this effect was most pronounced in animals anesthetized with chloralose urethane, it was also observed in the dial-urethane anesthetized animals. We frequently observed periods of apenusis with a duration in excess of 60 seconds. Onset of apneustic respiration ranged from 1 to 10 min after THC administration, and persisted for longer than 1 hour, often terminating in death. Coincident with reduced frequency of respiration and apneusis, arterial O_2 saturation was reduced by as much as 33%. Respiratory stimulants (doxapram, nikethamide, pentylenetetrazol) restored normal respiratory patterns for at least a brief period of time in every animal in which they were utilized. CNS depressants (diazepam, pentobarbital) increased both frequency and duration of apneustic periods. In cats pretreated with ethanol (500 mg/kg i.v.), a 1-mg/kg i.v. dose of THC induced marked apneusis in 5 of 6 cats studied.

It was possible to induce apneusis with THC in cats with the neuraxis transected posterior to the colliculi. In two of

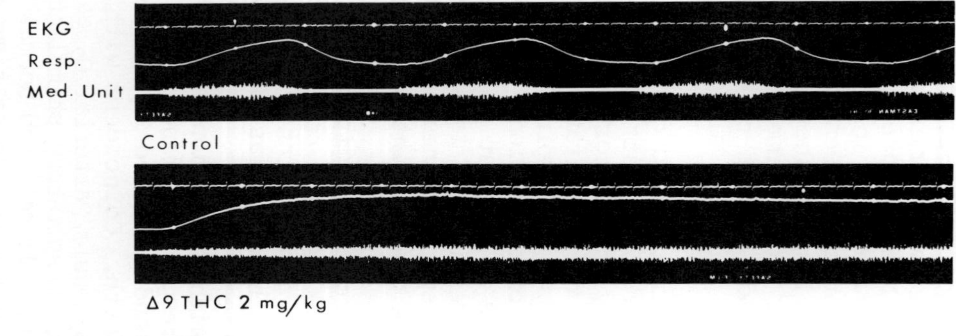
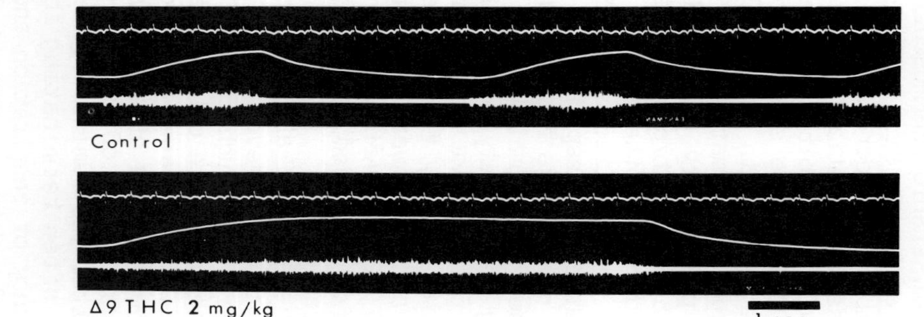
Δ9 THC on MEDULLARY "INSPIRATORY" NEURONS
THC-RC-15 ♂ 4·4 kg CU
EKG
Resp.
Med. Unit
Control
Δ9 THC 2 mg/kg
THC-RC-20 ♂ 2·3 kg CU
Control
Δ9 THC 2 mg/kg
1 sec.

these preparations, we were able to interrupt sustained inspiration by electrical stimulation of the "pneumotaxic center" (N. parabrachialis med.). Extracellular microelectrode recordings from medullary "inspiratory" and "expiratory" neurons were consistent with diaphragmatic EMG patterns.

Taken together, the data summarized here are consistent with and support our hypothesis that the primary autonomic effects of THC are mediated at caudal brainstem sites that are located for the most part between the levels of the midcolliculi and the first cervical segment.

ACKNOWLEDGMENT

The authors thank Mr. Michael Savio for his excellent technical assistance.

REFERENCES

1. Hosko, M. J., and Hardman, H. F., Evidence for a dual mechanism of action of cannabis on central cardiovascular control, in "Pharmacology of Marihuana" (M. C. Braude and S. Szara, eds.), pp. 239-253. Raven Press, New York, 1976.
2. Schmeling, W. T., and Hosko, M. J., Hypothermic effects of intraventricular and intravenous administration of cannabinoids in intact and brainstem transected cats, J. Neuropharmacol. 19:567-573 (1980).
3. Schmeling, W. T., Hosko, M. J., and Hardman, H. F., Potentials evoked in the intermediolateral column by hypothalamic stimulation-supression by delta-9-tetrahydrocannabinol, Life Sci. 29:673-680 (1981).
4. Schmeling, W. T., and Hosko, M. J., The effects of delta-9-tetrahydrocannabinol (THC) on centrally mediated homeostatic cardiovascular reflexes, Fed. Proc. 37:737 (1978).

FIGURE 7. Effect of THC on medullary respiratory neuron in two anesthetized, spontaneously breathing cats. The second trace in each panel (Resp.) goes up with inspiration. In both animals the post-THC records were obtained within 5 minutes of THc administration. The apneustic event illustrated in the second panel lasted longer than 90 seconds. The period of apneustic respiration in both animals had a duration longer than one hour.

5. Schmeling, W. T., and Hosko, M. J., Hypothermia induced delta-9-tetrahydrocannabinol in rats with electrolytic lesions of preoptic region, Pharmacol. Biochem. Behav. 5(1):79-83 (1976).
6. Hosko, M. J., Schmeling, W. T., and Hardman, H. F., Evidence for a caudal brainstem site of action for cannabinoid induced hypothermia, Brain. Res. Bull. 6:251-258 (1981).
7. Schmeling, W. T., and Hosko, M. J., Effect of delta-9-tetrahydrocannabinol on hypothalamic thermosensitive units, Brain. Res. 187:431-442 (1980).

THE EFFECTS OF DELTA-9-TETRAHYDROCANNABINOL INJECTIONS TO THE NUCLEUS ACCUMBENS ON THE LOCOMOTOR ACTIVITY OF RATS

Lisa H. Conti
Richard E. Musty

Department of Psychology
University of Vermont
Burlington, Vermont

I. INTRODUCTION

The nucleus accumbens (NA) is a forebrain structure innervated by A10 dopaminergic neurons descending the medial forebrain bundle (1,2). Apart from the caudate nucleus, the NA contains the highest concentration of dopamine (DA) in the rat brain (3). The dopaminergic system of the NA has been shown repeatedly to be involved in the mediation of locomotor activity. The direct application of DA to this nucleus produces an increase in such activity (4,5). Furthermore, this effect can be blocked by an i.p. injection of pimozide (a dopamine antagonist) (6). It has also been demonstrated that those drugs which act as dopamine receptor agonists, such as apomorphine, ADTN, and ergometrine, as well as amphetamine, produce an increase in locomotor activity when injected directly to the NA (6).

Within the NA, dopamine and its agonists produce their effects on locomotor activity by inhibiting the dopaminergic neurons in that area. The spontaneous firing rate of single neurons in the NA is decreased by the application of either DA, ADTN or ergometrine to that site (7). This decrease in neural activity causes the release from inhibition of those neurons in the globus pallidus which subserve locomotion (8).

Among the demonstrated behavioral effects of delta-9-tetrahydrocannabinol (THC) are those which it produces on locomotor activity. The systemic administration of low doses of THC has been shown to increase locomotor activity, while

ISBN 0-12-044620-0

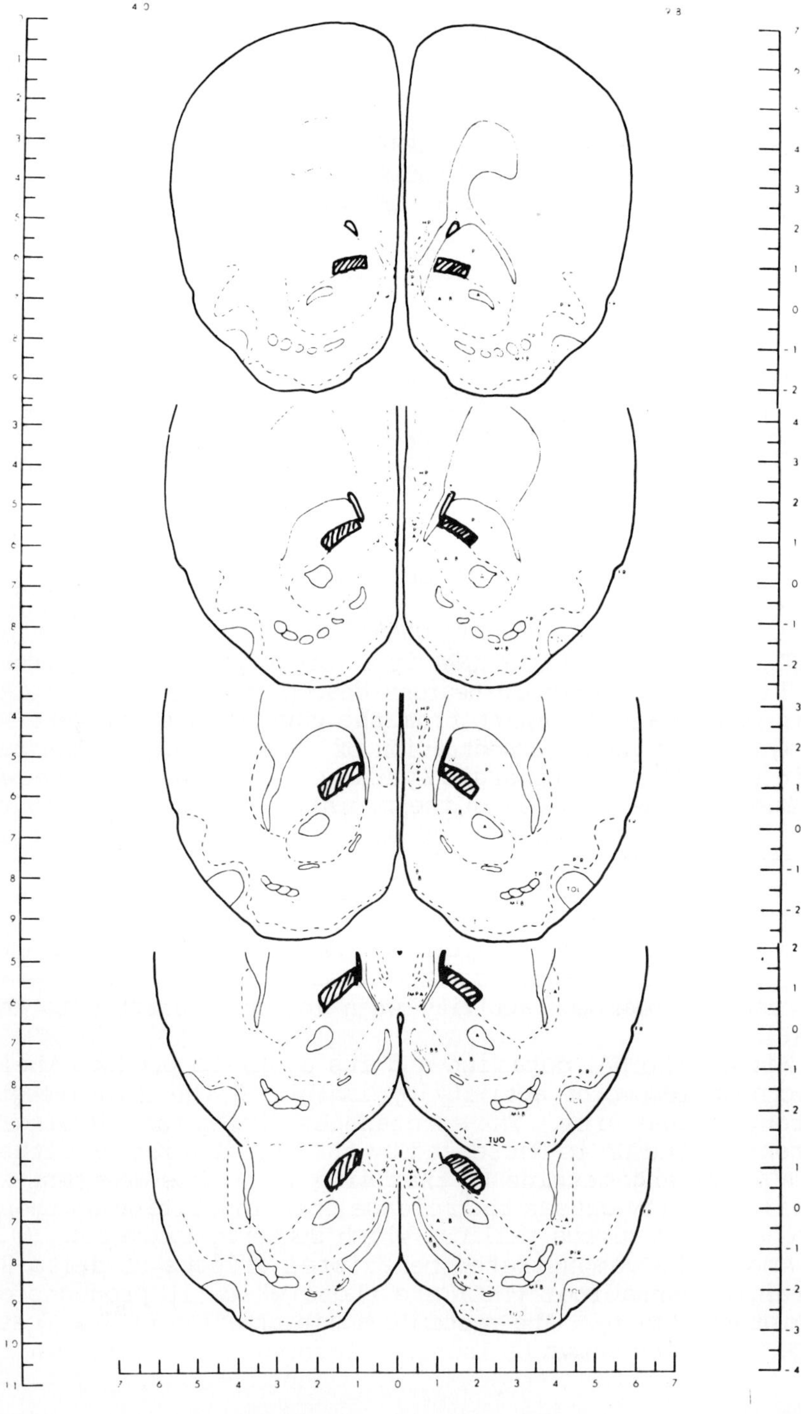

high doses have been demonstrated to decrease spontaneous locomotion (9–12).

The purpose of this study was to investigate whether THC is acting within the NA to produce its excitatory effects on locomotor activity. It can be hypothesized that locomotor stimulation produced by the application of a drug to the NA is mediated by the dopaminergic mechanism within the nucleus.

II. MATERIALS AND METHODS

Male, Long-Evans rats (Charles River Breeding Labs), weighing 250–350 g at the start of the experiment, were maintained on ad lib food and water until 24 hrs prior to surgery when they were deprived of food until post-surgery. The colony was on a 12 hr. light-dark cycle (7 a.m. – 7 p.m.).

Each rat was anesthetized with Sodium Pentobarbital and was administered Atropine Sulfate to maintain clear airways. Twenty-three gauge stainless-steel cannulae were bilaterally implanted to the nucleus accumbens at the stereotaxic coordinates of 3.4A, 1.5L, and 5.8V. Cannulae were kept patent with stainless-steel wire.

Seven to 10 days following surgery, the locomotor activity of each rat was assessed for a ten-minute, baseline period using a cylindrical activity chamber, which was housed in a sound-attenuating box containing a house light and ventilation system. The floor of the chamber was suspended on rubber mounts and vibrations of the floor were transduced by an accelerometer and converted into activity units. The cylinder measured 57 cm in diameter.

Immediately following the baseline period, the animal was taken from the chamber and injected with either one dose of THC (0.1, 0.5, 1.0, 2.0, or 10.0 mg/ml) or with vehicle solution (PVP) in a 1 mcl vol to each NA. Following the injection, each rat was tested in the activity chamber for a 50 min test session. Activity counts over the 50 min session were divided among 5 min bins on counters.

Animals were sacrificed for the purpose of histology. They were perfused with formal saline, and their brains were removed and kept in 10% formalin and saline for 24 hrs prior to being sectioned on a freezing microtone. Sections (50

FIGURE 1. Frontal sections of the rat brain taken from ref. 13. Cross hatched areas indicate areas of acceptable cannula placements, bilaterally. All placements outside these boundaries were rejected from the analysis.

microns) were mounted on microscope slides and stained. They were then read through a microscope in order to verify cannulae placements.

Activity counts during the 50 min test session were converted to a percentage of baseline activity for each rat. Grouppercentages were then submitted to a 2-way analysesof variance (drug dose x time). Appropriate t-tests were conducted following the analysis.

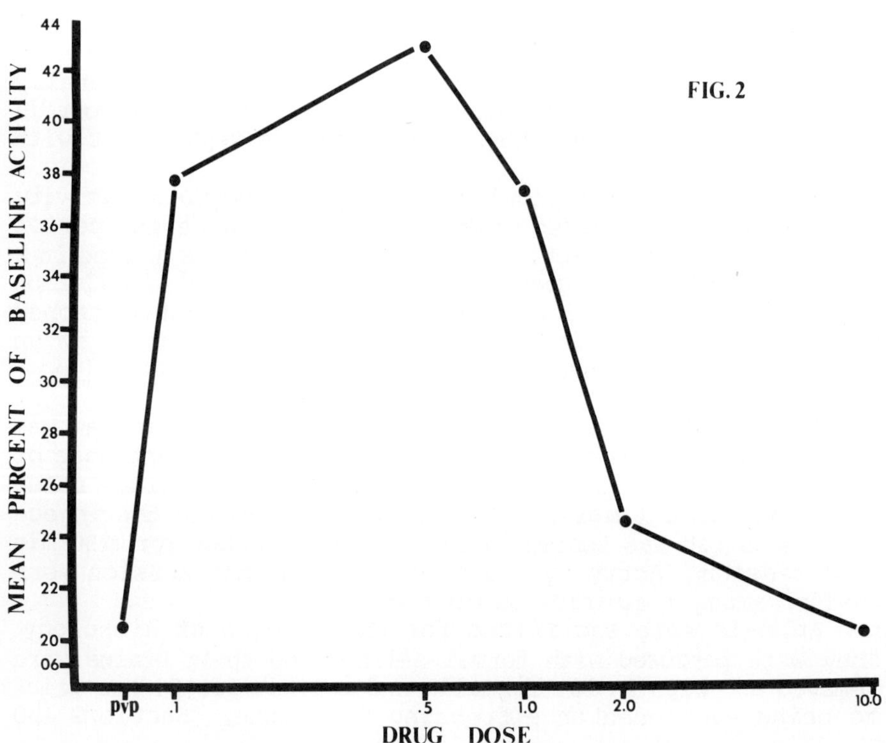

FIGURE 2. Mean percent of baseline activity plotted as a function of THC dose per cannula (two doses per animal). PVP is the vehicle alone. This control value is less than 100 per cent because activity decreases as a function of time.

III. RESULTS

The injection sites which were considered acceptable upon histology are circumscribed in Figurel. Those cannulae placements lying outside of these areas were not considered acceptable and the data from animals having such placements were not used in the analysis.

THC produced a significant increase in locomotor activity above that produced by vehicle injections for the first 20 min post-injection based on a 2-way analysis off variance (drug dose x time), $\underline{F}(5,36) = 3.34$, $p < 0.02$, (see Figure 2). The results of comparisons between drug doses revealed that the 0.5 mcg group had a significantly elevated locomotor activity score when compared to the vehicle control group, $\underline{t}(12) = 2.70$, $p < 0.01$, the 2 mcg group, $\underline{t}(12) = 2.04$, $p < 0.05$, and the 10 mcg group, $\underline{t}(12) = 2.22$, $p < 0.02$.

IV. DISCUSSION

Low doses of THC, bilaterally administered to the nucleus accumbens of rats, produced an increase in locomotor activity above that displayed by vehicle controls. The peak effect was observed at 20 min post-injection. While statistical analysis revealed that there was a significant difference among the groups at 25 min post-injection, the effect was of a lesser magnitude than that which was observed at 20 min post-injection.

The effect of injections of 10 mcg THC was virtually the same as the effect of the control injections. This suggests that higher doses administered directly to the nucleus accumbens produced a locomotor response similar to that produced by high doses upon systemic administration.

The increase in locomotor activity produced by THC in this study could be indicative of an effect upon dopaminergic mechanisms in the nucleus accumbens. Neurons with dopamine receptor sites in the NA project to the globus pallidus where they release GABA. Jones and Mogenson have shown that stimulation of the nucleus accumbens produces an inhibition of the firing of neurons in the globus pallidus (14). This inhibition is abolished by the application of picrotoxin (a GABAantagonist) to the globus pallidus. Furthermore, these investigators found that the application of GABA to the globus pallidus attenuates the increase in locomotor activity caused by the injection of dopamine to the nucleus accumbens.

Based on the evidence obtained in this study that low doses of THC are acting within the NA to produce an effect similar to that produced by dopamine agonists, investigations of the effects of THC application to the NA on the firing rate of single units there is warranted.

Those drugs which increase locomotor activity upon injection to the nucleus accumbens decrease the spontaneous firing rate of neurons there. The effect of inhibiting these neurons is to inhibit the transmission of GABA to the globus pallidus. Thus, the neurons in the globus pallidus which mediate locomotor activity are released from the inhibitory effect of GABA there.

Also of interest in the investigation of the site of action via which THC effects locomotor activity is the globus pallidus itself. Should local application of THC to the globus pallidus produce an effect on locomotion, it would seem possible that GABAnergic system there is directly involved in the effect. If however, no effect on locomotion results from the injection of THC to the globus pallidus the possibility that the drug is acting upon the dopaminergic neurons of the NA to produce its effects on locomotor activity would be reinforced.

Finally, further evidence that THC is acting upon dopamine receptors in the NA would be indicated if its effect on locomotor activity could be blocked by a dopamine receptor antagonist. Studies are being conducted in our laboratory to test these hypotheses.

REFERENCES

1. Nauta, W., Smith, G., Faull, R., and Domesick, V., Efferent connections and nigral afferents of the nucleus accumbens septi in the rat, Neuroscience 3:385-401 (1978).
2. Walass, I., and Fonnum, F., The effects of surgical and chemical lesions on neurotransmitter candidates in the nucleus accumbens of the rat, Neuroscience 4:209-216 (1979).
3. Palmer, G., and Chronister, R., The biochemical pharmacology of the nucleus accumbens, in "The Neurobiology of the Nucleus Accumbens". Haer Institute for Electro-physiological Research, Brunswick, Maine, 1981.
4. Costall, B., and Naylor, R., The behavioral effects of dopamine applied intercerebrally to areas of the mesolimbic system, Eur. Pharmacol. 32:87 (1975).
5. Jones, D., Mogenson, G., and Wu, M., Injections of dopaminergic, cholinergic, serotoninergic and GABA ergic drugs into the nucleus accumbens: Effects on locomotor activity in the rat, Neuropharmacol. (1980).

6. Jackson, D., Anden, J., and Dahlstrom, A., A functional effect of dopamine in the nucleus accumbens and some other dopamine-rich parts of the rat brain, Psychopharmacologia 45:139-149 (1975).
7. Woodruff, G., McCarthy, P., and Walker, R., Studies on the pharmacology of neurons in the nucleus accumbens of the rat, Brain Research 115:233-242 (1976).
8. Mogenson, G., and Yim, C., Electrophysiological and neuropharmacological-behavioral studies of the nucleus accumbens: Implications for its role as a limbic motor interface, in "The Neurobiology of the Nucleus Accumbens". Haer Institute for Electrophysiological Research, Brunswick, Maine, 1981.
9. Carlini, E., Santos, N., Claussen, U., Bienick, D., and Korte, F., Structure activity relationship of four tetrahydrocannabinols and the pharmacological activity of five semi-purified extracts of cannabis sativa, Psychopharmacologia 18:82-93 (1970).
10. Davis, W., Moreton, J., King, W., and Pace, H., Marijuana on locomotor activity: Biphasic effect and tolerance development, Res. Comm. Chem. Pathol. Pharmacol. 3:29-35 (1972).
11. Anderson, P., Jackson, D., Chesher, G., and Malor, R., Tolerance to the effects of delta-9-tetrahydrocannabinol in mice on intestinal motility, temperature and locomotor activity, Psychopharmacologia 43:31 (1975).
12. Evans, M., Harbison, R., Brown, D., and Forney, R., Stimulant actions of delta-9-tetrahydrocannabinol in mice, Psychopharmacology 50:245-250 (1976).
13. Pellegrino, L. J., Pellegrino, A., and Cushman, A. "A Stereotaxic Atlas of the Rat Brain." New York, 1980.
14. Jones, D., and Mogenson, G., Nucleus accumbens to globus pallidus GABA projection subserving ambulatory activity, Amer. J. Physiol. 238:65-68 (1980).

PEER AND MATERNAL SOCIAL INTERACTION PATTERNS IN OFFSPRING OF RHESUS MONKEYS TREATED CHRONICALLY WITH DELTA-9-TETRAHYDROCANNABINOL*

Mari S. Golub
E. N. Sassenrath
Gail P. Goo

California Primate Research Center
Davis, California

I. INTRODUCTION

Behavioral teratology studies assess the impact of developmental treatments on subsequent behavioral competence (1-3). The goal of such studies is to identify a detrimental effect on functional maturation of the nervous system and ultimately to define the mechanism by which this effect occurs.

Primate models in behavioral teratology are particularly valuable for identifying toxicity in adaptive systems relevant to humans, such as complex intellectual and social skills. These skills impact heavily on behavioral symptom complexes for which children are referred to physicians (developmental delay, learning disability, attention deficit disorder). The present study used a primate model (the rhesus monkey, <u>Macaca mulatta</u>) to assess the influence of chronic, low-level maternal delta-9-tetrahydrocannabinol (THC) treatment on early social behavior. In general, social behavior toward mother and peers was found to be adequate and within the range of the untreated control group. Some differences between THC offspring and untreated controls were identified in mother-infant interactions of late infancy and in the initial responseto entry into a social group with unfamiliar peers.

---

*Supported in part by NIDA grant DA-00135, NRSA award HD-05567, and NIH grants RR-00169 and RR-05684.

ISBN 0-12-044620-0

II. METHODS

A. Subjects

Five offspring (3 male and 2 female) of THC-treated rhesus dams (*Macaca mulatta*) were compared to nine controls (3 male, 6 female). Infants were born during two successive annual breeding seasons (See Table I for pregnancy outcome data). All dams were 5-8 years old and had been maintained according to the same experimental protocol during gestation and lactation and for at least two years prior to the study.

B. Housing and Maintenance

Dams and infants were maintained in individual indoor cages in the same cageroom. Care and maintenance met the guidelines of the Federal Animal Welfare Act and the Institute of Laboratory Animal Resources. Details of breeding procedures have been described (4). At 3.5 mos of age, infants were weaned and separated from the dam and began a behavioral test series (5). At 6 mos of age, infants were formed into small living groups of three or four animals each with one THC-treated animal per group.

C. Drug Treatment

A daily dose of 2.4 mg/kg THC was administered orally in a preferred food item. Alcohol solutions of THC (200 mg/ml)

TABLE I. Pregnancy Outcome in THC-treated Female Monkeys and Non-treated Controls in Two Successive Breeding Seasons*

	Non-treated		THC-treated	
	Year 1	Year 2	Year 1	Year 2
Liveborn, accepted by dam	5	5	3	2
Liveborn, nursery reared	1	2	0	1
Fetal death	1	0	1	1
Abortion	0	0	0	1

*Liveborn infants accepted by the dam served as subjects in the present experiment.

were obtained from the National Institute on Drug Abuse and injectedin to the food item. Independent studies have indicated that peak plasma concentrations of 200 to 300 ng/ml THC are reached within one to three hours of administration using this administration technique. Daily drug treatment began at least two years prior to conception and continued throughout gestation and lactation. Control dams received an undrugged food item according to the same schedule.

D. Behavioral Measures

Mother-infant behavior measures were obtained from five 20-min videotape sessions recorded during early infancy (10-20 days) and late infancy ((90-100 days of age). Tapes were scored for the duration of four arousal activity states and for the quality of mother-infant interaction (Table II) by trained observers who were unaware of the group assignments of the animals (see 4).

Peer interaction was recorded using a continuous, focal animal sampling technique with a 10-min daily sampling period per animal. For each social interaction, initiator, behavior and response were recorded (6).

E. Plasma Cortisol

Blood samples (0.5 ml) were obtained from the cephalic or femoral vein of the conscious, restrained animal within three minutes of capture. Samples were centrifuged immediately and plasma removed and frozen for subsequent determination of plasma cortisol using a protein binding assay (7).

III. RESULTS AND DISCUSSION

Various measures of maternal and infant behavior (Table II) were initially examined with analysis of variance using maternal drug treatment and sex of infant as independent variables. Measures reflecting a possible influence of the drug treatment variable (($p < 0.10$) were then examined in a multiple regression that included twelve other predictor variables relevant to perinatal influences on behavior. This procedure helps prevent false identification of the drug effect via confounding of drug with other factors affecting mother-infant behavior.

Measures of activity and arousal were not apparently affected by drug treatment. This is in agreement with other

TABLE II. Variables Considered in Regression Analysis

Major Independent Variables

Drug treatment of mother
Sex of infant

Background Variables

Age of mother
Social experience of mother
Mother bred in indoor or outdoor caging
Weight of mother prior to conception
Maximum weight gain of mother during pregnancy
Parity of mother
Infants raised previously by mother
Infants rejected previously by mother
Year of birth
Month of birth
Birth weight of infant
Weaning weight of infant

Dependent Variables (behavioral measures)

1. Duration of activity/arousal states
   a. Percentof total observation time of activity/arousal states
2. Frequency of occurrence of nonsocial behaviors
   a. Frequency of initiation
      1. social
      2. explore environment
      3. locomotion
      4. disturbance
3. Quality of mother-infant interaction
   a. Frequency of social categories
      1. minutes infant restrained by mother
      2. positive proximity behaviors by infant
      3. negative proximity behaviors by infant
      4. positive proximity behaviors by mother
      5. negative proximity behaviors by mother
   b. Relative proportion of all categories scored
      1. positive behaviors by infant
      2. positive behaviors by mother
   c. Totalnumberof social behaviorsrecordedin mother-infant pair
   d. Maternal rejection score

data suggesting that full behavioral tolerance to arousal-altering effects of this dosage level had developed in the chronically treated animals.

Several measures reflecting changes in the quality of mother and infant interaction from early to late infancy were associated with the drug treatment variable (Table III). Negative proximity behaviors, including primarily rejection of contact with the infant, increased more from early to late infancy in the THC-treated dams. At the same time, THC-infants increased the frequency of their attempts to gain contact with the dam. Such interaction patterns normally signal the onset of increased separation of mother and infant (8,9) and apparently were more intense, or earlier in appearance in THC-treated group. It should be noted that instances of neglect or physical abuse of infants were not recorded in either group. What is the potential significance of these alterations in mother-infant interaction in late infancy? Table IV demonstrates the intercorrelation in our data set

TABLE III. Behavioral Measures Associated with Maternal Drug Treatment[a]

	Predictor Variable	F	df	P
Decrease in maternal positive proximity behaviors (%)[b]	Maternal drug	5.01	1,12	< 0.05
	Weaning weight	6.96	1,11	< 0.025
Increase in infant positive proximity behaviors (%)[c]	Maternal drug	5.49	1,12	< 0.05
	Prior infants rejected	9.54	1,11	< 0.025
Increase in maternal negative proximity behaviors (%)[d]	Maternal drug	6.65	1,12	< 0.025
	Parity of mother	17.58	1,7	< 0.005
	Infant's birth weight	9.31	1,5	< 0.05

[a]"Maternal drug" entered the stepwise multiple regression first and accounted for a significant amount of variability in these measures. Other predictor variables with significant partial regression coefficients are also listed.

[b]Includes approach, retrieval, groom, restrain. Change from early to late infancy was measured.

[c]Includes approach, contact initiation, groom, play.

[d]Includes break contact, reject contact, punish.

between behavioral measures affected by drug and other measures reflecting mother-infant independence, such as amount of time spent by infant away from mother. These variables, as might be expected, increase from early to late infancy (Fig. 1). More detailed information about the growth of infant independence have been provided by Jensen and Bobbitt (8). Typically there is a dramatic increase in the level of infants physical activity while with the dam, followed by an increase in negative proximity behaviors by the dam and finally by an increase in physical separation of mother and infant. Apparently, in the present experiment, THC treatment influenced this transition between early dependence and later independence. It is not apparent whether the drug acted primarily on the dam or the infant in intensifying these transition behavior patterns.

Further information about mother-infant relationship was obtained by examining the response to separation. Plasma cortisol response to short-term separation from mother and to

TABLE IV. Product-moment Correlations Between Drug-related Variables and Variables Reflecting Strength of Mother-Infant Bond[a]

	Drug-related			Mother-infant Bond		
	1	2	3	4	5	6
1. Dam's negative behavior	-	.85[e]	.58[c]	.48	.88[e]	.66[d]
2. Dam's negative behavior (%)	-	-	.83[e]	.67[d]	.65[c]	.88[e]
3. Infant positive behavior (%)	-	-	-	.59[c]	.41	.84[e]
4. Infant's time away from mother	-	-	-	-	.34	.84[e]
5. Dam's behavior directed at infant	-	-	-	-	-	.42
6. Dam's "rejection score"[b]	-	-	-	-	-	-

[a]Based on 15 mother-infant pairs.
[b]Based on Hinde & Atkinson (2).
[c]$p < 0.05$
[d]$p < 0.01$
[e]$p < 0.001$

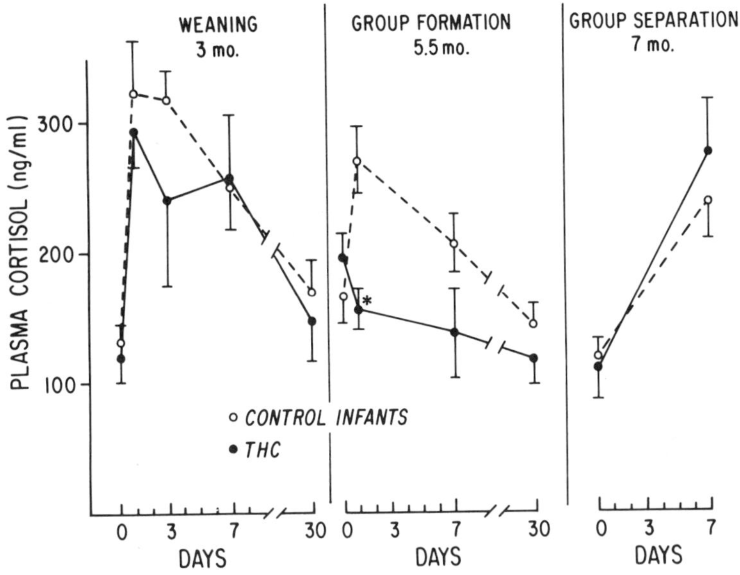

FIGURE 1. Changes in mother-infant behavior patterns from early to late infancy. Significant group differences are illustrated in Panel A. Related measures of activity level and mother-infant dependence are shown in Panels B and C.

weaning (Fig. 2) did not differ in THC and control offspring. This measure of response to separation is frequently used to assess the degree of mother-infant attachment in primates (10,11). Similarly, measures of heart rate, activity and vocalizations during a short term separation were similar in the two groups. This indicates that a normal degree of attachment had formed in the THC-treated mother-infant pairs. Group differences were apparent in the plasma cortisol response of THC infants to peer grouping (Fig. 2). While controls showed the expected increase in cortisol levels in response to this situation (12), THC infants maintained baseline values. Behavioral data supported a relative lack of stress-induced behavioral inhibition in THC offspring. Although the degree and type of social interaction varied widely from group to group, THC offspring consistently initiated more social interactions than any of their cagemates during the first three days of social grouping (Sign test, $p < 0.003$). Subsequently, initiation of social interaction was not associated with prior drug exposure, and plasma cortisol responses to later separation from the peer group were similar in the THC-treated and non-treated animals.

Taken together, these observations indicate that chronic low-level THC affects behavioral development on a relatively subtle level under controlled experimental conditions. This is consistent with our other evaluations of this sample of infants (4,6,13,14) and with the limited data available from other nonhuman primates (15) and from human infants (16). Similarly, behavioral evaluations of rats and mice exposed developmentally to THC and other cannabis preparations have not shown a clear cut pattern of severe developmental toxicity in terms of growth retardation, developmental delay or cognitive disorder (see review by Abel, 17). Social behavior was included in only one such evaluation. In an experiment using

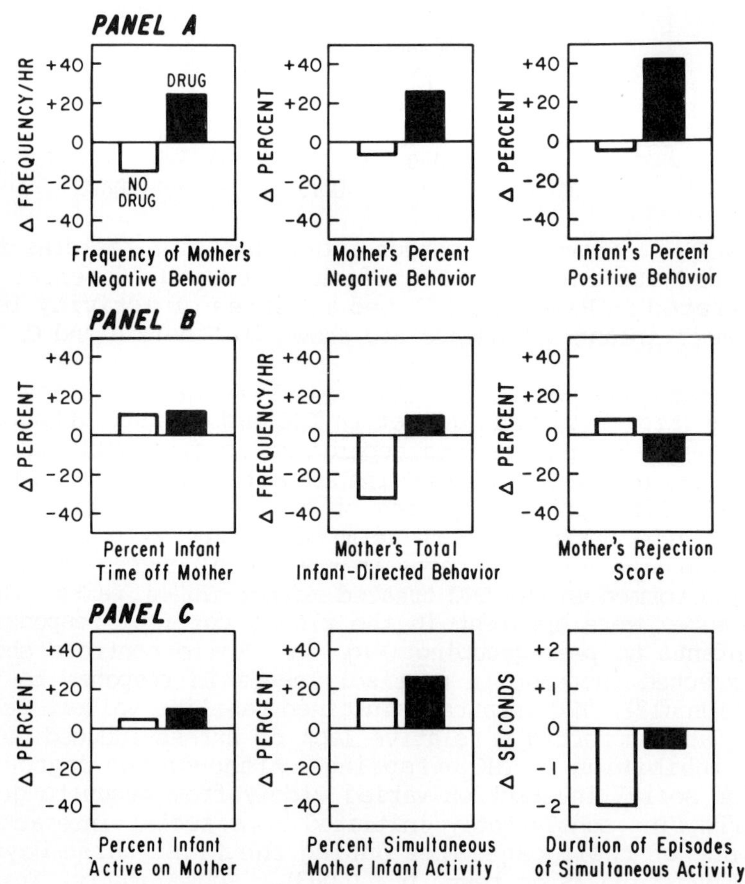

FIGURE 2. Plasma cortisol response of THC and control offspring to weaning (separation from dam), peer group formation and separation from peer group.

chronic, low-level treatments (2 mg/kg/day) throughout gestation, Vardaris et al. (18) demonstrated an increase in the number of treated rats gaining control of limited space in competition with another animal. This finding seems consistent with an interpretation of relative lack of inhibition in response to negative social cues in THC-treated monkey infants.

Certain precautions are appropriate in interpreting an experiment such as the one presented here. Behavioral changes in THC-treated infants are not necessarily attributable to an interaction between THC and developing neural tissues; indirect drug effects can occur via maternal behavior, maternal nutrition and physiology or environmental conditions created by the presence of the drugged dam. More complex designs involving fostering and artificial rearing would be necessary to establish these points.

Also, in a small sample experiment with a genetically heterogeneous population a chance confounding of drug treatment with some other relevant variable can occur. Careful subject selection and group assignment and detailed environmental control protocols are helpful in safeguarding against this possibility. In addition, the screening of identified drug effect with multiple regression, as illustrated above, is also useful.

With these precautions in mind, primate studies offer the exciting opportunity of examining a perinatal system very similar to humans in a controlled experimental setting. This is particularly important in the case of an agent, which like THC, cannot be evaluated for developmental toxicity in humans using a prospective design with random group assignment.

In conclusion, the present data, together with other studies, fails to support the hypothesis that severe morphological or functional disorders are likely to be identified after chronic low level developmental exposure to THC. However, limited behavioral changes may be detected under these circumstances.

ACKNOWLEDGMENT

The authors are grateful to Wilva Lathen and Ron Fitzgerald for technical assistance.

REFERENCES

1. Rodier, P. M., Behavioral teratology, in "Handbook of

Teratology", Vol. 4 (J.G. Wilson and F. C. Fraser, eds.), pp. 397-428. Plenum Press, New York, 1978.

2. Golub, M. S., and Golub, A. M., Behavioral teratogenesis, in "Advances in Perinatal Medicine" (A. Milunsky, E. Friedman and L. Gluck, eds.), pp. 2231-293. Plenum Press, New York, 1981.
3. Adams, J., and Buelke-Sam, J., Behavioral assessment of the postnatal animal: Testing and methods development, in "Developmental Toxicology" (C. A. Kimmel and J. Buelke-Sam, eds.), pp. 233-258. Raven Press, New York, 1982.
4. Golub, M. S., Sassenrath, E. N., and Chapman, L. F., Mother-infant interaction in rhesus monkeys treated chronically with delta-9-tetrahydrocannabinol, Child Development 52:389-392 (1981).
5. Golub, M. S., A primate model for detecting behavioral impairment in offspring after chronic parental drug exposure, Pharmacol. Biochem. Behav. 11:47-50 (1979).
6. Golub, M. S., Sassenrath, E. N., and Coo, G. P., Plasma cortisol levels and dominance in peer groups of rhesus monkey weanlings, Hormones and Behavior 12:50-59 (1979).
7. Murphy, B. E. P., Some studies of the protein-binding of steroids and their application to the routine micro and ultramicromeasurement of various steroids in body fluids by competitive protein-binding radioassay, J. Clin. Endocrinol. 27:973-990 (1967).
8. Jensen, G. K., and Bobbitt, R. A., On observational methodology and preliminary studies of mother-infant interaction in monkeys, in "Determinants of Infant Behavior", Vol. III (B. M. Foss, ed.), pp. 47-65, Methuen Co., London, 1964.
9. Hinde, R. A., and Atkinson, S., Assessing the roles of social partners in maintaining mutual proximity, as exemplified by mother-infant relations in monkeys, Animal Behav. 18:169-176 (1970).
10. Hill, S. D., McCormack, S. A., and Mason, W. A., Effects of artificial mothers and visual experience on adrenal responsiveness of infant monkeys, Developmental Psychobiol. 6:421-429 (1973).
11. Smotherman, W. P., Hunt, L. E., and McGinnis, L. M., Mother-infant separation in group-living rhesus macaques: A hormonal analysis, Developmental Psychobiol. 12:211-217 (1979).
12. Goo, G. P., and Sassenrath, E. N., Persistent adrenal activation in female rhesus monkeys after new breeding group formation, J. Med. Primatol. 9:325-338 (1980).
13. Golub, M. S., Sassenrath, E. N., and Chapman, L. F., Regulation of visual attention in offspring of female monkeys treated chronically with delta-9-tetrahydrocannabinol, Developmental Psychobiol. 14:507-512 (1981).

14. Golub, M. S., Sassenrath, E. N., and Chapman, L. F., An analysis of altered attention in monkeys exposed to delta-9-tetrahydrocannabinol during development, Pharmacol. Biochem. Behav. 4:469-472 (1982).
15. Kaplan, J. N., Maternal responsiveness in the squirrel monkey following chronic administration of delta-9-tetrahydrocannabinol, Pharmacol. Biochem. Behav. 11:539-544 (1979).
16. Fried, P. A., Marijuana use by pregnant women: Neurobehavioral effects in neonates, Drug and Alcohol Dependence 6:415-424 (1980).
17. Abel, E. L., Prenatal exposure to cannabis: a critical review of effects on growth development and behavior, Behav. Neurol. Biol. 29:137-156 (1980).
18. Vardaris, R. M., Weisz, D. J., Fazel, A., and Rawitch A. B., Chronic administration of delta-9-tetrahydrocannabinol to pregnant rats: Studies of pup behavior and placental transfer, Pharmacol. Biochem. Behav. 4:249-254 (1976).

Section VI CELLULAR ASPECTS

CELLULAR EFFECTS OF CANNABIS - SUPPORTING INTERFERENCE OF THE DRUG WITH ARGININE UTILIZATION AND/OR METABOLISM: A NEW HYPOTHESIS ON MECHANISM OF ACTION

Marietta R. Issidorides

Department of Psychiatry
University of Athens
Athens, Greece

I. INTRODUCTION

A single unifying mechanism by which cannabis exerts its many actions in a variety of tissues may not be a biological prerequisite. Data, however, obtained from cellular studies of chronic hashish users and matched controls, consistently indicated repercussions of the drug on arginine metabolic pathways in several functionally diverse cell populations. Analysis and interpretation of these data led to the formulation of the hypothesis that cannabis may act through a common metabolic denominator, namely arginine "depletion" (1). In the first studies (2), electron cytochemical methods (3,4) demonstrated a reduction of arginine-rich histones in the nuclei of lymphocytes and of arginine-rich protamines in the nuclei of spermatozoa. This reduction seemed counterbalanced by increased amounts of lysine-rich proteins in both cell types. Such altered histone ratios in the lymphocyte denotes over-repression of the genome (5), i.e., a reduced potential to respond to antigenic stimuli (6). In the sperm nucleus, however, the altered protein ratio denotes arrested maturation since during the late stages of spermiogenesis lysine-rich histones are shed and substituted by newly synthesized arginine-rich protamines (7) which endow: a) the sperm tail with motility, and b) the sperm chromatin with stability and resistance to noxious agents during its trajectory from testis to ovum (8). Clearly, the similarly altered histone ratio in lymphocytes and spermatozoa of chronic hashish users had entirely different implications for the functional capacity of

ISBN 0-12-044620-0

each cell type. Functional repercussions, predictable from the low levels of arginine-rich proteins in the lymphocytes and sperm, have been substantiated by the findings of inhibited cellular-mediated immunity (9) and of decreased motility and total sperm count (10) in heavy marijuana users. The causal relation of low protamine content to sperm functional impairment and oligospermia was established by Silvestroni and his collaborators in their studies of congenital fertility problems (11). Their findings would suggest that long-term cannabis use mimics the specific metabolic aberration, i.e. inhibition of protamine synthesis, that characterizes infertility or "idiopathic spermatidic arrest".

The dependence of normal spermatogenesis on the amino acid arginine was first reported by Holt and Albanese (12), who also demonstrated the experimental modulation of fertility solely by deprivation or supplementation of arginine in the diet, both in humans and rats. Subsequent studies established the therapeutic effectiveness of arginine administration in oligospermia (13) as well as its stimulatory action on sperm motility (14). Effects on sperm motility exactly opposite to those of arginine supplementation have been observed with the exposure of spermatozoa to THC (15). These data support our hypothesis that THC and arginine actions overlap at the same sites with opposite biochemical and functional effects.

In view of the mounting evidence that cannabis inhibits transcription in a variety of cellular systems (16, 17) we sought in cells of chronic hashish users morphological correlates of macromolecular synthesis inhibition, as those are defined in cell biology. Chromatin which is highly condensed, either as heterochromatin or as compact chromosomes of cell division, is transcriptionally inert (18). A wide spectrum of drugs and metabolic inhibitors induce structural changes in nuclei and these changes were found to have functional significance (19, 20). In previous studies with the electron microscope (EM) we had observed that structural changes, i.e., chromatin condensation, in leukocytes of patients after neuroleptic treatment paralleled clinical changes (21,22). These findings prompted the initiation of similar investigations on cells of chronic cannabis users and controls for the study of chromatin with a special EM method (23). The results showed significantly that in users the somatic cells (leukocytes) displayed highly condensed nuclear chromatin, while the germ cells (ejaculated spermatozoa) showed the opposite state: decondensed chromatin and undifferentiated nuclei (1). In a recent report (24) we demonstrated with the EM four types of sperm head abnormalities, in 50% of the spermatozoa of chronic hashish users, that exemplify the abnormalities classified by Holstein and Schirren (25) as indicative of infertility. It is well documented that sperm nuclear condensation during maturation is a process requiring the coordinated synthesis of arginine-rich proteins (26, 27). The different abnormalities in sperm nuclear condensation observed in the EM were, therefore, the natural consequence of the low protamine content, which distinguishes the sperm of chronic hashish users from that of controls (2). Similarly, the inappropriate excessive condensation of nuclear chromatin in somatic cells, observed in the leukocytes of the users, can rapidly be induced by deficiency of arginine in the medium (28). Arginine-poor media will also cause an arrest of DNA, RNA and protein synthesis (29), which also are well documented actions of cannabinoids (30). Other reports have shown that in the absence of arginine morphological disorganization of nuclei and fragmentation of chromosomes take place in cultured cells (31). Similar findings were reported by Leuchtenberger et al. (32) and Morishima et al. (33) in cultures exposed to cannabinoids, as well as in chronic hashish users (24), the neutrophils of which displayed in the EM protrusions of nucleus (drumsticks) and attached fragments of chromosomes in the cytoplasm (micronuclei). A synthesis of all these data reveals that a putative "depletion" of arginine by cannabis would suffice to explain both the chemical and the ultrastructural aberrations that we and others have observed in the cells of chronic hashish users and in cultures exposed to cannabinoids, respectively.

II. NEW FINDINGS

We pursued the concept of cannabis/arginine interaction further by examining in chronic hashish users and controls other cell types - known to be affected by cannabis -, where arginyl proteins have a major functional role.

The clinical group consisted of 16 chronic users and 10 matched controls. All were paid volunteers recruited from a larger population that was extensively used for a long-term controlled investigation of the effects of chronic cannabis use in man (34). Inclusion criteria in the users' group were 1) age below 58 years, 2) regular hashish use for more than 10 years continuing up to the day of testing, 3) no use of other addictive substances except for tobacco smoking and irregular social alcohol drinking, and 4) absence of gross neurological disorders or incapacitating physical illness. Controls had to match the users with respect to age, place of upbringing and residence, education and socio-economic level. They had also to be regular tobacco smokers and to never have used any addictive substances except alcohol irregularly and moderately. Data regarding hashish use by the group have appeared in detail elsewhere, (2,24). The material smoked by the subjects contained 4-5% delta-9-tetrahydrocannabinol (THC).

A. Chronic Effects of Hashish Smoking in Blood Platelets

In human platelets alpha-granules store basic proteins (Factor 4) with anti-herparin activity (35,36), which are released following stimulation by ADP or epinephrine (37,38). The precursor of these proteins is an immumologically identical more basic protein with essential arginines (39). Pellets of platelets from users and controls were prepared by the ammoniacal silver reaction for arginine (4) in order to localize this precursor at the ultrastructural level (24). The results showed that in control subjects all platelets contained numerous granular deposits of arginine-rich proteins, but in chronic users all platelets had suffered a 90% reduction of their granular arginine-rich deposits. This finding is consistent with the impaired ability of platelets from marijuana smokers to aggregate when stimulated by ADP _in vitro_ (40). The greatly reduced level of the arginine-rich protein in the platelets of chronic users justifies cannabis-induced impairment of aggregation potential since this protein _promotes_ clotting (38). We point out that polyamines, which are present in platelets (41) and modulate clotting by _inhibiting_ platelet aggregation induced by ADP (42), are also derivatives of arginine through the ornithine pathway. Given limited substrate levels, a diversion of arginine in the latter pathway would be adequate to explain both cannabis' inhibitory effect on ADP-stimulated aggregation (through polyamines?) and the observed depletion of arginyl proteins from their granulated stores.

B. Acute Effects of Marijuana Smoking in Erythrocytes

Five subjects were selected from the group of 16 on the basis of their continuous daily smoking during the previous 30-day period. They served as their own controls in a pilot study of the acute effects of cannabinoids on various ultrastructural and chemical parameters in blood (43). The subjects were instructed to abstain from cannabis smoking for 12 hours before testing. On the day of testing, each subject was allowed to smoke ad libitum within a period of 15 minutes home-made cigarettes containing 1 g active marijuana supplied by NIDA with a 2.6% THC content. Blood samples were obtained before smoking and again 30 minutes after smoking, i.e., at a time that coincides with the peak effect on heartbeat, with a subjective "high" and with the highest concentration of the drug in the blood (44).

We report the preliminary results obtained from blood smears (24), which were used to examine direct cannabis/arginine interations with the following rationale. The erythrocyte, which represents a well known target of cannabis actions (45-49), contains at least two membrane proteins rich in arginine residues. The first, enzyme acetylcholinesterase, is a major outer surface protein (50) with 31 arginine residues (51). The second, the structural band 3, is the preponderant transmembrane polypeptide of the human erythrocyte with 44 arginine residues (52), a certain of which is essential for cholride transport (53). Erythrocyte function relies heavily on lipoprotein associations in the membrane structure, especially on surface phospholipids, which are required also for the catalytic activity of (Na^+ + K^+) ATPase (54). Recent studies have provided clear and convincing evidence that arginine residues may play an important role in phospholipid-protein interactions by acting as binding sites for negatively charged phosphate groups in phospholipid molecules (55). This was demonstrated by the finding that modification of the phosphatidycholine-transfer (exchange) protein with butanedione and phenylglyoxal, which are arginine-specific dicarbonyl reagents, completely inactivated the enzyme. It has also been shown that the reactive arginines, essential for binding, are embedded in hydrophobic sequences of the protein (56), a property of the active site which favors strong anion binding (57) and for which THC would have special affinity (58).

In an earlier experimental trial, of a partly similar design, with a group of subjects drawn from the same population of users, it was shown that 30 minutes after heavy hashish smoking the concentration of phosphatidylcholine and of other membrane phospholipids decreases significantly in the erythrocytes (48). In light of Akeroyd's data (55) this acute effect of cannabis suggested a loosening by the drug of the phospholipid-protein association in surface molecules, presumably leaving the protein-bound arginyl residues unmasked. To test this particular eventuality we employed an arginine-specific ligand on formaldehyde-fixed blood smears collected from the five subjects before and after marijuana smoking. This reagent, phenanthrenequinone (PQ), is a non-fluorescent compound reacting specifically with arginine to form a condensation product, which exhibits strong fluorescence when viewed under ultraviolet light (59). The PQ reaction is an extremely sensitive and specific test for polypeptide-bound arginine in fixed smears (60) and in molecules with low arginine content such as hemoglobin (59). Because of these properties PQ is uniquely suitable for determining any acute changes in arginine availability in the erythrocytes following marijuana smoking. Staining and fluorescence microscopy were applied according to Magun and Kelly (60).

As expected, PQ/arginine condensation product was formed in the leukocytes (with histones) and the platelets (with basic proteins) and showed no changes at 30 minutes post-smoking. In contrast, the uniform diffuse fluorescence of the erythrocytes was blocked following marijuana smoking while intense fluorescence emerged along their membrane. These changes reveal cannabis/arginine interactions, an interpretation inherent in the PQ method employed. These results support first the presence of reactive arginyl residues at the erythrocyte surface following the presence of cannabis in the blood. Such a finding would be consistent with a perturbation in the lipoprotein structures and with the observed loss of phospholipids from the membrane (48). It is not clear from this experiment which of the membrane proteins is responsible for the cannabis-induced PQ-arginine fluorescence. Of the three proteins which have essential arginines at their active site, i.e. acetylcholinesterase (51), $(Na^+ + K^+)$ ATPase and band 3 at the chloride channel (53), the activity of the first two has been found to be inhibited by THC (62-64). Since phospholipids are required for the active ATPase configuration and for catalytic activity (54) it is reasonable to suggest that at least this protein would provide unmasked arginyl residues free to react with PQ after cannabis-induced phospholipid loss from the membrane.

The diffuse PQ fluorescence of the erythrocytes evident before smoking, but blocked after smoking, may tentatively be attributed to cannabis/hemoglobin interactions, without excluding alternative interpretations (24). Erythrocytes exhibit a lowered capacity to engage oxygen after cannabis use (46). Hemoglobin, which represents the major intracellular red cell protein shows decreased affinity for oxygen following modification of its arginyl residues by specific reagents (65). Furthermore, PQ generates intense fluorescence with the arginines in hemoglobin molecules (59). These data suggest that in our experiment the blocking of the diffuse PQ/arginine fluorescence in the erythrocytes 30 minutes post-smoking may be due to masking of the arginine residues in hemoglobin by a cannabis/arginine interaction, which produces hindrance to PQ attachment, and which would be in accord with both the chemical and physiological data.

C. Comment

The postulate that cannabis may produce its varied biological effects through interactions with arginine, in many cellular systems and pathways, does not appear to conflict with the data obtained from chronic or acute exposures to the drug. To test the validity of this hypothesis, however, we need to survey a wider spectrum of known biological effects of cannabis, as well as of known biological effects of arginine deficiency, deprivation, depletion or inactivation and, then, determine the degree of overlap by taking into account the proposed mechanism of action for each case. The review that follows is designed to serve this goal with no intent of being exhaustive.

III. REVIEW OF EXPERIMENTAL EVIDENCE SUPPORTING CANNABIS/ARGININE INTERACTIONS

Although limited to the discussion of our own findings, the previous sections have introduced some of the data defining the principles according to which THC, a highly lipophilic molecule, could modulate biological processes which are dependent upon the basic amino acid arginine. A comparatively recent realization in the field of protein chemistry is, that arginine, because of its unique molecular properties (66), has secured during evolution an important position in a broad spectrum of metabolic functions (67-69). The co-planarity of the three nitrogens and the central carbon atom enables the guanidium side chain of arginine to enter into extended patterns of hydrogen bonding that are unique, also a unique aspect of the side chain is its very high pKa; of all the common amino acids it is probably the only one whose charged nature can never be suppressed under physiological conditions (69). Present investigations emphasize important generality, that arginyl residues can serve as positively charged recognition sites for negatively charged substrates and anionic cofactors in enzyme active sites, and in all proteins that interact with anions (70). Arginine-specific reagents were unknown prior to benzil (71). The application of these alpha-dicarbonyl arginine-specific reagents (72), i.e. diacetyl or 2,3-butanedione (73), 1,2-cyclohexanedione (74) and phenylglyoxal (75) for the modification of arginyl residues opened up a rapidly progressing field and established the functional importance of essential arginines. Thirteen of the fourteen enzymes in the glycolytic pathway, in which all the intermediates are phosphoric acid esters, were shown to contain essential arginines at the active site (66). Arginyl residues are essential in carboxyl and nucleotide binding sites, as well as in dehydrogenases for binding of NADH and in kinases for binding of coenzymes (70). The functional importance of essential arginines also in strategic sites of other non-enzyme proteins is illustrated by hypophyseal pro-opiocortin, where arginine is essential for the processing of this molecule into its hormonally active subunits (76,77).

A. Macromolecular Synthesis

Nahas et al. (78, and refs. therein) were the first to introduce the notion of inhibition of macromolecular synthesis by cannabinoids _in vitro_. Jakubovic and McGeer (79) were the first to document extensively that under a variety of conditions THC brings about marked changes in the biosynthesis of key cerebral macromolecules. Experiments with isolated rat brain slices showed inhibition by THC of the incorporation of labeled leucine into protein fraction, while active transport of the amino acid into the cells was not affected. Similarly, THC inhibited incorporation of labeled uridine into nucleic acids, but also decreased uridine nucleotides in the soluble fraction, while the relative amount of labeled uridine was high. These results would imply that the decreased incorporation into nucleic acids was related to the reduced phosphorylation of the uridine. Another important finding was that a large amount of THC and/or metabolites was retained by brain slices during incubation which suggested the possibility of prolonged action in inhibiting the synthesis of cerebral macromolecules (79). Comparable results obtained with THC on rat testis (80) confirmed further that a general inhibition of protein synthesis occurs. It was found that _de novo_ synthesis of nucleic acids was inhibited as much as synthesis through the salvage pathway. The decreased biosynthesis of labeled RNA appears to be directly related to the inhibition of phosphorylation of the precursor of RNA. A severe reduction of TDP and TTP indicated the same mechanism for the inhibition of DNA synthesis. The authors suggested that "the reduced ATP levels in the cell and/or the phosphorylation or perhaps even direct inhibition or nucleic acid polymerases may be the principle steps at which cannabis derivatives act on nucleic acid synthesis".

Arginine or its metabolite(s) have been implicated in the regulation of DNA synthesis in cultured liver cells (81). These authors presented evidence that quiescent primary liver cells in culture can be induced by a) serum, b) ornithine or c) arginine to synthesize DNA and to divide, suggesting that low-molecular-weight nutrients might be involved in the control of DNA synthesis. In these experiments arginine seemed to be limiting for biochemical events which led to the initiation of DNA synthesis. When the pool size of arginine dropped below a certain level, the cells became arrested in the G_1 phase of the cell cycle. It was concluded that ornithine and/or arginine and/or their proximal metabolites have regulatory functions in the control of DNA synthesis, the latter being regulated by intracellular levels of these compounds. Alterations in liver nucleic acids and nucleotides in arginine-deficient rats were demonstrated by Hassan and Milner (82). A depression of approximately 30% in RNA and DNA synthesis in the livers of arginine-deficient rats were closely paralleled with growth depression, increased liver lipids and a 52% decrease in the concentration of ATP (82). In all these experiments the arginine deficiency increased total pyrimidine nucleotides while decreasing total purine nucleotides. Such altered ration of nucleotides leads to altered base ratios and concomitantly to altered nucleic acid synthesis.

Purine nucleoside phosphorylase has an important role in purine metabolism, probably in purine salvage. The enzyme from both human erythrocytes and calf spleen is inactivated by butanedione and phenylglyoxal through the covalent modification solely of arginine residues (83). In addition, each of the various classes of nucleotide polymerases has been reported to be inactivated by arginine modification (84-86). As in all other cases of enzyme inactivation by arginine-specific reagents, these inhibitions are reversible, and can be prevented by the simultaneous presence of the natural substrate of the enzyme in the test system; the substrate protects the active site arginine from reacting with the modifying agent. It is of interest that the results obtained by Jakubovic and McGeer (79, 80) from the exposure of brain and testis slices to cannabinoids were interpreted as being due to inhibition of phosphorylation, low ATP and, probably, to interference with the activity of nucleic acid polymerases, all of which could occur if cannabis interacted solely with arginine in these systems as described above.

Similar inhibition of macromolecular synthesis by THC has been observed not only in isolated mammalian cells such as normal human fibroblasts, human and mouse neuroblastoma cells (87), but also in the unicellular _Tetrahymena pyriformis_, where it resulted in depressed exponential growth (88). The reduction in DNA, RNA and protein synthesis in this unicellular organism was accompanied by effects also on the ribosomes. A reduction in the amount of polysomes was observed in cellular fractions obtained from THC-treated cells, while the amount of monosomes was the same in THC-treated and control preparations. Dissociation of polyribosomes _in vivo_ has been reported in electron microscopic studies in brain, both after chronic THC administration to adult monkeys (89) and after acute administration to infant rats (90). It is common knowledge that RNA synthesis from chromosomal DNA templates occurs in the nucleus, whereas translation occurs on cytoplasmic polyribosomes, Polyribosomes either in the cytoplasm or on the nuclear membrane are an index of attached mRNA emerging from the nucleus respectively. The dissociation of the polyribosomes entails interruption of these processes (91).

The reduction in nuclear membrane-attached ribosomes, following acute exposure to pharmacologically active cannabinoids, is dose-related and rapid, peaking at 30 min (90). This observation is important and relevant to our main thesis. A parallel is to be found in the modification of ribosomes with butanedione, which was accompanied by loss of mRNA-binding capacity and arrest of protein synthesis upon an incubation of 30 min (92). These experiments showed that arginine residues in ribosomal proteins are essential for the binding of mRNA through interaction of their positively charged guanidinium groups with the negatively charged phosphate moieties of the messenger nucleic acid. As in all other proteins discussed so far, these essential arginines are embedded in apolar sequences of the protein (57) and constitute sites of affinity for hydrophobic molecules (93). An essential condition for a putative interference by hydrophobic THC effects could have a documented common denominator, a cannabis/arginine interaction across a wide spectrum of tissues, species and phyla.

Although the data reviewed here are all consistent with such an interaction, it should be emphasized that it is far from clear how these interactions take place, especially since the necessary experiments have not been conducted. In the pursuit of the stated goal of this paper, i.e., to review the effects of THC and arginine on, as far as feasible, identical experimental systems, the HeLa S_3 human cell line constitutes a good model for analysis. In recent experiments (94, 95), it was demonstrated that cannabinoids depress in a dose-dependent way proliferative activity as well as incorporation of radiolabeled precursors into nucleic acids and proteins of HeLa S_3 cells growing in exponential cultures. These studies, as well as previous ones from the same group (30), demonstrated that the effects of cannabinoids on the intact cells could not be observed in _in vitro_ nuclear and chromatin transcription experiments. No alteration in the template activity of chromatin isolated from cannabinoid-treated cells was found when compared to that of chromatin from untreated cells. It was concluded that "the findings taken together could be explained by cannabinoid-induced modifications at the level of the cell membrane". Experiments with phenylglyoxal which reacts with arginine moieties in proteins, but does not enter intact cells, have shown that this reagent causes a dose-dependent inhibition of HeLa S_3 cell proliferation by chemically masking arginine moieties at the cell surface (96,97). With the use of labeled phenylglyoxal these authors demonstrated that there is a 24-fold increase in arginine at entry into G_1 from M when they propagate in mono-layer culture. Growth was inhibited by the chemical masking of arginine by phenylglyoxal only during the phases of the cycle when arginine-rich protein is exposed at the surface (96). Interaction of cannabinoids with the arginine-rich membrane protein in HeLa S_3 cells would be consistent with the findings, interpretations and conclusions of Stein et al. (30) and Mon et al. (94,95) based on their experiments with HeLa S_3 cells and cannabinoids. It is of further interest that this arginine enrichment at the cell surface has been implicated in cell surface-mediated growth control and/or transformed or tumor cell surface changes (98).

B. Steroids, Lipoproteins and Cholesterol

Diethyl stilbestrol bisphosphate, which has similar properties to estradiol and is commonly employed to control prostatic carcinoma, was recently found to interact directly with arginyl residues in protein substrates through binding to their guanidino group (99). Harris et al. (100) have emphasized that the binding of cannabinoids resembles that of steroids, on the basis of their strong spatial structural resemblance, their high lipid solubility and the absence of specific antagonists. Evidence was also presented that the cannabinoids may be interacting at steroid-specific sites (101). Carchman et al. (102) have shown that the cannabinoids can inhibit steroidogenesis both in normal adrenal and adrenal tumor cells. This inhibition was demonstrated to be very specific in that the cannabinoids had no significant effects on cell growth, O_2 consumption, etc. They proposed that this specific inhibition of steroid production involved early steps in the pathway, possibly cholesterol transport or cholesterol esterase, and attributed it to the strong structural and biological relationships between steroids and cannabinoids. A possible explanation may reside in the numerous lipid droplets, rich in cholesterol esters, present in the THC-inhibited cells (102). In the light of the section that follows, it is conceivable that cholesterol binding sites may be occupied by the cannabinoid.

Cholesterol in the adrenal gland is either converted into steroid hormones or esterified and stored in the intracellular lipid droplets, the hydrolysis of the esterified cholesterol being catalyzed by the cytoplasmic enzyme cholesterol esterase (103). A stepwise examination of the steroidogenic pathway in isolated Leydig cells for the purpose of locating the site of action of THC demonstrated that "virtually the only step inhibited" was the liberation by the esterase of "precursor" cholesterol from its lipid droplet storage (104). These studies demonstrated a direct effect of THC on steroid secreting cells. It has been suggested that the "inability to demonstrate reduced corticosteroid levels in animals treated with THC may reside in the ability of the animals to compensate physiologically, or pharmacologically by a secondary drug action, for reduced steroid synthesis with enhanced ACTH release" (101).

THC has a structural similarity to cholesterol (105). In the blood it is strongly bound to, and migrates in association with, lipoproteins (106). In electrophoretic experiments these authors showed that labeled THC in human plasma _in vitro_ is located in a peak in the albumin area and in a broad peak around the transferring; these two peaks which must be attributed to protein-bound THC amount to about 87% of the total radioactivity. Other experiments showed that THC and its 11-OH metabolite, which is also pharmacologically and psychologically active, are bound not only to albumin but also to $alpha_1$-lipoproteins and beta-lipoproteins (107). Arginine is known to be a constituent of beta- and prebeta-lipoproteins (108). Furthermore, there are arginine residues at or close to the strong hydrophobic anion-binding sites of bovine serum albumin (93). Chemical modification of the arginines in transferring with phenylglyoxal, 1,2-cyclohexanedione and 2,3-butanedione decreased iron binding activity by 50% (109) by modifying the guanidino group of arginine at the bicarbonate binding site. More importantly, very low density lipoproteins (VLDL) contain the arginine-rich apolipoprotein E, which is also found in HDL (110). Apoprotein E (apo-E) is a glycoprotein which occurs in several classes of lipoproteins of both humans and animals (111). Metabolically this apo-E is implicated in cholesterol transport in the plasma and mediates lipoprotein recognition and uptake by the liver. As a matter of fact, cyclohexanedione modification of arginine residues of LDL results in a retardation in plasma clearance, showing that the hepatocytes have a receptor for the arginines in apo-E (112). It has been shown that the guanidino groups of arginine (10%) in apo-E participate in cholesterol binding (113). This has been established by _in vitro_ experiments of cholesterol interaction with compounds containing guanidino groups (114). The unique importance of hydrophilic arginine residues interrupting an otherwise hydrophobic portion of a peptide, for effective cholesterol-protein interaction, has been established by recent experiments (115). It is evident that also in this general area of lipoproteins a unifying mechanism of cannabis effects may be envisaged, through interactions with arginine in many varied systems.

C. Chromosome Aberrations and Immune Function

Despite consistent evidence that THC and marijuana administrations induce immunological defects in experimental animals (116), the findings so far available in humans are conflicting (117). Two early papers dealing with the *in vitro* blastogenic responses of lymphocytes from long-term marijuana smokers exemplify the conflicting findings (9, 118). Subsequent experiments have established the strong dependence of such results upon culture media and culture conditions (119). It was shown that with serum concentrations of 0.5% in the culture medium, thymidine incorporation was nearly completely inhibited by THC, while with the same dose of THC, but in the presence of 10% serum concentration, thymidine incorporation was 90% of control. Analysis of the data indicated a direct interaction between THC and serum as well as the reversibility of the inhibition of thymidine incorporation by THC through washing the cells in RPMI medium and replacing them in culture. Cytogenetic analyses of lymphocyte cultures from chronic marijuana smokers have also yielded contradictory results (120) despite the fact that heavy doses of marijuana in humans (33), natural cannabinoids on normal human lymphocytes (121) and marijuana smoke in cultures (122) consistently induce hypoploidy and chromosomal aberrations. The questions arises whether the contradictory findings may not be attributed to the varied experimental designs. Aside from cannabis studies, probably in few other areas of cellular research have the methodological procedures played so important a role for the outcome of experiments as in cytogenetics (123) and in studies of the immune process using cell lines of diverse origins (124, and refs. therein).

Numerous studies initiated for the elucidation of the role of media and of culture conditions led to the unanimous conclusion that the main factor involved that determines the results obtained - and, under certain conditions, the artifacts produced - is the level of arginine in the experimental system. The many reasons why, and ways in which, this level may vary have been reviewed in the classic study of Freed and Schatz (31). Specifically, the chromosome damage resulting from arginine deprivation was initially observed in cultures recovering from inhibition of multiplication induced by liver extracts that inadvertantly contained arginase. The enzyme acted by degrading arginine in the culture medium thereby producing nutritional deficiency in the cells. Chromosome aberrations induced in cultured cells by infection of *Mycoplasma* appear also to stem from an arginine deficiency (29) since these organisms liberate arginine deaminase in the medium and consume the amino acid. Extracts prepared from mycoplasmas are inhibitory to the secondary production of antibody to rabbit lymph node fragments *in vitro* (125), to blastogenesis and to mixed lymphocyte culture reactions (126-128). These effects are due to the arginine depleting enzyme since they can be overcome by either adding excess arginine or eliminating the enzyme activity by heat or washing the cultures. Mitotic inhibition and increase in chromosome breakage have both been experimentally produced in arginine-deficient culture media and reversed again by addition of the amino acid (29). Cells cultured in limiting concentrations of arginine just adequate to produce multiplication, incur a significantly elevated level of chromosome abnormalities. The experiments showed that lack of any one of the essential amino acids was capable of inducing chromosome aberrations when the cells were "rescued" after a 24- or 48 h exposure. These findings suggested that "karyotype instability might stem from disparity between the amino acid requirement of the cells and the nutritional availability of these compounds" (31). Barile and Leventhal showed that only the species of mycoplasma which derive their energy from arginine utilization inhibit photohemagglutinin (PHA) - stimulated transformation of lymphocytes in cultures by their ability to deplete available arginine (129). Thus, PHA-induced lymphocyte transformation is inextricably linked to a normal level of arginine available in the culture medium, the lack of which inhibits the incorporation of thymidine into DNA (29). Lastly, it has been proposed that chromosome changes could be expected from the introduction into the culture of any drug tending to make an amino acid unavailable to the cell by whatever mechanism (31, and refs therein).

When the experiments and findings described above are taken into account, it becomes clear that an interaction of cannabis with arginine would suffice to explain a large number of the drug's effects in culture systems. Assuming that cannabis derivatives "deplete" available arginine, a given dose of the drug would cause a more effective inhibition in a 0.5% concentration of serum (which supplies the amino acid) than in a 10% concentration, which supplies a proportionally higher level of arginine to the same number of cells. Furthermore, the reversibility of THC inhibition of thymidine uptake by washing the cells in RPMI medium and resetting in fresh culture (78) would be equivalent to overcoming the metabolic block since the RPMI medium contains 200 mcg/ml arginine, i.e., much more than the 100 mcg/ml found required to abrogate inhibition caused by arginine deprivation (130). It is obvious, then, that media containing normally less arginine (Fisher's: 15 mcg/ml), if used, would lead to entirely different results and, probably, opposite conclusions. Cytogenetic experiments seem also to support a cannabis/arginine interaction at many levels. Stenchever et al. showed an increase in the incidence of chromosome breakage in marijuana smokers when their cells were placed in culture with nutritive media and PHA (131). No increase, however, in chromosome breakage was determined in normal lymphocytes when THC was added *in vitro* after PHA stimulation (132). Far from being contradictory these results support the experiments of Freed and Schatz (31), in which chromosomal breaks will appear *after* rescue from the deprivation of arginine (presumably occuring *in vivo* under marijuana smoking) when the cells are stimulated to enter mitosis, as in the Stenchever et al. experiment (131). On the other hand the addition of THC after PHA in a culture of lympocytes which have not been subjected to arginine depletion (those of non-smokers) will inhibit growth and block mitosis by acute arginine depletion (29) without evidence of chromosome aberrations, as in the Stenchever and Allen experiment (132). These results are consistent with the finding (31) that the frequency of chromosome aberrations increases with increasing periods of exposure of the resting cells to limiting levels of arginine, which may occur, as we proposed (1), in long-term cannabis users.

The impaired development of the F_2 generation of cannabis-treated pregnant rats (133) appears to support a mutagenic potential of THC. Limitation of available arginine is known to sensitize cells to the clastogenic activity of mutagens (134-136). Furthermore, death of a cell due to loss of genetic material may not be evident until later generations when the cell no longer possesses essential gene products, having depleted its intracellular pool (137). THC is capable of inducing segregational errors (121), which are studied in anaphase preparations of chromosomes obtained by omission of colchicine (138). These THC-induced anomalies were attributed to disruption of the spindle and of microtubule formation, a conclusion supported also by the findings of Leuchtenberger et al. (139). No other mechanism need be invoked for these effects than interference of cannabis with arginine. Modification of pig brain tubulin with the arginine specific reagent 2,3-butanedione results in a decrease of its microtubule formation capacity (140). These data suggested that at least one arginyl residue plays an essential role in tubulin polymerization through its interaction with the negatively charged moiety of GTP, which is required for tubulin polymerization. The preceeding analysis and critique of the experimental data does not exhaust the subject, but highlights fundamental mechanisms that may be operant in a wider spectrum of cannabis associated effects in development and in the modulation of central nervous system activity dependent upon microtubule function.

The health-related problem of whether cannabis consumption produces immune dysfunction in humans can be approached only indirectly. Conclusive evidence may prove elusive since cells *in situ* in a healthy subject may be protected by homeostatic mechanisms absent in cultures. One such approach is suggested by the observation of the interactive effects of nutrition and cannabis in experimental animals (141). This study showed that an enriched protein diet counteracted the effects of cannabis exposure. Although a relationship between nutritional status and cannabis induced immunosuppression in man is often mentioned no controlled studies have been carried out. However, modern concepts of the role of nutrition in the treatment of patients with tumors suggest that food intake plays a role in preventing or correcting the immune depression consequent to the tumor (142, and refs. therein). In healthy human volunteers eating their usual diets, supplemental arginine greatly enhances the in vitro blastogenesis of peripheral lymphocyte response to T-cell mitogens (143). In rodents with depressed immune function secondary to tumors or stress, dietary arginine supplementation can restore thymic weight, the number of thymic lymphocytes and in vitro thymocyte mitogenic response (142). Although the basal diet in the latter study contained 1.8% arginine and was therefore not arginine-deficient, the described restoration of function was observed only after supplementation of the diet and the drinking water with 0.5% arginine. Further experiments clearly showed for the first time that supplemental arginine improves thymic function also in animals with genetically decreased thymic function (144). Dietary arginine was also found to prevent thymic involution and adrenal hypertrophy due to stress or injury (142, 145). In experimental animals long-term and short term exposure to pure cannabinoids and crude marijuana extracts lead to adrenal weight increase and thymus weight decrease (146), while in humans several studies have failed to show any changes in adrenocortical function (120).

Taken together the foregoing studies emphasizes the opposite effects of cannabis and arginine in the intact organism and demonstrate the modulating role of nutritional state, i.e., dietary arginine, on immune function in man. Despite the lack of similar studies in long-term and short-term cannabis users, it seems valid to consider that plasma levels of arginine by some approximation could be a modifying factor in cannabis-induced immunosuppression in man, assuming that the in vitro effects of cannabis have functional significance for health. The reported reactivation of dormant genital herpes shortly after smoking of cannabis (147) could be explained by an arginine-depleting effect of cannabis. Actually, it has been shown that arginine deficiency can increase Herpes Simplex virus yields by inhibiting the induction of interferon (148). On the other hand Herpes Simplex virus fails to replicate and to produce extensive c.p.e. in human cell monolayer cultures exposed to THC (149); this effect of THC was observed only in the absence of serum from the culture since addition of 10% serum overcomes the inhibition in the presence of THC. This antiviral effect of THC in vitro is also consistent with a putative cannabis/arginine interaction since it is well documented that arginine is essential for the replication of *Herpes Simplex* virus (150). Absence of the amino acid from the culture medium prevents the formation of virions and addition of arginine immediately stimulated protein synthesis within 2 min which is followed by virus formation. Serum provides a high concentration of arginine (81) and, thus, may overcome the antiviral (arginine-depleting?) effect of THC as observed in the Blevins and Dumic experiments (149).

D. Carcinogenicity and Antineoplastic Activity

The data of the previous section on the effects of cannabis and on the role of arginine in immune function cover the main concepts that are also applicable to tumors. It is obvious, though, that the metabolic individuality of tumors, either in the transforming or in the proliferating state, will be a factor affecting the interaction of cannabis with these tissues. Available evidence indicates that cannabis has carcinogenic potential (122,151) as well as antineoplastic activity both *in vivo* and *in vitro* when added to certain cell cultures (117,153). From the data available in the literature it can be inferred that the various cell lines appear to react differently to the drug. The field is vast and complex, but some general considerations have emerged that permit us to examine cannabis/arginine interactions. The literature on the roles of arginine and arginase in cancer is voluminous and spans at least 35 years. An arbitrary sampling revealed that although the growth of some tumors is arrested by the administration of arginine (154-156), the growth of the majority of tumors or cell lines is arrested by the depletion of arginine by arginase (157-162). Far from being empirical this latter approach seems to simulate a natural defense mechanism of the organism. It has been shown that activated macrophages kill tumor cells by releasing arginase (130). The selective *in vitro* cytotoxic activity of zynosan or lipipolysaccharide (LPS) - activated rodent macrophages for cultured malignant cells is due to the lethal depletion of arginine mediated by arginase (163). Since arginine is present in high concentration throughout the extracellular fluid, arginase-mediated arginine deprivation of malignant cells "can be envisaged as a microenvironmental phenomenon occuring at or near the surface of the macrophage" (164). Arginine depletion of the extracellular fluid creates conditions inimical to the successful implantation and proliferation of the tumor. Effective arginine-degrading enzymes are currently being studied for use in cancer chemotherapy (165). The known inhibitory action of THC on macrophage function (47) would appear to support an *in vivo* enhancement by cannabis of cancerous growth, in those instances where macrophage _arginase_ is inhibitory to tumor growth. On the other hand, by the same mechanism (paralysis of macrophages) cannabis would arrest cancerous growth in those instances where _arginine_ is inhibitory to the tumor (154-156). It is evident that the metabolic idiosyncrasies of tumors introduce an ambiguity in the understanding of cannabis' effects. This is compounded by the fact that arginine may enter many alternative metabolic pathways (protein synthesis, urea cycle, production of creatine, proline, polyamines, etc.) subserving both growth and function, all of which are claimed by both host tissue and tumor tissue. Malignant cells are reported to require a higher concentration of arginine in the medium than their normal counterparts (163). Tumors obtain the amino acid from their host thus causing arginine depletion to healthy tissues (157), which results in immunosuppression as already discussed. We suggest that cannabis interaction with arginine in its different pathways could account for the apparent variability of the drug's effects in tumors.

E. Muscle and Nerve

Limitations to this review are set by the fact that not all areas of cannabis research have a counterpart in arginine investigations. Some new data in the literature, however, permit to close this paper by examining cannabis/arginine interactions in muscle and nerve. It has been reported that the hypotensive and cardiac slowing actions of THC in rats are not mediated by activation of parasympathetic nerves or by beta-adrenotropic blockade (166). It has also been shown that THC has a depressant effect on the beating of dissociated myocardial cells _in vitro_ (167). During muscle contraction myosin catalyzes, in the presence of actin, the hydrolysis of ATP. Mornet et al. have reported that phenylglyoxal reacts rapidly with isolated myosin heads and induces two successive and distinguishable effects on their enzymic properties: activation followed by inhibition (168). It was demonstrated that the sequential modification of two reactive arginyl residues is responsible for the observed activation-inhibition phenomenon. Furthermore, Johnson ad Blazyk demonstrated that modification of arginine-95 with 1,2-cyclohexanedione abolishes the ability of F-actin to interact with tropomyosin (169). Arginine-95, one out of 18 arginine residues per actin monomer, is part of the 'activated state' binding site. It is currently held (169, and refs. therein) that the interaction between one tropomyosin and seven adjacent actin molecules can control the interaction between actin and myosin for contraction. The tachycardia regularly observed as a consequence of cannabis smoking in humans and the bradycardia observed in animals could be reconciled by a cannabis/arginine interaction with species-dependent emphasis on the activation-inhibition phenomenon and on tropomyosin binding in the mechanism of muscle contraction described above.

The recent reports that muscle spasticity, associated with spinal cord injury or multiple sclerosis, improves after administration of marijuana strongly support a cannabis/arginine interaction in the urea cycle. Narayanareddy and Swami showed that there is a 100% increase in arginine during denervation in muscle (172). The atrophy process causes in addition a shift in ammonia metabolism. Although every enzyme in the urea cycle is subject to inherited abnormality and typical symptoms of hyperammonemia include lethargy, drowsiness and recurrent vomiting attacks (173), it is well documented that patients with arginase deficiency have an extreme degree of limb spasticity. This appears to be caused by some detrimental effect ofarginine accumulation since thespasticityis relieved by a low-arginine diet, which reduces blood arginine levels (174). The proposed depletion of arginine by cannabis (1) could cause the reduction of spasticity by reducing the amount of accumulated arginine. One report has been found to date that examines the question of THC effects on the urea cycle (175). Exposure of rabbits to hashish smoke every other day for a period of one month resulted in a marked increase in blood ammonia, not related to hepatic damage. Though behavioral data are not included in this study, still the biochemical findings offer the first direct roof of a cannabis/arginine interaction in, at least, one of the arginine pathways. Only during recent decades with the discovery of congenital hyperammmonemia in man has it been fully appreciated that ammonia at high levels can cause aberrant behavior, permanently damage the brain as well as inhibit growth (176, and refs. therein). This author stressed the fact that ammonia may have subtle but significant effects on metabolism, particularly in the brain, which are not apparent from neurological signs or blood ammonia concentrations, but which are responsible for abnormal neuro-transmission. The clinical symptoms of hyperammonemia: episodes of intermittent ataxia, irritability, lethargy and coma -- also observed with high doses of cannabis (177) -- can be reversed by dietary arginine (176, and refs. therein), which lowers blood ammonia levels (178). The above data taken together suggest that the results of Ghoneium et al. (175) give an important insight into the mechanismof action of cannabinoids and offer experimentalsupport to the working hypothesis of a cannabis/arginine interaction.

One of the most intriguing effects of cannabis on the nervous system is its biphasic action not only on behavior, but also on distinct neurochemical parameters (63,179,180).

In view of the consistently inhibitory action of cannabis on macromolecular synthesis in the brain, it is far from clear how these biphasic effects are produced. There is agreement that cannabis preparations interact with the cholinergic system (181, and refs. therein). Marijuana and THC affect human memory and cognition in ways that are always detrimental to the user (182). Neurochemical research suggests that these undesirable effects are related to a decrease in the release of neuronal acetylcholine (ACh) and its turnover in certain brain regions (181). The kinds of effects that marijuana can have on the memory process (183) are strikingly similar to those found in patients experiencing amnesia due to Herpes Simplex encephalitis (184), where cholinergic limbic pathways are disrupted (185). Physiological reactions as well as behavioral effects of cannabis are similar to those found with anticholinergic drugs (186). A number of studies have suggested that THC has antiepileptic effects; these effects appear paradoxical when THC has also produced epileptiform activity in hippocampus (183). Behavioral effects of cannabinoids can be blocked by anticholinesterase-type drugs (186). It has also been reported that THC has anticholinesterase-like activity (62). All these contradictory findings could stem from a common substrate assuming a cannabis/arginine interaction. Choline acetyltransferase, the enzyme involved in ACh synthesis, can be inactivated by butanedione and phenylglyoxal, the arginine specific reagents, through the modification of the coenzyme A binding active-site arginine residue (187). Acetylcholinesterase (AChE), the ACh degrading enzyme, can, however, also be inactivated by butanedione through the modification of one essential arginine residue which alters the conformation of the protein (51). Dose-dependent inhibition of choline acetyltransferase and/or AChE would have profound effects on the metabolism and turnover of ACh. An interaction of cannabinoids with active site arginines of these enzymes could account for their biphasic effects on the cholinergic system. Inactivation by phenylglyoxal of adenyl cyclase (188) and catechol-O-methyltransferase (189) extends the role of arginine into the catecholaminergic system. It has been reported that low doses of THC stimulate while high doses depress the noradrenergic and dopaminergic systems (179). This could be mediated through the antagonistic relationships between adenyl cyclase and ATPase activities (190). Interaction of cannabis with the active-site arginines of both enzymes (61,188) could disrupt feedback regulations. Furthermore, the well documented disrupting effect of THC and cannabis on microtubules (33,139) which mediate monoamine exocytosis (191) has also to be taken into account as a factor contributing to the drug's biphasic effects on neurotransmitters.

It is of interest that, also in this process, one arginyl residue of tubulin, the binding site of GTP, is essential for microtubule formation (140) and its modification with butanedione decreases the capacity of tubulin for polymerization. Thus, a putative interaction of cannabis with arginine would permit modulation of synaptic events at multiple sites through a common molecular mechanism. Other enzymes involved in neurotransmitter metabolism that possess essential arginine residues are glutamic decarboxylase (192) and gamma-aminobutyric acid (GABA) aminotransferase (193). Experiments with phenylglyoxal, which inactivates these enzymes, have shown that the decarboxylase, responsible for the biosynthesis of GABA, has essential arginine residues at both the glutamate and the pyridoxal phosphate binding sites; the transferase, responsible for GABA degradation, has an essential arginine at the pyridoxal phosphate binding site.

GABA is the main inhibitory neurotransmitter in the mammalian brain and excitability tends to vary inversely with GABA levels, so that increased brain GABA concentrations were thoughtto lead to protection against convulsions (194). The convulsant action of hydrazines was once attributed to a decrease in GABA, but it soon developed that seizures can occur in the absence of this change (195). It was later demonstrated that hydrazine interferes with the chloride channel "pumps" (196) thus causing postsynaptic disinhibition. THC enhances focal epileptic potentials and seizure activity, while cannabidiol has unique anticonvulsant properties (197) and marijuana has paradoxical anticonvulsant and convulsant effects (198). A differential interaction of cannabinoids with essential arginine in the GABA metabolizing enzymes as well as with the essential arginine in the chloride-channel protein (53) could well underlie their complex effects in convulsions. Roberts et al. have proposed the possibility that hydrazine might displace guanidino groups of arginyl residuesin proteins of nerve cell membranes from interacation with adjacently-located negatively-charged groups (199). This they assume to be the mechanism of hydrazine toxicity in convulsions, since arginine tested as a possible protective agent in hydrazine toxicity was found to be effective. That arginine may have a complex homeostatic role in the mechanisms of excitation/inhibition in the neuronal microenvironment is suggested by the finding that gamma-guanidinobutyric acid, a normal component of the brain, which is synthesized from GABA and arginine (200), inactivates inhibitory synapses (201) and may be important in the excitation of the central nervous system which leads to seizures (202). Chronic injections of THC increase the content of GABA in rat brain (203). Since the biphasic effects of cannabis suggest the interaction ofthe drug with homeostatic mechanisms of the brain, it would be consistent with these data to view the interaction as occuring via arginine involvement at the multiple sites described, where arginine appears to be essential to neuronal function.

Last, but not least, and relevant to THC's lipophilic nature, is the emerging role of arginine in the biochemistry of receptor binding. This role was anticipated by the work of Curtis and Watkins (204), predicted by Roberts et al. (199), elaborated by the hypothesis of Watkins (205), and is now supported by specific experiments (55, 206). Briefly, Watkins proposed that the pharmacological actions of ACh, GABA and glutamic acid result from dissociation of phospholipid-protein complexes contained in the membrane, and the ensuing permeability changes. He reached this conclusion after noting the similarity in the structure and charge distributions of ACh, GABA and glutamic acid with phosphatidyl-chlorine, phosphatidylethanolamine and phosphatidylserine respectively. The theory requires that receptor sites for GABA and glutamicacid should be ascribed to basic amino acid side chains in the protein. Confirmation of Watkins' hypothesis with respect to GABA was obtained when a preparation enriched in junctional complexes from rat cerebellum was incubated with labeled GABA, and binding was determined in the absence and presence of the enzyme that specifically hydrolyzes phosphatidylethanolamine (206). It was demonstrated that phospholipase C, in fact, enhanced the specific binding of GABA by 260% and, furthermore, that there was competition between GABA and the phospholipid for binding to the receptor. Hence, removal of the phospholipid unmasked a high affinity site for transmitter binding. Recent studies have now provided evidence that arginylresidues in proteins are the high affinity sites for negatively charged phosphate groups of phospholipid molecules (55). Other studies have established that the microenvironment of the binding-site arginines is always a hydrophobic sequence of the protein molecule (56), i.e., a locus for which THC has special affinity. Since the GABA is similarly a hydrophobic protein (206) a cannabis/arginine interaction at the receptor would be consistent with the data and may explain the observed increase in GABA content of rat cerebellum after chronic THC administration (203).

F. Comment

In the light of the data surveyed and analyzed from the published reports available in the literature it appears that the hypothesis of the cannabis/arginine interaction, as the common denominator of the drug's biological effects, remains valid. However, a hypothesis hovers around truth, it is not truth itself. It is hoped that the evidence offered in the present review in favor of the "common denominator" may stimulate the pertinent analytical disciplines into designing the crucial experiments that suggest themselves, and through which the hypothesis may claim reality status. The references cited may also generate a cascade of further contributory data, here witheld due to the limitation of space.

ACKNOWLEDGMENTS

The author thanks Mrs. Judy Ashmore of the Marine Biological Laboratory, Library, Woods Hole, Mass. for her invaluable help in collecting the literature. This study was supported by a grant of the National Research Foundation of Greece.

REFERENCES

1. Issidorides, M. R., Observations in chronic hashish users: nuclear aberrations in blood and sperm and abnormal acrosomes in spermatozoa, Adv. Biosci., 22 & 23: 377-388 (1979).
2. Stefanis, C. N., and Issidorides, M. R., Cellular effects of chronic cannabis use in man, in "Marihuana: Chemistry, Biochemistry and Cellular Effects" (G. G. Nahas, ed.) pp. 533-550, Springer-Verlag, New York, 1976.
3. Black, M. M., and Ansley, H. R., Histone specificity revealed by ammoniacal silver staining, J. Histochem. Cytochem. 14:177-181, 1966.
4. MacRae, E. K., and Meetz, G. D., Electron microscopy of the ammoniacal silver reaction for histones in theerythropoietic cells of the chick, J. Cell Biol., 45:235-345 (1970).
5. Littau, V. C., Burdick, C., Allfrey, V. G., and Mirsky, A. E., The role of histones in the maintenance of chromatin structure, Proc. Nat. Acad. Sci. USA 54:1204-1212 (1965).
6. Black, M. M., and Ansley, H. R., Antigen-induced changes in lymphoid cell histones. I. Thymus, J. Cell Biol., 26:201-208 (1965).
7. Vaughn, J.C., The relationship of the "sperm chromatophile: to the fate of displaced histones following histone transition in rat spermiogenesis, J. Cell Biol. 31:257-278 (1966).
8. Calvin, H. I., and Bedford, J. M., Formation of disulfide bonds in the nucleus and accessory structures of mamma-

lian spermatozoa during maturation in the epididymis, J. Reprod. Fert. Suppl. 13: 65-75 (1971).

9. Nahas, G. G., Suciu-Foca, N., Armand, J. P., and Morishima, A., Inhibition of cellular mediated immunity in marijuana smokers, Science, 183:419-420 (1974).

10. Hembree III, W. C., Nahas, G. G., Zeidenberg, P., and Huang, H. F. S., Changes in human spermatozoa associated with high dose marijuana smoking, Adv. Biosci., 22 & 23: 429-439 (1979).

11. Silvestroni, L., Frajese, G., and Fabrizio, M., Histones instead of protamines in terminal germ cells of infertile oligospermic men, Fertil Steril. 27:1428-1437 (1976).

12. Holt, L. E., and Albanese, A. A., Observations with amino acid deficiencies in man, Trans. Assoc. Amer, Physicians, 58:143-156 (1944).

13. Schachter, A., Friedman, S., Goldman, J. A., and Eckerling, B., The treatment of oligospermia with the aminoacid arginine, Int. Gynecol. and Ostet., 11:206-209 (1973).

14. Radany, E. W., and Atherton, R. W., Arginine-induced stimulation of rabbit sperm motility, Arch. Androl., 7:351-355 (1981).

15. Shahar, A., and Bino, T., In vitro effects of delta-9-tetrahydrocannabinol (THC) on bull sperm, Biochem. Pharmacol., 23:1341-1342 (1974).

16. Nahas, G. G. (ed.) "Marihuana: Chemistry, Biochemistry, and Cellular Effects". Springer-Verlag, New York, 1976.

17. Nahas, G. G., and Paton, W. D. M. (eds.) "Marihuana: Biological Effects, Analysis, Metabolism, Cellular Responses, Reproduction and Brain", Advances in Biosciences, Vol. 22 & 23, Pergamon Press, Oxford, 1979.

18. Dardick, I., and Setterfield, G., Volume of condensed chromatin in developing primitive-line erthrocytes of chick, Exp. Cell Res., 100:159-171 (1976).

19. Brasch, K., and Sinclair, G. D., The organization, composition and matrix of hepatocyte nuclei exposed to a-amanitin, Virchows Arch. B Cell Pathol., 27:193-204 (1978).

20. Harris, J. R., The biochemistry and ultrastructure of the nuclear envelope, Biochem. Biophys. Acta., 515:55-104 (1978).

21. Issidorides, M. R., Stefanis, C. N., Varsou, E., and Katsorchis, T., Altered chromatin ultrastructure in neutrophils of schizophrenics. Nature, 258:612-614 (1975).

22. Issidorides, M. R., Zioudrou, C., Lykouras, E., and Stefanis, C. N., Drug-induced changes in chromatin ultrastructure and nuclear basic proteins of the neutrophils of chronic schizophrenics, Prog. Neuro-Psychopharmacol.,

2:79-85 (1978).

23. Issidorides, M. R., and Katsorchis, T., Dispersed and compact chromatin demonstrated with a new EM method: Phosphotungstic acid hematoxylin block-staining, Histochemistry, 73:21-31 (1981).

24. Issidorides, M. R., Interaction of cannabis with arginine metabolism underlies biological effects: A new hypothesis on mechanism of action, in "Adverse Health and Behavioral Consequences of Cannabis Use. Working Paper for the ARF/WHO Scientific Meeting, Toronto, 1981", K. O. Fehr and H. Kalant, eds.) Addiction Research Foundation, Toronto, 1982.

25. Holstein, A. F., and Schirren, C., Classification of abnormalities in human spermatids based on recent advances in ultra-structure research on sermatid differentiation, in "The Spermatozoon: Maturation, Motility, Surface Properties and Comparative Aspects (D. W. Fawcett and J. M. Bedford, eds.), pp. 341-354. Urban & Schwarzenberg, Baltimore, MD, 1979.

26. Coelingh, J. P., Rozijn, T. H., and Monfoort, C. H., Isolation and partial characterization of a basic protein from bovine sperm heads, Biochem. Biophys. Acta., 188:353-356 (1969).

27. Fawcett, D. W., Anderson, W. a., and Phillips, D. M., Morphogenetic factors influencing the shape of the sperm head, Dev. Biol., 26:220-251 (1971).

28. Weissfeld, A. S., and Rouse, H., Arginine deprivation in KB cells, II. Characterization of the DNA synthesized during starvation, J. Cell Biol. 75:889-898 (1977).

29. Aula, P., and Nichols, W. W., The cytogenetic effects of mycoplasma in human leukocyte cultures, J. Cell Physiol., 70:281-29 (1967).

30. Stein, G. S., Mon, M. J., Haas, A. E., and Jansing, R. L., Cannabinoids: The influence on cell proliferation and macromolecular biosynthesis, in "Marihuana: Biological Effects: (G. G. Nahas and W. D. M. Paton, eds.) pp. 171-28. Pergamon Press, Oxford and New York, 1979.

31. Freed, J. J., and Schatz, S. A., Chromosome aberrations in cultured cells deprived of single essential amino-acids, Exp. Cell Res., 393-49 (1969).

32. Leuchtenberger, C., Leuchtenberger, R., Zbinden, I., and Schleh, E., Cytological and cytochemical effects of whole smoke and the gas vapor phase from marihuana cigarettes on growth and DN metabolism of cultured mammalian cells, in "Marihuana: Chemistry, Biochemistry, and Cellular Effects" (G. G. Nahas, ed.) pp. 243-256. Springer-Verlag, New York, 1976.

33. Morishima, A., Henrich, R. T., Jayaraman, J., and Nahas, G. G., Hypoploid metaphases in cultured lymphocytes of

marihuana smokers, Adv. Biosci., 22 & 23: 371-376 (1979).

34. Stefanis, C., Dornbush, R., and Fink, M., (eds.) "Hashish: Studies of Long-Term Use". Raven Press, New York, 1977.
35. Da Prada, M., Jakabova, M., Luscher, E. F., Pletscher, A., and Richards, J. G., Subcellular localization of the heparin-neutralizing factor in blood platelets, J. Physiol., 257:495-502 (1976).
36. Fukami, M. H., Niewiarowski, S., Rucinski, B., and Salganicoff, L., Subcellular localization of human platelet antiheparin proteins, Thromb. Res., 14:433-443 (1979).
37. Niewiarowski, S., Poplawski, A., Lipinsi, B., and Farbiszewski, R., The release of platelet clotting factors during aggregation and viscous metamorphosis, Exp. Biol. Med., 3:121-128 (1968).
38. Kaplan, K. L., Dauzier, M. J., and Rose, S., ADP and epinephrine-induced release of platelet fibrinogen, Blood, 58:797-802 (1981).
39. Holt, J. C., Harris, M., Lange, E., Rucinski, B., Henschen, A., and Niewiarowski, S., Platelet basic protein (PBP) is the precursor of low affinity platelet factor 4 (LA-PF_4) and b-thromboglobulin (BTG), Fed. Proc., 41:528 (1982).
40. Scgaefer, C. F., Brackett, D. J., Gunn, C. G., and Dubowski, K. M., Decreased platelet aggregation following marihuana smoking in man, J. Okla. State Med. Assoc., 72:435-436 (1979).
41. Cooper, K. D., Shukla, J. B., and Rennert, O. M., Polyamine distribution in cellular compartments of blood and in aging erythrocytes, Clin. Chem. Acta., 73:171-88 (1976).
42. Rennert, O. M., Buehler, B., Miale, T., and Lawson, D., Polyamines and platelet aggregation, Life Sci., 19:257-263 (1976).
43. Issidorides, M. R, et al., in preparation.
44. Miras, C., and Koutselinis, A., The distribution and excretion of tetrahydrocannabinol-C^{14} in humans, Med. Sci. Law., 11:197-199 (1971).
45. Raz, A., Schurr, A., and Livine, A., The interaction of hashish components with human erythrocytes, Biochem. Biophys. Acta., 247:269-271 (1972).
46. Rubin, V., and Comitas, L., "Ganja in Jamaica". Moulton Publ., The Hague, 1975.
47. Chari-Bitron, A., Effect of delta-9-THC on red blood cell membranes and on alveolar macrophages, in "Marihuana: Chemistry, Biochemistry and Cellular Effects" (G. G. Nahas, ed.) pp. 273-281. Springer-Verlag, New York, 1976.
48. Kalofoutis, A., and Koutselinis, A., Changes induced by hashish constituents on human erythrocyte phospholipids,

Pharmacol. Biochem. Behav., 11:383-385 (1979).
49. Kalofoutis, A., Koutselinis, A., Lekakis, J., and Miras, C., Levels of erythrocyte 2,3 DPG and ATP in heavy hashish smokers, Experientia. 36:897-898 (1980).
50. Martin, K., The effect of proteolytic enzymes on acetylcholinesterase activity, the sodium pump and choline transport in human erythrocytes, Biochem. Biophys. Acta. 203:182-184 (1970).
51. Mullner H., and Sund, H., Essential arginine residues in aceltylcholinesterase from Torpedo californica, FEBS Lett., 119:283-286 (1980).
52. Steck, T. L., Koziarz, J. J., Singh, M. K., Reddy, G., and Kohler, H., Preparation and analysis of seven major topographically defined fragments of band 3, the predominant transmembrane polypeptide of human erythrocyte membranes, Biochemistry, 17:1216-1222 (1978).
53. Zaki, L., Inhibition of anion transport across red cells with 1, 2-cyclohexanedione, Biochem. Biophys. Res. Commun., 99:243-251 (1981).
54. Goldman, S. S., and Albers, R. W., Sodium-potassium-activatedadenosine triphosphatase. IX The role of phospholipids, J. Biol. Chem., 248:867-874 (1973).
55. Akeroyd, R., Lange, L. C., Westerman, J., and Wirtz, K. W. A., Modification of phosphatidylcholine-transfer protein from bovine liver with butanedione and phenylglyoxal. Evidence for one essential arginine residue, Eur. J. Biochem., 121:77-81 (1981).
56. Norne, J. E., Hjalmarsson, S. G., Lindman, B., and Zeppezauer, M., Anion binding properties of human serum albumen from halide ion quadrupole relaxation, Biochemistry, 14:3401-3408 (1975).
57. Patthy, L., and Thesz, J., Origin of the selectivity of adicarbonyl reagents from arginyl residues ofanion-binding sites, Eur. J. Biochem. 105:367-393 (1980).
58. Paton, W. D. M., Concluding summary, in "Marihuana: Chemistry, Biochemistry, and Cellular Effects" (G.G. Nahas, ed.) pp. 551-552. Springer-Verlag, New York, 1976.
59. Yamada, S., and Itano, H. A., Phenanthrenequinone as an analytical reagent for arginine and other monosubstituted guanidines, Biochem. Biophys. Acta., 130:538-540 (1966).
60. Magun, B.E., and Kelly, J. W., A new fluorescent method with phenanthrenequinone for the histochemical demonstration of arginine residues in tissues, J. Histochem. Cytochem., 17:821-827 (1969).
61. Grisham, C. M., Characterization of essential arginyl residues in sheep kidney ($Na^+ + K^+$)-ATPase, Biochem, Biophys. Res. Commun., 88:229-236 (1979).
62. Brown, H., Possible anticholinesterase-like effects of trans (-)-delta-8 and delta-9-THC as observed in the

general motor activity of mice, Psychopharmacologia, 27:111-116 (1972).

63. Luthra, Y. K., Rosekrantz, H., Heyman, I. A., and Braude, M. C., Differential neurochemistry and temporal pattern in rats treated orally with delta-9-tetrahydrocannabinol for periods up to six months, Toxicol. Appl. Pharmacol., 32:418-431 (1975).
64. Toro-Goyco, E., Rodriguez, M. B., Preston, A., and Jering, H., Effect of (-)-delta-9-THC on ATPase systems from various sources, Adv. Biosci., 22 & 23: 229-242 (1979).
65. Kookkini, G., Stevens, V. J., Peterson, C. M., and Cerami, A., Modification of hemoglobin by ninhydrin, Blood, 56:701-705 (1980).
66. Riordan, J. F., McElvany, K. D., and Borders, Jr., C. L., Arginyl residues: anion recognition sites in enzymes, Science, 195:884-886 (1977).
67. Campbell, J. W., Comparative biochemistry of arginine and urea metabolism in invertebrates, Excerpta Med. Intnol. Congr. Series No. 195:48-68 (1968).
68. Jukes, T. H., The 'intruder' hypothesis and selection against arginine, Biochem. Biophys. Res. Commun., 58:80-84 (1974).
69. Wallis, M., On the frequency of arginine in proteins and its implication for molecular evolution, Biochem. Biophys. Res. Commun., 56:711-716 (1974).
70. Riordan, J. F., Arginyl residues and anion binding sites in proteins, Mol. Cell. Biochem., 26:71-92 (1979).
71. Itano, H. A., and Gottlieb, A. J., Blocking of tryptic cleavage of arginine bonds by the chemical modification of the guanido group with benzil, Biochem. Biophys. Res. Commun., 12:405-08 (1963).
72. Means, G. E., and Feeney, R. E., in "Chemical Modification of Proteins", pp. 194-18, Holden-Day, Inc. San Francisco, 1971.
73. Yankeelov, J., Jr., Kochert, M., Page, J., and Westphal, A., Reagent for the modification of arginine residues under mild conditions, Fed. Proc., 25:590 (1966).
74. Toi, K., Bynum, E., Norris, E., and Itano, H. A., Studies on the chemical modification of arginine I. The reaction of 1,2-cyclohexanedione with arginine and arginyl residues in proteins, J. Biol. Chem., 242:1036-1043 (1967).
75. Takahashi, K., The reaction of phenylglyoxal with arginine residues in proteins, J. Biol. Chem., 243:6171-6179 (1968).
76. Loh, Y. P., and Loriaux, L. L., Adrenocortiocotropic hormone, beta-lipotropin, and endorphin-related peptides in health and disease, J. Amer. Med. Assoc., 247:1033-1034 (1982).

77. Hook, V. Y. H., Eiden, L. E., and Brownstein, M. J., A carboxypeptidase processing enzyme for enkephalin precursors, Nature, 295:341-342 (1982).
78. Nahas, G. G., Desoize, B., Hsu, J., and Morishima, A., Inhibitory effects of delta-9-tetrahydrocannabinol on nucleic acid synthesis and proteins in cultured lymphocytes, in "Marihuana: Chemistry, Biochemistry, and Cellular Effects", (G. G. Nahas, ed.)pp. 299-312. Springer-Verlag, New York, 1976.
79. Jakubovic, A., and McGeer, P.L., Inhibition of rat protein and nucleic acid synthesis by cannabinoids in vitro, Can. J. Biochem., 50:654-662 (1972).
80. Jakubovic, A., and McGeer, P. L., In vitro inhibition of protein and nucleic acid synthesis in rat testicular tissue by cannabinoids, in "Marihuana: Chemistry, Biochemistry, and Cellular Effects", (G. G. Nahas, ed.) pp. 223-241. Springer-Verlag, New York, 1976.
81. Paul, D., and Walter, S., Initiation of DNA synthesis in primary fetal rat hepatocytes in cultures, Proc. Soc. Exp. Biol. Med., 145:456-460 (1974).
82. Hassan, A.S., and Milner J.A, Alterations in liver nucleic acids and nucleotides in arginine deficient rats, Metabolism, 30:739-744 (1981).
83. Jordan F., and Wu, A., Inactivation of purine nucleoside phosphorylase by modification of arginine residues, Arch. Biochem. Biophys. 190:699-704 (1978).
84. Borders, C. L., Jr., Riordan, J. F., and Auld, D. S., Essential arginyl residues in reverse transcriptase, Biochem. Biophys. Res. Commun. 66:490-495 (1975).
85. Armstrong, V. W., Sterbach, H., and Eckstein, F., Modification of an essential arginine in E. coli DNA-dependent RNA polymerase, FEBS Lett., 70:48-50 (1976).
86. Salvo, R. A., Serio, G. F., Evans, J. E., and Kimball, A. P., The affinity labeling of amino acids in or about the active enter of DNA-dependent polymerase I, Biochemistry, 15:493-497 (1976).
87. Blevins, R. D., and Regan, J. D., Delta-9-tetrahydrocannabinol: Effect on macromolecular synthesis in human and other mammalian cells, in "Marihuana: Chemistry, Biochemistry, and Cellular Effects", (G. G. Nahas, ed.) pp. 213-222. Springer-Verlag, New York, 1976.
88. Zimmerman, A. M., and Zimmerman, S., The influence of marihuana on eukaryote cell growth and development, in "Marihuana: Chemistry, Biochemistry, and Cellular Effects", (G. G. Nahas, ed.) pp. 195-204. Springer-Verlag, New York, 1976.
89. Myers, III, W. A., and Heath, R. G., Cannabis sativa: Ultra-structural changes in organelles of neurons in

brain septal region of monkeys, J. Neurosci. Res., 4:9-17 (1979).
90. Hattori, T., Jakubovic, A., and McGeer, P. L., The effect of cannabinoids on the number of nuclear membrane-attached ribosomes in infant rat brain, Neuropharmacology, 12:995-999 (1973).
91. Gierer, A., Function of aggregated reticulocyte ribosomes in protein synthesis, J. Mol. Biol., 6:148-157 (1963).
92. Hernandez, F., Lopez-Rivas, A., Pintor-Toro, J. A., Vazquez,D., and Palacian, E., Implication of arginyl residues in mRNA binding to ribosomes, Eur. J. Biochem. , 108:137-141 (1980).
93. Jonas, A., and Weber, G., Presence of arginine residues at the strong, hydrophobic anion binding sites of bovine serum albumin, Biochemistry, 10:1335-1339 (1971).
94. Mon, M. J., Haas, A. E., Sten J. L., and Stein, G. S., Influence of psychoactive and non psychoactive cannabinoids on cell proliferation and macromolecular biosynthesis in human cells, Biochem. Pharmacol., 30:31-43 (1981).
95. Mon, M. J., Haas, A. E., Steink, J. L., and Stein, G. S., Influence of psychoactive and nonpsychoactive cannabinoids on chromatin structure and function in human cells, Biochem. Pharmacol., 30:45-58 (1981).
96. Stein, S. M., and Berestecky, J. M., Inhibition of growth by masking of arginine moieties in protein at the cell surface, Cancer Res., 34:3112-3116 (1974).
97. Stein, S. M., and Berestecky, J. M., Exposure of an arginine-rich protein at surface of cells in S, G_2 and M phases of the cell cycle, J. Cell. Physiol., 85:243-250 (1975).
98. Mehrishi, J. N., Positively charged amino groups on the surface of normal and cancer cells, Eur. J. Cancer., 6:12-137 (1980).
99. Steven, F. S., Griffin, M. M., Hulley, T. P., and Brooman,P., Interaction of alpha,beta-stilbestrol-4,4'-bisphosphate with arginyl substrates resulting inapparent inhibition of typsin and thrombin, Eur. J. Biochem. 125: 305-309 (1982).
100. Harris, L. S., Carchman, R. A., and Martin, B. R., Evidence for the existence of specific cannabinoid binding sites, Life Sci., 22:1131-1138 (1978).
101. Warner, W., Harris, L. S., and Carchman, R. A., Inhibition of corticosteroidogenesis by delta-9-tetrahydrocannabinol, Endocrinology, 101:182101827 (1977).
102. Carchman, R. A., End, D. W., and Parker, M. R., Marihuana cell function, Adv. Biosci., 22-23:219-229 (1979).
103. Beins, D. M., Vining, R., and Balasubramaniam, S., The regulation of neutral cholesterol esterase and acetyl-Co

A:cholesterol acetyltransferase in the rat adrenal gland, Biochem. J., 202:631-637 (1982).
104. Burstein, S., Hunter, S. A., and Shoupe, T. S., Site of inhibition of Leydig cell testosterone synthesis by delta-1-tetrahydrocannabinol, Mol. Pharmacol., 15:633-640 (1979).
105. Gill, E. W., Jones, G., and Laurence, D. K., Chemical mechanisms of action of THC in "Cannabis and Its Derivatives: Pharmacology and Experimental Psychology" (W. D. M. Paton and J. Crown, eds.) pp. 76-87. London:Oxford University Press, 1972.
106. Wahlqvist, M., Nilsson, I. M., Sandberg, F., and Agurell, S., Binding of delta-1-tetrahydrocannabinol to human plasma proteins, Biochem. Pharmacol., 19:2579-2584 (1970).
107. Widman, M., Nilson, I. M., Nilson, J. L. G., Agurell, S., Borg, H., and Granstrand, B., Plasma protein binding of 7-hydroxy-delta-1-tetrahydrocannabinol: An active delta-1-tetrahydrocannabinol metabolite, J. Pharm Pharmacol., 25:453-457 (1973).
108. Fredrickson, D. S., Lux, S. E., and Herbert, P. N., Apolipoproteins, Adv. Exp. Med. & Biol., 26:25-56 (1972).
109. Rogers, T. B., Borresen, T., and Feeney, R. E., Chemical modification of argininein transferrins, Biochemistry, 17:1105-1109 (1978).
110. Havel, R. J., Lipoprotein biosynthesis and metabolism, Ann. N. Y. Acad. Sci., 348:16-29 (1980).
111. Weisgraber, K. H., Rall, S. C., Jr., and Mahley, R. W., Human E apoprotein heterogeneity, J. Biol. Chem., 256:9077-9083 (1981).
112. Mahley, R. W., Innerarity, T. L., and Weisgraber, K. H., Alterations in metabolic activity plasma lipoproteins following selective chemical modification of the apoproteins, Ann. N. Y. Acad. Sci., 348:265-280 (1980).
113. Titova, G. V., Kliueva, N. N., Kozhevnikova, K. A., and Klimov, A. N., Interaction of cholesterol with apoprotein E-An arginine-rich protein of very low density lipoproteins, Biokhimia, 45:51-55 (1980).
114. Klimov, A. N., Titova, G. V., Kozhenvnikova, K. A., Kliueva, N. M., and Smirnova, I. V., Interaction of cholesterol with polypeptides and amino acids, Biokhimia, 47:226-232 (1982).
115. Fukushima, D., Yokoyama, S., Kezdy, F. J., and Kaiser, E. T., Bindingof amphiphilic peptides to phospholipid/cholesterol unilamellar vesicles: A model for protein-cholesterol interaction, Proc. Natl. Acad. Sci. USA, 78: 2732-2736 (1981).
116. Levy, J. A., Munson, A. E., Harris, L. H., and Dewey, W.

L., Effects of delta-9-THC on the immune response of mice, Fed. Proc., 34:728 (1975).

117. Munson, A. E., and Fehr, K. O., Immunological effects of cannabis, in "Adverse Health and Behavioral Consequences of Cannabis Use. Working Papers for the ARF/WHO Scientific Meeting, Toronto 1981" (K. O. Fehr and H. Kalant, eds.). Addiction Research Foundation, Toronto, 1982.

118. White, S. C., Brin, S. C., and Janicki, B. W., Mitogen-induced blastogenic responses of lymphocytes from marihuana smokers, Science, 188:71-72 (1975).

119. Nahas, G. G., Morishima, A., and Desoize, B., Effects of cannabinoids on macromolecular synthesis and replication of cultured lymphocytes. FASEB Conference, "Organismal Response to the Environment", 60th Annual Meeting of FASEB, Anaheim, CA, April 15, 1976.

120. Bloch, E., Effects of marihuana and cannabinoids on reproduction, endocrine function, development and chromosomes, in "Adverse Health and Behavioral Consequences of Cannabis Use. Working Papers for ARF/WHO Scientific Meeting, Toronto, 1981". (K. O. Fehr and H. Kalant, eds.). Addiction Research Foundation, Toronto, 1982.

121. Henrich, R. T., Nogawa, T., and Morishima, A., In vitro induction of segregational errors of chromosomes by natural cannabinoids in normal human lymphocytes, Environmental Mutagenesis, 2:139-147 (1980).

122. Leuchtenberger, C., Effects of marihuana (cannabis) smoke on cellular biochemistry, utilizing _in vitro_ test systems, in "Adverse Health and Behavioral Consequences of Cannabis Use. Working Papers for the ARF/WHO Scientific Meeting, Toronto, 1981". (K. O. Fehr and H. Kalant, eds.). Addiction Research Foundation, Toronto, 1982.

123. Schempp, W., and Krone, W., Deficiency of arginine and lysine causes increases in the frequency of sister chromatid exchanges, Human Genet., 51:315-328 (1979).

124. Birke, C., Peter, H. H., Langenberg, U., Muller-Hermes, J. P., Peters, J. H., Heitman, J., Leibold, W., Dallugge, H., Krapf, E., and Kirchner, H., Mycoplasma contamination in human tumor cell lines: Effect of interferon induction and susceptibility to natural killing, J. Immunol., 127: 94-98 (1981).

125. Simberkoff, M. S., Thorbecke, G. L., and Thomas, L., Studies of PPLO infection: V. Inhibition of lymphocyte mitosis and anti-body formation by mycoplasma extracts, J. Exp. Med., 129:1163-1181 (1969).

126. Callewaert, D. M., Kaplan, J., Peterson, Jr., W. D., and Lightbody, J. J., Suppression of lymphocyte activation by a factor produced by _Mycoplasma arginini_, J. Immunol., 115:1662-1664 (1975).

127. Copperman, R., and Morton, H. E., Reversible inhibition

of mitosis in lymphocyte cultures by non-viable mycoplasma, Proc. Soc. Exp. Biol. & Med., 123:790-795 (1966).
128. Kaklamanis,E., and Pavlatos, M., The immunosuppressive effect of mycoplasma infection. I. Effect on the humoral and cellular response, Immunology, 22:695-702 (1972).
129. Barile, P. M., and Leventhal, B. G., Possible mechanism of Mycoplasma inhibition of lymphocyte transformation induced by phytohemagglutinin (PHA), Nature (Lond.), 219:758-759 (1978).
130. Currie, G. A., Activated macrophages kill tumour cells by releasing arginase, Nature (Lond.), 273:758-759 (1978).
131. Stenchever, M. A., Kunysz, T. J., and Allen, M., Chromosome breakage in users of marihuana, Amer. J. Obstet. Gynecol., 118-113 (1974).
132. Stenchever, M. A., and Allan, M., The effect of delta-9-THC on the chromosomes of human lymphocytes in vitro, Amer. J. Obstet. Gynecol., 114:891-821 (1972).
133. Fried, P. A., and Charlebois, A. T., Cannabis administered during pregnancy: First- and second-generation effects in rats, Physiol. Psychol., 7:307-310 (1979).
134. Carrano, A. V., Thompson, L. H., Lindl, P. A., and Minkler, J. L., Sister chromatid exchanges as an indicator of mutagenesis, Nature, 271:551-555 (1978).
135. MacRae, W. D., MacKinnon, E. A., and Stich, H. F., Effects of arginine deprivation upon chromosome aberrations, SCEs and survival of CHO cells treated with mutagenic agents, Mutat. Res., 62:495-504 (1979).
136. MacRae, W. D., MacKinnon, E. A., and Stich, H. F., Induction of sister chromatid exchanges and chromosomes alterations in CHO cells arrested in the cell cycle by arginine deprivation, In Vitro, 15:555-564 (1979).
137. Carrano, A. V., and Heddle, J. A., The fate of chromosome aberrations, J. Theor. Biol., 38:289-304 (1973).
138. Hsu, T. C., Editorial comments, Mammal. Chromo. Newslett., 17:1-7 (1976).
139. Leuchtenberger, C., Leuchtenberger, R., and Ritter, U., Effects of marihuana and tobacco smoke on DNA and chromosomal complement in human lung explants, Nature (Lond.) 242:403-404 (1973).
140. Maccioni, R. B., Vera, J. C., and Slebe, J. C., Arginyl residues involvement in the microtubule assembly, Arch. Biochem. Biophys., 207:248-255 (1981).
141. Charlebois, A. T., and Fried, P. A., Interactive effects of nutrition and cannabis upon rat perinatal development, Dev. Psychobiol., 13:591-505 (1980).
142. Rettura, G., Padawer, J., Barbul, A., Levenson, S. M., and Seifter, E., Supplemental arginine increases thymic cellularity in normal and murine sarcoma virus-inoculated mice and increases resistance to murine sarcoma virus

tumor, JPEN, 3:409-416 (1979).

143. Barbul, A., Sisto, D. A., Wasserkrug, H. L., and Efron, G., Arginine stimulates lymphocyte immune responsein healthy human beings, Surgery, 90:244-251 (1981).

144. Barbul, A., Sisto, D. A., Wasserkrug, H. L., Levenson, S. M., Efron, G., and Seifter, E., Arginine stimulates thymic immune function and ameliorates the obesity and hyperglycemia of genetically obese mice, JPEN, 5:492-495 (1981).

145. Barbul, A., Rettura, G., Levenson, S. M., and Seifter, E., Arginine, a thymotropic and wound-healing promoting agent, Surg. Forum., 28:101-103 (1977).

146. Block, E., Thysen, B., Morrill, G. A., Gardner, E., and Fujimoto, G., Effects of cannabinoids on reproduction and development, Vit. Hor., 36:204-258 (1978).

147. Juel-Jensen, B. E., Cannabis and recurrent herpes simplex, Brit Med. J., iv:296 (1972).

148. Manischewitz, J. E., Young, B. G., and Barile, M. F., The effectof mycoplasmas on replication and plaquing ability of Herpes Simplex virus, Proc. Soc. Exp. Biol. Med., 148: 859-863 (1975).

149. Blevins, R. D., and Dumic, M. P., Delta-9-tetrahydrocannabinol and Herpes Simplex, This volume, 1982.

150. Becker, Y., Olshevsky, U., and Levitt, J., The role of arginine in the replication of Herpes Simplex virus, J. Gen. Virol., 1:471-478 (1967).

151. Tennant, F. S., Jr., Clinical toxicology of cannabis use, in "Adverse Health and Behavioral Consequences of Cannabis Use. Working Papers for the ARF/WHO Scientific Meeting, Toronto, 1981", (K. O. Fehr and H. Kalant, eds.). Addiction Research Foundation, Toronto, 1982.

152. Munson, A. E., Harris, L. S., Friedman, M. A., Dewey, W. L., and Carchman, R. A., Antineoplastic activity of cannabinoids, J. Natl. Cancer Inst., 55:597-603 (1975).

153. Jering, H., and Toro-Goyco, E., Effect of delta-9-THC in nucleoside and amino acid uptake in Reuben H-35 hepatoma cells, Adv. Biosci., 22 & 23:161-169 (1979).

154. Milner, J. A, and Stepanovich, L. V., Inhibitory effect of dietary arginine on growth of Ehrlich ascites tumor cells in mice, J. Nutr., 109:489-494 (1979).

155. Cho-Chung, Y. S., Clair, T., Bodwin, J. S., and Hill, D. M., Arrest of mammary tumor growth in vivo by L-arginine: stimulation of NAD-dependent activation of adenyl cyclase, Biochem. Biophys. Res. Commun., 95:1306-1313 (1980).

156. Cho-Chung, Y. S., Clair, T., Bodwin, J. S., and Berghoffer, B., Growth arrest and morphological changes of human breast cancer cells by dibutyryl cyclic AMP and L-arginine, Science, 214:77-79 (1981).

157. Bach, S. J., and Lasnitzki, I., Some aspects of the role of arginine and arginase in mouse carcinoma 63, Enzymologia, 12:198-205 (1947).
158. Bach, S. J., and Maw, G. A., Creatine synthesis by tumour-bearing rats, Biochem. Biophys. Acta., 11:69078 (1953).
159. Bach, S. J., and Simon-Reuss, I., Arginase, an antimitotic agent in tissue culture, Biochem, Biophys. Acta., 11:369-402 (1953).
160. Storr, J. M., and Burton, A. F., The effects of arginine deficiency on lymphoma cells, Br. J. Cancer, 30:50-59 (1974).
161. Okabe, J., Hayashi, M., Honma, Y., and Houmi, M., Induction of differentiation of cultured mouse myeloid leukemic cells by arginase, Biochem. Biophys. Res. Commun., 89:879-884 (1979).
162. Scallan, C., Clynes, M., and Joyce, P., The effect of shark liver arginase on the growth of cells in culture, Biochem. Soc. Trans., 9:317 (1981).
163. Currie, G. A., and Basham, C., Differential arginine dependence and the selective cytotoxic effects of activated macrophages for malignant cells in vitro, Br. J. Cancer, 38:653-659 (1978).
164. Currie, G. A., Gyure, L., and Cifuentes, L., Microenvironmental arginine depletion by macrophages in vitro, Br. J. Cancer, 39:613-629 (1979).
165. Holcenberg, J. S., Enzyme therapy: problems and solutions, Ann. Rev. Biochem., 51:795-812 (1982).
166. Li, D. M., The lack of beta-adrenoreceptor involvement in the cardiac action of delta-1-tetrahydrocannabinol in rats, Clin. Exp. Pharmacol. Physiol., 7:23-29 (1980).
167. Choisy, H., Choisy, G., Millart, H., and Legris, H., Influence of delta-9-tetrahydrocannabinol on contraction rate and enzymatic activity of embryonic heart cells, Adv. Biosci., 22-23:265-277 (1979).
168. Mornet, D. Pantal, P., Audemard, E., and Kassab, R., Involvement of an arginine residue in the catalytic activity of myosin heads, Eur. J. Biochem., 100:421-431, (1979).
169. Johnson, P., and Blazyk, J. M., Involvement of an arginine residue of actin in tropomyosin binding, Biochem. Biophys. Res. Commun., 82:1013-1018 (1978).
170. Petro, D. J., and Ellenberger, Jr., C., Treatment of human spasticity with delta-9-tetrahydrocannabinol, J. Clin. Pharmacol., 21:413S-416S (1981).
171. Malec, J., Harvey, R. F., and Cayner, J. J., Cannabis effect on spasticity in spinal cord injury, Arch. Phys. Med. Rehabil. 63:116-118 (1982).

172. Narayanareddy, K., and Swami, K. S., Free aminoacid composition in the denervation atrophy of gastronemius muscle of the frog Rana hexadactyla, Indian J. Exp. Biol., 13:343-345 (1975).
173. Smith, I., The treatment of inborn errors of the urea cycle, Nature (Lond.), 291:38-380 (1981).
174. Snyderman, S. E., Sansaricq, C., Norton, P. M., and Goldstein, F., Argininemia treated from birth, J. Pediatr., 95:61-63 (1979).
175. Ghoneim, M. Th., Mikhal, M. M., Mahfouz, M., and Makar, A. B., Effect of hashish smoke on some blood and serum parameters in rabbits, Pharmazie, 35:226-228 (1980).
176. Visek, W. J., Ammonia metabolism, urea cycle capacity and their biochemical assessment, Nutr. Rev., 37:273-282 (1979).
177. Rosenkrantz, H., Cannabis marihuana and cannabinoid toxicological manifestations in man and animals, in "Adverse Health and Behavioral Consequences of Cannabis Use. Working Papers for the ARF/WHO Scientific Meeting, Toronto, 1981", (K. O. Fehr and H. Kalant, eds.), Addiction Research Foundation, Toronto, 1982.
178. Wergedal, J. E., and Harper, A. E., Metabolic adaptations in higher animals IX. Effect of high protein intake on amino acid nitrogen catabolism in vivo, J. Biol. Chem., 239:1156-1163 (1964).
179. Poddar, M. K., and Dewey, W. L., Effects of cannabinoids on catecholamine uptake and release in hypothalamic and striatal synaptosomes, J. Pharmacol. Exp. Ther., 214:63-67 (1980).
180. Fehr, K. O., and Kalant, H., Long-term effects of cannabis on cerebral function: A review of the clinical and experimental literature, in "Adverse Health and Behavioral Consequences of Cannabis Use. Working Papers for ARF/WHO Scientific Meeting, Toronto, 1981" (K. O. Fehr and H. Kalant, eds.), Addiction Research Foundation, Toronto, 1982.
181. Domino, E. F., Cannabinoids and the cholinergic system, J. Clin. Pharmacol., 21:2496-2556 (1981).
182. Ferraro, D. P., Acute effects of marihuana on human memory and cognition, in "Marihuana Research Findngs: 1980" (R.C. Peterson, ed.) pp. 98-119. NIDA Research Monograph 31, Department of Health and Human Services, NIDA, Rockville, MD, 1980.
183. Miller, L. L., Cannabis and the brain with special reference to the limbic system, Adv. Biosci., 22 & 23:539-566 (1979).
184. Rose, F. C., and Symonds, C. P., Persistant memory defect following encephalitis, Brain, 83:195-211.

185. Drachman, D. A., and Adams, R. D., Herpes Simplex and acute inclusion body encephalitis, Arch. Neurol., 7:61-79 (1962).
186. Brown, H., Some anticholinergic-like behavioral effects of trans (-)-delta 8-THC, Psychopharmacologia, 21:294-301 (1971).
187. Mautner, H. G., Pakula, A. A., and Merrill, R. E., Evidence for presence of an arginine residue in the coenzyme A binding site of choline acetyltransferase, Proc. Natl. Acad. Sci. USA 78:7449-7452 (1981).
188. Franks, D. J., Tunnicliff, G., and Ngo, T. T., Inactivation of adenylate cyclase by phenylglyoxal and other dicarbonyls. Evidence for the existence of essential arginyl residues, Biochem. Biophys. Acta., 611:358-362 (1980).
189. Tunnicliff, G., and Ngo, T. T., Involvement of arginyl residues in catalytic activity of catechol-O-methyltransferase, Gen. Pharmacol. 10:373-376 (1979).
190. Moszik, G., Some feedback mechanisms by drugs in the inter-relationship between the active transport system andadenyl cyclase system localized in the cell membrane, Eur. J. Pharmacol., 7:319-327 (1969).
191. Thoa, N. B., Wooten, G. R., Axelrod, J., and Kopin I. J., Inhibition of release of dopamine-beta-hydroxylase and norepinephrine from sympathetic nerves by colchicine, vinblastine, or cytochalasin-B, Proc. Natl. Acad. Sci. USA, 69:520-522 (1972).
192. Tunnicliff, G., and Ngo, T. T., Functional role of arginine residues in glutamic acid decarboxylase from brain and bacteria, Experientia, 34:989-900 (1978).
193. Tunnicliff, G., Essential arginine residue at the pyridoxal phosphate binding site of brain gamma-aminobutyrate aminotransferase, Biochem. Biophys. Res. Commun., 97:160-165 (1980).
194. Roberts, E., Prospectus. Epilepsy and antiepileptic drugs: A speculative synthesis, in "Antiepileptic Drugs: Mechanisms of Action" (G. H. Glaser, J. K. Penry and D. M. Woodbury, eds.) pp. 667-713. Raven Press, New York, 1980.
195. Stone, W. E., Action of convulsants: Neurochemical aspects, in "Basic Mechanisms of the Epilepsies" (H. H. Jasper, A. A. Ward, and A. Pope, eds.) pp. 184-193, Little Brown and Co., Boston, 1969.
196. Liebl, L., Convulsant action of hydraine:impairment of chloride-dependent inhibition in cat spinal motor neurons, Exp. Brain Res., (Suppl.) 23:125 (1975).
197. Karler, R., and Turkanis, S. A., Cannabis and epilepsy, Adv. Biosci., 22 & 23:619-641 (1979).

198. Feeney, D. M., Marihuana and epilepsy: paradoxical anti-convulsant and convulsant effects, Adv. Biosci., 22 & 23:643-657 (1979).
199. Roberts, E., Simonsen, D. G., and Roberts, E., Structural requirements of nitrogenous substances which have protective effects against acute hydrazine toxicity in mice, Proc. Soc. Exp. Biol. Med., 119:683-687 (1965).
200. Pisano, J. J., and Udenfriend, S., Formation of gamma-guanidino-butyric acid and guanidinoacetic acids in brain, Fed. Proc., 17:403 (1958).
201. Purpura, D., Girado, M., and Grundrest, H., Central synaptic effects of omega-guanidino acids and amino acid derivatives, Science, 127:1179-1181 (1958).
202. Jinnai, D., Sawai, A., and Mori, A., gamma-guanidinobutyric acid as a convulsive substance, Nature (Lond.), 212:617 (1966).
203. Edery, H., and Gottesfeld, Z., The gamma-aminobutyric acid system in rat cerebellum during cannabinoid-induced cataleptoid state, Br. J. Pharmacol., 194:74-81 (1975).
204. Curtis, D. R., and Watkins, J. C., The excitation and depression of spinal neurons by structurally related amino acids, J. Neurochem., 6:117-141 (1960).
205. Watkins, J. C., Pharmacological receptors and general permeability phenomena of cell membranes, J. Theoret. Biol., 9:37059 (1965).
206. Giambalvo, C. T., and Rosenberg, P., The effect of phospholipases and proteases on the binding of gamma-aminobutyric acid to junctional complexes of rat cerebellum, Biochem. Biophys. Acta., 436:741-756 (1976).

TRIGLYCERIDE/PHOSPHOLIPID PARTITIONING AND PHARMACOKINETICS OF SOME NATURAL AND SEMI-SYNTHETIC CANNABINOIDS: FURTHER EVIDENCE FOR THE INVOLVEMENT OF SPECIFIC RECEPTORS IN THE MEDIATION OF THE PSYCHOTROPIC EFFECTS OF DELTA-1-THC AND DELTA-6-THC

M. Binder, F.-J. Witteler
B. Schmidt, I. Franke

Institut fur Physiologische Chemie
der Ruhr-Universitat
Bochum, Germany

E. Bohnenberger
H. Sandermann, Jr.

Biologisches Institute II
der Universitat Freiburg
Freiburg, Germany

I. INTRODUCTION

Three hypotheses are discussed to explain the molecular mechanism of action of the psychotropic cannabinoids (3R,4R)-delta-1-tetrahydrocannabinol[1] (8, 1-THC) and (3R,4R)-delta-1(6)-tetrahydrocannabinol (9, 6-THC):

First, 1-THC (the same holds for 6-THC) might interact with the lipid phase of the neuronal membrane (1).

Second, 1-THC might act on one or several of the known neurotransmitter/receptor systems (2,3).

---

[1]The biogenetic nomenclature is used throughout this paper. 1-THC corresponds to delta-9-THC of the IUPAC nomenclature, 6-THC = delta-8-THC, 7-THC = delta-9(11)-THC.

ISBN 0-12-044620-0

Third, 1-THC might interact with a specific receptor of its own, implicating thus the existence of a physiological, i.e., endogenous THC agonist (4,5).

Careful evaluation of the experimental data gathered so far leads us to favor the third hypothesis (6).

In order to solve the question of the mechanism of action of 1-THC, specific molecular tools like THC antagonists or model compounds are required. While synthetic chemistry so far has failed to produce a THC antagonist, (3R,4R)-delta-1(7)-tetrahydrocannabinol (6, 7-THC),a semi-synthetic isomer of 1-THC has been proposed as a suitable model compound to differentiate between specific, receptor-mediated and nonspecific, lipophilicity-mediated effects of 1-THC (7). In the rhesus monkey, 7-THC in doses up to 5 mg/kg, which is 100 times the dose of 1-THC required to elicit behavioral changes, is devoid of psychotropic activity. The compound neither synergizes nor antagonizes the effects of 1-THC. Since 7-THC closely resembles 1-THC in structure, stereochemistry and physico-chemical properties, it was argued that this lack of psychotropic activity was due to the inability of the molecule to bind to the postulated THC receptor. In 7-THC, C(7) of the exocyclic methylidene group comes closer to the plane of the aromatic ring than C(7) of the corresponding methyl group of 1-THC. Thus by van der Waals contact to the receptor surface the formation of a hydrogen bond via the phenolic hydroxyl group, which we believe to be the key event in the binding of 1-THC to the receptor, is prevented. The stereochemical difference between 1-THC and 7-THC is illustrated in Fig. 1.

Alternative explanations for the psychotropic inactivity of 7-THC were suggested:

First, 7-THC could be metabolized, or, Second, excreted too quickly to compete with the potent 1-THC. Third, 7-THC might differ greatly in membrane affinity from 1-THC and 6-THC and thus not reach the receptor site.

The first question was answered by incubating 7-THC with a rat liver microsomal preparation and the isolation and identification of 20 metabolites have been reported (8). Compared to 1-THC, 7-THC is metabolized following essentially the same routes (i.e., allylic and aliphatic hydroxylation, epoxidation, etc.) but to a lower extent, the total amount of metabolites accounting only for 1/10 of those observed with 1-THC. This excludes the possibility that the inactivity of 7-THC is caused by rapid metabolism of the compound. Two independent studies on the *in vivo* metabolism of 7-THC in the mouse (9,10) gave similar results. To answer the questions of rapid excretion, i.e., pharmacokinetics and membrane affinity of 7-THC, 1-, 6- and 7-THC were synthesized in ^{14}C-labelled form. Brain levels were studied in the mouse and are expressed in % of the

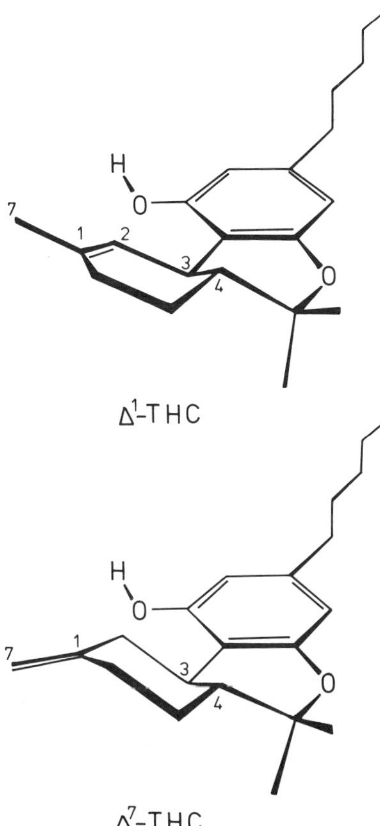

FIGURE 1. Steric formulae of 1-THC 8 and 7-THC 6 (adapted from ref. 6).

total of radioactivity administered. No corrections were made for the contribution of metabolites.

Since the usual water/octanol partitioning coefficients give only indications on the general lipophilicity of cannabinoids (which should not be confused with membrane affinity) we have employed a recently developed technique to measure the *in vitro* triglyceride/phospholipid partitioning of 1-, 6- and 7-THC (11). Though this system does not take into account transport phenomena across the blood/brain barrier, the results may be interpreted as a good approximation of membrane affinity vs adipose tissue solubility. Both, pharmacokinetics and triglyceride/phospholipid partitioning of 7-THC in regard to 1- and 6-THC should be seen as complementing each other and, therefore, are reported together. The *in vivo* and the *in* vitro experiment give a good indication concerning the actual distribution and membrane affinity of 7-THC, i.e., its concentration and availability at the site of the putative receptor.

Two novel cannabinoid model compounds, (3R,4R)-4"-carbomethoxy-delta-6-THC (15) and (3R,4R)-4"-methyl-delta-6-THC-5"-oic acid (16), synthesized as potential receptor probes (12,13) were included in both investigations. Pharmacokinetics and triglyceride/phospholipid partitioning are discussed with special regard to the THC receptor concept and to the role of 7-THC as a useful tool for THC receptor research.

II. MATERIALS AND METHODS

A. Syntheses of Radiolabelled Cannabinoids

1. [7-^{14}C]-1-, -6-, and -7-THC. The synthesis of [7-^{14}C]-1-THC, -6-THC, and -7-THC are summarized in Scheme I.

7-THC (2), obtained by photoisomerisation of 6-THC (1) was treated with CH_3I in dimethylformamide in the presence of K_2CO_3 to give methyl ether 3. In modifying the procedure of Nilsson et al. (14), 3 was reacted with OsO_4 in pyridine followed by addition of H_5IO_6 (15). Condensation of ketone 4 with [^{14}C]-methyl-triphenylphosphonium iodide (250 mcCi,0.38 mCi/mmol, NEN) in tetrahydrofuran in the presence of butyllithium yielded [7-^{14}C]-7-THC methyl ether 5 which was demethylated using potassium thiophenolate (15) to give [7-^{14}C]-7-THC (6) (0.29 mCi/mmol) in 7.4% yield calc. on 6-THC. Following the procedure of Petrazilka et al. (16), part of 6 was converted via the chloro compound 7 to [7-^{14}C]-1-THC (8) (0.34 mCi/mmol) and [7-^{14}C]-6-THC (9) (0.26 mCi/mmol). Compounds 6, 8 and 9 were stored in ethanol in the dark at -20°C.

2. [1",2"-^{3}H]-4"-Carbomethoxy-6-THC 15 and [1",2"-^{3}H]-4"-methyl-6-THC-5"-oic acid 16. The syntheses of compounds 15 and 16 are summarized in Scheme 2.

3,5-Bis(benzyloxy)benzaldehyde (10) was condensed with the triphenylphosphonium/salt 11 in dimethylformamide in the presence of potassium 2-methyl-2-butanolate to give the Wittig adduct 12, which was tritiated with 7.5 Ci T_2 in H_2 over Pd/C in ethyl acetate (NEN Tritiation Service). The substituted resorcinol 4 (2.5 Ci, 3.87 Ci/mmol) was reacted with p-menthadienol 13 (Firmenich) yielding [1",2"-^{3}H]-4"carbomethoxy-6-THC (15) (6.3% calc. on 10; spec. act. 2.46 Ci/mmol), part of which was hydrolyzed as described (12) to give acid 16. Ester 15 was stored in methanol at -20°C, acid 16 in benzene at 5°C in the dark.

B. Triglyceride/Phospholipid Partitioning

Egg phosphatidylcholine (Sigma) (3800 nmol in 30 mcl ethanol) and glycerol trioleate (Roth) 4170 nmol in 30 mcl hexane) was introduced in a 1 ml ultracentrifuge tube (Beckmann No. 354708). The following amounts of [7-^{14}C]-1-THC, [7-^{14}C]-6-THC, and [7-^{14}C]-7-THC, resp., were added to ethanolic solution (total radioactivity in parentheses): 12.6 nmol (9300 dpm 8, 7300 dpm 9, 8160 dpm 6); 38 nmol; 69 nmol; 131 nmol (each 28800 dpm 8, 222700 dpm 9 and 24500 dpm 6, resp.). Compound 15 added in amounts of 10.2 nmol (2.0 x 10^5 dpm), 25.5, 51.5, 77.5 and 103.3 nmol (4.85 x 10^5 dpm each), compound 16 in amounts of 10.6 nmol (2.0 x 10^5 dpm), 31.8, 54.5, 82.5 and 110.5 nmol (6 x 10^5 dpm each). Solvents were removed under N_2, 300 mcl of potassium phosphate buffer (0.1 mol/l, pH 6.6) and 200 mcl H_2O were added and the lipid film was dispersed by vibrating for 30 sec on a Vortex mixer. The sample was then shaken for 12 h at 25°C (in a water bath). After addition of 400 mcl H_2O and vibrating for 30 sec on the Vortex, the sample was centrifuged at 85000 x g at 20°C for 20 h. The tube was frozen in liquid nitrogen and cut into 5 slices. The radioactivity associated with each slice was assayed by liquid scintillation counting in 5 ml Rotiscint (Roth) containing 200 mcl H_2O.

C. Pharmacokinetics

Male HAN-NMRI mice (18-22 g) were obtained from the Zentral-institut fur Versuchstiere, Hannover.

Stock solutions of the labelled cannabinoids were prepared in poly-ethylene glycol/H_2O 4:1 (v/v) to give the following concentrations: [7-^{14}C]-1-THC, 2.06 mmol/l; [7-^{14}C]-6-THC (8), 2.89 mmol/l; [7-^{14}C]-7-THC (6), 3.5 mmol/l; [1",2"-^{3}H]4"-carbomethoxy-6-THC (15) 1.7 mmol/l; [1",2"-^{3}H]-4"-methyl-6-THC-5-oic acid (16), 2.29 mmol/l. All compounds were injected via the tail vein (Injection vol. 100 mcl; total amounts injected: 8, 64.8 mcg = 206 nmol = 154200 dpm; 9, 90.7 mcg = 289 nmol = 171400 dpm; 6, 111.7 mcg = 355 nmol = 228500 dpm; 15, 66.1 mcg = 177 nmol = 3436000 dpm; 16, 82.0 mcg = 229 nmol = 4440000 dpm). Animals were sacrificed after 5, 15, 30, 45, 60 and 120 min., resp., by cervical fracture and perfused with 30 ml 0.9% NaCl solution. Total brains removed, rinsed with NaCl solution, dried on filter paper and weighed. Following the method of Ohlsson et al. (17), each brain was digested in 4.0 ml tissue solubilizer (TS-1, Zinsser) at 50°C for 20 h and bleached after addition of 0.8 ml of 2-propanol and 0.8 ml of

Δ^6-THC **1**

$h\cdot\nu$

2

CH_3I/K_2CO_3

3

1. OsO_4
2. H_5IO_6

4

$\varphi_3P{=}\overset{\blacktriangle}{C}H_2$

5

φS^-K^+

$[7\text{-}^{14}C]\text{-}\Delta^7$-THC **6**

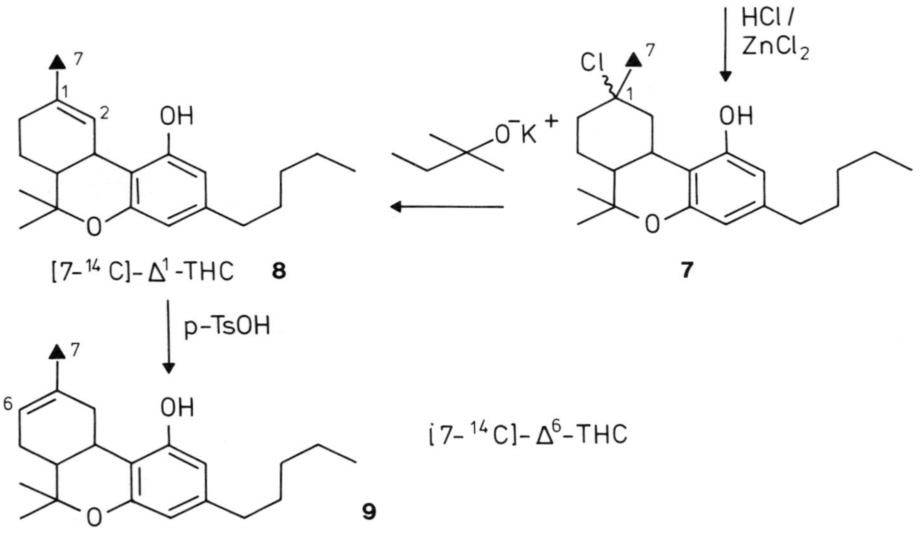

$HCl/ZnCl_2$

7

$[7-^{14}C]-\Delta^1$-THC **8**

p-TsOH

$[7-^{14}C]-\Delta^6$-THC **9**

SCHEME 1

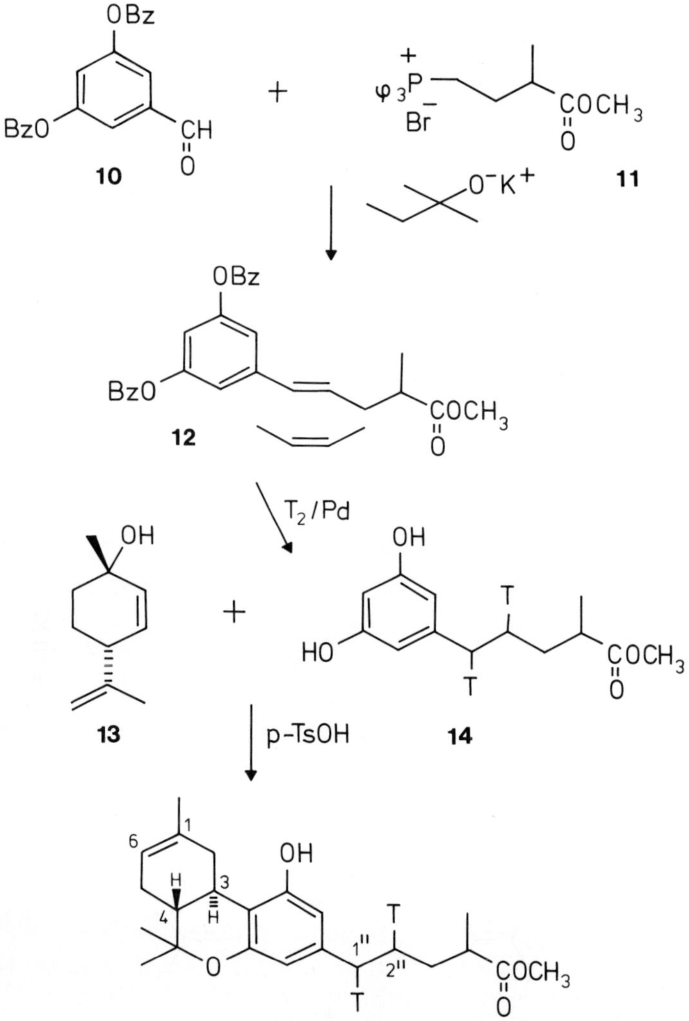

SCHEME 2

30% H_2O_2 at 40^oC for 30 min. Radioactivity was determined by counting samples of 1.0 ml in 10 ml Unisolve 1 (Zinsser); ^{14}C-samples were assayed shortly after addition of the scintillation cocktail, in case of the ^3H-samples strong chemoluminescence was observed and counting had to be repeated after 24, 48 and 96 hr. All values are corrected for quenching and counting efficiency.

III. RESULTS

A. Triglyceride/Phospholipid Partitioning

During the centrifugation of the partitioning mixture, glycerol trioleate accumulates at the top of the centrifuge tube, phosphatidyl choline at the bottom corresponding to slices No.1 and 5, resp. Due to the mutual solubility of the lipids the glycerol trioleate phase contains 150 nmol phosphatidyl choline, while the phosphatidyl choline phase contains 100 nmol glycerol trioleate leading to a total amount of 4220 nmol lipid in slice 1 and 3750 nmol lipid in slice 5. Based on these figures, the partitioning coefficients of the cannabinoids are expressed as mole fractions:

$K_{\text{glycerol } \underline{\text{tri}}\text{oleate}/\underline{\text{p}}\text{hosphatidyl } \underline{\text{c}}\text{holine}}$ ($K_{TRI/PC}$).

Figure 2 gives the results of the cannabinoid partitioning for all five compounds in % radioactivity per slice of total radioactivity added to each tube and the table summarizes the mole fractions.

Within the employed range the mole fractions are independent of concentration for all cannabinoids tested. This is illustrated in Fig. 3 where the $K_{TRI/PC}$ values for 7-THC and 4"-methyl-6-THC-5"-oic acid (<u>16</u>) are plotted vs their concentration.

With the exception of acid <u>16</u> the amount of cannabinoids in the aqueous zones (slices No. 2-4) is negligible. 1-THC (<u>8</u>) distributes almost equally between the two lipids ($K_{TRI/PC}$ = 0.88); 6-THC (<u>9</u>) and 7-THC (<u>6</u>) behave identically in showing a slight preference for the glycerol trioleate phase [$K_{TRI/PC}$ (<u>9</u>) = 1.4; $K_{TRI/PC}$ (<u>6</u>) = 1.3]. Ester <u>15</u> ($K_{TRI/PC}$ = 0.4) is found mostly in the phosphatidyl choline phase and acid <u>16</u> ($K_{TRI/PC}$ = 0.03) almost exclusively associates with the phospholipid.

B. Pharmacokinetics

Results are expressed in total brain radioactivity in % of the injected dose. Each value is averaged from six animals and corrections were made for deviations of single brain weights from the average brain weight of group. Figure 4 gives the total brain cannabinoid concentrations (including

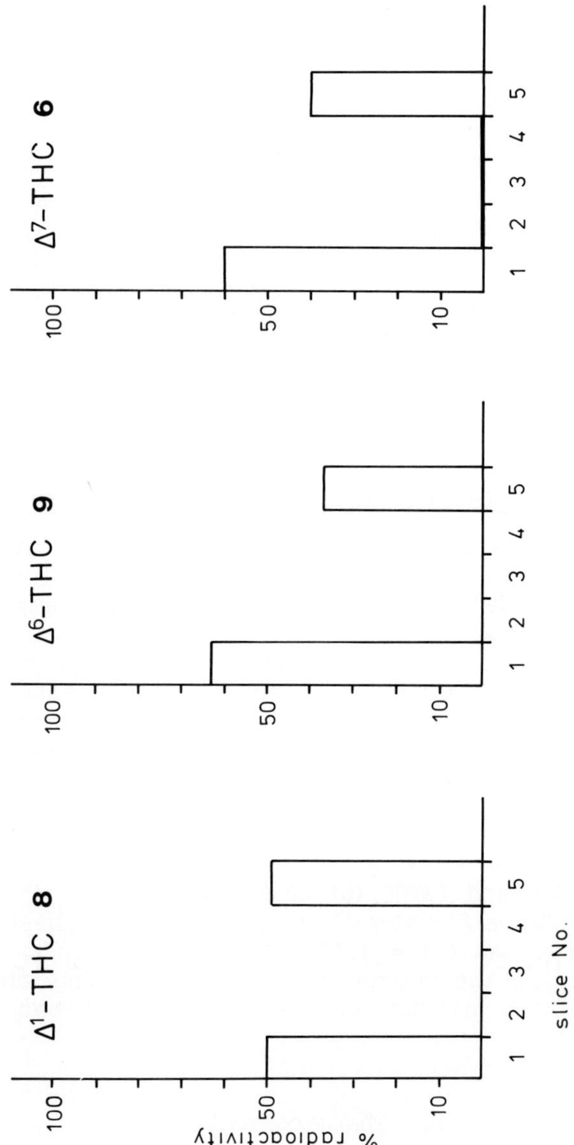

Δ^1-THC 8
Δ^6-THC 9
Δ^7-THC 6
% radioactivity
100
50
10
slice No.
1
2
3
4
5

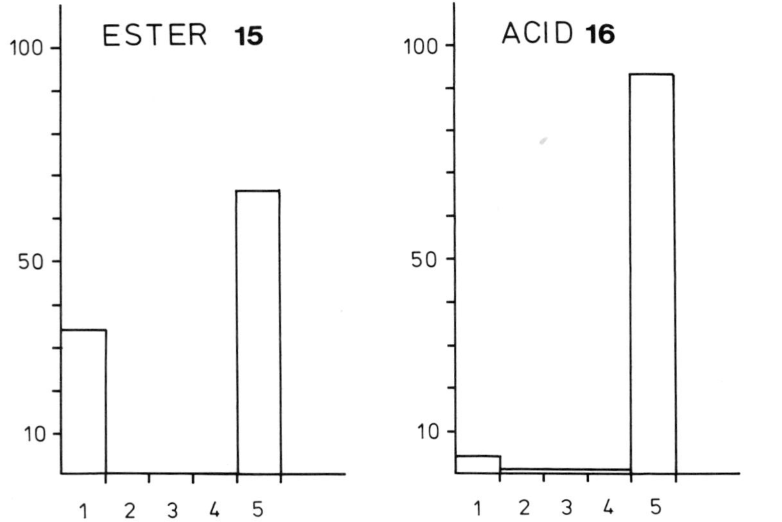

FIGURE 2. Distribution of radioactivity in the partitioning procedure. Values are plotted in % of total radioactivity vs slice number.

TABLE I. $K_{TRI/PC}$ Values

Conc. [nmol]	1-THC <u>8</u>	6-THC <u>9</u>	7-THC <u>6</u>	ESTER <u>15</u>	ACID <u>15</u>
10.2				0.52 0.57	
10.6					0.037 0.038
12.6	0.88 0.85	1.33 1.10	1.22 1.10		
25.5				0.47 0.36	
31.8					0.034 0.031
38.0	0.94 1.08	1.40 1.60	1.10 1.50		
51.5				0.42	
54.5					0.039 0.040
69.0	0.88 0.85	1.30	1.37		
77.5				0.48 0.38	
82.5					0.046
103.3				0.41 0.43	
110.5					0.028 0.030
131.0	0.71 0.88	1.40 1.60	1.30 1.30		

potential metabolites) and the lowest and highest value of each group.

Owing to the small amounts of cannabinoids reaching the brain (less than 1 mcg for 1-THC, 6-THC, and 7-THC and 0.4 mcg for ester <u>15</u> and acid <u>16</u>) no attempt was made to identify the radioactive material present in the brain or to differentiate between the original cannabinoids and their metabolites.

With 1-THC (<u>B</u>), 6-THC (<u>9</u>), and 7-THC (<u>6</u>), a rapid initial increase in brain radioactivity is observed. Peak concentrations are reached between 5 and 30 min (15 min values: 0.75%, 0.89% and 1.16% for <u>8</u>, <u>9</u> and <u>6</u>, resp.) followed by a decrease to 0.4-0.5% at 60 min and 0.2% at the end of the observation

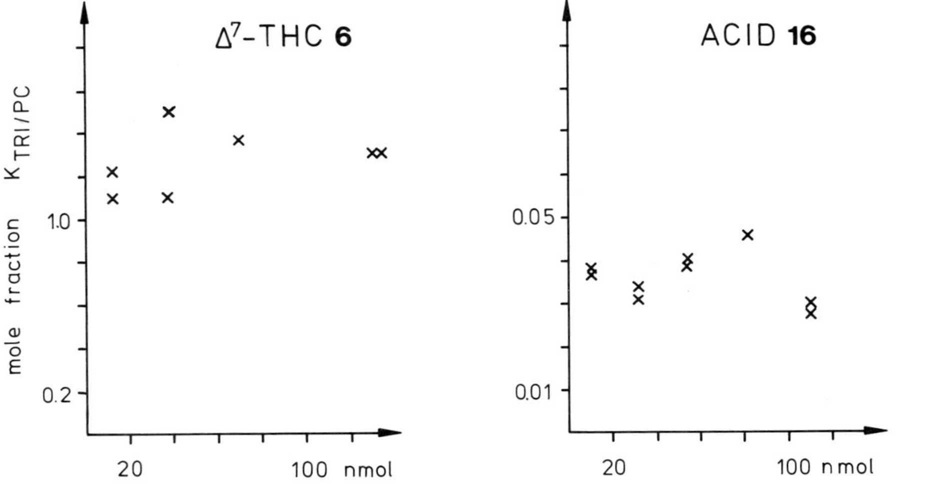

FIGURE 3. $K_{TRI/PC}$ values of 7-THC (<u>6</u>) and acid <u>16</u> at different concentrations.

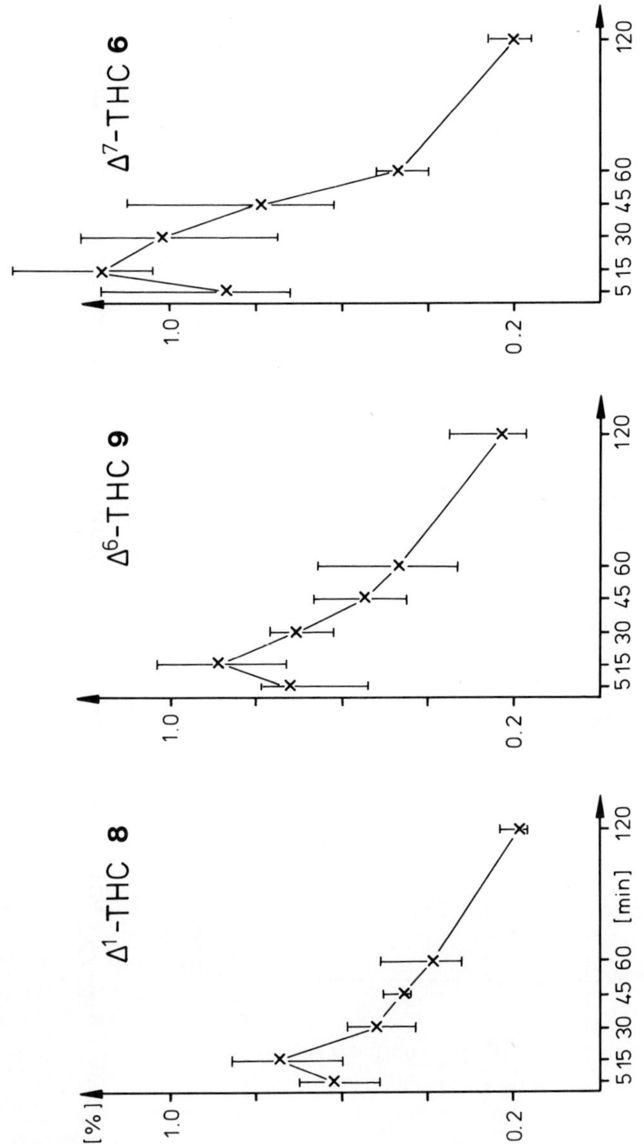

[%]
1.0
0.2
Δ1-THC 8
Δ6-THC 9
Δ7-THC 6
5 15 30 45 60
[min]
120

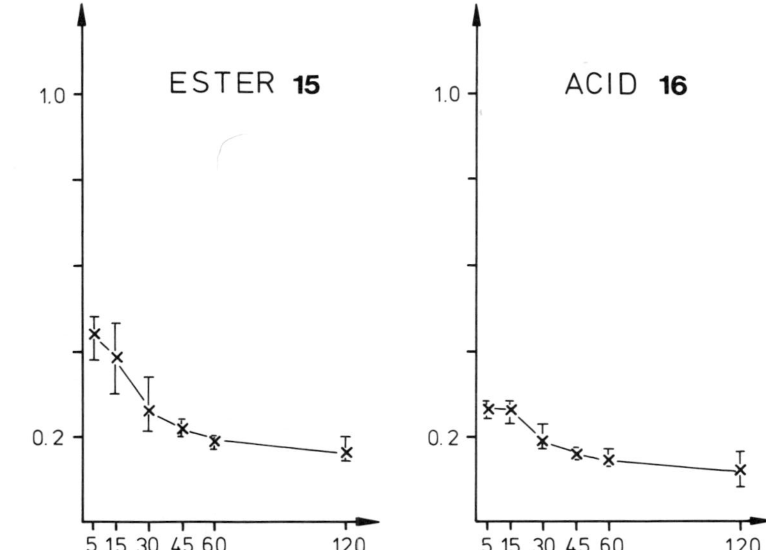

FIGURE 4. Brain levels of cannabinoids in % of total radioactivity administered. All values are averaged from 6 determinations. The highest and lowest values of each group are indicated.

period of 9120 min). All three cannabinoids exhibit remarkably similar pharmacokinetics. With ester 15 and acid 16 peak concentrations of 0.44 and 0.26% are reached within 5 min followed by a slow decrease to 0.19 and 0.14% at 60 min and 0.16 and 0.12% at 120 min. The similarity of the pharmacokinetics of compounds 15 and 16 is remarkable and will be discussed below.

IV. DISCUSSION

In order to be behaviorally active, a cannabinoid or cannabinoid-model compound must meet several conditions. First, it must penetrate the blood/brain barrier and, second, according to our hypothesis, it must exhibit affinity to the postulated receptor. From a study on the pharmacokinetics of 6-THC and several of its mono-oxygenated metabolites, Ohlsson et al. concluded, that psychotropic activity depends on the structure rather than on the pharmacodynamic properties of a given cannabinoid (17). After reaching the brain, a further requisite for psychotropic activity is the availability of the cannabinoid at the site of the putative receptor, i.e., its affinity to the neuronal membrane. It seems reasonable to postulate that a cannabinoid that reaches the brain and the neuronal membrane to the same extent as the active cannabinoids 1- and 6-THC and yet is psychotropically inactive, simply does not fit to the receptor. The objective of this investigation was to determine whether the model compound 7-THC (and ester 15 and acid 16) actually enters the brain and to compare its membrane affinity to 1- and 6-THC. Since it is difficult to measure *in vivo* membrane affinities, usually octanol/water partitioning coefficients are estimated (1,17). These coefficients, however, refer to the distribution of cannabinoids between water and an organic phase and do not differentiate between the "organic" phases available in a physiological environment, i.e., adipose tissue and membrane lipids. The partitioning procedure employed in this experiment gives information on the distribution of cannabinoids between atriglyceride, phospholipid and an aqueous phase simultaneously.

The $K_{TRI/PC}$ values should not be interpreted as absolute figures but should be seen as an indication to which extent the individual cannabinoids in relation to each other, after reaching the brain, will associate with membrane lipids. A combination of the brain levels of the cannabinoids and their $K_{TRI/PC}$ values gives their availability at the receptor site.

Brain levels of cannabinoids have been reported for 7-OH-1-THC (1), 1-THC and 7-OH-1-THC (18), 1-THC, 6-THC and 7-OH-6-

THC (19), 6-THC and seven mono-oxygenated metabolites (17) and 6-THC (20).

In our experiments 1-THC, 6-THC, and 7-THC behave very similar. Within experimental errors all three compounds reach the same brain levels and show a similar time curve for the decrease in brain radioactivity. There is an indication that 7-THC penetrates the blood/brain barrier slightly better than 1- and 6-THC but this finding is not statistically significant. This similarity holds for the triglyceride/phospholipid partitioning, where 7-THC behaves identically to 6-THC, both exhibiting a somewhat higher affinity over 1-THC for the triglyceride phase. Speculatively, the lower psychotropic activity of 6-THC compared to 1-THC (21) (6-THC is about 2/3 as potent as 1-THC) could be understood in terms of its lower affinity to the phospholipid phase, as reflected by the $K_{TRI/PC}$ values of 1.3 for 6-THC and 0.88 for 1-THC.

The fact, that 7-THC in both systems behaves identically to 6-THC, strongly indicates that the psychotropic inactivity of 7-THC can not be due to its pharmacodynamic properties or unspecific membrane effects, but must have a structural basis. This may be taken as further evidence for the THC receptor hypothesis. Simultaneously, the membrane hypothesis that was discussed initially is rendered highly improbable.

Since ester 15 and acid 16 are suited structurally for polar interactions both exhibit a markedly strong preference for the phospholipid phase, which is reflected in $K_{TRI/PC}$ values of 0.4 and 0.03. In spite of the difference in $K_{TRI/PC}$, brain levels and time curves of both compounds are very similar. In fact, the brain level curve for ester 15 may be a superposition of ester 15 and acid 16 since the ester is subject to rapid enzymatic hydrolysis.

V. CONCLUSION

We have demonstrated that the psychotropically inactive cannabinoid 7-THC exhibits essentially the same pharmacodynamic properties and phospholipid affinity as the psychotropically active compounds 1-THC and 6-THC. These observations support our view, that the molecular mechanism of action of 1-THC and 6-THC is not related to interactions with the lipid phase of the neuronal membrane but rather to interactions with a specific THC receptor.

ACKNOWLEDGMENTS

The syntheses of radiolabelled cannabinoids and the pharmacokinetic work was supported by a grant from the Deutsche Forschungsgemein-schaft which is gratefully acknowledged. The partitioning studies were supported by SFB 46, Freiburg.

REFERENCES

1. Gill, E. W., Jones, G., and Lawrence, D. K., Contribution of the metabolite 7-hydroxy-delta-tetrahydrocannabinol towards the pharmacological activity of delta-1-tetrahydrocannabinol in mice, Biochem. Pharmacol. 22:175-184 (1973).
2. Hershkowitz, M., and Szechtman, H., Pretreatment with delta-1-THC and psychoactive drugs: effects on uptake of biogenic amines on behaviour, Eur. J. Pharm. 59:267-276 (1979).
3. Poddar, M. K., and Dewey, W. L., Effects of cannabinoids on catecholamine uptake and release in hypothalamic and striatal synaptosomes, J. Pharm. Exp. Ther. 214:63-67 (1980).
4. Edery, H., Grunfeld, Y., Ben-Zvi, Z. and Mechoulam, R., Structural requirements for cannabinoid activity, Ann. N. Y. Acad. Sci. 191:40-53 (1971).
5. Binder, M., New psychotropic metabolites of delta-1-THC formed by microbial fermentation, Paper presented at the Conference on Psychotropic Drug Action with Special Reference to Cannabinoids, Arad, Israel, 1977.
6. Binder, M., and Franke, I., Is there a THC-Receptor? in: "Neuroreceptors". (F. Hucho, ed.), p.151. Walter de Gruyter, Berlin and New York, 1982.
7. Binder, M., Edery, H., and Porath, G., delta-7-tetrahydrocannabinol, a non-psychotropic cannabinoid: Structure-activity considerations in the cannabinoid series, in "Marijuana: Biological Effects", (G. G. Nahas and W. D. M. Paton, eds.), p. 71. Pergamon Press, Oxford and New York, 1979.
8. Binder, M., and Barlage, U., Metabolic transformation of (3R,4R)-delta-1-tetrahydrocannabinol by a rat liver microsomal preparation, Helv. Chim. Acta 63:255-267 (1980).
9. Harvey, D. J., Paton, W. D. M., The metabolism of deuterium-labelled analogues of delta-1-, delta-6-, and delta-7-THC and the use of deuterium labelling, Recent Dev. Mass. Spectrom. Biochem. Med. 2:127-147 (1979).

10. Harvey, D. J., Gill, E. W., Slater, M., Paton, W. D. M., Identification of the In vivo liver metabolites of (-)-delta-7-THC produced by the Mouse, Drug Metab. Dispos. 8:439-445 (1980).
11. Sandermann, Jr., H., Triglyceride/phospholipid partitioning and persistence of environmental chemicals, Chemosphere 8:499-508 (1979).
12. Franke, I., and Binder, M., Synthesis of cannabinoid model compounds, Part 2: (3R,4R)-delta-1(6)-tetrahydrocannabinol-5"-oic acid and 4"(R,S)-methyl-(3R,4R)-delta-1(6)-tetrahydrocannabinol-5"-oic acid, Helv. Chim. Acta 63:2508-2514 (1980).
13. Binder, M., and Franke, I., Synthese von cannabinoiden modellverbindungen, Paper presented at the Chemiedozenten-Tagung, Tubingen, Germany, 1981.
14. Nilsson, J. L. G., Nilsson, I. M., Agurell, S., Akermark, B., and Lagerlund, I., Metabolism of cannabis XI. Synthesis of delta-7-THC and 7-OH-THC, Acta Chem. Scand. 25:768-769 (1971).
15. Wildes, J. W., Martin, N. H., Pitt C. G., and Wall, M. E., The synthesis of (-)-delta-9(11)-trans-tetrahydrocannabinol, J. Org. Chem. 26:721-723 (1971).
16. Petrzilka, T., Haefliger, W., and Sikemeier, C., Synthese von Haschisch-Inhaltsstoffen (4. Mitteilung), Helv. Chim. Acta 52:1102-1134 (1969).
17. Ohlsson, A., Widman, M., Carlsson, S., Ryman, T., and Strid, C., Plasma and brain levels of delta-6-THC and seven mono-oxygenated metabolites correlated to the cataleptic effect in the mouse, Acta pharmacol. et toxicol. 47:308-317 (1980).
18. Ford, R. D., Balster, R. L. Dewey, W. L., and Beckner, J. S., Delta-9-THC and 11-OH-delta-9-THC: behavioural effects and relationship to plasma and brain levels, Life Sci. 20:1993-2004 (1977).
19. Ho, B. T., Estevez, V. S., and Engler, L. F., The uptake and metabolic fate of cannabinoids in rat brains, J. Pharm. Pharmacol. 25:488-490 (1973).
20. Nahas, G. G., Leger, C., Tocque, B., and Hoellinger, H. The kinetics of cannabinoid distribution and storage with special reference to the brain and testis, J. Clin. Pharmacol. 21:208S-214S (1981).
21. Mechoulam R., and Edery, H., Structure-activity relationship in the cannabinoid series in "Marijuana: Chemistry, Pharmacology, Metabolism and Clinical Effects", (R. Mechoulam, ed.) p. 101. Academic Press, New York, 1973.

THE ROLE OF PROSTAGLANDINS IN THE ACTIONS OF THE CANNABINOIDS

Sumner Burstein
Sheila A. Hunter

Department of Biochemistry
University of Massachusetts Medical School
Worcester, Massachusetts

I. INTRODUCTION

The molecular events surrounding the interactions of cannabinoids with various tissues remain ill-defined despite more than a decade of intense activity by many investigators. A number of hypotheses have arisen during this period (1), however, many of the observed pharmacological effects of the cannabinoids still are lacking a molecular model. Several of the proposed sites of action involve membrane-bound enzymes and it has been suggested that the cannabinoids exert their effects by changing the nature of the lipid environment surrounding these enyzmes. Data from our laboratory has given rise to the possibility of an additional membrane site for cannabinoid action (2).

Our findings have pointed to the activation of phospholipases as a likely primary site for the initiation of events (3) that could result in the production of a number of mediators with a spectrum of activities (4). This involves the release of phospholipid-bound arachidonic acid which then becomes available for bioconversion to a variety of potent regulatory substances, such as, prostaglandins (PGs), prostacyclin, leukotrienes, etc.; this process has acquired the name, the arachidonic acid cascade. Phospholipases are thought to be involved as physiological regulators in these

*Supported by NIDA Research Scientist Award DA-00043 and grants DA-02043 and DA-02052.

ISBN 0-12-044620-0

bioconversions, in particular, phospholipase A_2 has been implicated in the synthesis of PGs in several systems. An alternate mechanism has recently been suggested known as the "PI" hypothesis (4). In this type of regulation, phospholipase C acts on phosphatidylinositol to generate a diacylglyceride, which is then enzymically converted to the monoglyceride and free arachidonic acid. The two mechanisms seem to be either tissue specific or agonist specific and could account for the physiological and pharmacological specificity observed with the arachidonic acid cascade.

Observations from several laboratories using invivoor other complex systems suggested that the cannabinoids were able to stimulate the production of PGs. An interesting set of experiments has been reported by Fairbairn and Pickens using THC induced catalepsy in the mouse as an endpoint (5). They found that the cataleptic effect of the drug could be blocked by pretreating the mice with aspirin or other inhibitors of PG synthesis. If the animals were then injected with PGE_2, the catalepsy could be restored. In another study they reported that mice raised on a diet deficient in essential fatty acids did not respond to the delta-9-tetrahydrocannabinol (THC), however, the administration of arachidonic acid rapidly restored the cataleptic response (6).

We have demonstrated an analogous effect using THC induced hypotension in dogs as the test system (7). Table I shows that pretreatment of pentobarbital anesthetized dogs with aspirin greatly reduces the hypotensive action of THC. A likely explanation for these findings is that THC is stimulating the synthesis of an arachidonate-derived vasodilator, such as prostacyclin, either in the lungs or the peripheral vascular bed. Aspirin is known to effectively block this process (8), thereby preventing THC released arachidonate from being converted to prostacyclin.

A role for prostaglandins in the cannabinoid effects on the pituitary-testicular axis in mice has been suggested by Dalterio et al (9). Under specific conditions, they found that both PGE and PGF synthesis in the pituitary and testis were stimulated by THC, CBD, and CBN. The data were obtained by immunoassays for the PGs from incubation of the tissues following in vivo drug treatment.

Direct measurement in the rat brain of "PGE_2-like" material following THC using a bioassay procedure was reported by Coupar and Taylor (10). They found no changes in most brain regions except the hypothalamus where there was a small decrease. Considerable methodological difficulties have been reported in measuring brain levels of PGs (11), so that these results should be viewed with some caution. A number of earlier reports on cannabinoid-PG effects have been reviewed already (1) and will not be discussed here.

TABLE I. Inhibition of THC-induced Hypotension by Aspirin

	Decrease in mean arterial blood pressure (+/- S.D.) (mm Hg)			
Time[a]	THC[b]	Aspirin-THC[c]	%I[d]	P
5	38.5 (23)	7.25 (4.6)	81	< 0.0005
10	62.3 (22)	17.5 (12)	72	< 0.0005
15	71.8 (23)	27.8 (17)	61	< 0.005
20	75.0 (18)	38.5 (15)	49	< 0.005
30	67.0 (13)	42.5 (19)	37	< 0.05
40	60.5 (14)	39.3 (19)	35	> 0.05

[a] Post THC injection times.
[b] Intravenous dose of 0.45 mg/kg in 0.45 ml EtOH; N = 4.
[c] Intravenous dose of 50 mg/kg in 5 ml H_2O at pH 7.3, 30 min prior to THC; N = 4.
[d] Percent inhibition of the hypotensive effect by aspirin.
Ref.: 20.

For some time now we have been studying PG-cannabinoid interactions in an attempt to describe the biochemical basis of the effect. Our earlier studies using cell culture systems suggested that THC somehow activated a phospholipase, releasing arachidonic acid which then was converted to PGs (3). These experiments were done primarily with Hela cells although some data was obtained using suspensions of mouse Leydig cells. The data demonstrated that THC was effective in releasing ^{14}C-arachidonate from labelled phospholipid pools, and that this could be blocked by the use of lipase inhibitors such as mepacrine (12). The precise identity of the phospholipid(s) involved is not known nor has its cellular location been determined. These points are of obvious mechanistic importance and will be the subject of future studies.

More recently, we have utilized a different cell line for this investigation, namely, the WI-38 human lung fibroblast (13). This choice was governed by several considerations. Preliminary experiments had shown that these cells were highly sensitive to THC at 3.2 mcM giving an 80% increase of arachidonate release over control values (3). Moreover, these cells were of human origin from an organ where cannabinoids are known to concentrate making them relevant to *in vivo* effects. Finally, they are a well-established easily maintained system about which a great deal is known, especially the effects of THC on c-AMP metabolism (14).

II. DISCUSSION

The dose-response relationship for PGE stimulation by THC in the WI-38 fibroblast is shown in Figure 1 (7). It can be seen that, even at the rather modest dose of 1.6 mcM, a two-fold elevation of PGE levels over base line was observed. The exact shape of the curve represents the average of several experiments. In this same report we also showed that the stimulation of PGE levels could be blocked by either aspirin or mepacrine pretreatment. Both of these drugs are well known inhibitors of PG synthesis, the former acting on cyclooxygenase (8) and the latter on phospholipase (12,15).

Our current experiments have centered around the effect of cannabinoid structural features on the release of arachidonate and the subsequent elevation of PG levels (16). We have con-

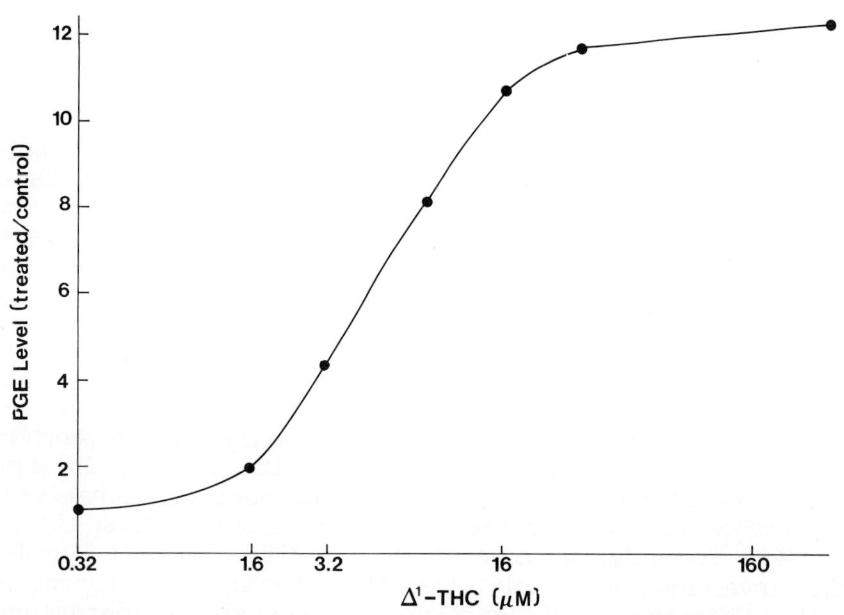

FIGURE 1. Effect of increasing concentrations of THC on PGE_2 levels in monolayer cultures of WI-38 human lung fibroblasts. The cells were grown and treated as described in Ref. 7. Each data point is the mean of six determinations. The stimulated cells were significantly different from controls at the $P < 0.0005$ level using Student's t-test ($N = 6$) at each dose level tested.

tinued to use the WI-38 cells as before and have measured the drug effects by both the radiolabelled precursor method and immunoassay measurement of the release of endogenous PGE. The effect of the cannabinoids on cell viability was also studied since visual observation had suggested that high doses caused such changes. Figure 2 gives several examples of the relationship of drug dose to DNA content, which was our criterion for cell viability. The three primary cannabinoids THC, CBN, and CBD, caused marked changes in viability starting at around 8mcM; by contrast, the 7-hydroxy metabolite of THC had no measurable effect on the cells even at 32 mcM.

The effect of metabolic changes in THC structure on PGE levels is rather interesting and is summarized in Figure 3. Unmetabolized THC is the most potent while the 7-carboxy

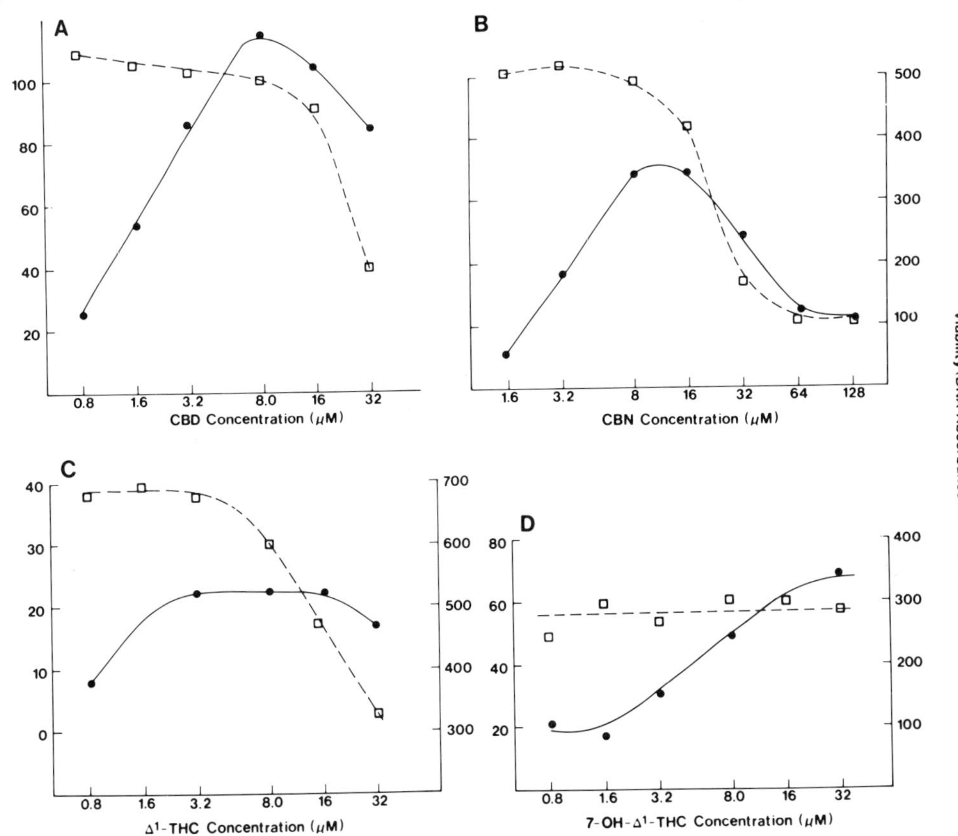

FIGURE 2. Cannabinoid effects of fibroblast viability compared with PGE production.

derivative, a metabolic end product, is essentially inactive. The other products give a spectrum of intermediary activities. This parallels in an approximate fashion some of the *in vivo* activities of the substances (17-19). These results suggest that the prostaglandin effect is related to cannabinoid actions *in vivo*, or that they are each mediated by similar molecular events.

If the release of arachidonic acid by the cannabinoids is responsible for the stimulation of PG synthesis, there should be a good correlation between their individual potencies in both effects. Figure 4A shows that this is indeed the case for every substance tested except cannabicyclol (CBCy). The data were obtained by measuring released ^{14}C-arachidonic acid and released ^{14}C-PGE$_2$ following separation by thin layer chromatography. The nonconformity exhibited by CBCy may be related to the fact that it is the only compound of the group which cannot assume a planar conformation.

Figure 4Bshows similar results on a smaller series of cannabinoids which probably accounts for a somewhat less perfect correlation (R = 0.849). In this experiment, ^{14}C-arachidonate is compared with PGE measured by immunoassay. The latter would arise from the endogenous pool(s) of arachidonate

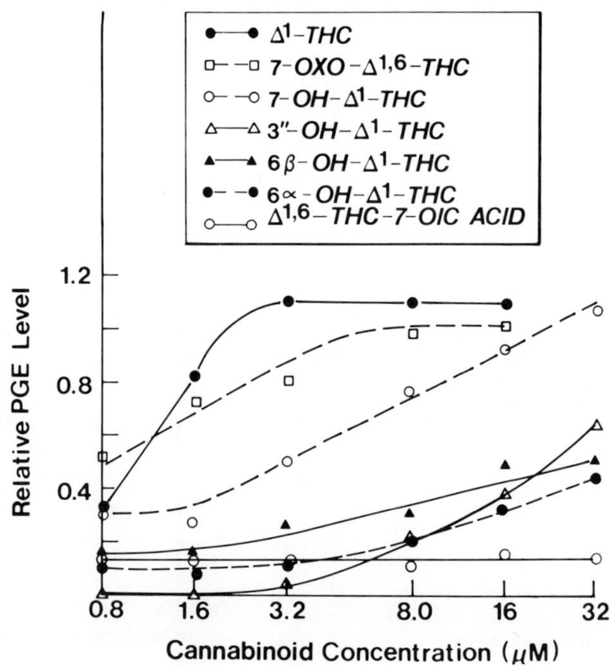

FIGURE 3. The effect of metabolism on cannabinoid stimulation of PGE synthesis in fibroblasts.

indicating that the radiolabelled precursor method accurately monitored the actual cell response.

The order of activites of the primary cannabinoids we observed is unrelated to their known *in vivo* actions. At this time we have no explanation for this, however, it may well be related to distribution and metabolism considerations. It is worth noting that White and Tansik have also observed cannabinoid mediated stimulation of arachidonate and PG release in ^{14}C-labelled platelets (16). Interestingly, they also found that CBD was about 1.5 times more potent than THC.

The question of what role, if any, the prostaglandins may have as mediators of cannabinoid action(s) can now be approached with relative certainty in view of the data discussed above. These reports from other laboratories as well our own allow several conclusions to be made. First, there is strong evidence that central nervous system effects, such as, catalepsy and pituitary secretion involve PGs as mediators. Secondly, effects on the cardiovascular system, in particular arterial blood pressure, can be explained by cannabinoid induced stimulation of vasodilatory products of the arachidonic acid cascade, such as prostacyclin. Thirdly, drugs, such as aspirin and other nonsteroidal anti-inflammatory agents, should be clinically effective anti-cannabinoids. Mepacrine may also exhibit this property due to its phospholipase inhibition. Finally, *in vitro* systems such as cells in culture or other systems which contain membrane assemblies seem to provide relevant models for studying cannabinoid action at the molecular level.

Of the many actions of the cannabinoids, the mood altering effect of the tetrahydrocannabinols presents the greatest interest in terms of cannabis use and abuse. At this point it is not possible to say whether prostaglandins do, in fact, play a role in this behavioral response in which man is the only truly valid model. It would be of interest to see whether some of the findings discussed above can be brought to bear on this problem. For example, does aspirin usage have any effect on the nature or intensity of the marijuana "high"?

ACKNOWLEDGMENTS

We are grateful to Kent Ozman for technical assistance and to John Cruz, Jr. for preparing the cells used in our studies.

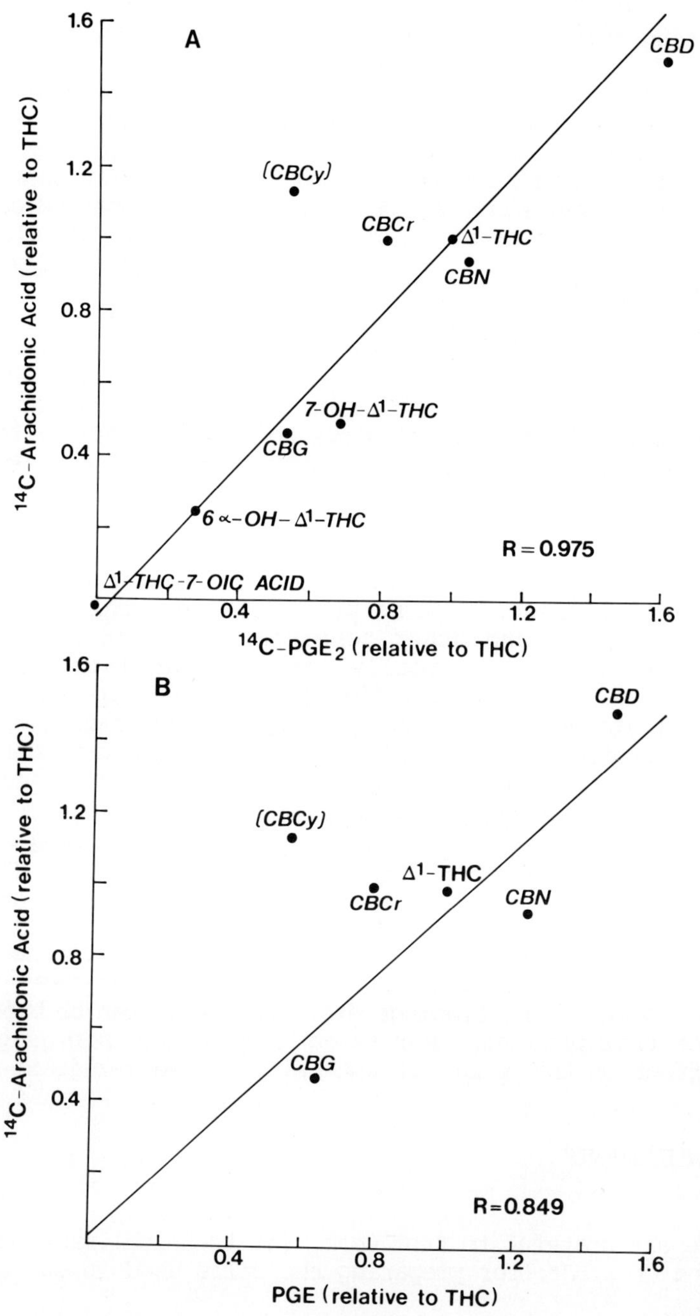

FIGURES 4A & 4B. Comparison of arachidonic acid release and PGE synthesis in fibroblasts.

REFERENCES

1. Burstein, S., and Hunter, S. A., The biochemistry of the cannabinoids, Revs. Appl. Pharmacol. Sci. 2:155-226 (1981).
2. Burstein, S., and Hunter, S. A., Prostaglandins and cannabis - VI. Release of arachidonic aid from Hela cells by THC and other cannabinoids, Biochem. Pharmacol. 27:1275-1280 (1978).
3. Burstein, S., and Hunter, S. A., Prostaglandins and cannabis - VIII. Elevation of phospholipase A_2 activity by cannabinoids in whole cells and subcellular preparations, J. Clin. Pharmacol. 21:2405-2485 (1981).
4. Wolfe, L. S., Eicosanoids: prostaglandins, thromboxanes, leukotrienes, and other derivatives of carbon-20 unsaturated fatty acids, J. Neurochem. 38:1-14 (1982).
5. Fairbairn, J. W., and Pickens, J. T., The oral activity of delta-9-THC and its dependence on PGE_2, Brit. J. Pharmacol. 67:379-385 (1979).
6. Fairbairn, J. W., and Pickens, J. T., The effect of conditions influencing endogenous prostaglandins on the activity of delta-1-THC in mice, Brit. J. Pharmacol. 69:491-493 (1980).
7. Burstein, S., Hunter, S. A., Sedor, C., and Shulman, S., Prostaglandins and cannabis - XI. Stimulation of prostaglandin E_2 synthesis in human lung fibroblasts by delta-1-THC, Biochem. Pharmacol. 31:2361-2365 (1982).
8. Preston, E. F., Whipps, S., Jackson, C. A., French, J. A., Wyld, P. J., and Stoddard, C. T., Inhibition of prostacyclin and platelet thromboxane A_2 after low-dose aspirin, N. E. J. Med. 304:76-79 (1981).
9. Dalterio, S., Bartke, A., Harper, M. J. K., Huffman, R., and Sweeny, Effects of cannabinoids and female exposure on the pituitary - testicular axis in mice: possible involvement of prostaglandins, Biol. Repro., 24:315-322 (1981).
10. Coupar, I. M., and Taylor, D. A., Alteration in the level of endogenous hypothalmic prostaglandins induced by delta-9-THC in the rat, Br. J. Pharmacol. 76:115-119 (1982).
11. Poddubiuk, F. M., Blumberg, J. B., and Kopin, I. J., Brain Prostaglandin content in rats sacrificed by decapitation vs. focused microwave irradiation, Experentia 38:987-988 (1982).

12. Blackwell, C. J., Flower, R. J., Nijkamp, F. P., and Vane, J. R., Phospholipase A_2 activity of guinea pig isolated perfused lungs: stimulation and inhibition by anti-inflammatory steroids, Brit.J.Pharmacol. 62:79-80 (1978).
13. Hayflick, L., and Moorhead, P. S., The serial cultivation of herman diploid cell strains, Exp. Cell. Res. 25:585-621 (1961).
14. Kelly, L. A., and Butcher, R. W., The Effects of delta-1-THC on c-AMP levels in WI-38 fibroblasts, Biochem. Biophys. Acta. 320:540-544 (1973).
15. Yorio, T., and Bartly, P. J., Phospholipase A and the mechanism of action of aldosterone, Nature 271:79-81 (1978).
16. Burstein, S., Hunter, S. A., and Ozman, K., Prostaglandins and cannabis - XII. The effect of cannabinoid structure on the synthesis of prostaglandins by human lung fibroblasts, Mol. Pharmacol. 23: in press (1983).
17. Mechoulam, R., and Edery, H., Structure-activity relationships in the cannabinoid series, in "Marijuana" (R. Mechoulam, ed.), pp. 101-133. Academic Press, New York, 1973.
18. Perez-Reyes, M., Timmons, M. C., Lipton, M. A., Christensen, H. D., David, K. H., and Wall, M.. E., A comparison of the pharmacological activity of delta-9-THC and its monohydroxylated metabolites in man, Experentia 29:1009-1010 (1973).
19. Hollister, L. E., Structure-activity relationships in man of cannabis constituents and homologs and metabolites of delta-9-THC, Pharmacol., 11:3-11 (1974).
20. Burstein, S., Ozman, K., Burstein, E., Palermo, N., and Smith, E., Biochem. Pharmacol. 31:591 (1982).

THE EFFECT OF A SINGLE INJECTION OF DELTA-9-TETRAHYDROCANNABINOL ON THE FRACTIONAL SODIUM AND POTASSIUM EXCRETION IN THE DOG: A PRELIMINARY STUDY

J. Santos-Martinez

Department of Physiology and Pharmacology
School of Medicine
Universidad Central del Caribe
Cayey, Puerto Rico

M. A. Gonzalez-Castillo
E. Toro-Goyco

Departments of Pharmacology and Biochemistry
University of Puerto Rico School of Medicine
San Juan, Puerto Rico

I. INTRODUCTION

Since the isolation of (-)-delta-9-tetrahydrocannabinol (THC), the active principle of marijuana, by Gaoli and Mechoulam in 1964 (1), and its synthesis by Farenholtz et al. (2), intensive studies on the physiological actions of this compound have been performed. The interest of investigators have ranged widely. In the past few years interest has been placed on its action at the cellular level. The compound has been found to inhibit "in vitro" membrane bound enzymes, amongst them the Na^+-K^+ dependent ATPases (3-5). Based on these findings, a hypothesis has been advanced ascribing several of THC's physiological effects to its Na^+-K^+ ATPase inhibitory activity. An appropriate "in situ" system to study this effect would be the kidney. Were we to expect THC to be an ATPase inhibitor, detectable changes in the urinary output of Na^+ (Na) and K^+ (K) would take place. Although extensive studies on the identification of THC, its metabolites and

ISBN 0-12-068380-6

analogs in urine have been conducted (6-8), information on the role played by these agents on the modification of the composition of the urine is nonexistent. With these considerations in mind, we decided to study the effects of single intravenous injections of THC on the urinary excretion of Na and K in dogs.

II. MATERIALS AND METHODS

Experiments were performed on mongrel dogs weighing 7-15 kg, anesthesized with 25 mg/kg sodium pentobarbital i.v. Since the excretion of Na and K may be influenced by changes in glomerular filtration rate and this in turn by changes in systemic arterial pressure below 80-90 mm Hg, systemic arterial pressure was recorded continuously from the right femoral artery by means of a pressure transducer (Statham, P23AC), which in turn was connected to a 5PI Grass polygraph. The right and left ureters were exposed by a ventral laparotomy and catherterized for urine collection. A priming solution containing 0.5 g inulin in 20 ml saline was administered prior to the start of a maintenance solution containing inulin in adequate concentrations for clearance determination and 15g mannitol per deciliter of a 0.85% saline solution so as to maintain adequate urine flow. The maintenance solution was infused at a rate of 0.76 ml per minute by means of a Harvard infusion pump. Arterial blood samples were taken into heparinized syringes at approximately midpoint of the clearance periods from the catheter inserted into the right femoral artery. Urine samples were withdrawn separately from each kidney through the catheters inserted into the respective ureters and volumes obtained were pooled for clearance determination purposes.

The THC used in this work was obtained from NIDA. The preparation was essentially free of impurities as determined by one dimensional thin-layer chromatography using two different solvent systems: hexane:diethyl ether-acetic acid (90:15:1) and chloroform-methanol-water (65:25:4), and by high pressure liquid chromatography (Bondapack column) with acetonitrile-water (90:10) used as eluant.

A constant dose of THC, 20 mg, was used throughout the experiments. Because of the insolubility of THC in aqueous medium, several vehicles were used for dissolving it prior to injection. One procedure consisted in the solution of 100 mg THC in 0.5 ml acetone, i.e., 200 mg/ml. Plasma was removed from the experimental dog to be tested. One tenth ml of THC solution in acetone was mixed with 2 ml of plasma, agitated to get a homogeneous mixture and injected i.v. This procedure was used in three experimental animals. In three more dogs, acetone-aqueous solutions (1:1, v/v) containing 20 mg/ml THC were prepared and 1 ml injected intramuscularly. In a single experiment, 2 ml of a solution of THC in ethanol containing 10 mg/ml was injected to a dog intramuscularly.

Control clearance periods were performed using the standard priming and maintenance solutions previously described. In the experiment in which ethanol was used as vehicle for dissolving the THC, a sham control was performed in which the vehicle was injected by the same route as the THC solution. Likewise, since to our surprise, acetone-saline mixtures were found to alter the Na and K excretion in urine, sham controls were run after i.m. injection of saline. One to one and a half hours elapsed between sham clearances and clearance periods in which THC or acetone were administered. Recordings started 5 min after injection of the THC solution whenever it occurred by the i.v. route; 30 min after injection by the i.m. route.

Inulin determination in urine and in arterial plasma were performed by the anthrone method as described by Fuhr et al. (9). Sodium and potassium were determined by flame photometry (Beckman) using lithium as the internal standard (10).

From the data gathered, the fractional sodium (FE_{Na}) and potassium (FE_K) excretions were determined as follows:

$$FE_{Na} = \frac{U_{Na} \cdot V}{C_{In} \cdot P_{Na}} (100) \quad \text{and} \quad FE_K = \frac{U_K \cdot V}{C_{In} \cdot P_K} (100)$$

where $U_{Na} \cdot V$, $U_K V$, $C_{In} \cdot P_{Na}$ and $C_{In} \cdot P_K$ denote urinary sodium and potassium excretion rates, and filtered loads of sodium and potassium, respectively.

III. RESULTS

Results of selected individual experiments are shown in Tables I, II and III. Fig. 1, which summarizes the results of the three experiments of which the data in Table I are a representative sample, shows that 20 mg of THC, when dissolved in a 20:1 plasma-acetone mixture, caused a significant decrease in the FE_{Na} when compared to control values ($p < 0.001$), but change in FE_K is not statistically significant ($p > 0.2$) most probably because of large deviations between measurements. Likewise Fig. 2, which summarizes results of the experiments

TABLE I. Data of an Experiment Showing the Effect of Delta-9-THC Dissolved in Plasma on Fractional Sodium and Potassium Excretion

Value (+/- S.D.)	Sodium		Potassium	
	Control	THC	Control	THC
P, mEq/L	141.3 (0.3)	142.2 (0.4)	4.4 (0.1)	4.8 (0.1)
C_{In}, ml/min	27.1 (1.1)	23.4 (0.6)	27.1 (1.1)	23.4 (0.6)
C_{In} x P, uEq/min	3832.4 (192.8)	3331.3 (107.5)	118.5 (5.0)	113.0 (4.4)
U, mEq/L	76.2 (2.1)	28.8 (0.9)	101.8 (3.2)	118.0 (1.9)
V, ml/min	0.37 (0.02)	0.31 (0.01)	0.37 (0.02)	0.31 (0.01)
U x V, uEq/min	28.2 (1.5)	8.94 (0.17)	37.5 (0.07)	36.8 (1.3)
FE, %	0.74 (0.03)	0.27 (0.01)[a]	31.76 (0.87)	32.81 (1.87)[b]

[a] $P < 0.001$ from control.
[b] N. S. from control.

TABLE II. Data of an Experiment Showing the Effect of Acetone on Fractional Sodium and Potassium Excretion

Value (+/- S.D.)	Sodium		Potassium	
	Control	Acetone	Control	Acetone
P, mEq/L	133.0 (0.8)	138.6 (0.7)	3.3 (0.0)	3.3 (0.0)
C_{In}, ml/min	22.2 (2.6)	16.2 (0.8)	22.2 (2.6)	16.2 (0.8)
C_{In} x P, uEq/min	2943.8 (303.8)	2255.1 (106.7)	73.2 (7.9)	53.6 (3.0)
U, mEq/L	133.0 (3.3)	50.5 (3.9)	68.2 (4.7)	104.6 (6.9)
V, ml/min	0.17 (0.01)	0.14 (0.01)	0.17 (0.01)	0.14 (0.01)
U x V, uEq/min	22.3 (1.5)	6.1 (0.8)	11.5 (1.2)	14.2 (1.1)
FE, %	0.82 (0.11)	0.31 (0.04)[a]	17.34 (3.03)	27.5 (2.2)[b]

[a] $P < 0.001$ from control.
[b] $P < 0.02 > 0.01$ from control.

TABLE III. Data of One Experiment Showing the Effect of Delta-9-THC Dissolved in Ethanol on Fractional Sodium and Potassium Excretion

Value (+/- S.D.)	Sodium		Potassium	
	Control	THC in EtOH	Control	THC in EtOH
P, mEq/L	149.0 (0.8)	146.2 (0.2)	4.0 (0.1)	4.3 (0.6)
C_{In}, ml/min	2.6 (1.1)	25.9 (1.1)	27.6 (1.1)	25.9 (1.1)
C_{In} x P, uEq/min	4115.2 (168.6)	3873.2 (1.1)	111.4 (4.7)	111.6 (4.8)
U, mEq/L	124.3 (11.8)	58.5 (6.1)	46.3 (6.1)	62.6 (4.2)
V, ml/min	0.30 (0.01)	0.27 (0.01)	0.30 (0.01)	0.27 (0.01)
U x V, uEq/min	36.5 (3.4)	16.1 (2.2)	13.6 (0.5)	16.8 (3.2)
FE, %	0.97 (0.13)	0.43 (0.06)[a]	12.43 (0.97)	15.16 (0.69)[b]

[a] $P < 0.01 > 0.001$ from control.
[b] $P < 0.05 > 0.02$ from control.

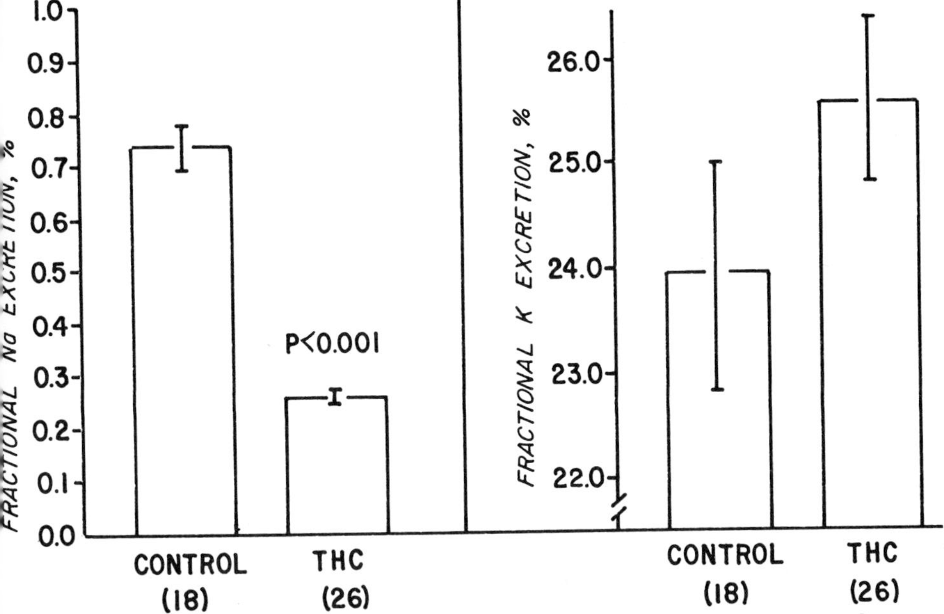

FIGURE 1. Effects of a single i.v. injection of THC dissolved in plasma on the fractional excretion of Na and K. Controls were the same experimental animals prior to injection. Numbers in parenthesis indicate number of determinations.

of which the data in Table II is a representative sample, show that acetone per se causes a significant decrease in FE_{Na} ($p < 0.001$) and a significant increase in FE_K ($p < 0.02$). In these experiments, the amounts of acetone injected (i.m.) were 10-fold higher than the amount of acetone added to plasma and used to dissolve THC for the i.v. injections. Notice, however, that the diminution in FE_{Na} caused by such a big dose of acetone is smaller (from 0.78% down to 0.48%) than that caused by THC dissolved in a 20:1 saline-acetone mixture (from 0.7% down to 0.26%).

Table III summarizes the data of the individual experiment in which ethanol was used as a vehicle for dissolving the THC. It is apparent that when compared to the sham control, the observed effect of THC is to significantly increase both the FE_{Na} ($p < 0.01$) and FE_K ($p < 0.05$).

Table IV summarizes the tendency of a number of relevant parameters to either increase or diminish after injections of THC dissolved in plasma, acetone per se, or THC in ethanol. The highest percent changes were in the total amount of Na in the urine (U_{Na} x V) and therefore on the FE_{Na}. In comparison, changes in urine flow (V) were smaller and so were the diminu-

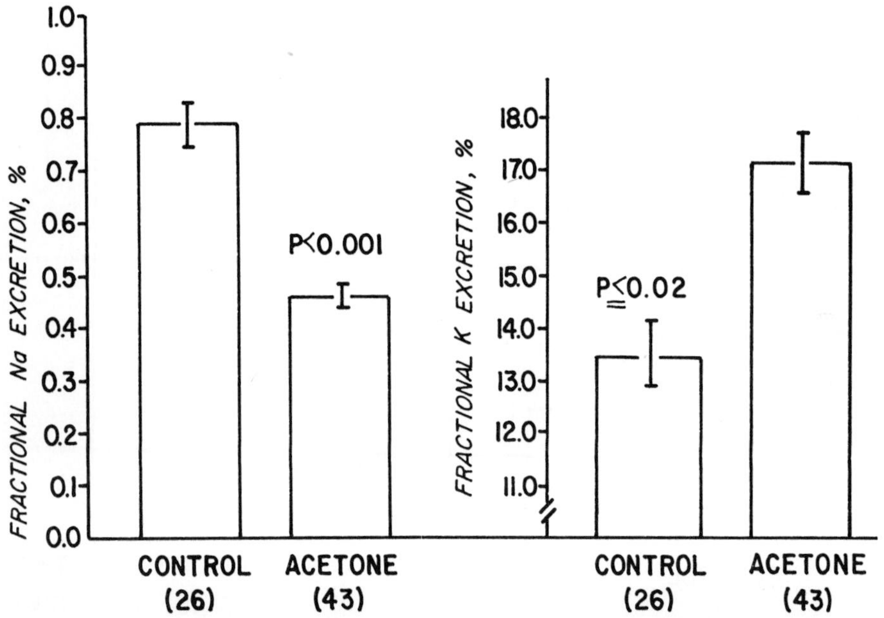

FIGURE 2. Effects of a single i.m. injection of two ml of a 1:1 acetone-saline mixture on the fractional excretion of Na and K. Controls received saline prior to injection of the mixture. Numbers in parenthesis indicate number of determinations.

tions in glomerular filtration rates. The latter changes definitely do not seem to account for the pronounced alterations in Na and K excretion.

IV. DISCUSSION

Since it is a well known fact that Na-K dependent ATPase is instrumental in the transport of Na across epithelial membranes (11), and renal epithelium is no exception (12), we designed these experiments in the hope of developing an "in situ" model for the study of ATPase inhibition by THC. A logical consequence of ATPase inhibition would be increased excretion of Na, because of a block in its reabsorption. This is the effect that has been observed with ouabain and digoxin, where doses which block up to 85% of the enzyme activity of the kidney block from 25-35% of the renal sodium reabsorption (13). This apparent quantitative discrepancy may be explained by the fact that there is a significant fraction of the Na reabsorption in the kidney that is independent of ATPase activity (14). An alternate explanation could be that the remaining enzyme activity would be enough to account for most of the renal Na reabsorption (15). The observed results, however, were contrary to our expectations. THC caused a significant increase in the retention of Na, as is apparent from the results presented in Fig. 1 and Tables I and III.

A factor that contributes to make these preliminary findings on Na retention still more meaningful is the fact that in order to maintain adequate urine flows during the experiments, we used maintenance solutions containing mannitol. It has been established that Na reabsorption is inhibited during mannitol diuresis (16), that is, mannitol causes an increase in Fe_{Na}.

As has already been mentioned in the section on Results (Table IV), the slight changes observed in GFR and urine flow do not account for the changes in urinary Na concentration (U_{Na}) and urinary sodium excretion (U_{Na} x V). Neither do changes in systemic arterial pressure, which were found to be negligible during these experiments.

A valid explanation must exist for the diminished sodium excretion. If the suggestion that THC binding to membranes causes them to become leaky (17) has any basis in fact, it can then be speculated that THC binding at the tight junction in the proximal tubules of the nephron causes leakage of Na from the lumen into the extracellular fluid and back into the system. This would not be surprising, since even under normal conditions the tight junction can become leaky to Na and water (18). This explanation, however, fails to give a satisfactory

TABLE IV. Per Cent Changes From Control Values in Tables I - III

Table:	I THC	II Acetone	III THC in ETOH
GFR	13.1 dec*	27.0 dec	0.6 dec
V	16.2 dec	17.6 dec	10.0 dec
U_{Na}	62.2 dec	62.0 dec	53.0 dec
U_K	13.7 inc	36.7 inc	25.2 inc
U_{Na} x V	68.3 dec	72.6 dec	55.1 dec
U_K x V	2.0 dec	23.5 inc	25.8 inc
FE_{Na}	63.5 dec	62.2 dec	55.6 dec
FE_K	3.2 inc	58.5 inc	21.9 dec

*Indicates decrease (dec) or increase (inc) change.

answer to the observed changes in K, that although not statistically significant because of the large variations in observed measurements, seem to be real.

It is a well known phenomenon that increases in aldosterone levels show effects that are identical to the ones observed and reported here for THC (19). We may speculate that THC triggers, in some unknown fashion, an increased activity of aldosterone. Alterations on other steroid hormone, namely testosterone, has been reported (20) although the data of a latter report by the same group of investigators fail to show a convincing effect (21).

In evaluating the FE_{Na} and FE_K, caution must be exerted. FE_{Na} is as a rule, in the absence of renal disease, a fairly constant value. On the other hand, FE_K is a highly variable value, depending to a large extent on the nutritional status of the animals used. This can be easily observed from the results presented in Tables I and II. The FE_K for controls in Table I significantly higher than that of control animals in Table II.

An interesting and unexpected finding in this preliminary study, was the effect of acetone in Na and K excretion. Increased electrolyte excretion is one of the problems in ketoacetosis. Acetone is a product of decarboxylation of the main ketone body, acetoacetic acid. A teleological explanation for the production of acetone may be that the acetone produced, besides being electrically uncharged, puts into action a mechanism that tends to compensate for the loss of electrolytes. This certainly deserves further study.

The dose of THC used throughout these experiments was constant (20 mg). Thus, because of differences in weight among the experimental animals, it varied between 1 and 2 mg/kg. This dose is within the range of the dosages used by innumerable investigators in their "in vivo" experiments with other mammals.

Assuming the mechanism of action of THC is identical in dog and in man, it would be important to find out what would be its effect on fluid volumes and on electrolyte concentrations in habitual users of marijuana, specially in those already showing increased Na retention.

ACKNOWLEDGMENTS

We thank Mrs. Maria M. Rivera and Mrs. Esther Torres for the typing and Mr. Carlos Marin for the illustration.

REFERENCES

1. Gaoni, Y., and Mechoulam, P., J. Amer. Chem. Soc. 86:1646 (1964).
2. Farenholtz, K. E., Lurie, M., and Dierstead, R. W., J. Amer. Chem. Soc. 88:2709 (1966).
3. Toro-Goyco, E., Rodriguez, M. B., and Preston, A. M., Mol. Pharmacol. 14:130 (1978).
4. Toro-Goyco, E., Rodriguez, M. B., Preston, A. M., and Jering, H., in "Marihuana: Biological Effects" (G. G. Nahas and W. D. M. Paton, eds.), p. 229. Pergamon Press, New York, 1979.
5. Huzlar, L. A., Greenburg, J. H., and Mellors, A., Mol. Pharmacol. 13:1086 (1977).
6. Williams, P. L., and Moffat, A. C., J. Chromatogr. 186:595 (1979).
7. Nordqvist, M., Lindreen, J. E., and Agurell, S. J., Pharm. Pharmacol. 31:231 (1979).
8. Kanter, S. L., Hollister, L. E., and Loeffler, K. O., J. Chromatogr. 150:233 (1978).
9. Fuhr, J., Kaczmarczyk, J., and Kruttgen, C. D. Klin. Wochenschr. 33:729 (1955).
10. Santos-Martinez, J., Laboy-Torres, J. A., Aviles, T. A., and Lopez, J. E., Res. Comm. Pathol. Pharmacol. 5:345 (1973).
11. Skou, J. C., Physiol. Rev. 45:596 (1965).
12. Martinez-Maldonado, M., Allen, J. C., Eknoyan, G., Suki, W., and Schwartz, A., Science 165:807 (1969).
13. Brady, J. M., and Nechay, B. R., J. Pharmacol. Exp. Ther. 190:346 (1974).
14. Giebisch, G., New Eng. J. Med. 287:913 (1972).
15. Lewy, P. R., Quintanilla, A., Levin, N. W., and Kessler, R. H., Ann. Rev. Med. 24:365 (1973).
16. Seely, J. F., and Dirks, J. H., J. Clin. Invest. 48:2330 (1969).
17. Blevins, D. R., and Regan, J. D., in "Marihuana: Chemistry Biochemistry and Cellular Effects" (G. G. Nahas, W. D. M. Paton, and Idanpaan-Heikkila, eds.), p. 213. Springer-Verlag, New York (1976).
18. Mercer, P. F., Maddox, D. A., and Brenner, B. M., West. J. Med. 120:33 (1974).
19. Ganong, W. F., and Mulrow, P. J., Amer. J. Physiol. 195:337 (1958).
20. Dalterio, S., Bartke, A., and Mayfield, D., Science 213:581 (1981).
21. Dalterio, S., Badr, F., Bartke, A., and Mayfield, D., Science 216:315 (1982).

RESPONSE OF SALMONELLA TYPHIMURIUM MUTANTS TO DELTA-9-TETRAHYDROCANNABINOL AND IN CONJUNCTION WITH KNOWN MUTAGENS

R. D. Blevins
M. S. Shelton

Department of Biological Sciences
Health Sciences Division
East Tennessee State University
Johnson City, Tennessee

I. INTRODUCTION

Marijuana, a preparation made from an annual herbaceous plant *Cannabis sativa*, is being increasingly used and abused by many in this country and throughout the world (1), but information on the potential hazards and long term effects of marijuana is limited (2). In fact, marijuana is the most widely used of the illicit drugs, and this fact has spawned cannabinoid research in the biological, chemical, pharmacological, and medical sciences (3). Delta-9-tetrahydrocannabinol (THC) is the major psychoactive compound in marijuana (1,4), and there is a growing amount of literature which suggest that THC may interfere with DNA structure and chromosome morphology. But when tested in the Ames Salmonella/microsomal assay, THC proved to be non-mutagenic (3-5). However, smoke condensates from marijuana smoke have been found to contain organic bases that are frameshift mutagens in the Ames assay. Since tobacco smoke condensates also contain frameshift mutagens, no correlation between these mutagenic bases and THC have been shown to exist (2,6).

The effects of THC on HeLa cells and herpes simplex virus have been studied by Blevins and co-workers (7-10), and has been shown to retard cell division by depressing the process of nucleic acid synthesis (9).

The present study was undertaken to examine the ability of THC to reduce spontaneous mutation as well as mutations in the

ISBN 0-12-044620-0

presence of known mutagens. In an unpublished work from the laboratory of Blevins, THC was shown to have depressed DNA synthesis in *Pseudomonnas aeruginosa*. With this in mind, different concentrations of THC were employed in combination with known mutagens that are used for positive controls in the Ames bioassay. This was done to see if THC can in fact slow down the mutation rate of any of the five mutant strains of *Salmonella typhimurium*, or at least the phenotypic expression of mutation (growth on minimal media). Several concentrations of THC were initially employed in the presence and absence of S-9 mix to determine the optimum concentrations to use in conjunction with the known mutagens. Also, a growth study was done to determine the toxicity level of the dose employed.

II. MATERIALS AND METHODS

A. Preparation of the Solutions

Dilutions of THC were prepared for incorporation tests and growth studies. The THC was obtained as an alcohol solution in a 2 mg/ml (6.36×10^{-3}M) sample. Dilutions of 10^{-3}M, 10^{-4}M, and 10^{-5}M were made and employed in the testing.

B. Preparation of Mutagen Solutions

Mutagenic solutions were prepared with special precautions. Solutions of the chemicals were prepared by putting a few milligrams of the mutagen compound in a preweighed glass vial. The vial was then capped and reweighed. The amount of solvent needed for the appropriate concentration of each compound was then determined and added to the vial under the hood. The mutagens used are routinely employed as positive controls in the Salmonella/microsomal assay. Dimethyl sulfoxide (DMSO) was the solvent for 2-aminoanthracine and 4-nitro-o-phenylene diamine, absolute ethanol was the solvent for 9-aminoacridine, and double distilled water was the solvent for sodium azide.

C. Preparation of S-9 Mix

Supernatant from homogenized rat livers (S-9) was used to activate 2-aminoacridine from a promutagen to a mutagen. The S-9 was prepared by Litton Bionetics Laboratories (Kensington,

TABLE I. Characteristics of the Mutant Tester Strains and Chemicals Used for Positive Controls

Strain	Mutation Detected	Chemical Used For Positive Control: -S9	Chemical Used For Positive Control: +S9	Histadine Mutation	uv Repair Mutation	R Factor	Accepted Range for Spontaneous Revertants[a]
TA1535	Base Pair Substitution	SA	2AA	hisG46	$uvrB^-$	-	5 - 50
TA1537	Frameshift Mutation	9AAC	2AA	hisC3076	$uvrB^-$	-	3 - 25
TA1538	Frameshift Mutation	4NPD	2AA	hisD3052	$uvrB^-$	-	5 - 40
TA100	Base Pair Substitution	SA	2AA	hisG46	$uvrB^-$	-	60 - 220
TA98	Frameshift Mutation	4NPD	2AA	hisD3052	$uvrB^-$	-	15 - 75

*Range of spontaneous revertants per plate considered acceptable in eight laboratories.

SA = Sodium azide; 9AAC = 9-aminoacridine; 4NPD = 4-nitro-o-phenylene diamine; 2AA = 2-aminoanthracine.

Maryland) using the procedure described by Garner et al. (11). The S-9 was stored in 4 ml portions in a Revco freezer at -80°C until used to prepare the S-9 mix on the day of each test.

D. Bacterial Strains

Five mutant strains of <u>Salmonnella</u> <u>typhimurium</u> LT2 -- hisTA98, hisTA100, hisTA1535, hisTA1537, and hisTA1538 -- were selected for use in this research because of their ability to revert to protrophy in the presence of a broad spectrum of mutagens, and their sensitivity to mutagens (12). Characteristics of the five Salmonnella strains and their expected spontaneous reversion rates are shown in Table I. Each strain contains three mutations (12,13). One is a histidine mutation which makes each strain auxotrophic for histidine. The other two mutations effect losses of the excision repair mechanisms and the lipopolysaccharide portion of the cell wall. The mutagenicity assays were performed as described by Ames et al. (12) and as performed in our laboratory (14-16).

E. Plate Incorporation Testing

The incorporation tests were performed by melting 100 ml of sterile top agar and placing it in a 45° water bath. Ten milliliters of sterile 0.5 m<u>M</u> histidine HCl - 0.5 m<u>M</u> biotin was poured into the top agar and mixed. The top agar was added in 2 ml portions to sterile 13 x 100 mm test tubes using a sterile syringe dispensor. The different concentrations of THC were added in 0.1 ml proportions to the respective test tubes, followed by the addition of 0.1 ml of the mutagen solutions used for testing of each bacterial test strain. To each test tube was added 0.1 ml of a 16 hour nutrient broth culture and 0.5 ml of the S-9 mix. The test tubes were removed from the 45°C water bath as quickly as possible, mixed individually for 2 seconds on a Vortex mixer, and poured onto minimal glucose agar plates that were appropriately labeled. The plates were slightly swirled in a figure-8 fashion to evenly distribute the top agar. Three concentrations of THC were tested in all five bacterial test strains and in at least four independent tests. Duplicate plates were made for each strain and each concentration. The plates were incubated for 48 hours at 37°C in a dark incubator and counted on a Quebec colony counter. Each plate was examined for the "background lawn", or unreverted bacteria by the use of a microscope on low power.

F. Controls

Controls were run in each test and included negative controls, positive controls, and sterility controls. The negative control plates were prepared with and without S-9 mix and included plates containing only bacteria, and plates containing bacteria and 0.1 ml of the solvent used for each of the chemicals. Sterility control plates were prepared for each chemical, solvent, top agar, S-9, and for each concentration of THC used. Positive control plates were prepared for each of the mutagen chemicals used in the test.

G. Growth Study Procedure

A growth study using different concentrations of THC was carried out to see if the level of toxicity upon the Salmonella typhimurium mutants was dependent upon the dose of THC employed. Nutrient top agar was prepared by dissolving 1.55 g nutrient agar in 100 ml double distilled water. After autoclaving for 15 min at 15 pounds, the melted agar was dispensed in 3.0 ml portions into 13 x 100 mm test tubes and stored at $4^{o}C$ until used. A 16 hour culture of each of the Salmonella strains (containing approximately 10^6 to 10^7 organisms/ml) was diluted by adding 0.1 ml of the nutrient broth containing the bacteria to 99.9 ml of sterile water (1:100 dilution). A 0.1 ml sample of the 1:100 bacterial dilution was then added to a second 9.9 ml of sterile water (1:10,000 dilution). A 0.1 ml sample of the 1:10,000 bacterial dilution was added to 0.9 ml of sterile water (1:100,000 dilution) containing the various quantities (ranging from 6.36×10^{-3}M to 1×10^{-5}M) of THC. A 1.0 ml aliquot of the 1:100,000 bacterial dilution was added to sterile petri dishes in triplicate for each Salmonella strain. Melted nutrient agar (25 ml/plate) was poured onto the petri dishes and was well mixed. After the agar hardened the plates were incubated at $37^{o}C$ for 48 hour, with the resulting colonies being counted.

II. RESULTS

A. Controls

Positive and negative control plates were made for each plate incorporation test; the results are presented in Table II. Negative controls both with and without S-9 mix were used to determine the spontaneous reversion rate for each strainof Salmonella as well as to determine the effect (if any) of the

TABLE II. Positive and Negative Control Values

Compound or solvent[b]	Amount per Plate	S9[c]	TA1538
Negative control	(mcl)		
Spontaneous	0	-	7 ± 2 (6)
	0	+	12 ± 2 (4)
Water	100	-	15 ± 4 (3)
	100	+	16 ± 1 (3)
Ethanol	100	-	7 ± 2 (3)
	100	+	11 ± 4 (3)
DMSO	100	-	10 ± 3 (3)
	100	+	10 ± 2 (3)
Positive controls	(mcg)		
2-AA in DMSO	5	-	19 ± 7 (4)
		+	146 ± 61 (4)
4-N-o-PA in DMSO	50	-	451 ± 31 (4)
NaAz in water	50	-	
9-AA in ethanol	50	-	

[a]Meanplusor minus standard deviation for(N) observations.

[b]Water is double distilled; DMSO = dimethylsulfoxide; 2-AA = 2-aminoanthracine; NaAz = sodium azide; 9-AA = 9-aminoacridine.

[c]Rat liver homogenate added (+).

solvents on the spontaneous reversion rates. The results showed that the solvents used in this study had no significant effects on the number of reverted colonies for any of the tested Salmonella strains when compared to the spontaneous revertant colonies were observed in all plates receiving S-9 mix. This supports similar findings reported by Ames et al. (12).

Positive control results are also shown in Table II. Fifty micrograms per plate of 4-nitro-o-phenylene diamine produced a 45-fold revertant increase in Salmonella strain TA1538 and a 207-fold increase in strain TA98 when compared to the solvent (dimethyl sulfoxide) values. Strain TA1537 was treated with 50mcg/plate of the mutagen 9-aminoacridine.

Number of colonies/plate[a]			
TA1537	TA1535	TA100	TA98
9 ± 3 (6)	20 ± 6 (6)	96 ± 17 (6)	24 ± 6 (6)
13 ± 2 (4)	26 ± 22 (4)	118 ± 29 (4)	45 ± 8 (4)
13 ± 2 (3)	29 ± 6 (3)	97 ± 13 (3)	40 ± 3 (3)
28 ± 5 (3)	29 ± 11 (3)	104 ± 12 (3)	45 ± 16 (3)
9 ± 4 (3)	20 ± 5 (3)	97 ± 18 (3)	25 ± 5 (3)
10 ± 0 (3)	15 ± 5 (3)	109 ± 5 (3)	47 ± 5 (3)
8 ± 1 (3)	24 ± 9 (3)	85 ± 9 (3)	25 ± 8 (3)
8 ± 2 (3)	12 ± 5 (3)	84 ± 13 (3)	33 ± 8 (3)
20 ± 7 (4)	24 ± 7 (4)	150 ± 39 (4)	31 ± 5 (4)
164 ± 38 (4)	539 ± 145 (4)	4034 ± 643 (4)	1745 ± 623 (4)
			5181 ± 589 (4)
	2865 ± 92 (4)	4585 ± 83 (4)	
3572 ± 482 (4)			

Table II shows that the incidence of TA1537 revertants was 447-fold greater than solvent (ethanol) alone. Strains TA1535 and TA100 were both treated with 50 mcg/plate of the mutagen sodium azide. Salmonella strain TA1535 exhibited a 110-fold increase in revertants and strain TA100 increased 47-fold when compared to the plates receiving only the solvent (double distilled water). The increased rate of reverted colonies when treated with the known mutagens confirmed that all of the Salmonella strains were responding properly.

Plate counts in the presence of 5 mcg/plate of the promutagen 2-aminoanthracine but without S-9 mix were essentially the same as the plate counts resulting from treatment with only the solvent dimethyl sulfoxide (Table II). However, plates containing both S-9 mix (0.5 ml/plate) and 5 mcg/plate of 2-aminoanthracine exhibited a revertant increase of 15-fold for TA1538, 70-fold for TA98, 21-fold for TA1537, 22-fold for TA1535, and 47-fold for TA100. This demonstrated that the S-9 mix had the capacity to activate promutagens to mutagens in each of the tests performed.

The sterility control plates for all solvents, top agar, S-9 mix, THC, and known mutagens showed no contamination for any of the results obtained in this research.

B. THC Concentrations

Incorporation tests in the presence of various quantities of THC were performed to determine the degree of toxicity of THC on the Salmonella strain and thus arrive at the optimal concentration of THC to be used in conjunction with the known mutagens. The results, presented in Table III, show that 100 mcg of 6.36 x 10^{-3}M of THC/plate as well as 100 mcl of 1 x 10^{-3}M/plate of THC dilutions were toxic for all five Salmonella strains. Either the complete absence of a background lawn or a greatly diminished number of small colonies in the background lawn were viewed as being toxic. However, 100 mcl/plate of either 1 x 10^{-4}M or 1 x 10^{-5}M THC dilutions demonstrated no toxicity to the background lawn; therefore, these dilutions were employed throughout this study. Table III shows that 100 mcl/plate of 1 x 10^{-4}M THC with strain TA1538 produced a 43% reduction in the number of spontaneous revertants when compared to the negative control results. One hundred microliters per plate of 1 x 10^{-5}M THC produced a 29% reduction in the spontaneous revertant colonies with TA1538. Strain TA1537 showed a 33% reduction in revertant colonies when treated with 100 mcl/plate of 1 x 10^{-4}M THC and a 33% reduction when 100 mcl/plate of 1 x 10^{-5}M THC was employed. Strain TA1535 exhibited a 10% reduction in reverted colonies when treated with 100 mcl/plate of 1 x 10^{-4}M THC and a 2% reduction with 100 mcl/plate of 1 x 10^{-5}M THC. Strain TA98 exhibited a 21% reduction in the number of reverted colonies when treated with 100 mcl/plate of 1 x 10^{-4}M THC and an 8% reduction when 100 mcl/plate of 1 x 10^{-5}M THC was employed. These data are shown graphically along with the solvent (ethanol) control values in Figures 1, 2, and 3.

C. Incorporation Tests with Known Mutagens

Results of incorporation tests with non-toxic levels of THC being employed in conjunction with known concentrations of mutagens are shown in Table IV. Strains TA1538 and TA98 were insulted with 50 mcg/plate of 4-nitro-o-phenylene diamine in conjunction with THC. With 100 mcl/plate of 1 x 10^{-4}M THC, strain TA1538 showed a 20% reduction in revertant colonies, and strain TA98 exhibited a 4% reduction, when compared to mutagen control plates having received no THC. With 100 mcl/plate of 1 x 10^{-5}M THC, TA1538 showed a 12% reduction in

TABLE III. Delta-9-THC Concentration Values

THC Concentration	Amount per plate (mcl)	Number of colonies/plate[a]				
		TA1538	TA1537	TA1535	TA100	TA98
6.36×10^{-3}	100	T[b]	T	T	T	T
1.00×10^{-3}	100	T	T	T	T	T
1.00×10^{-4}	100	4 +/- 3 (4)	6 +/- 2 (4)	18 +/- 4 (4)	82 +/- 21 (4)	19 +/- 2 (4)
1.00×10^{-5}	100	5 +/- 2 (4)	6 +/- 1 (4)	24 +/- 5 (4)	94 +/- 21 (4)	22 +/- 5 (4)

[a]Mean plus and minus standard deviation for (N) observations.
[b]Toxic - background lawn was sparce or absent.

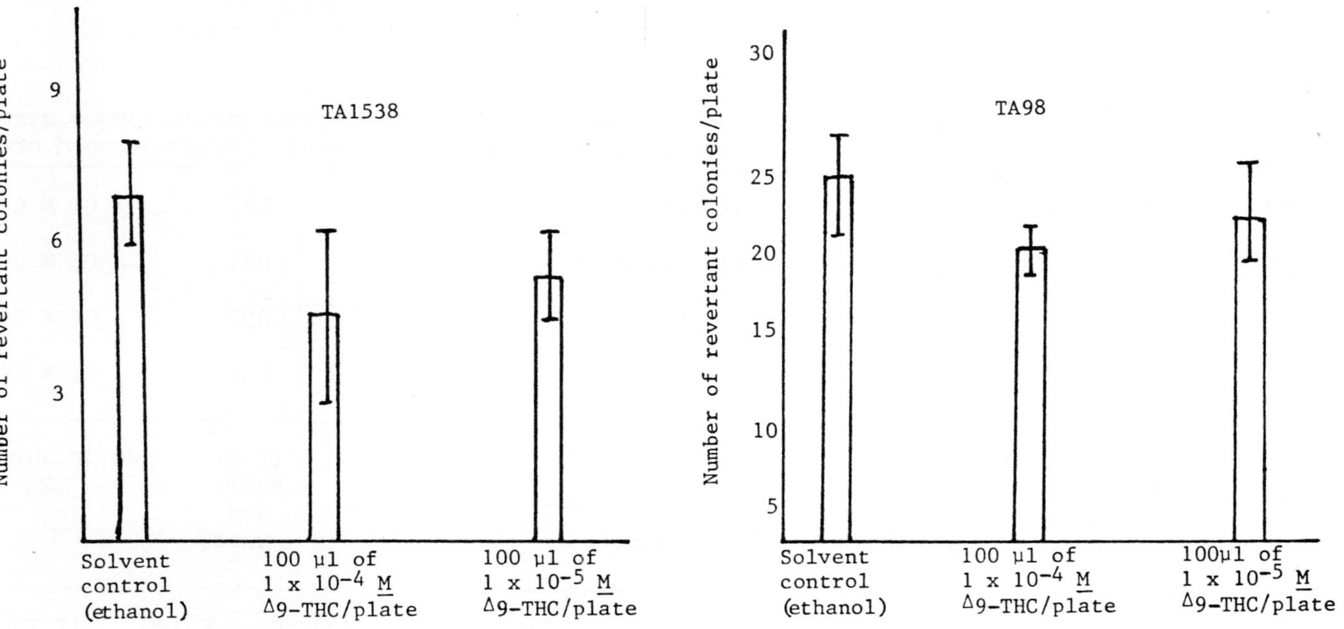

FIGURE 1. THC concentration values compared to negative control values with strains TA1538 and TA98. Brackets indicate +/- standard error of the mean.

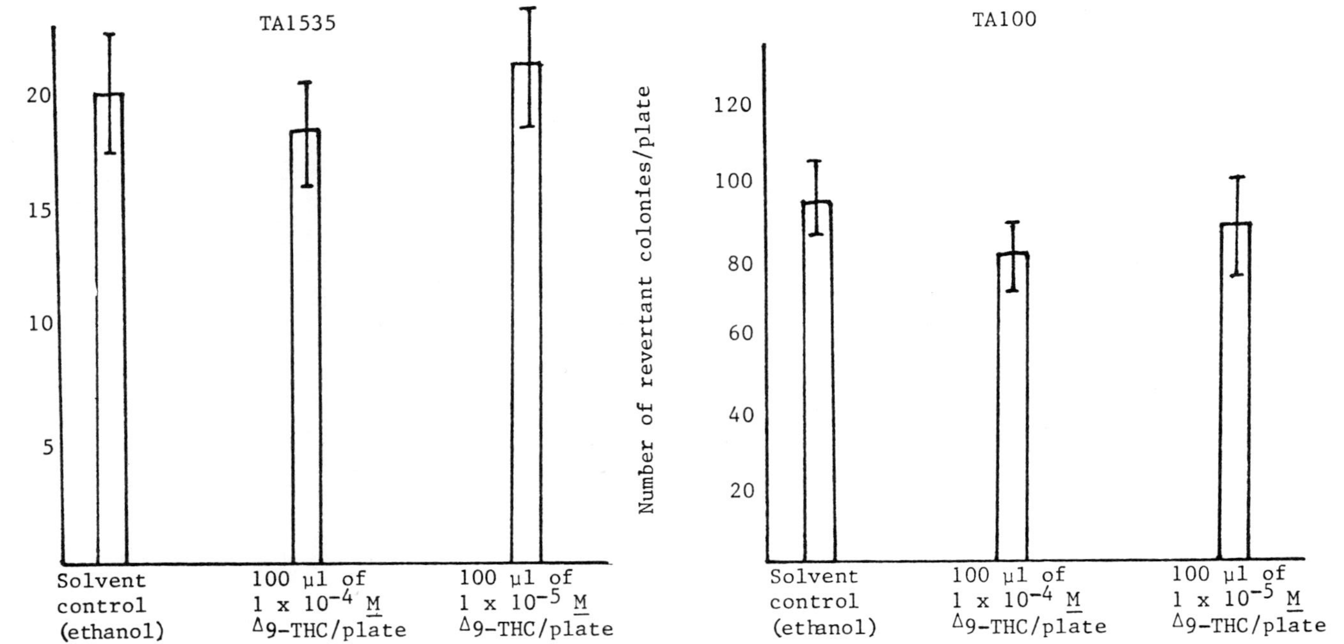

FIGURE 2. THC concentration values compared to negative control values with strains TA1535 and TA100. Brackets indicate +/- standard error of the mean.

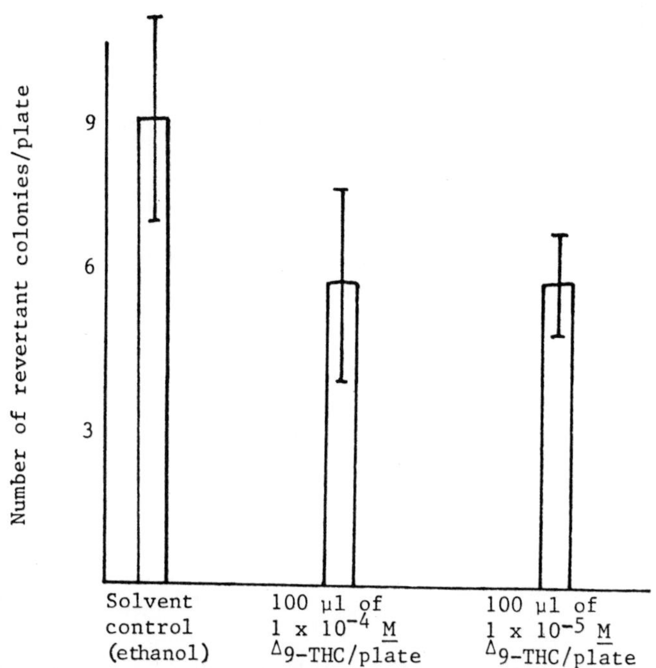

FIGURE 3. THC concentration values compared to the negative control values with strain TA1537. Brackets indicate +/- standard error of the mean.

revertant colonies, and TA98 showed a 1% reduction, when compared to positive control values.

Salmonella strains TA1535 and TA100 were exposed to 50 mcg/ plate of sodium azide in conjunction with THC. With 100 mcl/ plate of 1 x 10^{-4}M THC, strain TA1535 showed a 18% reduction in the number of revertant colonies, and strain TA100 exhibited a 10% reduction when compared to positive controls. When 100 mcl/plate of 1 x 10^{-5}M THC was employed, TA1535 showed no reduction, while TA100 showed a 7% reduction in the number of revertant colonies when compared to positive control values.

Salmonella strain TA1537 was treated with 50 mcg/plate of 9-aminoacridine in conjunction with THC. With 100 mcl/plate of 1 x 10^{-4}M THC, 1537 exhibited a 5% reduction in the number of revertant colonies, and with 100 mcl of 1 x 10^{-5}M THC, TA1537 experienced no reduction in the number of revertant colonies when compared to positive control values. These data are shown graphically along with the positive control values in Figures 4, 5, and 6.

TABLE IV. Delta-9-Concentration in Conjunction with Known Mutagen Values

		Number of colonies/plate[a]				
Compound[b]	THC[c]	TA1538	TA1537	TA1535	TA100	TA98
4-N-o-PA	1.00×10^{-4}	359 +/- 63				4989 +/- 190
	1.00×10^{-5}	395 +/- 67				5108 +/- 291
Sodium azide	1.00×10^{-4}			2493 +/- 251	4104 +/- 118	
	1.00×10^{-5}			2863 +/- 310	4270 +/- 136	
9-AA	1.00×10^{-4}		3387 +/- 225			
	1.00×10^{-5}		3585 +/- 300			

[a]Mean plus and minus standard deviation for four observations.
[b]50 mcg added per plate; 4-N-o-PA = 4-nitro-o-phenylenediamine; 9-AA = 9-aminoacridine.
[c]Delta-9-THC concentration added in 100 mcl per plate.

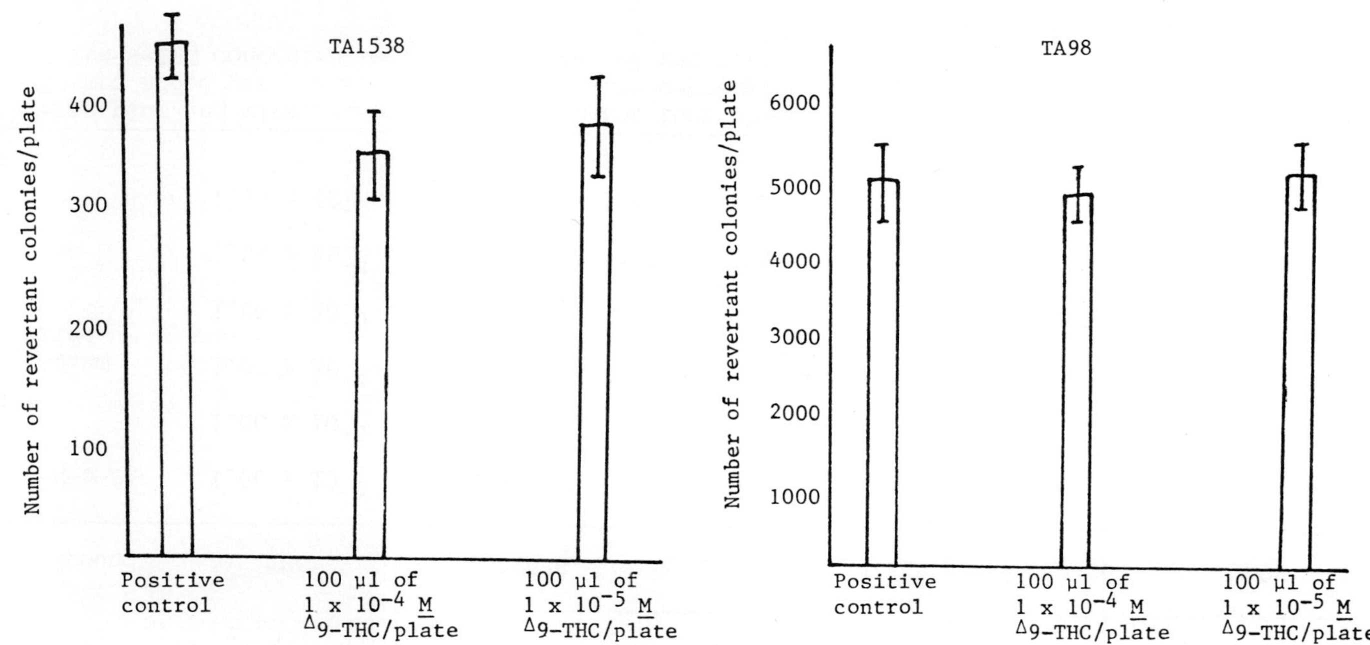

FIGURE 4. THC concentrations in conjunction with 4-nitro-o-phenylene diamine compared to positive control values with strains TA1538 and TA98. Brackets indicate +/- standard error of the mean.

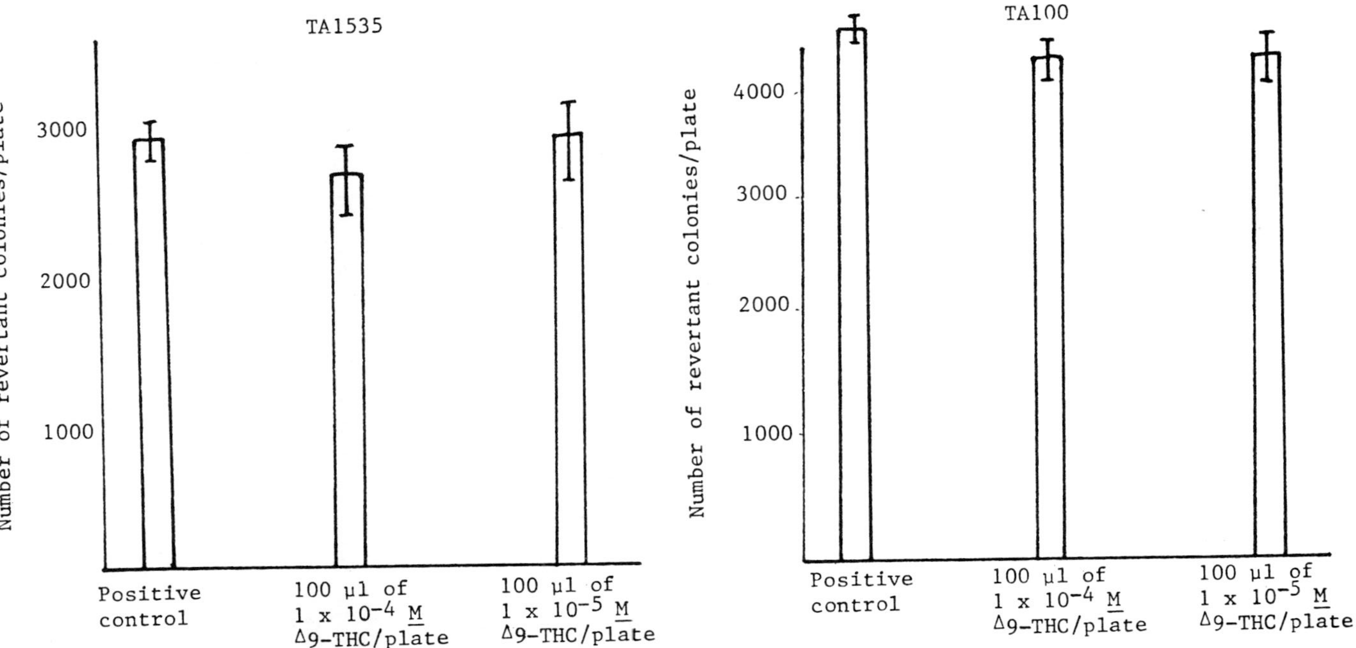

FIGURE 5. THC concentrations in conjunction with sodium azide compared to positive control values with strains TA1535 and TA100. Brackets indicate +/- standard error of the mean.

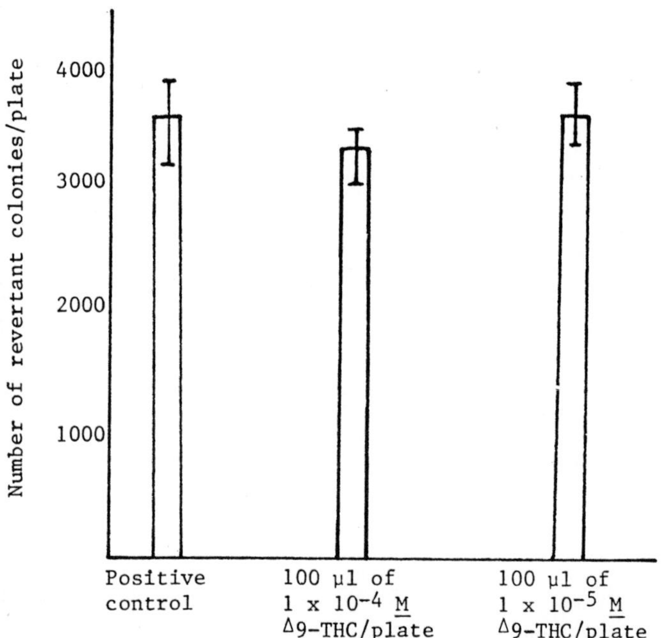

FIGURE 6. THC concentrations in conjunction with 9-aminoacridine compared to positive control values with strain TA1537. Brackets indicate +/- standard error of the mean.

The only statistical reductions (P = 0.05, Student t-Test) in the number of revertant colonies on the THC and mutagen treated plates when compared to the positive control plates receiving mutagens but no THC were with strains TA1538 and TA1535. Salmonella strain TA1538 demonstrated a 20% reduction in the number of revertant colonies when 100 mcl/plate of 1×10^{-4} M THC was employed in conjunction with 50 mcg/plate of 4-nitro-o-phenylene diamine; whereas, TA1535 plates showed a 18% reduction in the revertant colony counts when 100 mcl/plate of 1×10^{-4}M THC was employed simultaneously with 50 mcg/plates of sodium azide. All other experimental results when utilizing Salmonella strains TA1537, TA100, and TA98 were not statistically different from positive control values. However, the experimental results from these Salmonella strains suggested some suppression of mutagenicity.

D. Incorporation Tests Using S-9 Mix

Five micrograms per plate of 2-aminoanthracine, a promutagen, was used in conjunction with THC and 0.5 ml/plate of S-9 mix for all five bacterial test strains. Results are shown in Table V. With 100 mcl/plate of 1 x 10^{-4}M THC, strain TA1538 exhibited a 27% increase in the number of revertant colonies as compared to positive control plates receiving only 2-aminoanthracine and S-9 mix and a 14% increase when 100 mcl/plate of 1 x 10^{-5}M THC was employed. TA1537 showed a 23% increase in the number of revertant colonies when 100 mcl/plate of 1 x 10^{-4}M THC was used and a 1% increase when 100 mcl/plate of 1 x 10^{-5}M THC was employed as compared to the positive control values. Strain TA100 gave colony counts that were 24% lower than the positive control values when 100 mcl/plate of 1x 10^{-4}M THC was administered; a 2% reduction in revertant colonies was observed when 100 mcl/plate of 1 x 10^{-5}M THC was used. Strain TA98 showed a 4% decrease in the number of reverted colonies when 100 mcl/plate of 1 x 10^{-5}M THC was used. These results are compared with the positive control values for 2-aminoanthracine with S-9 mix in Figures 7, 8, and 9.

The THC seemed to have an unusual effect on strains TA1538 and TA1537 when 2-aminoanthracine and S-9 mix was employed in that they gave colony counts slightly higher than positive controls. This could be the result of cumulative effect of all these agents (THC, 2-aminoanthracine, and S-9 mix). However, strains TA1535, TA100, and TA98 gave colony counts slightly lower than the positive control values. None of these results when utilizing S-9 mix and THC using the promutagen were statistically different from the positive control plates (P = 0.05, Student t-Test) due to the wide variation of colony counts from one observation to another.

E. Growth Studies with THC

A growth study using different concentrations of THC was done to see if the level of toxicity upon the *Salmonella typhimurium* mutants was dependent on the dose of THC employed. Results presented in Table VI show that as the concentrations of THC being used was diminished, the number of bacteria that grew into colonies were higher, thus showing that the level of toxicity of THC is dependent upon its dosage being employed with all five strains of *Salmonella typhimurium* being used in the Ames Salmonella/microsomal testing being performed.

IV. DISCUSSION

Mutagens are thought to alter DNA; thus it is feasible to use bacteria in testing for mutagenicity (17). Dr. Bruce Ames

TABLE V. Delta-9-THC Concentrations in Conjunction with 2-Aminoanthracine and S-9 Mix[a]

Compound	THC[c]	Number of colonies/plate[b]				
		TA1538	TA1537	TA1535	TA100	TA98
2-AA[d]	1.00×10^{-4}	185 +/- 28	215 +/- 29	415 +/- 36	3076 +/- 867	1670 +/- 86
	1.00×10^{-5}	167 +/- 29	213 +/- 30	474 +/- 43	3969 +/- 406	2035 +/- 503

[a] Rat liver homogenates containing enzymes for promutagen activation (0.5 ml/plate).
[b] Mean plus and minus standard deviation for four observations.
[c] Delta-9-THC concentration added in 100 mcl per plate.
[d] 2-AA = 2-aminoantracine with 0.5 ml S-9 mix per plate.

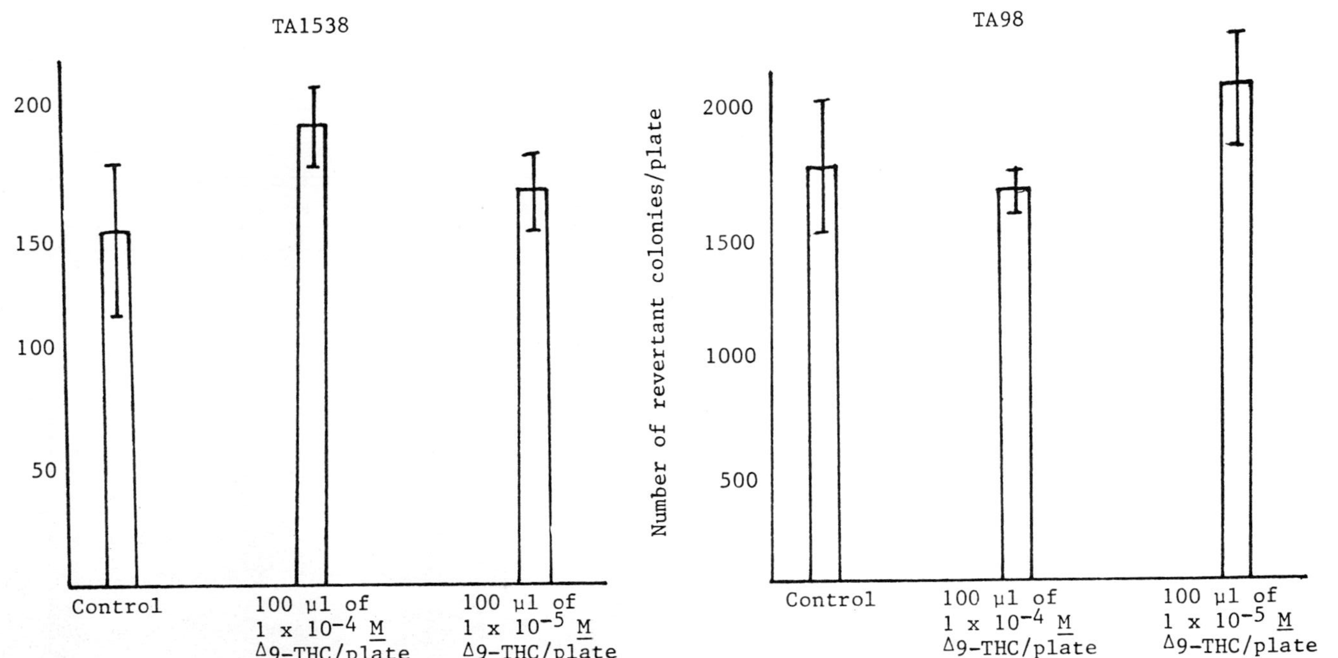

FIGURE 7. THC concentrations in conjunction with 2-aminoanthracine and S-9 mix (rat liver homogenates containing enzymes for promutagen activation, 0.5 ml/plate) compared to control values with strains TA1538 and TA98. Brackets indicate +/- standard error of the mean.

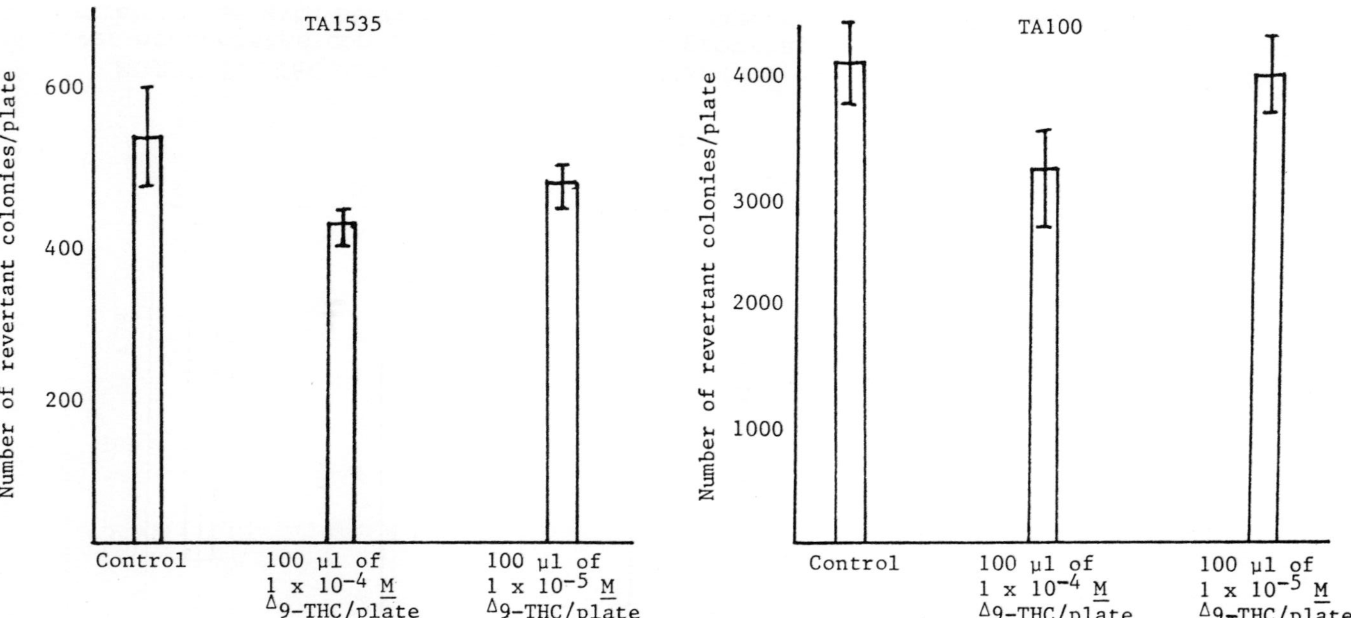

FIGURE 8. THC concentrations in conjunction with 2-aminoanthracine and S-9 mix (rat liver homogenates containing enzymes for promutagen activation, 0.5 ml/plate) compared to control values with strains TA1535 and TA100. Brackets indicate +/- standard error of the mean.

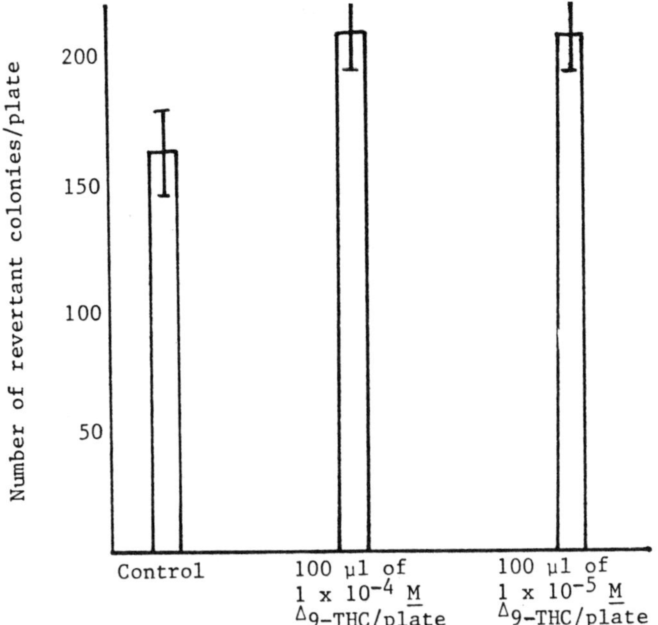

FIGURE 9. THC concentrations in conjunction with 2-aminoanthracine and S-9 mix compared to control values with strain TA1537. Brackets indicate +/- standard error of the mean. S-9 mix: rat liver homogenates containing enzymes for promutagen activation (0.5 ml/plate).

and co-workers have developed a method for detecting mutagens (and thus carcinogens) by using mutants of *Salmonella typhimurium* to observe reversion of a histidine-requiring auxotrophic mutant to a non-histidine requiring prototroph (12). An enzyme-activated liver homogenate, termed S-9 mix, can be employed to better stimulate a mammalian system that either can activate promutagens to mutagens or can produce nonmutagenic metabolites from that which was originally mutagenic. Many of the established carcinogens have been found to be mutagenic (18). About 90% of the known carcinogens tested in the Ames Salmonella/ microsomal system have been found to be mutagenic (12, 18).

Since the early 1960's the use of marijuana and other illicit drugs have increased at an alarming rate (19). Delta-9-tetrahydrocannabinol (THC), the major psychoactive compound in marijuana, has been shown to inhibit the incorporation of radioactively labeled precursors of DNA in HeLa cells, human fibroblastic cells, human neuroblastoma cells, and mouse fibroblastic cells by as much as 50% (8,20). By diminishing DNA synthesis the incorporation of radioactively labeled precursors of RNA and protein were also significantly diminished.

TABLE VI. Results of THC Dose-Dependent Growth Study.

Condition	Number of colonies/plate[a]				
	TA1538	TA1537	TA1535	TA100	TA98
Control	34	23	167	111	102
Ethanol[b]	59	28	153	125	156
6.36×10^{-3}[c]	3	7	14	0	0
1.00×10^{-3}	10	8	21	3	30
1.00×10^{-4}	22	21	34	11	45
1.00×10^{-5}	37	24	48	53	63

[a]Numbers represent the average from triplicate plates.
[b]Ethanol, 100 mcl/plate, added as solvent control.
[c]Delta-9-THC concentration added in 100 mcl per plate.

Also, THC has been shown to substantially decrease the number of spontaneous revertants of Salmonella typhimurium mutants in the Ames Salmonella/microsomal bioassay system (4,5,14).

The research presented in this study shows that THC not only decreased the number of spontaneous revertants of the five Salmonella mutant strains tested but also the ability to diminish the rate of mutation in two of the Salmonella mutant strains when used in conjunction with known mutagens. When 100 mcl/plate of 1×10^{-4}M THC was used in conjunction with 50 mcg/plate of 4-nitro-o-phenylene diamine, the number of revertant colonies in Salmonella strain TA1538 was reduced by 20% when compared to the positive control plates. When 100 mcl/plate of 1×10^{-4}M THC was employed in conjunction with 50 mcg/plate of sodium azide, the number of revertant colonies in Salmonella strain TA1535 was reduced by 13% when compared to the positive control plates. Since strain TA1538 is a frameshift mutant and TA1535 is a base-pair substitution mutant, these results indicate that THC may have the ability to suppress the action of some frameshift and base-pair substitution mutagens in bacterial systems to some extent. Salmonella strains TA1537, TA100, and TA98 also were repressed to some degree, depending on the amount of THC employed, but these values were not satistically different ($P = 0.05$) from the positive control values. The growth study performed showed that the toxicity of THC on the Salmonella typhimurium mutants is dependent upon the amount employed.

The mechanistic action of THC regarding repression of nucleic acid synthesis is not well understood. Blevins and

Smith (8) showed that THC did not prevent membrane uptake of radioactively labeled precursors of DNA, RNA and proteins, and proposed that one way in which THC could suppress DNA synthesis was by decreasing DNA pool sizes. However, subsequent studies revealed that DNA pool sizes were not adversely affected (21). This had led some researchers to propose that THC's effect on repression growth is at the level of enzymatic synthesis of DNA (8,22). Other studies have shown that very low concentrations of THC may stimulate the enzyme adenylate cyclase, involved in the synthesis of cyclic adenosine 3'-5' monophosphate (cyclic AMP), which in turn is associated with reduced cellular growth (23).

REFERENCES

1. Abel, E. L., "The scientific study of marijuana". Nelson-Hall Publishers, Chicago, 1976.
2. Busch, F. W., Seid, D. A. and Wei, E. T., Mutagenic activity of marijuana smoke condensates, Cancer letters 6:319-324 (9179).
3. Glatt, H., Ohlsson, A., Gurell, A., and Oesch, F., delta-9-tetrahydrocannabinol and la,2a-epoxyhexahydrocannabinol: Mutagenicity investigation in the Ames test, Mutat. Res. 66:329-335 (1979).
4. Zimmerman, A. M., Stich, H., and San, R., 1978. Nonmutagenic action of cannabinoids in vitro, Pharmacol. 16:333-343 (1978).
5. Lee, M. R., 1976. Mutagenicity screening of pesticides, nitrosocarbamates, and hallucinogens using Salmonella typhimurium mutants, p. 32. Thesis, East Tennessee State University, Johnson City, Tennessee, 1976.
6. Kier, L. D., Yamasaki, E., and Ames, B., Detection of mutagenic activity in cigarette smoke condensates, Proc. Natl. Acad. Sci. 71:4159-4163 (1974).
7. Sholes, T. E., Effects of pharmacologically active chemicals on HeLa cell numbers, nucleic acids and protein, p. 31. Thesis, East Tennessee State University, Johnson City, Tennessee, 1974.
8. Blevins, R. D., and Smith, D., Effects of delta-9-tetrahydrocannabinol on cultured HeLa cell growth and development, Growth 44:133-138 (1980).
9. Smith, D. P., The effect of delta-9-THC, nitrosocarbaryl and lysergic acid diethylamide of DNA and cytoplasmic RNA fractions in HeLa cells, p. 29. Thesis, East Tennessee State University, Johnson City, Tennessee, 1977.
10. Blevins, R. D., and Dumic, M., The effect of delta-9-tetrahydrocannabinol on herpes simplex virus replication, J. Gen. Virol. 49:427-431 (1980).

11. Garner, R. C., Miller, E. C., and Miller, J. A., Liver microsomal metabolism of aflatoxin B_1 to a reactive derivative toxic to _Salmonella typhimurium_ TA1530, Cancer Res. 32:2058-2066 (1972).
12. Ames, B. N., McCann, J., and Yamasaki, E., Methods for detecting carcinogens and mutagens with the Salmonella/ mammalian microsome mutagenicity test, Mutat. Res. 31:347-364 (1975).
13. Malling, H. V., in "Handbook of Teratology", Volume 4, (J. Wilson and F. Fraser, eds.), pp. 35-39. Plenum Press, New York, 1978.
14. Blevins, R. D., Lee, M., and Regan, J., Mutagenicity screening of five methyl carbamate insecticides and their nitroso derivatives using mutants of _Salmonella typhimurium_ L2, Mutat. Res. 56:1-6 (1977).
15. Blevins, R. D., Crenshaw, R., Hougland, A., and Clark, C., The effects of microwave radiation and heat on specific mutants of _Salmonella typhimurium_ LT2, Rad. Res. 82:511-517 (1980).
16. Blevins, R. D., and Taylor, D. E., Mutagenicity screening of 25 cosmetic ingredients with Salmonella/microsome test, J. Enviro. Sci. Health A17:217-239 (1982).
17. Ames, B. N., The detection of chemical mutagens with enteric bacteria, in "Chemical mutagens: Principles and methods for their detection". Vol.1 (A. Holiaender, ed.), pp. 267-282. Plenum Press, New York, 1971.
18. McCann, J., Choi, E., Yamasaki, E., and Ames, B., Detection of carcinogens as mutagens in the Salmonella/microsome test Assay of 300 chemicals, Proc. Natl. Acad. Sci. 72:5135-5139 (1975).
19. Cohen, S., "The drug dilemma". McGraw-Hill Book Company, St. Louis, 1969.
20. Blevins, R. D., and Sholes, T., Response of HeLa cells to selected pesticides and hallucinogens, Growth 42:478-485 (1978).
21. Blevins, R. D., and Smith, D., Effects of delta-9-tetrahydrocannabinol on cultured HeLa cell growth and development, Growth 44:133-138 (1980).
22. Pringle, H. L. and Bradley, S., Mechanism of the antimicrobial action of delta-9-tetrahydrocannabinol on _Naegleria fowleri_. Developments in Industrial Microbiology 22:789-796 (1981).
23. Maugh, T. H., II., Marijuana: New support for immune and reproductive hazards, Science 190:865-867 (1975).

Section VII THERAPEUTIC ASPECTS

RECENT ADVANCES IN THE USE OF CANNABINOIDS AS THERAPEUTIC AGENTS

R. Mechoulam

Hebrew University
Jerusalem, Isreal

N. Lander, M.Srebnik, I. Zamir
A. Breuer, B. Shalita, S. Dikstein

Hebrew University Pharmacy School
Jerusalem, Isreal

E. A. Carlini, J. Roberto Leite

Department of Psychobiology
Escola Paulista de Medicina
Sao Paulo, Brazil

H. Edery, G. Porath

Isreal Institute for Biological Research
Sackler School of Medicine
Tel Aviv University
Ness Ziona, Isreal

I. INTRODUCTION

The search for therapeutically active cannabinoids is going on in numerous laboratories throughout the world. The main thrust has been in trying to dissociate the undesirable CNS side effects (typical THC-type effects) from the potentially useful antiemetic, antiglaucoma, anticonvulsive and analgetic effects (1-3).

The Cannabinoids: Chemical,
Pharmacologic, and Therapeutic Aspects

ISBN 0-12-044620-0

The main psychotropic component of hashish and marijuana, delta-1-tetrahydrocannabinol (THC) (or delta-9-THC by an alternative nomenclature), which we isolated, identified and synthesized in the sixties (4), is already in wide experimental clinical use as an antiemetic during cancer chemotherapy. However, the side effects caused by THC prevent its use in other pharmaceutical areas at present.

In the last few years we have devoted considerable amount of effort towards dissociating, by molecular modification, the CNS side effects from the anti-convulsive, antiglaucoma and analgetic effects in this series. We wish to report now on some of our results. A few of these have been disclosed in patents.

II. PHARMACOLOGICAL STUDIES

A. Anticonvulsant Activity

The anticonvulsant action of natural (-)-CBD in animals and in man is well documented (5-8). It seemed of interest to determine the structure-activity relationships in these series in order to explore the possibility of increasing the potency

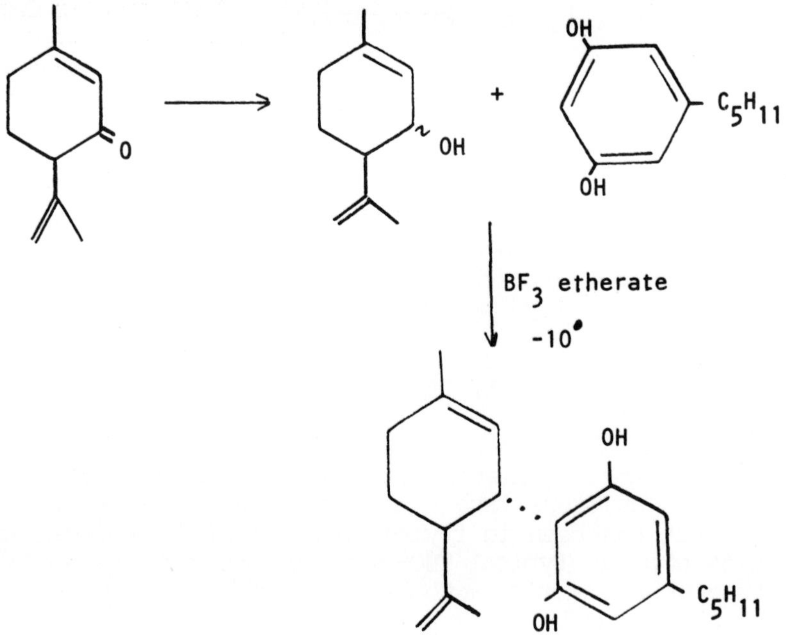

FIGURE 1. Synthesis of (+)-CBD.

as well as to obtain initial clues as to the mechanism and site of action. Some years ago, we reported on the activity of several simple derivatives of CBD (6). Most derivatives were active in the transcorneal electroshock test at approximately the same dose levels as CBD itself.

It is generally believed that the unique stereospecificity seen in biological systems is due to a complementary three dimensional interaction between a drug and an assymetric receptor site (9). The actual equivalence of activity of CBD and its analogs observed by us previously (6) led us to suspect that CBD acts on a system which does not involve a receptor site, but rather a less specialized system. In order to verify this hypothesis we synthesized the (+)-enantiomer of the active natural (-)-CBD. We assumed that a high stereospecificity in the action of CBD could indicate the existence of a three dimensional receptor or site of action. The synthetic route is described in Fig. 1. The method used is applicable to both enantiomers as the starting material is available in

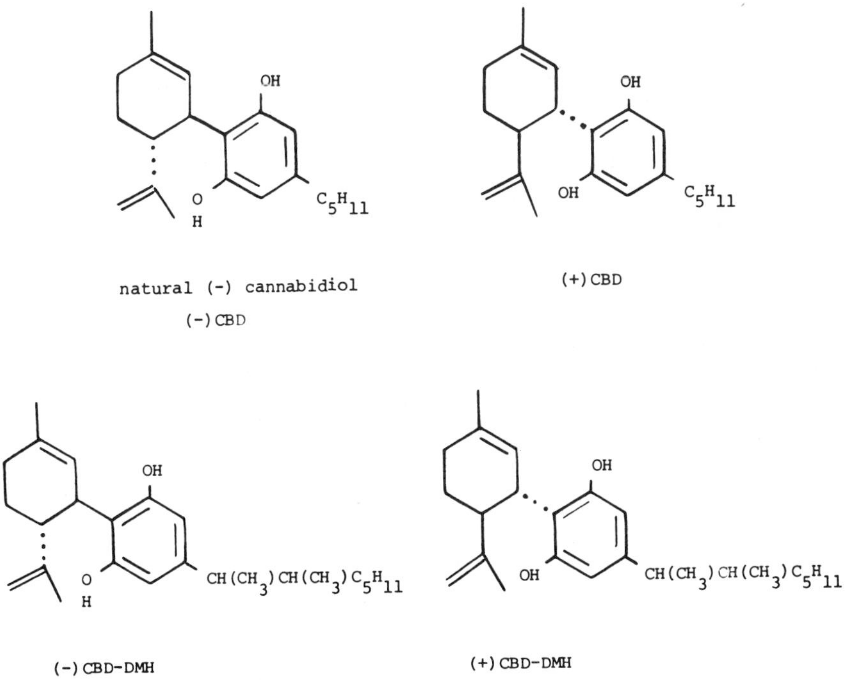

FIGURE 2. CBD and analogs tested in the anticonvulsant test described in the text and in the legend to Fig. 3.

both the 4S and the 4R isomers. In addition, the side-chain 1,2-dimethylheptyl (DMH) homologs of both enantiomers were prepared (Fig. 2). This particular modification was chosen as in the tetrahydrocannabinol (THC) series as such a chemical change was known to greatly increase the psychotropic potency.

1. Maximal Electroconvulsive Seizures (MES). After convulsive current 99.9% (C.C 99.9%) was established, groups of ten animals were injected i.p. with the cannabinoid suspensions. At several time intervals after the injection, the animals were submitted to the test. It consisted in applying a convulsive current transcorneally. The time of hindlimbs extension and frontlimbs flexion ratio were recorded and expressed as to ratio extension/flexion (6).

2. Pentobarbitone Sleeping-Time. Groups of 10 animals each were injected with suspensions of the cannabinoids or with saline solution. Forty five minutes later, the animals received a pentobarbitone solution, 40 mg/kg, i.p. The interval between loss and recovery of righting reflex was recorded as being the sleeping-time.

3. Results. Fig. 3 shows that the (+)- and (-)-isomers of CBD are essentially equally active in the MES test. The DMH homologs of both isomers are also essentially equipotent, although they are somewhat more active than the CBD isomers.

The two CBD isomers, as well as the two CBD-DMH isomers, potentiated pentobarbitone sleeping time. At some dose levels the (+)-isomers were somewhat more potent.

The above results tend to support our assumption that CBD does not act on a specific receptor, but rather on a less specialized system.

Some years ago Banerjee et al. (10) showed that CBD inhibited the rate of cerebral cortex synaptosomal uptake of GABA. It should be a considerable challenge to correlate this finding with the apparent lack of stereospecificity of CBDaction reported now.

B. Dissociation of the Psychotropic and Analgetic Effects in a Synthetic Cannabinoid

Delta-1-tetrahydrocannabinol (THC) and several of its synthetic analogs have been found to cause analgesia in animals and man (for formula of THC and analogs, see Fig. 4). As cannabis does not have a high addiction potential, an analgetic drug based on the cannabinoid skeleton can be of pharmaceutical importance, if dissociation between the psychotropic and analgetic effects is achieved as discussed above. Indica-

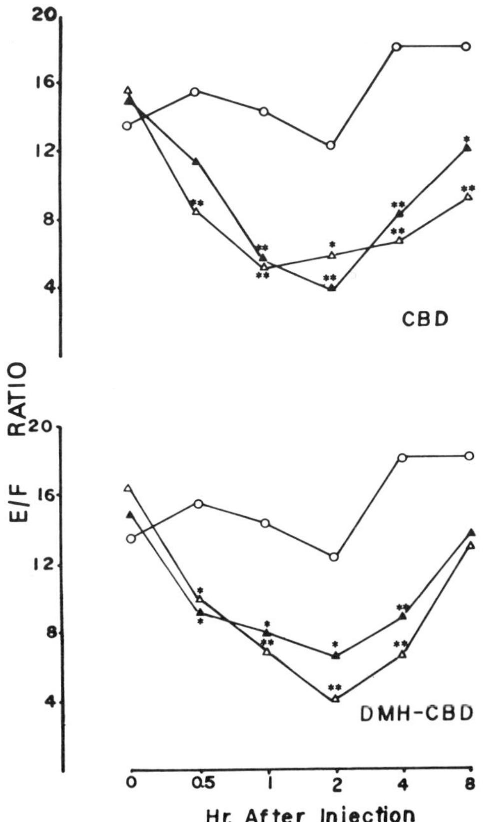

FIGURE 3. Influence of dextro (open triangles) and levo (solid triangles) isomers of CBD (100 mg/kg) and DMH-CBD (50 mg/kg) on the extension of flexion time ratio (E/F ratio). Control mice injected with the vehicle are represented by open circles. (* $p < 0.05$; ** $p < 0.01$; Student's t-test)

tions that these two effects are inherently separable have been published (11).

As part of a program aimed at achieving such a dissociation we have synthesized and tested a series of cannabinoids. The complete results will be published elsewhere. We wish to report now that in preliminary pharmacological tests the THC analog I has been found to have approximately retained the analgesic activity of the parent drug but to be at least 20 times less psychotropic than THC (12).

The most salient feature of the new analog I is that its two chiral centers (at C-3 and C-4) have a configuration oppo-

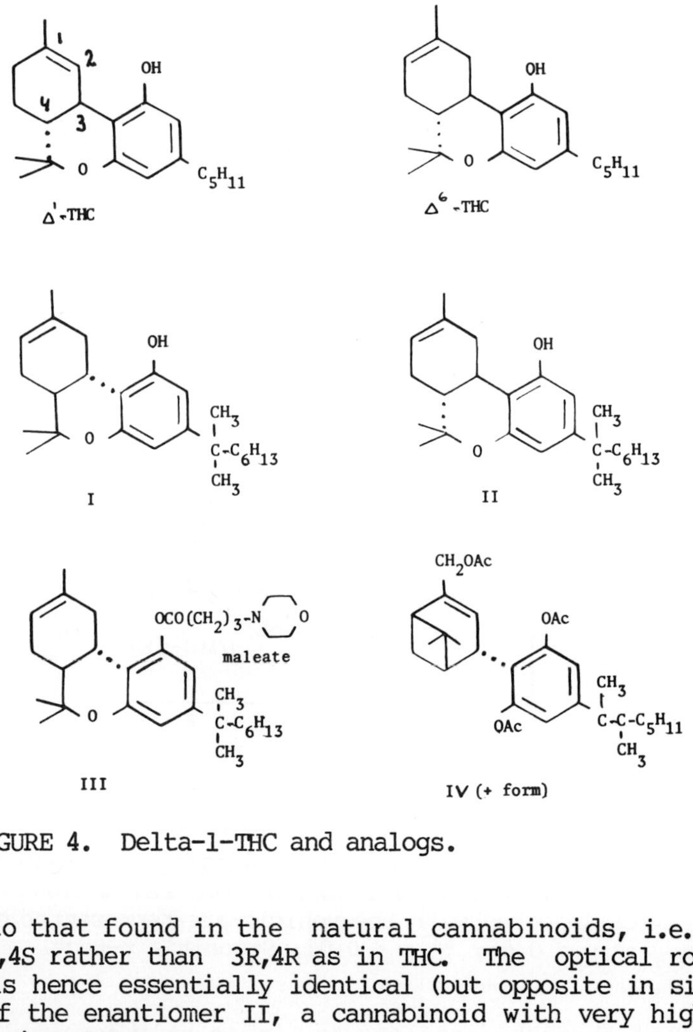

FIGURE 4. Delta-1-THC and analogs.

site to that found in the natural cannabinoids, i.e., they are 3S,4S rather than 3R,4R as in THC. The optical rotation of I is hence essentially identical (but opposite in sign) to that of the enantiomer II, a cannabinoid with very high psychotropic potency.

1. Synthesis. We have followed the general route previously developed by us (4b) for 3S,4S cannabinoids (Fig. 5). The optical purity of I (and consequently the level of psychotropic activity) obviously depends on the optical purity of the starting material (+)-pinene from which verbenol is obtained. In our best preparation, starting from (+)-pinene (a) + 51.4^{o}, we obtained I, $[a]_D$ + 218°. Enantiomer II, in which the chiral centers correspond to those in the natural series showed $[a]_D$-2122°.

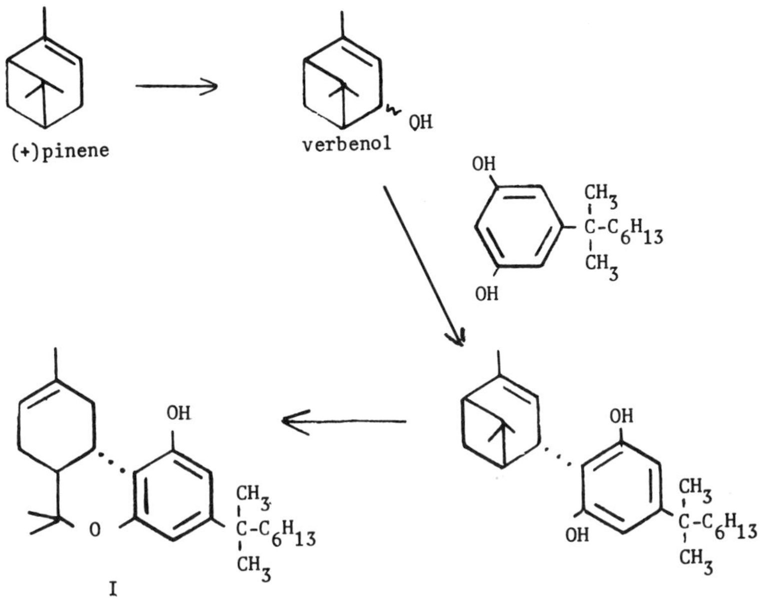

FIGURE 5. Synthesis of THC analog I.

2. Analgetic tests. All compounds were administeredas fresh suspension (0.1-0.2 ml) orally to mice. The test compound was dissolved in propylene glycol and a solution of 2% gun accacia was gradually added to form the suspension. The final concentration of propylene glycol was never above 5%. The tests were carried out at least on 3 dose levels in order to calculate the dose response lines.

a. Acetic acid induced writhing test. Six mice perdose level were examined. Thirty minutes after administration of the drug 0.6% acetic acid (0.25 ml) was injected i.p. The numberof abdominal contractions per animal was counted for 25 minutes (13).

b. Tail flick test. Ten mice per dose level was examined. The mouse was held in the standard receptacle. The tail was immersed into water at 58°C and immediately withdrawn on jerk. If no response occurred up to 5 sec., the tail was withdrawn. After a 5 sec. rest the procedure was repeated for a total of

10 times. The percentage of negative responses were noted and statistically evaluated. We found that counting the negative responses gave more reproducible data than measuring the time of the response as the original paper (14).

3. Psychotropic Tests. The psychotropic activity of cannabinoids has been tested in a number of laboratory animals including dogs, mice, rats, gerbils and monkeys. A comparison of the major somatic and behavioral effects by a THC in man and in rhesus monkey shows a reasonable similarity: close threshold effective doses (ca. 50 mcg/kg), dose dependent effects, impairment of motor coordination, redness of conjuctivae, pseudoptosis, loss of muscle strength, heart rate increase, decline of aggression, sleepy state, impairment of performance, etc. Some of these symptoms such as redness of conjunctivae and pseudoptosis, seem to be specific for primates. Hence the rhesus monkey test has been found the most suitable (15).

The compounds were administered i.v.; the solvent used was propylene glycol. Injections were made into the saphenous vein at a maximum volume of 0.1 ml/kg. The observers were unaware of the nature of the compounds being tested. At least two animals were used for the testing of each compound at every dose. The estimation of the psychotropic effects is semiquantitative. The effects were monitored and rated as previously described (16).

C. Results and Discussion

A significant difference between the enantiomers I and II is observed (see Table I). The (-)-enantiomer II, in which the chiral centers correspond to those of the natural cannabinoids, causes a cataleptoid state in mice at the analgetic dose range of THC, thus preventing any meaningful evaluation of an analgetic dose response curve. The analgetic effect of the (+)-enantiomer I in both tests is at the range of THC and delta-6-THC; its dose response lines do not significantly deviate from the parallel lines of morphine. The (+)-enantiomer I is ca 20 times less psychotropic than THC; the (-)-enantiomer II is more potent than THC.

A point of interest is that the analgetic activity of cannabinoids administered orally is better manifested in the writhing pain test than in the tail test. As writhing pain is assumed to be mediated by prostaglandin formation, it seems possible that the analgetic effect reported now is due to this inhibition (18).

It must be taken into account, however, that the optical purity of I depends on the optical purity of the starting

TABLE I. Mouse Analgesia and Monkey Behavioral Tests[a]

Compound	Mouse ED_{50}[b]		Monkey Psychotropic Activity	
	Writhing	Tail Flick	mg/kg	rating
Delta-1-THC	5	50	0.05	(+/-)
			0.10	(++)
			0.25	(++)
			0.50	(+++)
Delta-6-THC	7	>80	0.1-0.3	(+)
			0.4-0.9	(++)
			1.0-2.0	(+++)
Compound I	9	60	1.0	(-)
			2.0	(+)
			4.0	(++)
Compound II	P[c]	P	0.02	(-)
			0.05	(+)
			0.10	(+++)
			0.25	(+++)[d]
Compound IV			1.0	(-)
+ isomer	10	50	4.0	(-)
- isomer	10	30	5.0	(-)
Morphine	4	20		

[a]For experimental conditions see text.

[b]Expressed in mg/kg and calculated according to Lichfield and Wilcoxon (17). The dose-response curves did not deviate from parallel.

[c]P, denoted psychotropic activity, due to which analgesia could not be determined.

[d]The behavioral changes were remarkably intense and lasted for three days.

material which is seldom absolute. Hence a low percentage (1-2%) of II may be present in the tested samples of I. A possible pharmacological interaction between I and II cannot be excluded.

The observation that the analgetic and psychotropic activity are separable may be of considerable importance in the development of new analgetics.

III. NOVEL CANNABINOID ANTIGLAUCOMA AGENTS

Interest in using cannabis for the treatment of glaucoma was first stimulated by the observation of Hepler et al. (19) that intraocular pressure decreased when healthy human subjects smoked cannabis (see ref. 20 for extensive reviews). A considerable amount of research has been published on this topic. Smoking or ingestion of marijuana or THC definitely causes reduction of intraocular pressure in both healthy humans and those with glaucoma. However, intraocular administration has not led to definite results and consistent effects have not been observed (21).

Ideally a preparation that could be applied topically to the eye would be most desirable for humans because this would allow for self-administration and would limit the action to the eye. One would also look for cannabinoids which do not cause CNS side effects.

We assumed that THC showed inconsistent results when administered topically due to the extremely low water solubility. Hence we decided to prepare water soluble derivative of cannabinoids which showed no 'hashish' effects when administered to monkeys. In part 'A' of this presentation, we described the synthesis of (+)-delta-6-THC-DMH (I) and presented data showing that it has a low 'hashish' effect on monkeys. Hence we decided to prepare its water soluble maleate salt III, and test it for antiglaucoma effect. The synthesis is straightforward from compound I and follows related preparations by Pars et al. (22).

TABLE II. Reduction of Intraocular Pressure in Glaucomatic Rabbits Treated with Compound III*

Time of Treatment	Intraocular Pressure (mm Hg)
0	29
15 min	18.5
30 min	19.5
60 min	22.0
90 min	21.5
6 hr	22
22 hr	24

*For description of method see text and ref. 23.

The maleate salt III was tested by topical application into an eye of a glaucomatic rabbit of 0.2 ml of a 0.3% aqueous solution. The glaucoma was induced by administration of Betsovet (Glaxo, betamethasone adamantoate and betamethasone sodium phosphate) as described by Bonomiet al. (23). The results are presented in Table II.

We assumed that the water soluble ester III is rapidly hydrolyzed to compound I when absorbed into the eye and is not washed away by the tears due to its lipid solubility. We expect this to be the case in humans as well, and as compound I has very low 'hashish' type activity we expect no CNS side effects.

We have demonstrated here that dissociation can be achieved between the antiglaucoma and typical 'THC-like' effects and, as in the case of analgesia, we believe that this observation may lead to the development of new antiglaucoma drugs.

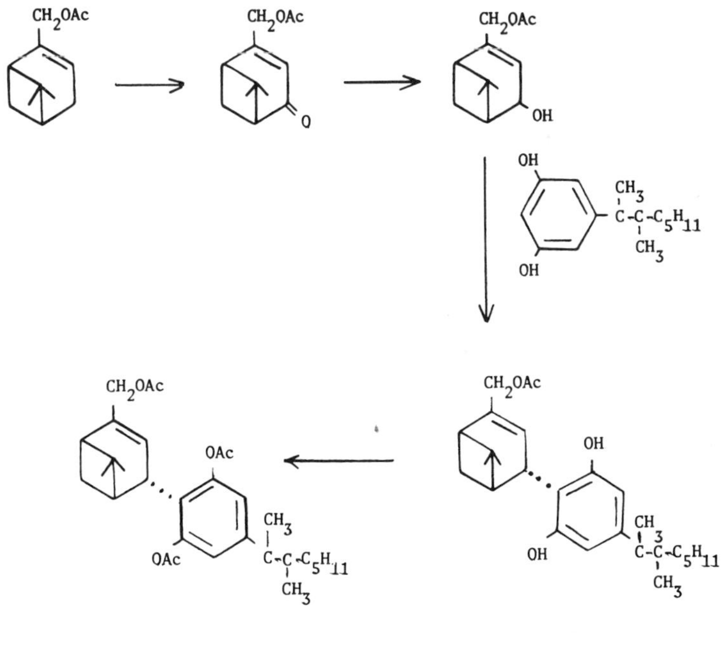

CH_2OAc → CH_2OAc (O) → CH_2OAc (OH)

OH, OH, CH_3, C-C-C_5H_{11}, CH_3

CH_2OAc, OAc, OAc, CH_3, C-C-C_5H_{11}, CH_3 ← CH_2OAc, OH, OH, CH_3, C-C-C_5H_{11}, CH_3

IV (+ form)

FIGURE 6. Synthesis of cannabinoid IV, lacking a pyran ring.

D. Is a Pyran Ring Needed for Cannabinoid Analgetic Activity?

As mentioned above, numerous THC-type cannabinoids have been found to possess analgetic activity. All these cannabinoids possess a pyran ring. It seemed of possible interest to find cannabinoids in which major structural changes were made and yet have retained some of their pharmacological properties. We wish to report now that compounds such as acetate IV, which do not possess a pyran ring and retain the analgetic properties of THC yet show no THC-type psychotropic activity. These observations have been reported in a patent (24).

The synthesis of compound IV is described in Fig. 6. The results of the analgetic tests and the psychotropic test in monkeys are given in Table I.

Compound IV [in both the (+) and the (-) form] is about as active as THC in the writhing test but is at least 50 times less active than THC in the psychotropic test.

The observation that a pyran ring is not an absolute requirement for analgetic activity (although it may be one for THC-type activity) is of considerable importance and may lead to the eventual development of clinically useful analgetics.

E. THC Augments Opioid Activity

Both cannabis, in its various forms, and opium are widely used in Indian traditional medicine. Frequently they are used together suggesting a possible synergism. The potentiation of morphine activity by crude cannabis has indeed been documented (25). It seemed of interest to find out whether a synergistic

TABLE III. Analgesia Produced by Analgetics Administered Orally[a]

Compound	ED_{50} (mg/kg)[b]
Morphine hydrochloride	4
Codeine phosphate	17
Acetyl salicylic acid	330
(-)-delta-1-THC	5
(-)-delta-6-THC	7
Phenylbutazone	180

[a]For experimental conditions see text.
[b]Calculated according to ref. 17.

effect does indeed exist between cannabinoids and opiates. The existence of such an effect could eventually make possible the use of lower doses of opiates than those in a clinical setting, generally administered today, thus avoiding side effects.

We would like to report now on the effects of THC and delta-6-THC on various analgetics.

The acetic acid writhing test was employed as described above. Initially we tested the potency of several analgetics administered orally. The results are presented in Table III and are compatible to those in the literature.

Then we administered mixtures containing ED_{20} doses of THC and the appropriate analgetic. We found that ED_{50} doses of the analgetic tested were reduced 4-6 fold (Table IV). These results are better expressed in graphic form in Fig. 7 and 8.

These results show that the potency of certain analgetics, including opiates, can be increased considerably by the addition of low amounts of either delta-1- or delta-6-THC. These observations, if valid for man, can be of considerable importance. Thus, if the increase in potency of codeine is not paralleled by an increase in dependence liability (which for codeine is much lower than that of morphine), this relatively safe compound may find a new, very important place in the clinic. The same applies to phenylbutazone. The possibility of using doses of morphine in the clinic lower than those generally employed today is also an intriguing one.

Is it possible to augment analgetics using non-psychotropic cannabinoids? We do not have a definite answer yet but preliminary evidence is encouraging.

TABLE IV. Potentiation of Action Analgetic Agents by Delta-1- or 6-THC[a]

Compound A	Compound A[b]	Compound B[c]	Synergism
Acetylsalicylic acid	50	1-THC	6-fold
Codeine phosphate	3	1-THC	5-fold
Codeine phosphate	3	6-THC	5-fold
Morphine HCl	1	1-THC	4-fold
Phenylbutazone	40	1-THC	5-fold
Phenylbutazone	40	6-THC	5-fold

[a]For method employed see text.
[b]Dose, ED_{50} in mg/kg.
[c]Dose, ED_{20} = 3 mg/kg.

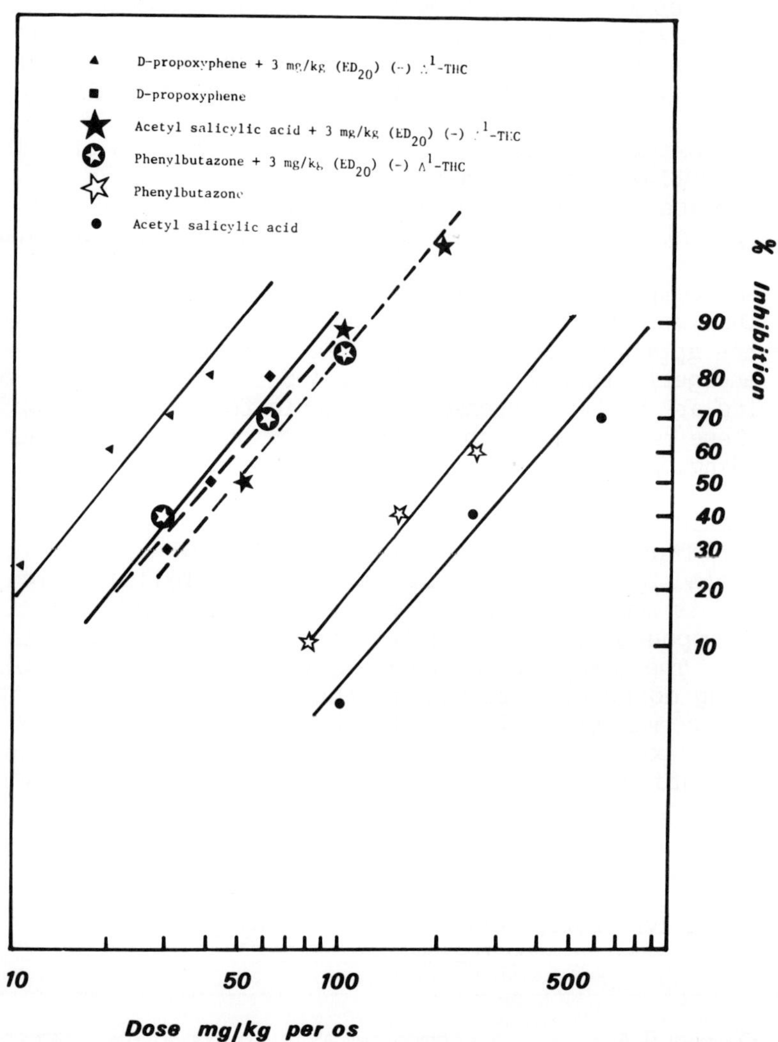

FIGURE 7. Potentiation of non opiate analgetics by THC. See text for details.

REFERENCES

1. Cohen, S., and Stillman, R. C., (eds.), "The Therapeutic Potential of Marihuana". Plenum, New York and London, 1976.

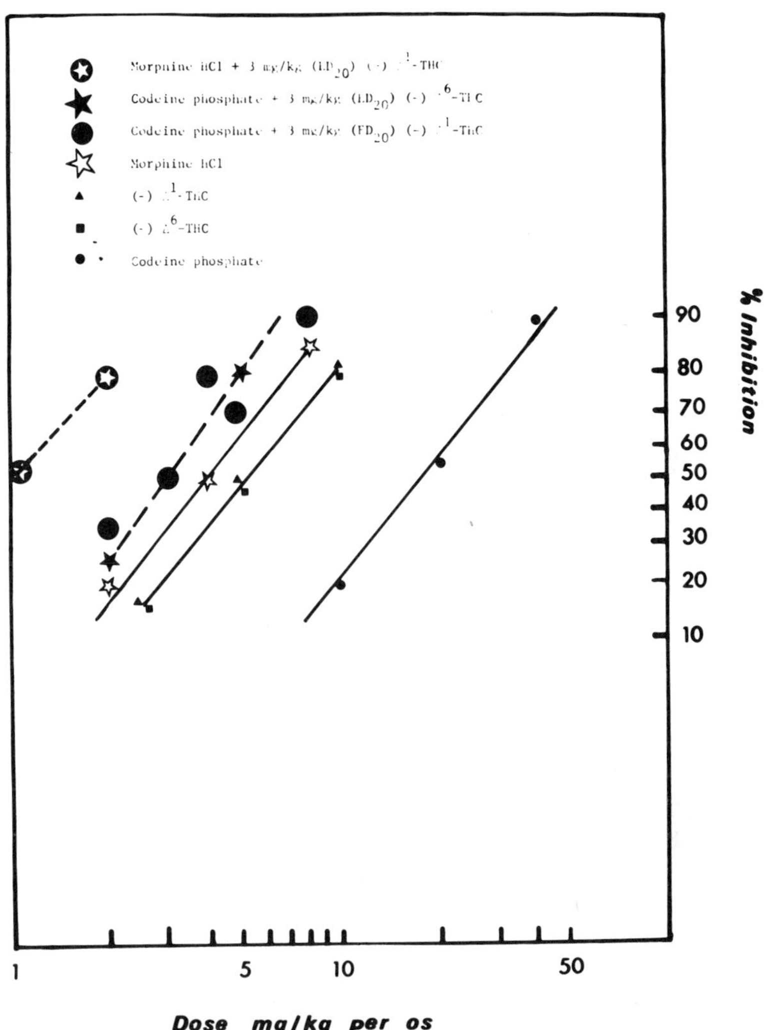

FIGURE 8. Potentiation of opiate analgetics by delta-1- and -6-THC. See text for details.

2. Mechoulam, R., and Carlini, E. A., Naturwissenschaften 65:174 (1978).
3. Milne, G. M., Johnson, M. R., Wiseman, E. H., and Hutcheon, D. E., (eds.), "Therapeutic Progress in Cannabinoid Research". Pfizer Biomedical Research Symposia, J. Clin. Pharmacol. 21, Nos 8 and 9, Supplement (1981).

4. a. Gaoni, Y., and Mechoulam, R., J. Amer. Chem. Soc. 86:1646 (1964); b. Mechoulam, R., Braun, P., and Gaoni, Y., Amer. Chem. Soc., 89:4552 (1967) and 94:6159 (1972); c. Mechoulam, R., Shani, A., Edery, H., Grunfeld, Y., Science 169:611 (1970).
5. Cunha, J. M., Carlini, E. A., Pereira, A. E., Ramos, O. L., Pimentel, C., Gagliardi, R., Sanvito, W. L., Lander, N., and Mechoulam, R., Pharmacology 21:175 (1980).
6. Carlini, E. A., Mechoulam, R., and Lander, N., Res. Commun. Chem. Pathol. Pharmacol. 12:1 (1975).
7. Karler, R., and Turkanis, S. A., J. Clin. Pharmacol. 21:437S (1981).
8. Consroe, P., Martin, A., and Singh, V., J. Clin. Pharmacol, 21:428S (1981).
9. Patil, P. W., Miller, D. D., Trendelenburg, U., Pharmacol. Rev. 26:323 (1975); Humbler, C., and Marshall, G. R., Ann. Rep. Medic. Chem. 15:267 (1980).
10. Banerjee, S. P., Snyder, S. H., and Mechoulam, R., J. Pharmacol. Exp. Therap. 194:74 (1975).
11. Wilson, R. S., May, E. L., Martin, B. R., and Dewey, W. L., J. Med. Chem. 19:1165 (1976); Milne, G., Koe, B. K., Johnson, M. R., in "Problems Drug Depend. Proc. 41 Annual Meeting" (L. S. Harris, ed.), p. 84. Dept. Health, Education, and Welfare, Washington, D. C., 1979.
12. Compound I was first disclosed by us in a patent (US Patent 4,179,517, 1979). The same compound I, as well as its enantiomer II, were later independently reported by Archer et al., J. Org. Chem. 42:2277 (1977), but no biological data were discussed.
13. Sofia, R. D., Nalepa, S. D., Harakal, J. J., Vassar, H. B., J. Pharmacol Exp. Ther. 186:646 (1973).
14. Grotton, M., and Sulman, F. G., Arch. Int. Pharmacodyn. 170:257 (1967).
15. Grunfeld,Y., and Edery, H., Psychopharmacologia, 14:200 (1969).
16. Mechoulam, R., and Edery, H., in "Marijuana, Chemistry, Pharmacology, Metabolism and Clinical Effects" (R. Mechoulam, ed.), pp. 101-136. Academic Press, New York, 1973.
17. Litchfield, J.T., and Wilcoxon, F., J. Pharmacol. Exp. Ther. 96:99 (1949).
18. Burstein, S., Levin, E., Varanelli, C., Biochem. Pharmacol. 22:2905 (1973); Jackson, D. M., Malor, R., Chesher, G. B., Starmer, G.A., Welburn, P. J., Bailey, R., Psychopharmacology 47:187 (1976).
19. Hepler, R. S., and Frank, I. M., J. Amer. Med. Assoc., 217:1392 (1971).
20. Green, K., in "Current topics in eye research" (J. A. Zadunaisky and H. Davson, eds.), p. 175. Acad. Press,

New York, 1979. Korczyn, A.D., Gen. Pharmacol. 11:419 (1980).
21. Merritt, J. C., Perry, D. D., Russell, D. N., and Jones, B. F., J. Clin. Pharmacol. 21:467S (1981).
22. Pars, H. G., Razdan, R. K., and Howes, J. F., Adv. Drug. Res., 11:97 (1977).
23. Bonomi, L., Perfetti, S., Noya, E., Bellucci, R., and Massa, F., v. Graefes Arch. Klin. Exp. Ophthal. 210:1 (1979).
24. Mechoulam, R., Lander, N., and Distein, S., Israel Patent 55.274 (1978); U.S. Patent 4,282,248 (1981).
25. Ghosh, R., and Bhattacharya, S. K., Ind. J. Med. Res., 70:275 (1979).

POSSIBLE ANXIOLYTIC EFFECTS OF CANNABIDIOL

Richard E. Musty

Department of Psychology
University of Vermont
Burlington, Vermont

I. INTRODUCTION

Cannabidiol (CBD) has anti seizure effects as demonstrated by several techniques, e.g., electroshock induced seizures (1), kindled seizures (2), pentylenetetrazol induced seizures (1), and in a small sample of human epileptics (3). In addition, CBD has sedative properties since it increases pentobarbital-induced sleeping time and decreases the ED50 of naloxone-induced withdrawal from morphine (4). While CBD seems to share some of these properties with delta-9-tetrahydrocannabinol (THC), differences between these marijuana constituents are also apparent. CBD depresses spontaneous motor activity much less than THC (4), and produces much less depression of lever-pressing behavior on a variable interval schedule of reinforcement (5). Finally, CBD does not produce a psychological "high" in human subjects (3,6-8). Likewise rats can discriminate THC from Tween-80/saline control solution, while they can discriminate CBD from the THC but cannot discriminate CBD from the same control solution (9).

In addition to these data, reviews of historical uses of cannabinoids have suggested that marijuana has been used for analgesic, antispasmodic, anti-hypertensive, and sleep-induction effects. Furthermore, on the basis of clinical observation the author has clinical reports that marijuana can block spasmodic-toritcolus and relieve situational anxiety. While none of these reports is clearly experimental nor do they separate the effects of one cannabinoid molecule from another, these reports are suggestive enough to warrant experimental investigation of cannabinoid effects in animal experiments which may reflect anxiolytic properties of such molecules. The present experiments were designed to test the effects of

ISBN 0-12-044620-0

CBD on body tremor and seizures during withdrawal from alcohol intoxication in mice, on active avoidance acquisition in mice, on lick-suppression in rats and on ulcerogenesis in mice. If CBD has effects which are similar to known anxiolytic drugs on these tests, such data would suggest further examination of CBD for anxiolytic effects.

II. EXPERIMENT I: Effects of CBD, THC and Clonidine on Alcohol Withdrawal Symptoms in Mice.

Since anti-anxiety-type compounds are often recommended for their calming effects during alcohol withdrawal, the present investigation was designed to test the effectiveness of THC and CBD during alcohol withdrawal in mice. In addition, recent human studies have suggested that clonidine (an alpha-2-adrenergic blocker) has anti-anxiety properties (12). It is anti-hypertensive, in both animals (13-15) and man (16) and has calming effects during withdrawal from opiates in animals (17-18) and in man (19). Finally, clonidine is effective in reducing symptoms during withdrawal from alcohol in man (20). Thus the present study was also designed to test the relative efficacy of clonidine during alcohol withdrawal.

A. METHOD

1. Subjects. A total of 450 naive male C57BL/6J mice (23-268) (a high alcohol preference strain) were obtained from Jackson Laboratory, Bar Harbor, Maine. They were maintained on a 12-hour light-dark cycle at 21°C. Animals were given food and water ad libitum and were group housed until the experiment was started, at which time they were placed in single cages for the duration of the experiment.

2. Drugs. The following drugs and doses were used: 1) Delta-9-tetrahydrocannabinol (THC): of 0.5, 2.0 and 4.0 mg/kg; 2) Cannabidiol (CBD): 20, 40, and 80 mg/kg; 3) Clonidine, 4, 40 and 80 mg/kg; 4) Tween-80 + saline placebo (control); 5) No drug (sham injection control).

THC and CBD were obtained from the National Institute on Drug Abuse (NIDA). Clonidine was obtained fromBoehringer Ingleheim, Inc. All drugs were prepared in a 0.6% Tween-80 in 9% physiological saline solution and injected as a constant volume concentrations. Drugs were administered intraperitoneally (i.p.) at three consecutive times during with withdrawal period; since the duration of the effect of each drug may have been short, due to rises and falls in blood levels of the drugs, we decided to inject each at 1.0, 2.5, and 4.0 h after the beginning of the measurement period.

3. Experimental Design. Twelve to 16 mice were withdrawn from alcohol and injected with one of the 9 drugs by dose combinations or 2 control injections in each of 20 replications across 40 weeks. In each replication, the injection of drug or control treatments were randomized. The final number of animals in each treatment group was 16.

4. Intoxication Procedure. The intoxication and withdrawal procedures were adapted from those of Freund (21,22); since our procedures are significantly different from his, they are described in detail. Mice were weighed and then placed on a feed deprivation schedule for 4 days. Each mouse was fed once daily for 1 hour. Water was available *ad libitum*. On the fifth day, each mouse was given a liquid diet dispensed in a 30 ml plastic syringe with a stainless steel drinking tube attached to it (23). The diet was a mixture of Sustacal, alcohol, and water and was the sole source of food and water during the phase of the experiment. Diet was prepared daily and given to the animals at 0900 h. Liquid diet consumption was measured at 0900, 1400 and 1900 h daily. The degree of intoxication was rated at the same times that diet consumption was recorded, as follows: *Stage 1*: ataxic, with rapid gait; *Stage 2*: grossly impaired gait or body movements, falling to the side, with the righting reflex intact; *Stage 3*: no righting reflex or comotose. After four days mice which had reached an intoxication criterion of Stage 2 or greater for in two-thirds of all daily ratings were used for withdrawal. Approximately 60% of the mice in each replication reached this criterion in 4 days, while about 20% died and 20% did not reach criterion.

5. Behavioral Measures of Withdrawal Data Recordings. Trained observers recorded the frequency and duration of two withdrawal signs: 1. tremors, which were defined as tremor of the hindquarters, or the whole body; 2. seizures, which were defined as tonic-clonic behavioral convulsions. Recording of these behaviors was accomplished by the observer depressing a switch at the beginning of each behavioral event and releasing the switch upon its termination. Switches were connected to an ABLE-40 computer (New England Digital Corporation), which recorded the frequency and durations of tremors and seizures in 5-min time blocks. The data were stored on diskettes, for subsequent reduction and analysis. Each observer recorded tremors and seizures for 4 mice simultaneously, in 3.5 h shifts. Interrater reliability was periodically

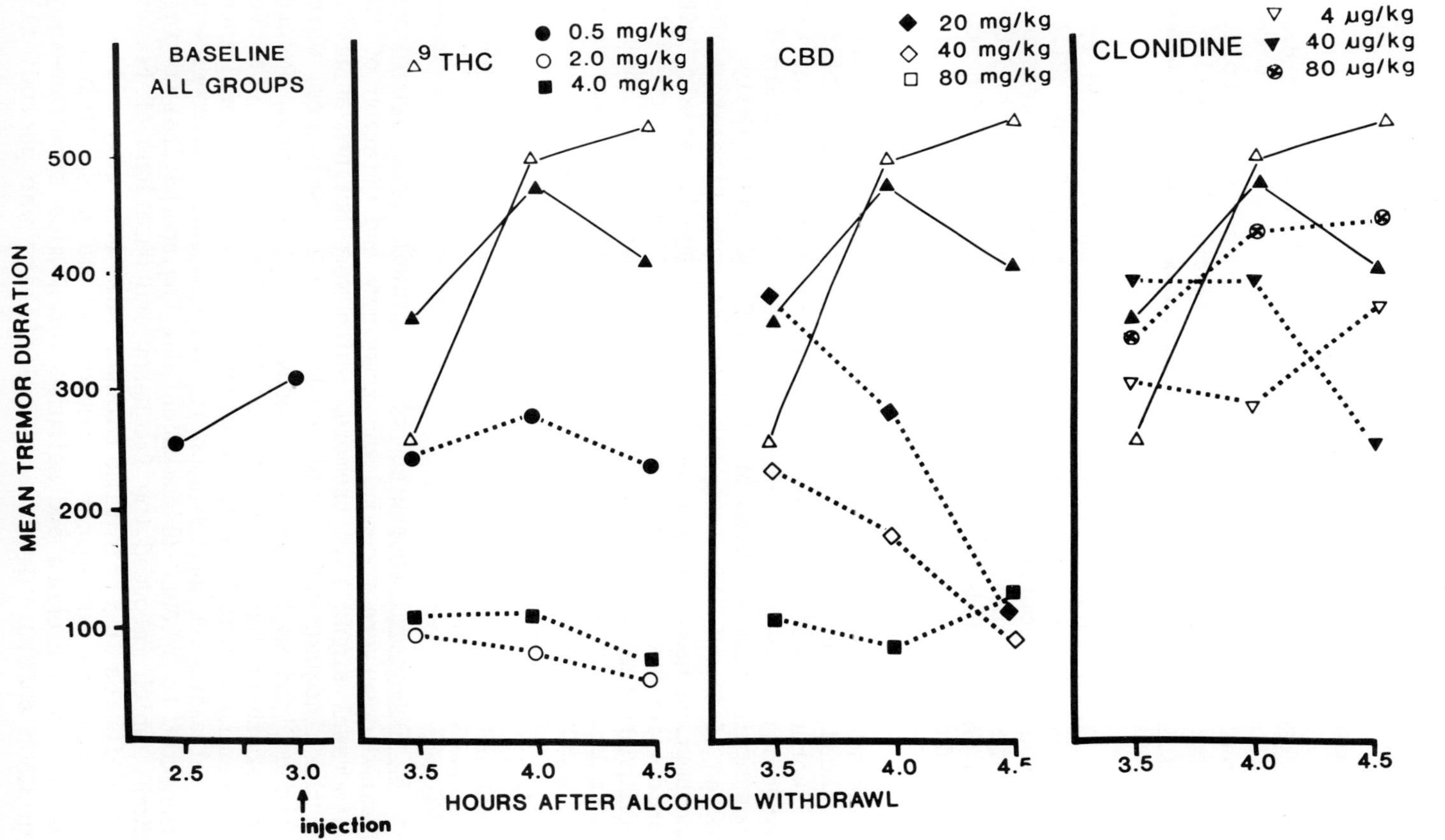

BASELINE
ALL GROUPS
Δ9 THC
0.5 mg/kg
2.0 mg/kg
4.0 mg/kg
CBD
20 mg/kg
40 mg/kg
80 mg/kg
CLONIDINE
4 µg/kg
40 µg/kg
80 µg/kg
MEAN TREMOR DURATION
500
400
300
200
100
2.5
3.0
injection
3.5
4.0
4.5
3.5
4.0
4.5
3.5
4.0
4.5
HOURS AFTER ALCOHOL WITHDRAWL

checked throughout the experiment and was considerably 0.90 or better.

6. Withdrawal Procedure. On the fifth day, the alcohol diet was withdrawn at 0800 h. A diet of Sustacal and water was provided during the subsequent 9 h withdrawal period. At 1100 h, observation of withdrawal symptoms began, for a baseline period of 1 h. At this point, the appropriate drug or control solution was injected, using a double blind procedure. Recording continued for 6 additional hours (9 hours after withdrawal of the alcohol diet).

7. Audiogenic Seizure Tests. In addition to recording spontaneous seizures, tests for audiogenic seizures were conducted at 1.5, 3.0, 4.5 and 6.0 h after the beginning of the measurement period. These times correspond to 30 min after each drug injection and 2.0 h after the last drug injection. (Seizures were elicited by sounding a fire alarm bell for 90 sec at each of the above times.) The sound intensity was measured as 100 db at 2 cm above the cage floor.

8. Data Analysis. The data for each drug were analyzed against the control injection conditions using two-way analyses of variance with repeated measures on one factor, on all behavioral measures. *Post hoc* comparisons were conducted only if main effects or interactions were significant, as recommended by Winer (24). For these comparisons, Simple-effects analyses and Newman-Keuls analyses were used (24). Initial analyses were conducted using drug x 5 min time blocks, and subsequent analyses were made in 30 min time blocks. All data are presented in reduced 30 min form.

B. RESULTS

1. Tremors. Figure 1 shows the effects of THC, CBD and clonidine on the duration of tremors during baseline and the 1.5 h period following the first injection of each drug. THC produced significant decreases in tremor duration at all

FIGURE 1. Mean tremor duration plotted as a function of the first 4.5 hours after alcohol withdrawl. Baseline shows the mean of all groups prior to injection. Appropriate drug injections occurred at 3.0 hours after withdrawl. Control groups are no injection (open triangles) and Tween-80 and saline injection (closed triangles) in each panel. Each drug group is shown in panels to the right of the baseline plot.

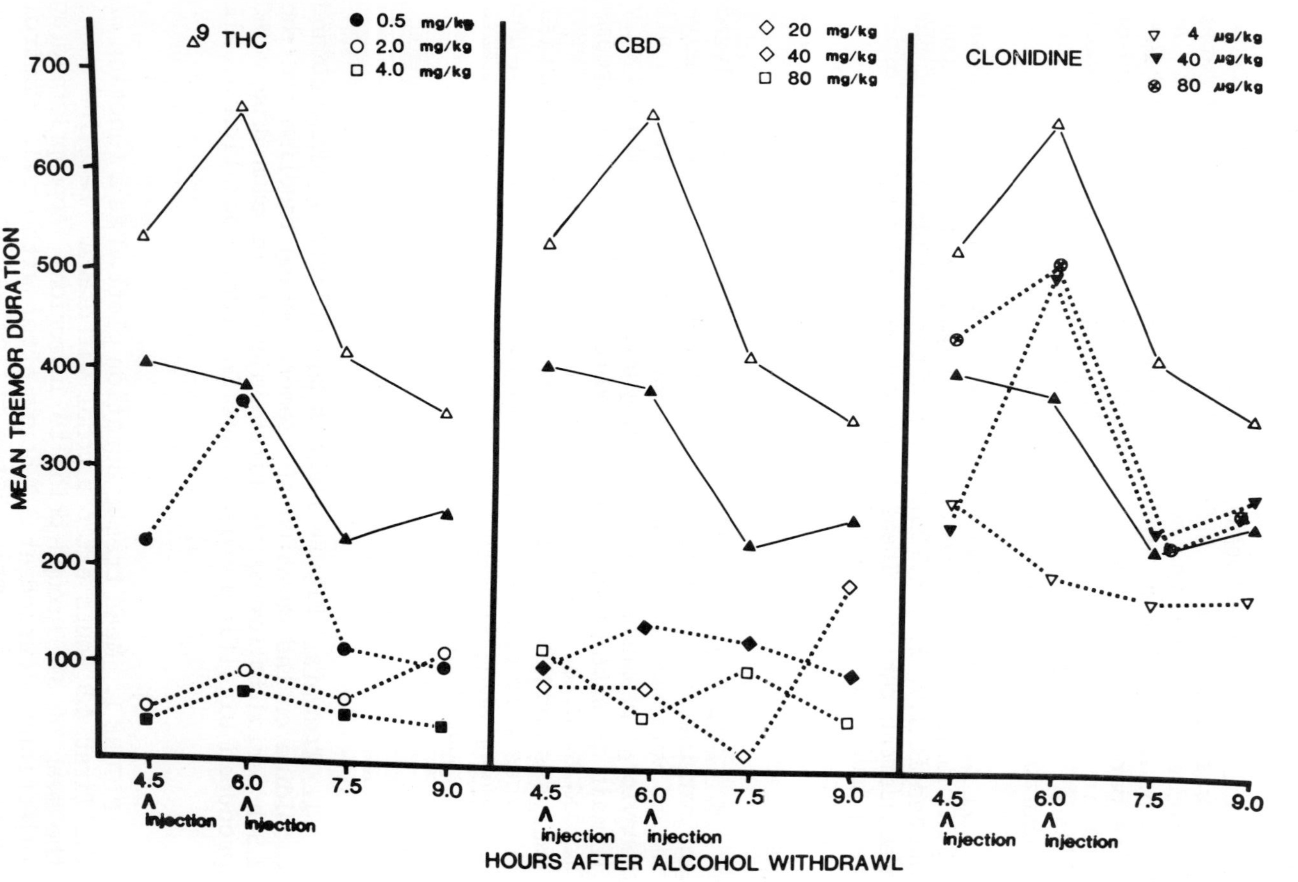
Δ9 THC
● 0.5 mg/kg
○ 2.0 mg/kg
□ 4.0 mg/kg
CBD
◇ 20 mg/kg
◇ 40 mg/kg
□ 80 mg/kg
CLONIDINE
▽ 4 μg/kg
▼ 40 μg/kg
⊗ 80 μg/kg
MEAN TREMOR DURATION
700
600
500
400
300
200
100
4.5
6.0
7.5
9.0
injection
injection
HOURS AFTER ALCOHOL WITHDRAWL

doses, when each dose was compared with the control groups (Newman-Keuls tests $p < 0.01$ for all comparisons). The two higher doses produced a significantly greater suppression of the tremors than the low dose (Newman-Keuls, $p < 0.01$). Control groups did not differ from each other. Simple-effects tests for each dose or control (condition) across that 1.5 h period (hours 3.0-4.5 after withdrawal) demonstrated that tremor durations increased significantly in both control groups and decreased in all THC groups ($p < 0.0001$ forall tests). CBD produced a significant decrease in tremor durations at all doses (Newman-Keuls, all tests, $p < 0.01$). CBD produced a dose related decrease in tremor at the 4.0 h point, but by 4.5 h, all doses were equally effective in reducing tremor durations. Simple-effects tests across the 1.5 h period indicate that the 20 and 40 mg/kg doses of CBD produced linear decreases in tremor duration, but the 80 mg/kg dose did not. (All tests, $p < 0.001$). With regard to clonidine, no significant changes in tremor duration were found at any dose (simple effects tests) during the 1.5 h period following injection.

Figure 2 illustrates the results of the second and third drug injections given during withdrawal. Simple-effects analyses demonstrated that subsequent injections of THC significantly suppressed tremor duration during the remainder of the test session. The two higher doses almost eliminated tremors entirely (Newman-Keuls, $p < 0.01$, all tests). The low dose of THC, however, produced significant decreases only in the last part of the test period (7.5 and 9.0 h after withdrawal). CBD, at all three doses, produced significant reductions in tremor durations (Simple effects, $p < 0.01$). No dose differences were found (Newman-Keuls). Clonidine significantly suppressed tremor durations only at the 6.0 and 7.5 h marks (Simple effects, $p < 0.01$). This effect was due solely to the 4.0 mg/kg dose. (Newman-Keuls, $p < 0.01$).

2. Seizures. Figure 3 illustrates the mean seizure frequencies for each half hour period following the presentations of the bell. Newman-Keuls analyses for each drug against control groups demonstrated that THC, CBD, and clonidine significantly suppressed seizure frequencies at the 3.5 and 6.0 h measurement periods. The frequency of seizures declined significantly in the control groups (Simple effects, $p < 0.01$).

FIGURE 2. Mean tremor duration plotted as a function of hours 4.5-9.0 after withdrawl from alcohol. Injections were made at 4.5 and 6.0 hours as indicated. Control groups are as in Fig. 1. Each drug group is shown in panels of the figure.

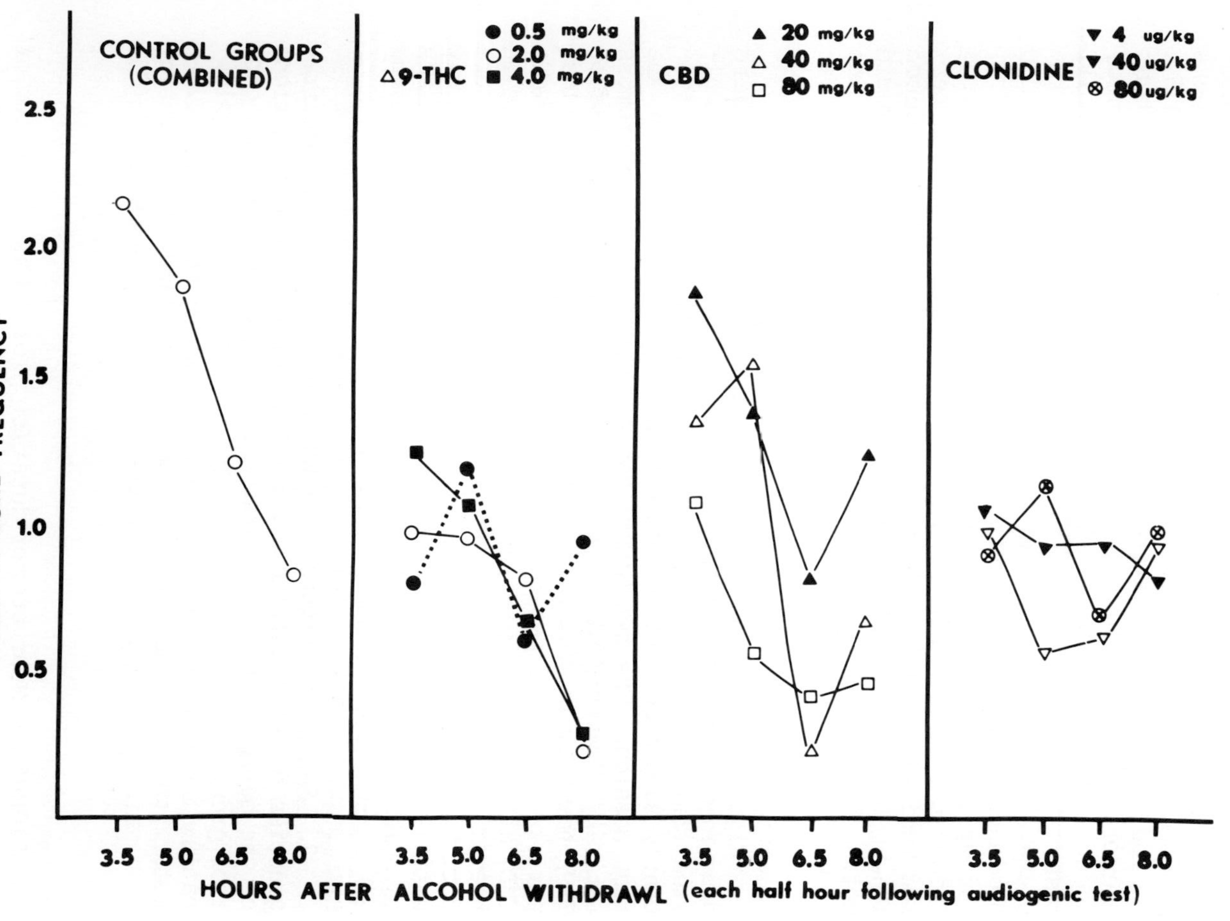
CONTROL GROUPS
(COMBINED)
Δ9-THC
● 0.5 mg/kg
○ 2.0 mg/kg
■ 4.0 mg/kg
CBD
▲ 20 mg/kg
△ 40 mg/kg
□ 80 mg/kg
CLONIDINE
▼ 4 ug/kg
▼ 40 ug/kg
⊗ 80 ug/kg
MEAN SEIZURE FREQUENCY
2.5
2.0
1.5
1.0
0.5
3.5 5.0 6.5 8.0
HOURS AFTER ALCOHOL WITHDRAWL (each half hour following audiogenic test)

Thus, when drug groups were tested against the control groups at the 6.5 and 8.0 h measurement periods, no significant differences were found, for any of the drugs. No significant effects of drug doses were found for THC or clonidine. With CBD, a significantly lower frequency of seizures was found between the 80 mg/kg dose and the 20 and 40 mg/kg dose at the 4.5 and 6.0 h measurement periods. The two lower CBD doses were not significantly different from controls.

III. EXPERIMENTS II: Effects of CBD, THC, and Diazepam on Active Avoidance Acquisition in Mice.

Anti-anxiety drugs have been shown to improve active avoidance behavior (25). Similarly, THC improves the acquisition of two-way active avoidance in rats (26). Thus, the present experiment was designed to compare the effects of CBD, THC, and diazepam (DZP) on active avoidance and acquisition in mice.

A. Methods

1. Subjects. Subjects were 78 C57Bl6J mice bred in our colony at the University of Vermont, from breeding stock obtained from the Jackson Laboratory, Bar Harbor, Maine. They were maintained in group cages of six mice per cage.

2. Drugs and Experimental Design. Ten groups of mice were run in the following conditions (numbers in each group are shown in parentheses): Tween 80 (0.06%) + normal saline, control injection (8); CBD: 20 (5) and 40 (9) mg/kg; THC: 1 (8), 2 (8), and 4 (8) mg/kg; and diazepam: 2.5 (8), 5.0 (8) and 10.0 (8) mg/kg. All drugs were mixed daily and administered in constant volume injections of 1.0 mg/100 g of body weight.

3. Procedure. A plexiglass running wheel for mice was used. Shock was delivered at 0.25 mA by a Grason Stadler shock source. A mouse was placed in the running wheel. Five

FIGURE 3. Mean seizure frequency for each half hour following the presentation of bell-sound to elicit audiogenic seizures. See text for further explanation. Groups are plotted separately in panels as indicated.

seconds after being placed in the wheel a 0.25 mA shock was delivered continuously until the mouse ran and turned the wheel at least one-half revolution. Once this had occurred shock was terminated for 20 seconds. If the mouse continued to run, each half revolution delayed subsequent shock for 20 seconds. If, however, the mouse remained motionless for 20 seconds, shock reoccurred. Each mouse was run on this schedule for 30 minutes.

Data recorded were: The number of shocks received per 5 min interval and the number of half revolutions per 5 min interval. Since there is a very high correlation between these measures, the number of shocks received are reported here.

B. Results

Figure 4 displays the number of shocks received by each test group during the 30-minute session plotted as a function of the dose of drug administered. CBD produced a significant decrease in the number of shocks received ($F = 3.64$, $df = 2,19$; $p < 0.0001$), as did THC ($F = 4.21$, $df = 3,28$; $p < 0.01$), and DZP ($F = 2.85$, $df = 3,28$; $p < 0.05$).

IV. EXPERIMENT III:
Effects of CBD and Diazepam (DZP) on Lick Suppression in Rats.

It has been demonstrated that benzodiazepines reduce the suppression of a learned response when that response is punished (27,28). Thus, the present experiment was designed to compare the effects of CBD and DZP in a punished response paradigm.

A. Method

1. Subjects. Seventy male, hooded rats weighing 200-225 g from Charles River Breeding Laboratories were used. They were maintained in cages in groups of two.

2. Drugs. Seven groups of rats were run in the following drug conditions (number of rats in each group are shown in parentheses): Tween 80 (0.6%) and normal saline, control injection (8); CBD: 15 (9), 30 (9), and 60 (9) mg/kg; DZP: 2.5 (10), 5 (10), and 10 (9) mg/kg. All drugs were mixed in

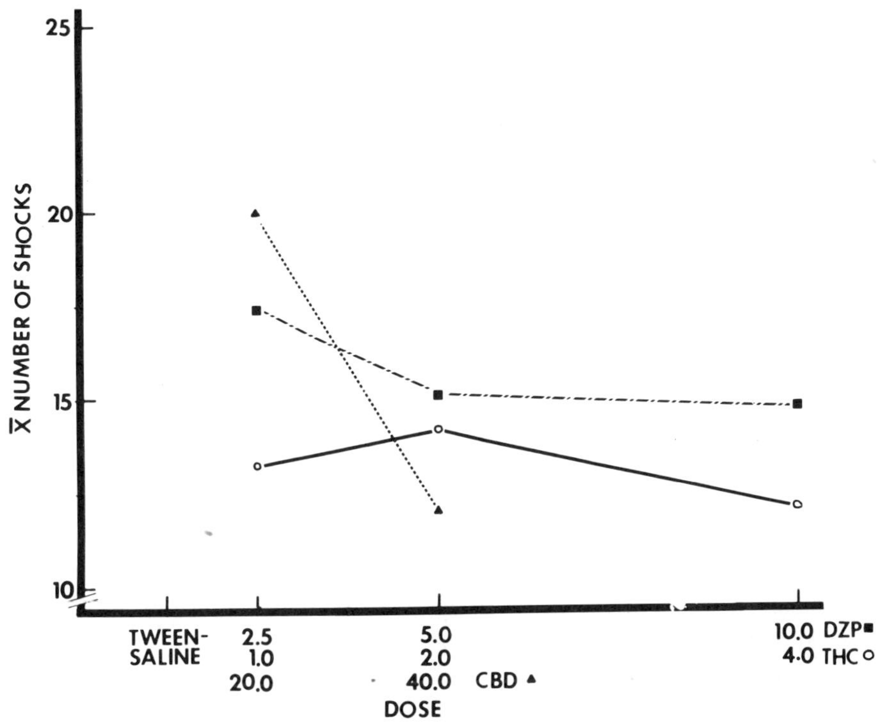

FIGURE 4. Mean number of shocks received in the running wheel avoidance task plotted as a function of control solution (Tween-80 + saline) and doses of diazepam (DZP), THC, and cannabidiol (CBD) as indicated on the abscissa.

Tween 80 - saline daily and were administered in constant volume injections of 1.0 ml/kg of body weight.

3. Procedure. A standard operant conditioning chamber with a stainless steel grid floor was used. On one wall a 20 ml syringe of water with a ball-point drinking tube projected into the chamber. Rats were first trained to drink from these tubes using the following procedure. On Day 1, the rats were deprived of water for 23 hours. Following this, they were allowed to drink in their home cage for one hour. This procedure was repeated for three consecutive days. On the fourth through the seventh days, each rat was allowed one hour to drink from the tube in the operant conditioning chamber. On

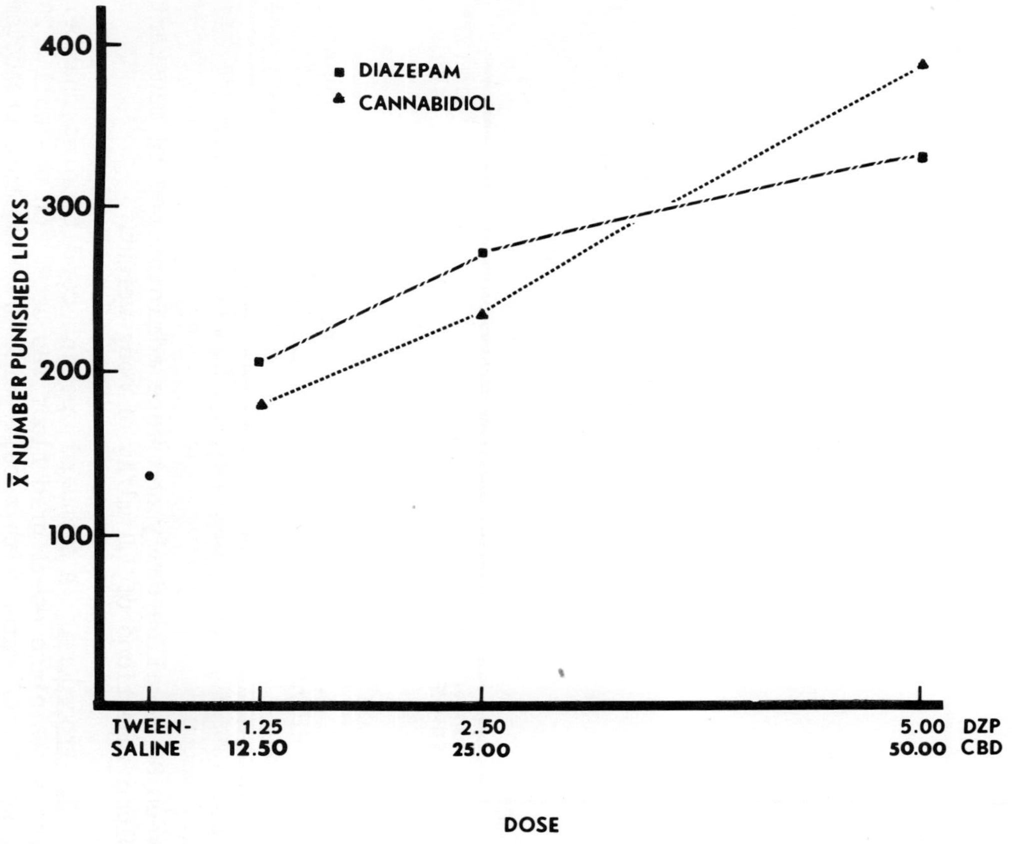

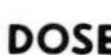

DIAZEPAM
CANNABIDIOL
$\bar{X}$ NUMBER PUNISHED LICKS
400
300
200
100
TWEEN-
SALINE
1.25
12.50
2.50
25.00
5.00 DZP
50.00 CBD
DOSE

the eighth day, each rat was placed in an operant conditioning chamber 20 min after the injection of CBD, DZP, or the Tween-80/saline control solution. The rat was allowed 1 min in which to freely drink water, during which time the number of licks was recorded using a Lehigh Valley lickometer circuit. From the end of the first minute for 9 additional minutes, the water spout was electrified with a mild shock (Grason-Stadler shock source 0.016 mA between the water spout and the grid floor). During this time, a lick was punished by electrical shock to the tongue of the rat. During this time, the number of punished licks (licks associated with shock) was recorded.

4. Data analysis. Data (number of punished licks) were analyzed by analysis of variance for each drug group.

B. Results

Figure 5 shows the results. Both CBD and DZP produce dose-related increases in the number of licks during the period in which drinking was punished (CBD: $F = 4.80$, $df = 3,37$, $p < 0.006$; and DZP: $F = 3.76$, $df = 3,39$, $p < 0.019$).

V. EXPERIMENT IV: Effects on CBD, THC and DZP on Stress Induced Ulcers in Mice.

The benzodiazapine chlordiazepoxide has been demonstrated to protect the rat against restraint induced ulcers (29). Glavin has presented evidence that experimentally induced ulcers is a valuable model for examining the relationship between stress and peptic ulcer disorder (30). Thus, the present experiments were designed to test the effects of CBD, THC, and DZP on the development of ulcers. In this experiment, we tested the effects of CBD and THC on ulcer development in mice.

FIGURE 5. Mean number of punished lick responses during the shock phase of a lick suppression test, plotted as a function of control solution (Tween-80 + saline) and doses of diazepam (DZP, squares) and cannabidiol (CBN, triangles) as indicated on the abscissa.

1. Subjects. Subjects were 70 male, CD-1 mice bred in our own colony at the University of Vermont from breeding stock obtained from Charles River Laboratories.

2. Drugs. Ten mice were tested in each of the following drug conditions: Tween-80 (0.6%) in saline, control injection; 2, 4, and 8 mg/kg THC; and 20, 40, or 80 mg/kg CBD. All drugs were mixed daily and administered in constant volume injections of 1.0 ml/100 g of body weight.

3. Procedure. In this paradigm, mice were administered the appropriate drug of control injection and placed in cylindrical chambers made of metal mesh 2 cm in diameter and 10 cm long and which were mounted on a board. An electrode was attached to the tail of the mouse after the technique of Weiss (31) and shocks of 0.24 mA were delivered to the feet of the mouse using a Grason-Stadler shock source. Shocks were automatically programmed to be delivered on a Variable-Interval, 60-second schedule for a period of 18 h. After this procedure, each mouse was returned to its home cage for 6 h without food and water being available. After this, each mouse was sacrificed by ether anesthesia and the stomach was removed, washed, and examined under a dissecting microscope for ulceration. Each ulcer was counted, the preparation photographed and later an independent observer recounted the ulcers to check the original observations.

B. Results

Figure 6 shows the results for this experiment. Both THC and CBD produced significant decreases in the frequency of ulcers (Chi square test, $p < 0.01$ for each drug).

VI. DISCUSSION

In the present series of experiments, we have demonstrated that cannabidiol: 1) reduces tremor and seizure activity associated with withdrawal from alcohol addiction, 2) facilitates the acquisition of an active avoidance behavior, 3) reduces the suppression of a punished response, and 4) reduces the development of stress induced ulcers. Several details about the comparative efficacy of cannabidiol require further discussion. First, in all of the tests used, CBD produced effects which were of equal or greater magnitude than various comparison drugs. In the alcohol withdrawal experiment, CBD and THC suppressed body tremor equally at the highest dose of

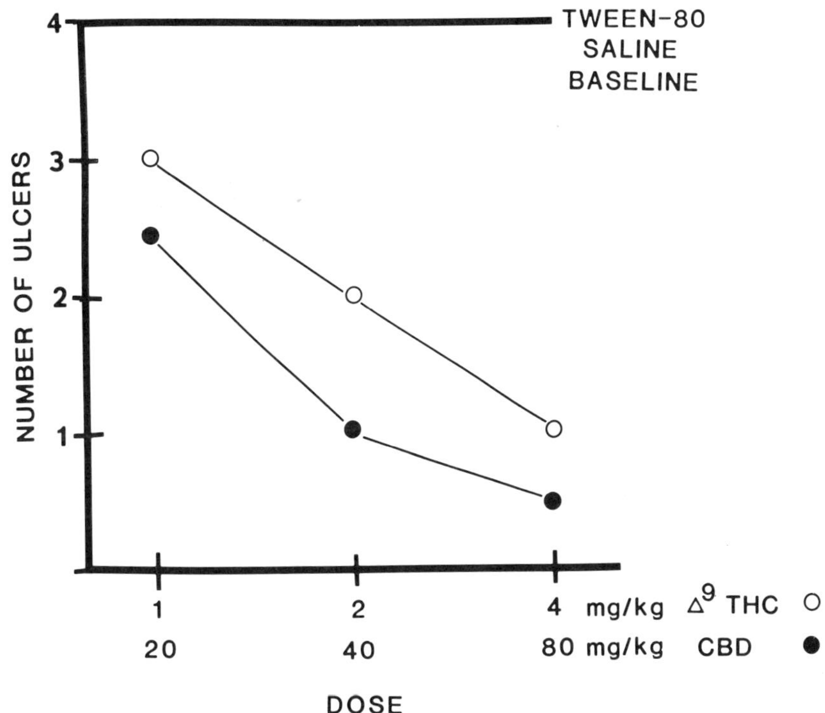

FIGURE 6. Mean number of ulcers which developed, plotted as a function of THC and CBD as shown on the abscissa. Mean number of ulcers in the control-injected group (Tween-80 + saline) is shown as a solid black line at the top of the plot.

each of the two drugs, and clonidine, the comparison drug, was also effective in reducing body tremor. With regard to seizures, drugs appeared to have seizure suppressing qualities and all were approximately equal in their efficacy in reducing the seizures, but dose response effects were not entirely clear. With regard to acquisition of active avoidance in the running wheel, CBD, THC, and DZP produced improved avoidance learning. Again, peak effects of each drug were not statistically different from each other. Similarly, in the lick-suppression test, both CBD and DZP produced a lack of response suppression and peak effects were not statistically different between the two drugs tested. Finally, both CBD and THC produced significant reductions in ulcerogenesis and were not different in the degree to which each drug reduced ulcers.

The consistency of these data strongly suggest that CBD can produce changes in anxiety-like responses which are at least equal to the changes seen with the various comparison drugs. Secondly, CBD is not as potent as either THC, clonidine, or DZP in the various experiments. These CBD doses are similar to those which produce measurable effects in various behavioral pharmacological tests of CBD, e.g., suppression of electroshock induced seizures (6,32). Thirdly, CBD seems to produce dose response effects in all of the tests used suggesting that the observed effects are not attributed to non-specific effects of CBD. Thus, it is safe to conclude that CBD produces pharmacological effects which are similar to drugs that have been established as having anxiolytic properties in both animals and man, e.g., clonidine (17-19) and DZP (33-35).

A short analysis of the behavioral paradigms used in this series of studies on CBD is appropriate. There are no direct tests of human anxiety in animal behavioral pharmacology because there are both cognitive and affective components to the anxiety state in the human. The anxiety state in humans, however, is often related to a recognizable different state, that of fear. Thus behavioral pharmacologists have often used fear conditioning or performance (avoidance conditioning or performance and the conditioned emotional response) as models to study fear states in animals and as tests oftranquillizers (36). In the experiments reported here, the running wheel avoidance task is a learning task in which the animal is learning to run to avoid shock. The benzodiazepine diazepam clearly facilitates the learning, presumably due to the anxiolytic properties of the drug, which presumably reduce arousal in the fear or anxiety situation. In the conditioned suppression paradigm, punishment (e.g., shock) is used to suppress an ongoing response (e.g., licking for water). Again diazepam seems to act via anxiolytic properties, as demonstrated by the fact that response suppression does not occur under the influence of the drug. In the alcohol withdrawal syndrome in man, anxiety and agitation are highly correlated symptoms. The remarkable calming effect of clonidine on agitation and anxiety in human alcoholics withdrawing from alcohol suggested that an animal model using body tremor (a component of motor agitation) and seizures might reveal anxiolytic properties of drugs. At least partial support for this approach was found with clonidine. Finally, we employed a stress-induced model in animals since stress-ulcers seem to reflect a symptom that is a well known consequence of stress and anxiety. Taken together, these four very divergent tests bear a logical relationship to anxiety states at both the human-behavioral and physiological level as a complex of multifactored consequences of anxiety-like effects. This approach seems to provide a valuable composite analysis of the anxiolytic properties of drugs.

Thus, we conclude that these behavioral pharmacological approaches provide a reasonable basis on which to posit anxiolytic properties of cannabidiol. Further research on cannabidiol analogs may reveal more potent or effective compounds which might later be tested in humans.

REFERENCES

1. Carlini, E. A., Lette, J. R., Tannhauser, M., and Berardi, A. C., Cannabidiol and cannabis sativa extract protect mice and rats against convulsive agents, Pharm. Pharmacol. 25:664-665 (1973).
2. Izuierdo, I., and Tannhauser, M., The effect of cannabidiol on maximal electroshock seizure in rats, J. Pharm. Pharmacol. 25: 916-917 (1973).
3. Cunha, J. M., Carlini, E. A., and Pereira, A. E., Chronic administration of cannabidiol to healthy volunteers and epileptic patients, Pharmacol. 21:175-185 (1980).
4. Carlini, E. A., Mechoulam, R., and Lander, N., Anticonvulsant activity of four oxygenated cannabidiol derivatives, Res. Comm. Chem. Pathol. Pharmacol. 12(1):1-15 (1975).
5. Musty, R. E., and Sands, R., Effects of marijuana extract distillate and cannabidiol on variable interval performance as a function of food deprivation, Pharmacol. 16:199-205 (1978).
6. Karniol, I. G., and Carlini, E. A., Pharmacological interaction between cannabidiol and delta-9-tetrahydrocannabinol, Psychopharmacol. (Berl.) 33:53-70 (1973).
7. Lemberger, L., Dalton, B., Martz, R., Rodda, B., and Forney, R., Clinical studies on the interaction of psychopharmacologic agents with marijuana, Ann. Acad. Sci. 281:219-228 (1976).
8. Hollister, L. E., Cannabidiol and cannabinol in man, Experientia 29:825-826 (1973).
9. Zuardi, A. W., Finkelfarb, E., Bunco, O. F. A., Musty, R. E., and Karniol, I. G., Cannabidiol effects on discriminative responses between delta-9-tetrahydrocannabinol and control solution in rats, Arch. Int. Pharmacodyn. Ther. 249:137-146 (1981).
10. Bhargave, H. N. Potential therapeutic applications of naturally occurring synthetic cannabinoids, Gen. Pharmacol. 9:195-213 (1978).
11. Mechoulam, R., and Carlini, E. A., Toward drugs derived from cannabis, Naturwissenschaften 65:174-179 (1978).
12. Redmond, 1977.

13. Chen, Y. H., and Chan, S. H. H., Clonidine-induced hypothesion and bradycardia in cats: The role of medial medullary reticular alpha-adrenoceptors and vagus nerve, Neurosci. Abstr. 4:18 (1978).
14. Chen, Y. H., and Chan, S. H. H., The involvement of medial medullary reticular formation in cardiovascular effects of clonidine in experimentally-induced hypertensive cats, Neurosci. Abstr. 5:39 (1979).
15. Reid, J. L., Clonidine and central noradrenaline turnover. In "Central Action of Drugs in Blood Pressure Regulation" (D. S. Davies and J. L. Reid, eds.), pp. 194-204. Pitman Medical, Tunbridge Wells, 1975.
16. Connolly, M. E., Clonidine in the treatment of hypertension, in :Central Action of Drugs in Blood Pressure Regulation" (D. S. Davies and J. L. Reid, eds.), pp. 268-276. Pitman Medical, Tunbridge Wells, 1975.
17. Tseng, L. Fu, Loh, H. H., and We, E. T., Effects of clonidine on morphine withdrawal signs in the rat, Eur. J. Pharmacol, 30:93-99 (1975).
18. Lipman, J. J., and Spencer, P. S. J., Clonidine and opiate withdrawal, The Lancet 2:521 (1978).
19. Gold, M. S., Redmond, Jr., D. E., Kleber, H. D., Clonidine blocks acute opiate-withdrawal symptoms, The Lancet, 599-602 (1978).
20. Bjorkquist, S. E., Clonidine in alcohol withdrawal, Acta. Psych. Scand. 52:256-263 (1975).
21. Freund, C., Alcohol withdrawal syndrome in mice, Arch. Neur. 21:315-320 (1969).
22. Freund, G., Animal models of ethanol withdrawal syndromes and their relevance to pharmacology, in "Biological and Behavioural Approaches to Drug Dependence" (H. D. Cappell and A. E. LeBlanc, eds.), pp. 13-25. Alcoholism and Drug Addiction Research Foundation of Ontario, Toronto, Canada, 1975.
23. Musty, R. E., Homeostatic drives and consummatory behavior: Hunger and thirst, in "Motivation, an Experimental Approach" (E. D. Ferguson, ed.). Holt, Rinehart and Winston, New York, 1976.
24. Winer, B. J., "Statistical Principles in Experimental Design." McGraw Hill, New York, 1971.
25. Heise, G. A., and Boff, E., Continuous avoidance as a base-line for measuring behavioral effects of drugs, Psychopharmacol. 3:264-282 (1962).
26. Pandina, R. J., and Musty, R. E., Effects of delta-9-tetrahydrocannabinol on active avoidance acquisition and passive avoidance retention in rats with amygdaloid lesions, Pharmacol. 13:297-308 (1974).
27. Geller, I., and Seifter, J., The effects of meprobamate, barbiturates, d-amphetamine and promazine on experimen-

tally induced conflict in the rat, Psychopharmacol. 1:482-492 (1960).

28. Stein, L. , Wise, C. D., and Berger, B. D., Antianxiety action of benzodiazepines: Decrease in activity of serotonin neurons in the punishment system, in "The Benzodiazepines" (S. Garattini, E. Mussini, and L. O. Randall, eds.), pp. 299-326. Raven Press, New York, 1973.
29. Hoat, J. B., Djahanguiri, Richelle, et M., Action protectrice du chloridazepoxide sur l'ulcere de contrainte chex le rat, Arch. int. Pharmacodyn. 148:557-559 (1964).
30. Glavin, G., Restraint ulcer: History, current research and future implications, Brain Res. Bull. 5:51-58 (1980).
31. Weiss, J. M., Effects of coping behavior in different warning signal conditions on stress pathology in rats, J. Comp. Physiol. Psychol. 77:1-13 (1971).
32. Consroe, P. F., and Wolkin, A. L., Cannabidiol-antiepileptic drugs. Comparisons and interactions in experimentally induced seizures in rats, J. Pharmacol. Exp. Ther. 201:26-32 (1977).
33. Miczek, K. A., Effects of scopolamine, amphetamine and benzodiazepines on punishment, Psychopharmacologia 28:373-389 (1973).
34. Miczek, K. A., Effects of scopolamine, amphetamine and benzodiazepines on conditioned suppression, Pharmacol. Biochem. Behav. 1:401-411 (1973).
35. Rickels, K., Benzodiazepines: Clinical use patterns, in "Benzodiazepines: A Review of Research Results, 1980" (S. Szara and J. P. Ludford, eds.), pp. 43-60. NIDA Research Monograph 33, DHHA Publication Number (ADM) 81-1052, Rockville, MD, 1981.

TETRAHYDROCANNABINOL EFFECTS ON EXTRAPYRAMIDAL MOTOR BEHAVIORS IN AN ANIMAL MODEL OF PARKINSON'S DISEASE*

D. E. Moss
S. P. Montgomery
A. A. Salo

Department of Psychology
The University of Texas at El Paso
El Paso, Texas

R. W. Steger

Department of Obstetrics and Gynecology
The University of Texas Health Science Center at San Antonio
San Antonio, Texas

I. INTRODUCTION

Although delta-9-tetrahydrocannabinol (THC) and related cannabinoids have been studied for several years, no clear functional relationship between a specific neurotransmitter effect and an important influence on behavior has been discovered. The key to understanding the functional effect of cannabinoids on behavior would require that: 1) the neuroanatomical substrate for the behaviors being studied must be relatively known, 2) the neurotransmitters interacting in the system must be at least partially identified, and 3) the behavior being studied should be very sensitive to cannabinoid effects as well as easily and reliable measured. A behavioral model which meets the above criteria and which may be useful in elucidating behaviorally significant neurotransmitter effects of the cannabinoids is the reserpine animal model of Parkinson's disease. In this model, monoamines in the extrapyramidal system are depleted by pretreatment with reserpine.

*Supported in part by the National InstituteofMental Health and a MBRS Program, DRR, NIH, grant RR-08012.

ISBN 0-12-044620-0

The resulting behavioral syndrome includes the classic Parkinsonian symptoms of muscular rigidity and hypokinesia (1). These behavioral effects are easily and reliably measured as well as exquisitely sensitive to cannabinoid effects (2).

Creveling et al. have established that the main symptoms of rigidity and hypokinesia observed in the reserpine syndrome are due to depletion of dopamine, as in Parkinson's disease (3). For example, these investigators were able to demonstrate a dramatic "awakening" of reserpinized animals by administration of L-DOPA but not by 3,4-dihydroxyphenylserine, a compound decarboxylated directly to norepinephrine in the brain. In addition, Anden and Johnels found that apomorphine, a dopaminergic agonist, injected directly into the corpus striatum (caudate/putamen) and related extrapyramidal areas of reserpine-treated rats caused a marked reduction in reserpine-induced rigidity and hypokinesia (4). Furthermore, because of the extensive studies of extrapyramidal disorders, the neurotransmitters that interact with the major dopamine systems related to the control of extrapyramidal motor behaviors are relatively well known. These include very important interactions between dopamine and acetylcholine, gamma-aminobutyric acid (GABA), glutamic acid, 5-hydroxytryptamine, norepinephrine, and other minor neurotransmitters (for reviews, see 5-7). The reserpine syndrome, as an animal model of Parkinson's disease, is therefore, relatively well understood particularly with regard to the origin of the symptoms of hypokinesia and rigidity.

II. EXPERIMENTS AND RESULTS

A. Experiment 1. The Effects of THC and Other Cannabinoids on Reserpine-induced hypokinesia in a Model of Parkinson's Disease

In view of the information regarding the origin of the behavioral effects observed in the reserpine syndrome, it was of particular interest that Moss, McMaster and Rogers reported that THC produces a remarkable potentiation of reserpine-induced hypokinesia in the rat (2). In these experiments, rats were pretreated with 7.5 mg/kg reserpine 24 hours prior to behavioral tests for hypokinesia. In addition, part of these animals were also give 10 mg/kg THC by gavage 4 to 5 hours before the behavioral tests. This method of THC administration was selected because it produces a large and reliable decrease in rectal temperature that peaks at 4 to 5 hours after administration (8). In these experiments, reserpine-induced hypokinesia was measured by the bar test (2,9). In the bar test, the rat is placed with its front paws resting on a small horizontal rod (i.e., a "bar") elevated 9 cm above a small platform upon which the rear paws are placed. The bar test simply measures the amount of time required for the animal to get down from the bar. It is a very reliable measure of unwillingness or inability to move (i.e., hypokinesia). As shown in Figure 1, control animals (i.e., undrugged animals that received vehicle only) and animals treated only with THC remove themselves from the bar with an average time of less than 3 seconds. The bar test results obtained with reserpine, however, show significant hypokinesia with an average bar time of about 40 seconds. This hypokinesia was expected as one of the Parkinsonian-like symptoms observed in this animal model. The most striking results were obtained, however, when animals were given both reserpine and THC. In this case, the animals required an average of more than 15 minutes to remove themselves from the bar. Insofar as an arbitrary maximum time of 30 minutes was allowed for the bar test, this effect was partially limited by a ceiling effect. Although muscular rigidity was not objectively measured in these experiments, informal observations suggested that there was no difference between reserpine-alone pretreated rats and THC/reserpine pretreated rats with regard to this particular reserpine-induced

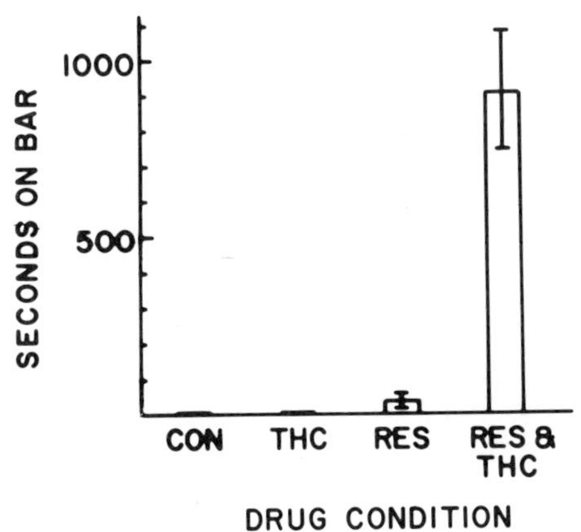

FIGURE 1. Effect of THC (10 mg/kg) on reserpine-induced hypokinesia. Comparison of the reserpine treated animals (RES) and the THC/reserpine treated animals (RES & THC) shows the magnitude of the THC potentiation of reserpine-induced hypokinesia. All groups contained 8 animals and the error bars represent one SEM. The main effect of RES and the interaction between RES and THC were both highly significant ($p < 0.001$). [Reproduced from Moss et al. (2) with permission].

effect. In spite of the severe hypokinesia observed in these tests, the THC/reserpine treated animals were able to show immediate and well organized righting reflexes as well as locomotor responses to footshock.

Using the same procedures reported above, the effects of 10 mg/kg (orally by gavage) of cannabichromene, cannabidiol, and levonantradol, a synthetic analog of THC, on reserpine-induced hypokinesia were also studied in the rat. Cannabichromene had no detectable effect, cannabidiol was less potent than THC, and levonantradol was extremely powerful relative to THC. In fact, all 6 of the animals tested with the combination of levonantradol and reserpine stood motionless at the bar for the maximum recorded time of 30 minutes. Actually, some of the animals remained on the bar more than an hour and one exceeded 2 hours.

Because of the extreme interaction observed between THC and reserpine in the rat as described above, it was important to determine if this effect could be expected in primates as well as rodents, and furthermore, to determine if THC would potentiate the hypotensive effect of reserpine. The latter effect, if it occurred, could have significant health-related potential. Therefore, a 15 Kg male 12 year old stump tailed macaque (M. arctoides) was trained to present his arm to the experimenters for food reward so that his blood pressure could be measured using a sphygmomanometer. A predrug baseline systolic and diastolic pressure was established at 138/78 mm Hg (S.E.M. = 5 mm Hg). Thereafter, the monkey was given increasing doses of reserpine orally twice a day until a drop in both systolic and diastolic pressures were observed. Thedose determined by this procedure was 2 mg/kg, which caused a peak drop in blood pressure to 86/44 mm Hg (S.E.M. = 7 mm Hg)3 hours after the reserpine. THC was then administered orally (1 mg/kg) in an oil solution on a cookie at the beginning of the reserpine-induced hypotension and blood pressure was measured regularly for the following 7 hours. THC had no reliable effect on reserpine-induced hypotension and, in addition, there were no differences observed 24 hours later on the first drug-free recovery day following each replication of the experiment.

Even though there were no differences in blood pressure produced by adding THC to reserpine, there were very clear behavioral differences that corroborate the effects observed earlier in rats. In the no drug condition, this monkey was very active and aggressive. With 2 mg/kg reserpine, he was much less active and was generally cooperative and submissive. When THC was added to the reserpine treatment, however, he became very unresponsive and cataleptic (i.e., he spentseveral periods of an hour or longer in peculiar positions without movement). He frequently sat with his face propped into the corner of his cage. One time he hung upside down by all four feet from the top of his cage for well over an hour without moving. In the THC/reserpine condition, he could be rolled out of his cage and positioned for his blood pressure measurements. Because of his extreme cataleptic condition, he would maintain positions established by the experimenters for long periods of time. The behavioral effects of adding THC to reserpine were quite dramatic and none of these peculiar behaviors were ever observed in the THC-alone or reserpine-alone conditions.

The results obtained in Experiment 1 show that THC greatly increases reserpine-induced hypokinesia in rats and primates. However, THC does not increase all effects of reserpine insofar as THC had no detectable effect on reserpine-induced hypotension.

B. Experiment 2. Dose Response and Time Course of the THC Effect in Reserpinized Rats

In order to obtain more information about the THC/reserpine-induced hypokinesia observed in Experiment 1, this experiment was conducted to determine the effect of dose of THC and the duration of its potentiation of reserpine hypokinesia. Figure 2 shows that THC potentiation of reserpine-induced hypokinesia, in fact, follows a well defined time course. In this experiment, 7.5 mg/kg reserpine was administered 24 hours before the bar test for all animals. The administration of THC was, however, varied so that it preceded the bar test in each independent group by the time shown in the figure. The bar tests were conducted at the same time of day for all groups to control for possible circadian effects on behavior. Figure 2 also shows that THC/reserpine hypokinesia is dependent on the dose of THC administered up to 10 mg/kg, the highest dose tested in these experiments. It is interesting to note that the time course of the THC effect revealed in these experiments on motor behaviors is similar to the time course reported for the euphoric effects of marijuana after oral administration in humans (10). In addition, because of the distinct time course revealed in this experiment, it appears that THC might be producing its motor effects observed in these experiments through a specific and well defined neurotransmitter effect.

C. Experiment 3. The Effect of Administering Reserpine after THC-Pretreatment

In the experiments reported above, reserpine was always

administered 24 hours prior to the behavioral tests so that the behavior was studied during a steady state of monoamine depletion. Fischer and Heller also observed that the behavioral effects of reserpine develop shortly after injection and remain unaltered for longer than 24 hours and then gradually diminish to a practically normal state by 48 hours (11). However, if THC was having its effect by alteration of the rate of turnover of affected neurotransmitters or the rate or extent of depletion, there might be a significantly different effect early in the development of the reserpine syndrome. Therefore, the effect of THC on reserpine-induced hypokinesia was studied at a constant 4 to 5 hours after THC administration as in the above experiments but only two hours after reserpine administration. The results were quite remarkable. Although the reserpine-alone animals showed severe hypokinesia and rigidity, the THC/reserpine treated animals showed a much more extreme effect. Bar tests were not administered because their bodies were so rigidly fixed in a curled posture (e.g., a "bean" appearance) that it was impossible to place them on the bar. The THC/reserpine treated animals showed no righting reflex and showed no response when their rigid bodies were tapped gently on a table. This extreme effect lasted only between 2 and 3 hours after reserpine administration. The results of this experiment emphasized the importance of examining the effect of THC on reserpine-induced depletion of the monoamines.

D. Experiment 4. The Effects of THC on Reserpine-Induced Monoamine Depletion

In this experiment, rats were pretreated with reserpine and THC exactly in accordance with the procedures used in the first THC/reserpine experiments reported above. Specifically, the animals were pretreated with reserpine (7.5 mg/kg) or a placebo control injection either 2 or 24 hours prior to being sacrificed for biochemical analysis of the caudate/putamen. in addition, half of the reserpine pretreated and half of the control animals were further treated with 10 mg/kg THC by gavage approximately 4 hours before being sacrificed. There were 8 animals in all drug conditions. All animals were also given tests for hypokinesia immediately before sacrifice in order to confirm that the biochemical data were collected during the extreme behavioral effects observed earlier. The animals were then decapitated, the brain was rapidly removed and cooled, and the caudate/putamen dissected out of the brain. The caudate/putamen was then rapidly frozen on dry ice and maintained frozen until analysis. The monoamines and two related metabolites were separated by high performance liquid

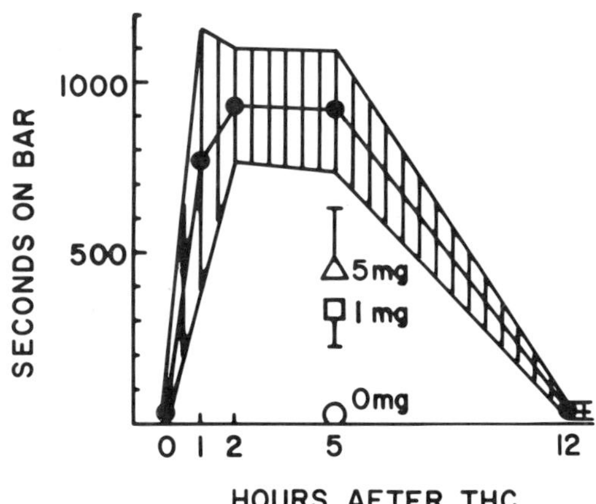

FIGURE 2. Dose- and time-dependence of THC effect on reserpine-induced hypokinesia. All animals were pretreated with 7.5 mg/kg reserpine. The shaded area (mean +/- SEM) represents the time-dependent effect at 10 mg/kg THC. The open symbols at 5 hours show the effect of various doses of THC. Animals were tested at only one time or dose group. The results obtained at 24 hours were identical to those obtained at 0 and 12 hours and are, therefore, not shown. All groups contained 4 animals except those at 5 hours which contained 8 animals. The effects of time and dose were both highly significant ($p < 0.01$). [Reproduced from Moss et al. (2) with permission].

chromatography and quantified by electrochemical detection. Dopamine, norepinephrine and the dopamine metabolite 3,4-dihydroxyphenylacetic acid (DOPAC) were assayed according to the procedure of Steger, Bartke and Goldman (1982). 5-Hydroxytryptamine and the metabolite 5-hydroxyindoleacetic acid (5-HIAA) were measured according to the method of Steger and Bartke (12,13). The results are shown in Figures 3 and 4.

Figures 3 and 4 demonstrate that THC has no effect on reserpine induced depletion of the monoamines in the caudate/putamen at either 2 or 24 hours after reserpine. The finding that there was no apparent effect of THC at either 2 or 24 hours after reserpine and, in addition, THC had no effect on the content of DOPAC and 5-HIAA suggests that THC also probably did not affect turnover rates of the monoamines being studied.

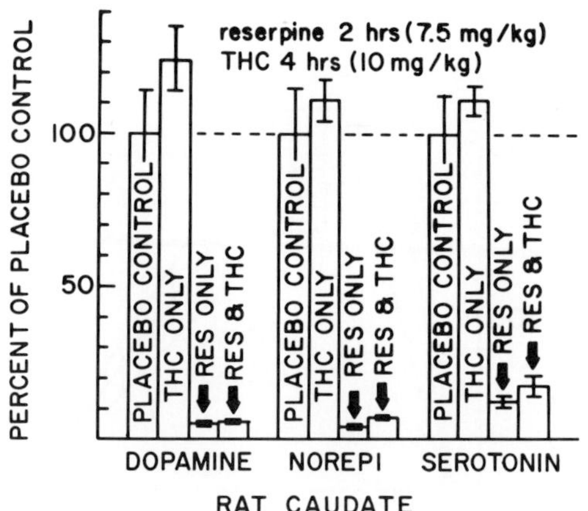

FIGURE 3. The effects of reserpine (RES) and THC on rat caudate/putamen monoamine content at 2 hours after reserpine. The THC and/or reserpine treated animals received THC (10 mg/kg) 4 hours and/or reserpine (7.5 mg/kg) 2 hours prior to being sacrificed for assays. The 100% control values taken from placebo treated animals are 6194 ng/gm dopamine, 2602 ng/gm norepinephrine, and 450 ng/gm 5-hydroxytryptamine. There were 8 animals in each group and the error bars represent one SEM.

E. Experiment 5. The Effects of THC on Haloperidol- and Chlorpromazine-induced Hypokinesia

Insofar as THC had no apparent effect on monoamine depletion induced by reserpine, an additional experiment was conducted to determine if hypokinesia induced by other, more specific dopaminergic antagonists is also increased by concurrent administration of THC. These results, obtained with haloperidol (a representative butyrophenone) and chlorpromazine (a representative phenothiazine), are shown in Figure 5. It is interesting to note the striking difference between the effects of THC on the hypokinesia induced by these two dopaminergic antagonists. Although the reason for the difference in the effects observed with these two compounds is completely obscure, it may be due to the alpha-adrenergic effect of the chlorpromazine which is largely absent in the haloperidol (14).

In spite of the inconsistent effect obtained with chlorpromazine in this experiment, our working hypothesis is that the THC influence on extrapyramidal motor function is normally

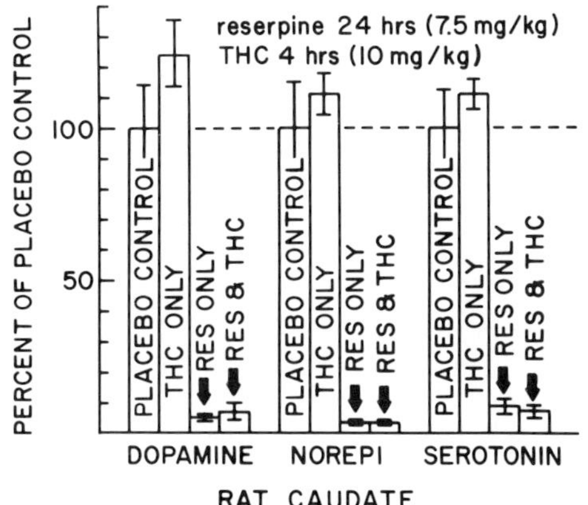

FIGURE 4. The effect of reserpine (RES) and THC on rat caudate/putamen monoamine content 24 hours after reserpine. The THC and/or reserpine treated animals received reserpine (7.5 mg/kg) 24 hours and/or THC (10 mg/kg) 4 hours prior to being sacrificed for assays. This experiment was conducted concurrently with that shown in Fig. 3 and, therefore, the 100% values determined in the undrugged control animals are the same for Figs. 3 and 4. There were 8 animals in each group and the error bars represent on SEM.

a minor subtle effect, probably on a nondopaminergic system, that is masked by the function of the major extrapyramidal dopamine system. In the absence of the regulatory effect of the main dopamine system, however, the normally occult effect(s) of THC become observable.

F. Experiment 6. The Effects of THC on KCl-Induced Inactivation of the Striatum

The purpose of Experiment 6 was to determine if, in contradiction to the working hypothesis presented above, nonspecific inactivation of the striatum would be a sufficient condition for observing the THC effect on extrapyramidal motor behaviors. This was a particularly important experiment because of the earlier work by Gough and Olley (9).

Gough and Olley reported inducing "catalepsy" (hypokinesia) in rats by intracranial injection of THC and 11-OH-THC into the caudate/putamen of rats through chronically in-dwelling cannulae (9). In addition, they observed catalepsy in similarly prepared rats which received THC systemically even though no injections were made through the cannulae. Catalepsy was never observed in control rats (i.e., not prepared with cannulae) when THC was administered systemically. This "cannula" effect, in particular, suggested that nonspecific disruption of striatal function is sufficient for THC-induced hypokinesia.

It is important to note that Gough and Olley used a bar test virtually identical to that used in our experiments except that they placed the rats on the bar once a minute for several minutes until catalepsy was observed (9). In contrast, in our experiments, the bar tests are separated by at least 30 minutes and administered a maximum of 3 times. In fact, some experiments we conducted suggested very strongly that the "catalepsy" observed by Gough and Olley (9) was due to learning to stand at the bar (for example, to avoid being handled, etc.) or some other nonspecific effect induced by excessive testing. However, the report of the "cannula" effect suggested that THC might produce hypokinesiawhenever striatal function was disrupted. In this case, the specific dopamine involvement suggested in our working hypothesis presented above might be unfounded. Therefore, Experiment 6 was completed to test the hypokinetic effect of THC when normal striatal function was disrupted by intracranial injection of KCl.

In this experiment, seven rats were prepared with chronically indwelling cannulae directed into the dorsal caudate/putamen according to the coordinates of Gough and Olley (9). In the first part of this experiment, the inactivation of the striatum by KCl injection was confirmed by the procedure of Anden and Grabowska-Anden (15). In this control experiment,each animal was injected intracranially with 1 mcl of 25% KCl on one side and an equimolar amount of NaCl (1mcl of 20%) simultaneously on the other side. Immediately following these intracranial injections, the animals were injected i.p. with apomorphine, a dopamine agonist. The extent to which the KCl injection inactivated the striatum was then measured behaviorally but the number of rotations observed during the next 45 minutes. In accordance with the desired effect of inactivating the striatum, after the first few minutes, all of the animals showed rotation ipsilateral to the KCl injection site.

The control experiment described above confirmed that the location of the cannulae and the injections of KCl were sufficient to produce nonspecific functional disruption of striatal function. In the second part of the experiment all animals were then injected bilaterally with 1 mcl of 25%KCl or, in the control condition, 1 mcl of 20% NaCl and tested for hypokinesia using the bar test procedure of Moss et al. (2). with and without an additional administration of 10 mg/kgTHC (gavage). All of the subjects were subjected to all condi

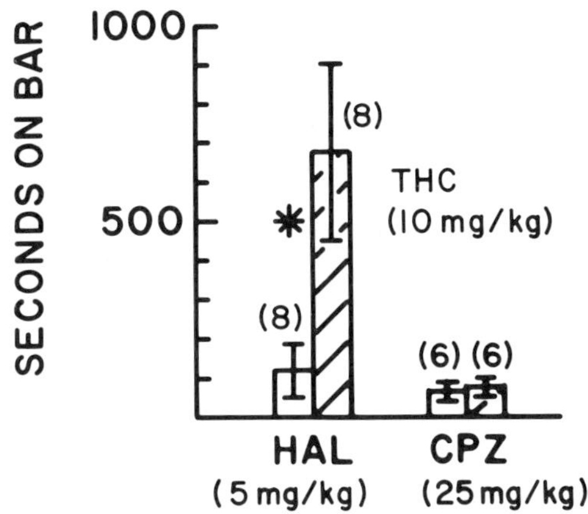

FIGURE 5. The effect of THC (10 mg/kg) on haloperidol (HAL) or chlorpromazine (CPZ) induced hypokinesia. THC or a placebo was administered 4 hours prior to and either HAL or CPZ was administered i.p. 30 minutes prior to the bar tests. The number of animals in each group is shown in parentheses and the error bars represent one SEM. The effect of THC on HAL-induced hypokinesia was significant ($p < 0.05$).

tions in a counterbalanced order so that they served as their own controls. In addition, the entire experiment was replicated so that there were two different observations taken on each animal in each drug condition. Tests under different drug conditions were separated by a minimum of one week. The animals were tested with THC placebo and NaCl intracranial injections (placebo control), 10 mg/kg THC and NaCl intracranial injections (THC only condition), THC placebo and KCl intracranial injections (KCl only condition), and 10 mg/kg THC and KCl intracranial injections (THC/KCl condition). The results of this experiment were very clear. There was no hypokinesia observed in the control condition, the KCl only condition, THC only condition, and, furthermore, there was no hypokinesia observed in the THC/KCl condition. The average bartimes for these four drug groups ranged from 7 to 14 seconds. After the behavioral data were collected, frozen section histologies were performed on all subjects and the locations of the cannulae were confirmed. This experiment demonstrated that nonspecific disruption of striatal function is not a sufficient condition for the observation of THC effects on extrapyramidal motor behaviors.

G. Experiment 7. The Interaction of Cholinergic Drugs with THC as Measured in Motor Behaviors

Because of the very important cholinergic/dopaminergic interactions in the striatum and the effects of cholinergic drugs on the symptoms of Parkinson's disease, the effects of cholinergic drugs on reserpine-alone and THC/reserpine-induced hypokinesia were tested in this model. The results showed that reserpine-alone and THC/reserpine hypokinesia could be only slightly enhanced by 0.5 mg/kg physostigmine salicylate, a dose sufficient to produce 80% inhibition of brain cholinesterase (Moss, unpublished experiments). Even though the effect of physostigmine on reserpine alone as well as THC/reserpine hypokinesia was statistically significant, the behavioral effect was not at all dramatic and appeared to be a small, strictly additive effect. In addition, the interaction of THC with the cholinergic system was further studied by determining if the THC/reserpine hypokinesia could be reduced or blocked by 2 mg/kg scopolamine HBr, a muscarinic receptor antagonist, and 30 mg/kg ethopropazine (Parsidol), an anticholinergic antiparkinsonian drug. The THC/reserpine hypokinesia was not significantly reduced by the traditional muscarinic antagonist scopolamine but it was dramatically reduced by the administration of ethopropazine (2). The results of these experiments are, therefore, in general agreement with the effects of cholinergic drugs on Parkinson's disease. Specifically, the symptoms of this disease are moderately exacerbated by physostigmine, relatively unchanged by scopolamine, and reduced fairly effectively by ethopropazine.

The results of the experiments reported above using cholinergic drugs suggests that the cholinergic system does not have a major functional role in mediating the effect of THC on these extrapyramidal motor behaviors. It should be pointed out, however, that the effect of relatively specific nicotinic drugs has not been tested in this model. Although some of the effects were statistically significant, the magnitude ofthe behavioral changes was only modest and apparently insufficient to explain the large effect of THC on reserpine-induced hypokinesia.

III. CONCLUSIONS

Although the purpose of these experiments was to conduct basic research into the mechanisms of action of the cannabinoids, the results reported may have some potential clinical significance. The profound effects of THC and levonantradol on extrapyramidal motor behaviors suggest that patients taking monoamine depleting or dopamine blocking drugs, or those who are suffering Parkinson's disease might experience untoward effects from the use of marijuana. On the other hand, THC or a related cannabinoid might be used to increase the clinical efficacy of drugs used in hyperkinetic motor disorders. For example, reserpine was one of the first agents to be employed in the treatment of various hyperkinetic choreiform disorders (16), and it has been shown to be of benefit in tardive dyskinesia (17,18), and Huntington's disease (19,20). In addition, it is interesting to note that patients with torsion dystonia have mentioned that marijuana use produces therapeutic effects comparable to those obtained with diazepam, a drug used in the treatment of that disorder (21). It appears, therefore, that selected cannabinoids may have some therapeutic value in the treatment of certain motor disorders. The series of experiments reported here, however, suggests that the most productive direction for future research may be related to the effects of cannabinoids on gamma-aminobutyric acid and other amino acid neurotransmitters or peptides that have functional significance in extrapyramidal motor control.

In the research related to marijuana and the cannabinoids, there seems to be an increasing interest in determining a relatively specific mechanism of action. It also seems quite likely that a class of drugs like the cannabinoids will, in fact, be discovered to have many mechanisms of action related to their diverse effects. The main disadvantage of studying the effects of the cannabinoids in this animal model of Parkinson's disease is that the cannabinoids must be studied as an interaction with other drugs. The other behavioral effects of cannabinoids are, however, usually extremely subtle and difficult to measure reliably. On the other hand, the relatively complete understanding of this model of Parkinson's disease afforded by extensive research on the extrapyramidal motor diseases and the exquisite sensitivity of these behaviors to certain cannabinoids may provide an unusual opportunity to discover at least one mechanism of action of the cannabinoids that has important functional significance for the nervous system and behavior.

REFERENCES

1. Carlsson, A., Pharmacol. Rev. 11:490-493 (1959).
2. Moss, D. E., McMaster, S. B., and Rogers, J., Pharmacol. Biochem. Behav. 15:779-783 (1981).
3. Creveling, C. R., Daly, J., Tokuyama, T., and Witkop, B., Biochem. Pharmacol. 17:65-70 (1968).

4. Anden, N. E., and Johnels, B., Brain Res. 133:386-389 (1977).
5. Hassler, R., J. Neurol. Sci. 36:187-224 (1978).
6. Butcher, L. L., (ed.), "Cholinergic-Monoaminergic Interactions in the Brain." Academic Press, New York, 1978.
7. Divac, I., and Oberg, R. G. E., (eds.), "The Neostriatum". Pergamon Press, New York, 1979.
8. Moss, D. E., Peck, P. L., and Salome, R., Pharmacol. Biochem. Behav. 8:763-765 (1978).
9. Gough, A. L., and Olley, J. E., Neuropharmacol. 17:137-144 (1978).
10. Jaffe, J. H., in "The Pharmacological Basis of Therapeutics". 6th ed., (A. G. Gilman, L. S. Goodman, and A. Gilman, eds.), pp. 535-584. Macmillan, New York, 1980.
11. Fischer, E., and Heller, B., Nature 216:1221-1222 (1967).
12. Steger, R. W., Bartke, A., and Goldman, B. D., Biol. Reproduction. 26:437-444 (1982).
13. Steger, R. W., and Bartke, A., Endocrinol. in press.
14. Nickerson, M., in "The Pharmacological Basis of Therapeutics", 4th ed., (A. G. Gilman and L. S. Goodman, eds.), pp. 549-584. Macmillan, New York, 1970.
15. Anden, N. E., and Grabowska-Anden, M., Adv. Neurol. 24:235-246 (1979).
16. Weber, E., Schweiz. med. Wschr. 84:968-974 (1954).
17. Villeneuve, A., and Boszormenyi, A., Lancet 1:353-354 (1970).
18. Soto, S., Daly, R. and Peters, H., Dis. Nerv. Syst. 32:680-685 (1971).
19. Kempinsky, W. H., Boniface, W. R., Morgan, P. P., and Busch, A. K., Neurobiol. 10:38-42 (1960).
20. Klawans, H. L., Eur. Neurol. 4:148-163 (1970).
21. Marsden, C. D., in "Disorders of Movement, Current Status of Modern Therapy", Vol. 8, (A. Barbeau, ed.). Lippincott Co., Philadelphia, 1981.

BEHAVIORAL PHARMACOGENETIC STUDIES OF CANNABINOIDS: DEVELOPMENTAL EFFECTS IN TETRAHYDROCANNABINOL-SEIZURE SUSCEPTIBLE RABBITS

Paul Consroe*
Barbara Schneiderman Fish

Department of Pharmacology and Toxicology
College of Pharmacy
University of Arizona
Tucson, Arizona

I. INTRODUCTION

Marijuana, by virtue of its major active ingredient, delta-9-tetrahydrocannabinol (THC), produces a rather unique spectrum of objective (tachycardia, conjunctival injection) and subjective (mental) effects. Of the latter, an extremely wide range of effects such as stimulation (anxiety, heightened perceptions, euphoria), sedation (sleepiness, dreamlike states), and psychotomimetic effects (altered perceptions, cognitive dysfunctions, depersonalization, visual illusions, and pseudo-hallucinations) have been reported (1). While it is clear that mood changes following marijuana or THC administration may vary widely from purportedly desired states (e.g., euphoria, dream-like state) to those that are clearly dysphoric, there is considerable debate as to the major reasons for this variability.

Both pharmacological factors, such as dose and route of administration (1,2) and psychosocial factors, such as subject expectancy (2,3), environmental setting (3,4), personality (5), and previous experience with marijuana (3) and/or other drugs (5), have been deemed important in determining the subjective response to marijuana or THC. Recent evidence indicates that complex interactions between the dose of THC and

---

*Supported by NIDA grant DA-01448.

ISBN 0-12-044620-0

personality characteristics, notably extroversion and neuroticism, of the subjects are important in determining the effects of THC (6). The fact that the degree of extroversion and neuroticism may play a dominant role is salient since these personality characteristics have been reported to be highly heritable in comparison to other personality dimensions (7,8). It would then appear that in addition to the above mentioned environmental factors, the element of genetics should be included among the influences on the overall expression of THC-induced effects.

Genetic polymorphisms occur in humans (and infra-human species), and many of these have important biological implications, e.g., for drug metabolism, drug sensitivity, and/or etiology of some psychiatric diseases (9,10). Further, it is well known that genetics can act as powerful determinants of the behavioral effects of many types of psychotropic drugs (11,12). Although there are no direct corollary data concerning marijuana's effects in humans, it is, perhaps, significant that findings of two human studies may implicate genetic determinants in the psychopharmacological effects of the drug (13,14). Additionally, studies in mice (15,16) and in rabbits (17) have clearly shown that genetic factors can significantly influence the behavioral effects of THC.

With respect to the latter findings, our research at the University of Arizona over the past several years has led to the serendipitous discovery, and the development and maintenance of a genetically unique animal stock, the THC-seizure-susceptible (THC-SS) rabbit (18). THC-SS rabbits exhibit non-fatal, convulsive-like behaviors when injected intravenously (i.v.) with THC and other cannabinoids that are known to be psychoactive in humans (18). THC-SS rabbits fail to convulse when given non-psychoactive cannabinoids (18), non-cannabinoid psychoactive drugs (18) or non-pharmacological sensory stimuli known to have convulsive-inducing potential (19). Based upon the specificity of response, numerous rabbit-human parallels and various practical and theoretical considerations as previously outlined (18-24), we have hypothesized that the THC-SS rabbit may be a useful animal model of marijuana-induced psychoactivity in humans.

Our previous findings indicate that a single, autosomal, recessive gene (thc) mechanism of inheritance is responsible for THC-produced seizure susceptibility in our rabbit colony (17). Depending upon the segregation pattern of the thc gene, rabbits are either phenotypically THC-SS or THC-seizure resistant (-SR). THC-SS rabbits consist of either a thc/thc (affected) genotype and THC-SR rabbits consist of either a thc/+ (carrier) or +/+ (normal) genotype. The (affected) genotype-mediated phenotype is fully penetrant in THC-SS rabbits who are 39 postnatal days of age (PN) or older (25). That is, every THC-SS rabbit tested at these PN exhibited behavioral convulsions with THC given in doses of 0.1 mg/kg, i.v., or greater (17,25). However, THC (0.1 mg/kg, i.v.) failed to elicit convulsions in THC-SS rabbits at PN 15-23, and produced convulsions in less than 85% of THC-SS rabbits at PN 24-38 (25). These findings indicate age-related differences in the pharmacogenetic response to THC, and as such, provide preliminary information concerning the behavioral responsiveness of the developing animal to the stimulant effects of the cannabinoid.

The present study was undertaken to investigate, further, the effects and potential mechanisms of action of psychoactive cannabinoids during the early development (PN 15-42) of THC-SS rabbits. In the first experiment, the dose-response behavioral effects of THC were studied in the offspring derived from THC-SS *inter-se* matings in order to characterize, in more detail, the onset of THC seizure susceptibility. In addition, the behavioral responses to two active THC metabolites, 11-OH-delta-9-THC and 11-OXO-delta-8-THC were studied. This was done to investigate the possibility that the ontogeny of THC responsiveness was associated with the maturation of liver metabolic capacities. The second experiment was designed to ascertain the potential influence of some early environmental factors (maternal, paternal and sibling effects) on the behavioral response to THC in the developing THC-SS rabbits. For this purpose the behavioral effects of THC were evaluated in THC-SS offspring derived from breeding various combinations of the paternal genotypes.

II. MATERIALS AND METHODS

A. Experiment I

Individual rabbits (279) ranging from PN 15 to 42 were used in the study. The rabbits were housed with their mothers until weaning at PN 42. Nest boxes were supplied until the offspring were no longer making use of them. Food and water were available *ad libitum*. The animals were maintained on an automatic 12 hour photoperiod. The rabbits were derivedfrom THC-SS *inter-se* matings. On the basis of our genetic findings (17), all were expected to be THC-SS (*thc*/*thc*) rabbits. For identification purposes, rabbits were marked with picric acid according to a predetermined numbering scheme. There were weighed to the nearest gram and administered drug preparations via the marginal ear vein. Two experimenters, who were unaware of the specific preparations administered, were required for injection of each rabbit since it was necessary to hold the animal, preventing it from moving during the injection. The rabbits were administered THC, 11-OH-delta-9-THC or 11-OXO-delta-8-THC. Each cannabinoid was prepared in a 10% polysorbate (Tween) 80 and 90% distilled water vehicle. This vehicle permits the incorporation of cannabinoids into a suitable preparation for i.v. injection but does not, by itself, cause convulsions or any other overt behavioral response in our rabbits (20,23). In order to assure accuracy, injection volumes were 0.1 ml/100 g in animals weighing less that 1 kg. Those weighing more than 1 kg were injected with 0.1 ml/kg. The doses of cannabinoids used (mg/kg) were 0.1, 0.5 and 5.0 for THC and 11-OXO-delta-8-THC, and 0.04, 0.2 and 2.0 for 11-OH-delta-9-THC. These doses were chosen on the basis of data from adult THC-SS rabbits indicating that THC and 11-OXO-delta-8-THC were equipotent and 11-OH-delta-9-THC was 3-4 times more potent than the former in causing convulsions (18,24). Thus, the doses used in the present study were approximately equipotent among the 3 cannabinoids. The occurrence of a convulsion was recorded if the rabbit exhibitedthe following endpoints: limb extension where limbs (fore- and/or hind-limbs) are rigid and tonically extended; clonus, characterized by a series of rapid rhythmic contractions and relaxations of the limbs; and thrashing or swinging about of the body from side to side flailing and violent motion. These endpoints are the major identifying criteria ofcannabinoid convulsions in adult THC-SS rabbits (18,20,24).

In accordance with our earlier studies (25), the youngest age at which the rabbits were tested was PN 15. Rabbits were assigned to a particular cannabinoid dose and were administered this dose at weekly intervals. This is the interdrug interval which precludes the development of tolerance to the convulsive effect of THC in adult THC-SS rabbits (21).

For each drug dose administered at a given PN, the proportion (number responding/number tested) and percentage of rabbits convulsing were calculated. A perusal of the data suggested that, depending on the drug and/or dose, there were five distinct periods of seizure-susceptibility, i.e., PN 15-20, 21-23, 24-26, 27-38, and 39-42. The data within each of these periods were combined for analyses. The Fisher exact probability test (26) was used to compare the incidence of seizures between any 2 age periods and between any 2 doses. A probability level of 0.05 was adopted to reject the null hypothesis.

Additionally, the data within PN 15-26 (the fastest rising portion of the dose-response curves) were combined for each dose of each cannabinoid. With these data, the median convulsant doses (CD50's) and 95% confidence limits (CL) of each cannabinoid were determined by profit analysis (27). Comparison of dose-response slopes of regression lines and CD50 potencies of cannabinoids were then made by the method of Litchfield and Wilcoxon (28).

B. Experiment II

Rabbits (200) ranging from PN 27-45 were used. Of this total, 55 offspring were derived from mating female THC-SS x male THC-SR carrier (thc/+) parents, and 70 offspring from mating female THC-SR carrier x male THC-SS parents. These progeny were expected to be both THC-SS and THC-SR genotypes with general physical characteristics indistinguishable from one another (17). The 75 offspring of THC-SS parents mated *inter-se* are the same rabbits obtained and tested in Experiment I and, as explained previously, were expected to be all THC-SS (17). Housing and other conditions were the same as described in Experiment I.

Rabbits within the litters were randomly selected, marked with picric acid, and weighed. Rabbits were PN 27-38 at the time of initial testing, a period when THC-SS rabbits are subsensitive to the convulsant effects of 0.1 mg/kg of THC (0.1 mg/kg) during PN 42-45 in order to determine which rabbits were THC-SS and THC-SR carrier genotypes. That is, the THC would be expected to cause convulsions in every THC-SS rabbit and fail to cause the response in every THC-SR rabbit over PN 39-548 (25).

For each type of parental mating, the number of convulsing offspring at PN 27-38 and at PN 42-45 were determined. The resultant ratios (number convulsing THC-SS offspring at PN 27-38/number convulsing THC-SS offspring at PN 42-45) were compared among the 3 types of parental crosses by the Fisher exact probability test (26).

III. RESULTS

A. Experiment I

The ontogenetic data of the first experiment are presented in Table I. The data for each cannabinoid were analyzed separately by making multiple pair-wise comparisons across PN periods for each dose, and multiple, pair-wise comparisons across doses for each PN period. A summary of the resultant, statistically significant contrasts is presented in Table II. These data and their reliability estimates yield a numberof general trends. First, for each dose of each cannabinoid, the incidence of seizures increased as the age of the rabbit increased. Generally, this increase in seizure susceptibility was more gradual and protracted with lower doses than with higher doses of a given cannabinoid. Second, within a given age range, the incidence of seizures increased as the dose of cannabinoid increased. This was particularly evident at younger ages (PN 15-26) where maximal seizure susceptibility had not, as yet, developed. Third, by PN 39-42, THC-SS rabbits had attained maximal, or near maximal, susceptibility to cannabinoid-produced convulsions over the range of doses tested. Finally, there was no age period of complete nonsusceptibility to cannabinoid-produced convulsions. Even at the earliest ages tested (PN 15-20), some THC-SS rabbits exhibited convulsions at the highest doses of each drug.

From the data in Table I, dose-response curves were constructed and analyzed for each cannabinoid by collapsing the data across PN 15-26 for each dose (PN 15-26 was generally the fastest rising, the most linear, portion of each age-effect

TABLE I. Ontogeny of Cannabinoid-induced Convulsions in THC-SS Rabbits[a]

Drug and Dose[b]	Postnatal Days of Age				
	15-20	21-23	24-26	27-38	39-42
delta-9-THC					
0.1	0/27 (0)	0/21 (0)	8/16 (50)	61/75 (81)	24/24 (100)
0.5	0/15 (0)	8/11 (73)	7/10 (70)	15/17 (88)	15/15 (100)
5.0	3/4 (75)	4/4 (100)	8/8 (100)	8/8 (100)	8/8 (100)
11-OH-delta-9-THC					
0.04	0/14 (0)	22/47 (47)	15/20 (75)	13/13 (100)	13/13 (100)
0.2	0/7 (0)	4/7 (57)	9/9 (100)	26/26 (100)	26/26 (100)
2.0	4/5 (80)	8/8 (100)	9/9 (100)	9/9 (100)	9/9 (100)
11-Oxo-delta-8-THC					
0.1	0/8 (0)	1/5 (20)	4/7 (57)	6/10 (60)	8/10 (80)
0.5	0/7 (0)	4/4 (100)	4/4 (100)	4/4 (100)	8/8 (100)
5.0	4/6 (67)	4/4 (100)	10/10 (100)	8/8 (100)	8/8 (100)

[a]Ratios refer to the number of rabbits convulsing/number of rabbits tested (= %).
[b]Units are in mg/kg, i.v.

TABLE II. Summary of Fisher Exact Probability Tests for Age Periods (1-5) and Doses of Cannabinoids (A-I) Used in THC-SS Rabbits*

Drug and dose (mg/kg, i.v.)	Postnatal Days of Age 15-20 (1)	21-23 (2)	24-26 (3)	27-38 (4)	39-42 (5)
delta-9-THC					
0.1 (A)	1-3;1-4 1-5:A-C	2-3;2-4 2-5:A-B A-C	3-1;3-2 3-4:3-5 A-C	4-1;4-2 4-3;4-5	5-1;5-2 5-3;5-4
0.5 (B)	1-2;1-3 1-4;1-5 B-C	2-1;B-A	3-1;3-5	4-1	5-1;5-3
5.0 (C)	C-A;C-B	C-A	C-A		
11-OH-delta-9-THC					
0.04 (D)	1-2;1-3 1-4;1-5 D-F	2-1;2-4 2-5;D-F	3-1	4-1;4-2	5-1;5-2
0.2 (E)	1-3;1-4 1-5;E-F	2-4;2-5	3-1	4-1;4-2	5-1;5-2
2.0 (F)	F-D;F-E	F-D			
11-OXO-delta-8-THC					
0.1 (G)	1-3;1-4 1-5;G-I	G-H;G-I	3-1:G-I	4-1	5-1
0.5 (H)	1-2;1-3 1-4:1-5 H-I	2-1;H-G	3-1	4-1	5-1
5.0 (I)	I-G;I-H	I-G	I-G		

*Data, obtained from Table I, were analyzed separately for each cannabinoid; only statistically significant contrasts (two-tailed) are shown above.

curve). The resultant CD50's (and 95% CL) in mg/kg were: 0.614 (0.135-2.79) for THC, 0.061 (0.004-0.927) for 11-OH-delta-9-THC, and 0.398 (0.054-2.92) for 11-OXO-delta-8-THC. Analyses of slope ratios indicated that the 3 dose-response curves did not differ significantly from parallelism. Further analyses of relative (CD50) potencies indicated that 11-OH-delta-9-THC was 10.1 times more potent than THC and 6.5 times more potent than 11-OXO-delta-8-THC, and each of these differences was statistically significant. While the CD50 of 11-OXO-delta-8-THC was 1.5 times less than that of THC, this difference in potency was not statistically significant.

B. Experiment II

The results of the second experiment are presented in Table III. When the parental THC-SS rabbits were mated _inter-se_, all the progeny tested at PN 42-45 were THC-SS. However, despite their affected genotype, only 81% of the rabbits convulsed to THC during PN 27-38 (these same data are also shown in Table I). With parental matings of THC-SS and THC-SR carrier genotypes, offspring at PN 42-45 were a mixture of THC-SS and THC-SR phenotypes. Of the total offspring with the THC-SS (affected) genotype, the incidence of convulsions at PN 27-38 was 71% in the offspring derived from mating a female THC-SR (carrier) and a male THC-SS parental genotype. Pair-wise (two-tailed) comparisons of these ratios indicated that 81% and 71% did not differ statistically ($p = 0.389$), but that 95% was significantly different from 71% ($p = 0.009$) and from 81% ($p = 0.048$).

IV. DISCUSSION

The results of the present two experiments provide evidence that the behavioral response of THC-SS rabbits to THC is influenced by developmental and environmental factors. This is to be expected since the behavior genetic literature is replete with examples of the dependence of the genotypis expression of phenotype on the developmental status of, and environmental influences on, an individual (7,29).

We have previously found that THC, 11-OH-delta-9-THC and 11-OXO-delta-8-THC, each given in the doses employed in Experiment I, will cause convulsions in 100% of THC-SS rabbits who are PN 39 or older (18,24). The results of the first experiment indicate that seizure susceptibility of young THC-SS rabbits is dependent on the dose of cannabinoid employed and the age of developing offspring. In general, seizure susceptibility increased as a function of increasing age and as a function of increasing dose. Susceptibility increases were most pronounced over PN 15-26. Potencies among cannabinoids, based upon comparisons of dose-response curves over this latter age span, indicated the following ranking: 11-OH-delta-9-THC > THC = 11-OXO-delta-8-THC. These dose-response and potency relationships agree with those previously found in adult THC-SS rabbits (18,2,24). Thus, the major characteristics of the young THC-SS rabbits, compared with older animals, is a subsensitive response to cannabinoids.

The drug responsiveness of infant animals is frequently found to be less than that of older animals (30), and this subsensitivity is more often associated with stimulant drugs, including convulsants, than with depressant drugs (31,32). With respect to THC, reports of the mouse locomotor response and shuttle box avoidance learning (15,16) and the chicken hypothermic response (33) indicate age-related differences in drug responsiveness. Although the effects seen after acute injections were more pronounced in the younger, compared to the older animals, the reversal of this was found after chronic injections (15,16,33). The behavioral effects of acute injections of THC in the THC-SS rabbits are in the opposite direction from these earlier reports of age-related effects of THC. However, the species and type of response

TABLE III. Convulsant Effects of Delta-9-THC in Rabbit Offspring Derived From Mating THC-SS with THC-SS or THC-SR Carrier Parents[a]

Parental Matings	No. Convulsing Offspring/No. Tested		% of THC-SS Offspring at PN 27-38[b]
Female x Male	PN-27-38	PN 42-45	
THC-SS X THC-SS	61/75	75/75	81.3[c]
THC-SS x THC-SR	17/55	24/55	70.8%
THC-SR x THC-SS	40/70	42/70	95.2%

[a]Delta-9-THC dose, 0.1 mg/kg, i.v.

[b]Number of THC-SS offspring convulsing at PN 27-38/number of THC-SS offspring convulsing at PN 42-45.

[c]The offspring obtained and tested from this type of parental mating are the same rabbits used in Experiment I; these data are also shown in Table 1.

monitored may be critical variables that influence the ontogenetic effects of THC.

Many factors are potentially responsible for differences in the responsiveness to drugs at different ages. To take an example, an incomplete development of liver metabolic capacities could account for the reduced degree of genetic penetrance of the THC seizure susceptible trait in the young THC rabbits in comparison to older THC-SS rabbits. Considerable scientific debate has revolved around the putative biological importance of THC metabolites oxidized at the 11-position (34,35). Both THC and delta-8-THC are converted by liver enzymes to their respective 11-OH-THC metabolites (34,35), and the latter are pharmacologically active across species (34-36). Further oxidation yields 11-OXO-THC metabolites (37,38). Although corollary data are apparently not available for 11-OXO-delta-9-THC (including the present study since this metabolite was unavailable to us), 11-OXO-delta-8-THC is very active in a variety of pharmacological tests (39,40). Subsequent oxidation results in carboxylic acid metabolites (i.e., the THC-11-oic acids or the 11-nor-9-carboxy-THC's) which are pharmacologically inactive (24,39). If the pharmacological effects of THC are largely attributable to the 11-OH and 11-OXO metabolites as previously suggested (34,39) thenthe reduced seizure susceptibility in the present study may be due, in part, to decreased liver metabolism of THC. Although we have no direct data in our THC-SS rabbits, it is known that liver enzyme functioning is not fully mature until the end of the first neonatal month in other rabbits (41). Also, the high degree of convulsant activity of the THC metabolites, especially 11-OH-delta-9-THC, in the present study offer some support for the pharmacological importance of liver metabolism of THC in our rabbits.

If an immaturity in liver metabolism was totally responsible for the subsensitive response of the young THC-SS rabbits, then 100% of these rabbits should exhibit convulsions after administration of maximally effective, adult doses of the metabolites. That is, doses of 11-OH-delta-9-THC (0.04, 0.02 and 2 mg/kg) and 11-OXO-delta-8-THC (0.1, 0.5 and 5 mg/kg) produce convulsions in 100% of THC-SS rabbits of PN 42 and older, and should produce the same incidence of convulsions in all of the younger THC-SS rabbits. However, the absence of this finding in the present study suggests that an immaturity of liver metabolism (i.e., conversion of THC to its 11-OH and 11-OXO metabolites) cannot be solely responsible for the observed subsensitive, behavioral response. Therefore, other factors may also be of importance. For example, the THC-SS rabbit, because of its unique genome, may have a neuroanatomical or neurochemical substrate in the brain which renders it susceptible to cannabinoid-produced convulsions.

While being fully developed in adult THC-SS rabbits, the appropriate substrate(s) in the brain may be immature in the younger, affected rabbits. Although data are unavailable for THC-SS rabbits, it is known that, in other rabbit stocks, the central nervous system undergoes gradual maturation during the postnatal period studied in the present experiment (42-44). Additional factors which might amount for the decreased stimulant properties of THC in the young THC-SS rabbits include immaturity in the mechanisms associated with plasma protein binding, distribution and rate of tissue uptake of the parent drug or its metabolites.

Obviously, the specific mechanism(s) responsible for the subsensitivity, and for the underlying convulsant effect of cannabinoids in THC-SS rabbits, remain to be determined. In any event, the data of the present study clearly indicate an ontogenetic effect of cannabinoid reactivity in our rabbits. Although there is an attenuation of cannabinoid response, the young, developing THC-SS rabbits are still capable of exhibiting the same qualitative pattern of behavioral stimulation as are the adult THC-SS rabbits. Additional studies are required to determine whether THC-SS rabbits will respond to highdoses of the cannabinoids prior to PN 15, the earliest age which we have investigated.

In the second experiment, THC-SS rabbit offspring were obtained from different parental combinations of THC-SS and THC-SR carrier genotype matings in order to assess potential parental- and sibling- genotype interactions. With each type of parental mating, the THc-SS rabbit offspring at PN 27-38 are subsensitive, compared with older THC-SS rabbits, to the convulsive effects of THC. That is, a dose (0.1 mg/kg) of THC that is effective in 100% of THC-SS rabbits at PN 42-45 produced incidences of convulsions in less that 100% of THC-SS rabbits at the earlier ages. These findings corroborate and extend our previous findings (25) that THC-SS progeny derived from THC-SS parents mated <u>inter-se</u> are subsensitive to the convulsant effects of THC (0.1 mg/kg) when tested between PN 24 and 38.

The present data also show that THC-produced seizure susceptibility of THC-SS offspring varies with the particular type of parental mating employed. When a female THC-SS parent was mated with a male THC-SS or a male THC-SR (carrier) parent, the resulting incidences of convulsing offspring (at PN 27-38) were not reliably different. However, when a female THC-SR (carrier) parent was mated with a male THC-SS parent, the resultant incidence of convulsing offspring was significantly higher than the other incidences. The sibling genotypes resulting from the 2 matings in which the incidences of convulsion were similar, were either only THC-SS, or THC-SS and THC-SR (carrier). This finding in combination with the differing paternal genotypes in these matings suggests that the critical factor may be the maternal rabbit. It appears that environmental factors associated with the THC-SR (carrier) mother enhanced the expression of THC seizure susceptibility in the developing THC-SS rabbits. Whether the maternal effect occurred during the postnatal period and/or in utero must be determined by further study. While the supposition of an interaction between a maternal factor and an inherited, phenotypic response to THC is novel, maternal-behavioral genetic interactions are well known for other types of drugs (12,45,46).

In conclusion, the results of these studies suggest that the genetically mediated stimulant response of THC-SS rabbits to cannabinoids is dependent on specific subject (age) and environment (maternal influence) variables. The extent to which these findings may generalize to a human situation is unknown. With respect to genetic factors, one study has reported a high frequency of dysphoric reactions to THC among patients with unipolar depression (13). Since putative genetic determinants of depressive disorders have been advanced (47), it could be speculated that THC produced a specific pharmacogenetic effect in the above population. Another study reported prolonged depersonalization after marijuana use, and this unusual reaction appeared to be genetically mediated (14). Additionally, many human studies indicate that various types of environmental factors can influence the subjective response to THC (1-6). The interpretation of these human studies in conjunction with results from the present study and results from studies of inbred strains of mice (15,16) raise the intriguing possibility that genetic-environmental interactions might be important determinants of the behavioral effects of marijuana across species. Further, while an age-dependency of marijuana responsiveness in humans has not been investigated, the results of the present study suggest that an appropriate dose of THC will induce behavioral effects in very young organisms. This may have serious ramifications in conjunction with the rather prevalent usage patterns of marijuana in adolescents (48) and in pregnant women (49,50). It is hoped that further study of the ontogenetic characteristics of the THC-SS rabbit will yield appropriate generalizations about the response of the developing human to the effects of the psychoactive cannabinoids.

ACKNOWLEDGMENT

The authors wish to thank the National Institute on Drug Abuse for the supply of cannabinoids.

REFERENCES

1. Hollister, L. E., Clinical pharmacology of marijuana, in "Research Advances in Alcohol and Drug Problems", Vol. 1 (R.J. Gibbons, Y. Israel, H. Kalant, R. E. Popham, R. E., W. Schmidt, and R. G. Smart, eds.), pp. 243-266. John Wiley and Sons, New York, 1974.
2. Hollister, L. E., Overall, J. E., and Gerger, M. L., Marijuana setting, Arch. Gen. Psychiat. 32:789-801 (1975).
3. Jones, R. T., Marijuana-induced "high". Influenceof expectation, setting and previous drug experience, Pharmacol. Rev. 23:359-369 (1971).
4. Rossi, A. M., Kuehnle, J. E., and Mendelson, J. H., Marijuana and mood in human volunteers, Pharmacol. Biochem. Behav. 8:447-453 (1978).
5. McAree, C.P., Steffenhagen, R. A., and Zheutlin, L. S., Personality factors and patterns of drug usage in college students, Amer. J. Psychiat. 128:890-893 (1972).
6. Ashton, H., Golding, J., March, U. R., Millina, J. E., and Thompson, J. W., The seed and the soil. Effect of dosage, personality and starting state on the response to delta-9-tetrahydrocannabinol in man, Brit. J. Clin. Pharmacol. 12:705-720 (1981).
7. Fuller, J. L., and Thompson, W. R., "Foundation of Behavior Genetics". The C. V. Mosby Company, St. Louis, 1978.
8. Kessler, S., and Noble, M., Behavior genetics, in "Principles of Psychopharmacology" (W. G. Clark and J. del Giudice, eds.), pp. 371-385. Academic Press, New York, pp. 371-385, 1978.
9. Vesell, E.S., Twin studies in pharmacogenetics, Human Genet. Suppl. 1:19-30 (1978).
10. Stabenau, J. R., Genetic and other factors inschizophrenic, manic-depressive and schizo-affective psychoses, J. Nerv. Ment. Dis. 164:149-167 (1978).
11. Eleftheriou, B. E., "Psychopharmacogenetics". Plenum Press, New York, 1975.
12. Broadhurst, P. L., "Drugs and the Inheritance of Behavior". Plenum Press, New York, 1978.
13. Ablon, S. L., and Goodwin, F. K., High frequency of dysphoric reactions to tetrahydrocannabinol among depressed patients. Amer. J. Psychiat. 131:448-453 (1974).
14. Szymanski, H. V., Prolonged depersonalization after marijuana use, Amer. J. Psychiat. 138:231-233 (1981).
15. Radouco-Thomas, S., Magnan, F., Grove, R. N., Singh, P., Garcin, F. and Radouco-Thomas, C., Effects of chronic administration of delta-1-tetrahydrocannabinol on learning and memory in developing mice, in "The Pharmacology of

Marijuana", Vol. 2 (M.C. Braude and S. Szara, eds.), pp.487-498. Raven Press, New York, 1976.

16. Radouco-Thomas, S., Magnan, F., and Radouco-Thomas C., Pharmacogenetic studies on cannabis and narcotics: Effects of delta-1-tetrahydrocannabinol and morphine in developing mice, in "Marijuana: Chemistry, Biochemistry and Cellular Effects" (G. G. Nahas, ed.), pp. 481-494. Springer-Verlag, New York, 1976.
17. Fish, B. S., Consroe, P., and Fox, R. R., Inheritance of delta-9-tetrahydrocannabinol seizure susceptibility, J. Hered. 72:215-216 (1981).
18. Consroe, P., and Fish, B. S., Rabbit behavioral model of marijuana psycho-activity in humans, Med. Hypotheses 7:1079-1090 (1981).
19. Fish, B. S., Consroe, P., and Fox, R. R., Convulsant-anticonvulsant properties of delta-9-tetrahydrocannabinol (THC), Behav. Genet., accepted for publication (1982).
20. Consroe, P. and Fish, B. S., Behavioral pharmacology of tetrahydrocannabinol seizure susceptible rabbits, Comm. Psychopharmacol. 4:287-291 (1980).
21. Fish, B. S., and Consroe, P., Tolerance to, and symmetrical cross-tolerance between, cannabinol and delta-9-tetrahydrocannabinol, Experientia 31:295-296 (1981).
22. Consroe, P., and Martin, P., EEG profile of tetrahydrocannabinol seizure susceptible rabbits, Proc. West. Pharmacol. Soc. 24:11-13 (1981).
23. Consroe, P., Martin, P., and Eisenstein, D., Anticonvulsant drug antagonism of delta-9-tetrahydrocannabinol-induced seizures in rabbits, Res. Comm. Chem. Path. Pharmacol. 16:1-13 (1977).
24. Consroe, P., Martin, A. R., and Fish, B. S., The use of a potential rabbit model for structure-behavioral activity studies of cannabinoids, J. Med. Chem. 25:596-599 (1982).
25. Fish, B.S., and Consroe, P., The ontogeny of delta-9-tetrahydrocannabinol responsiveness in the rabbit, Develop. Psychobiol., accepted for publication (1982).
26. Siegel, S., "Nonparametric Statistics for the Behavioral Sciences". McGraw-Hill, New York, 1956.
27. Finey, D.J., "Probit Analysis". Cambridge University Press, London, 1962.
28. Litchfield, J. T., and Wilcoxon, F., A simplified method of evaluating dose-effect experiments, J. Pharmacol. Exp. Ther. 95:99-113 (1949).
29. McClearn, G. E., and DeFries, J. C. "Introduction to Behavioral Genetics". W. H. Freeman & Co., Publishers, 1973.
30. Spear, L. P. The use of psychopharmacological procedures to analyze the ontogeny of learning and retention:

Issues and concerns, in "Ontogeny of Learning and Retention" (N. E. Spear and B. A. Campbell, eds.), pp. 135-156. Lawrence Erlbaum Associates, Hillsdale, New Jersey, 1979.

31. Pylkko, O. O., and Woodbury, D. M., The effect of maturation on chemical induced seizures in rats, J. Pharmacol Exp. Ther. 131:185-190)1961).
32. Yeary, R. A., Benish, R. A., and Finkelstein, M., Acute toxicity of drugs in newborn animals, J. Pediat. 69:663-667 (1966).
33. Abel, E. L., McMillan, D. E., and Harris, L. S., Tolerance to the hypothermic effects of delta-9-tetrahydrocannabinol as a function of age in the chicken, Br. J. Pharmacol. 47:452-456 (1973).
34. Lemberger, L., McMahon, I., and Archer, R., The role of metabolic conversion on the mechanism of actions of cannabinoids, in "Pharmacology of Marijuana", Vol. 1 (M. C. Braude and S. Szara), pp. 125-133. Raven Press, New York, 1976.
35. Hollister, L. E. and Gillespie, B. A., Action of delta-9-tetrahydrocannabinol: An approach to the active metabolite hypothesis, Clin. Pharmacol. Ther. 18:714-719 (1975).
36. Paton, W. D. M., and Pertwee, R. G., The pharmacology of cannabis in animals, in "Marijuana Chemistry, Pharmacology, Metabolism and Clinical Effects" (R. Mechoulam, ed.), pp. 191-284. Academic Press, New York, 1973.
37. Ben-Zvi, Z., and Burstein, S., 7-OXO-delta-1-tetrahydrocannabinol: A novel metabolite of delta-1-tetrahydrocannabinol, Res. Comm. Chem. Pathol. Pharmacol. 8:223-229 (1974).
38. Watanabe, K., Yamamoto, I., Oguri, K., and Yoshimura, H., Microsomal oxygenase catalyzed oxidation of 11-hydroxy-delta-1-tetrahydrocannabinol to 11-OXO-delta-1-tetrahydrocannabinol, Biochem. Biophys. Res. Comm. 88:178-182 (1979).
39. Watanabe, K., Yamamoto, I, Oguri, K., and Yoshimura, H., Comparison in mice of pharmacological effects of delta-8-tetrahydrocannabinol and its metabolites oxidized at 11-position, Eur. J. Pharmacol. 63:1-6 (1980).
40. Yamamoto, I., Watanabe, K., Oguri, K., and Yoshimura, H., Anticonvulsant activity of 11-hydroxy-delta-8-tetrahydrocannabinol and 11-OXO-delta-8-tetrahydrocannabinol against pentylenetetrazol-induced seizures in the mouse, Res. Comm. Subst. Abuse 1:287-298 (1980).
41. Fouts, J. R., and Adamson, R. H., Drug Metabolism in the newborn rabbit, Science 129:897-898 (1959).
42. Pscheidt, G. R., Schweigerdt, A., and Himwich, H. E., Effects of some psychoactive drugs on electroencephalo-

gram and brain amines of immature rabbits, Life Sci. 4:1333-1343 (1965).

43. Harel, S., Watanabe, K., Linke, I., and Schain, R. J., Growth and development of the rabbit brain, Biol. Neonate 21:381-399 (1972).
44. Tennyson, V. M., Development of the substantia nigra, pars compacta and neostriatum, in "Progress in Neuropathology", Vol. 3 (H. M. Zimmerman, ed.), pp. 359-381. Grune and Stratton, New York, 1976.
45. Randall, C. L., and Lester, D., Alcohol selection by DBA and C57BL mice arising from ova transfers, Nature 255:147-148, 1975.
46. Randall, C. L., and Lester, D., Cross-fostering of DBA and C57BL mice: Increase in voluntary consumption of alcohol by DBA weanlings, J. Stud. Alcohol 36:973-980 (1975).
47. Weitkamp, L .R., Stancen, H. C., Persad, E., Flood, C., and Guttormsen, S., Depressive disorders and HLA: A gene on chromosome 6 that can affect behavior, N. Engl. J. Med., 305:1301-1306, 1981.
48. Hendin, H., Pollinger, A., Ulman, R., and Carr, A. C., "Adolescent Marijuana Abusers and Their Families", NIDA Research Monograph 40, National Institute on Drug Abuse, Rockville, Maryland, 1981.
49. Fried, P. A., Marijuana use by pregnant women: Neurobehavioral effects in neonates, Drug Alcohol Depend., 6:415-424 (1980).
50. Fried, P. A., Watkinson, B., Grant, A., and Knights, R. M., Changing patterns of soft drug use prior to and during pregnancy: A prospective study, Drug Alcohol Depend 6:323-343, 1980.

ELECTROPHYSIOLOGICAL MECHANISMS OF DELTA-9-TETRAHYDROCANNABINOL'S CONVULSANT ACTIONS*

Stuart A. Turkanis
Ralph Karler

Department of Pharmacology
University of Utah School of Medicine
Salt Lake City, Utah

I. INTRODUCTION

Delta-9-tetrahydrocannabinol (THC) elicits a complex mixture of central excitatory and depressant properties (1,2). Central excitation, however, represents a major facet of the drug's pharmacological profile, which ranges from vocalization to overt convulsions (3). Its propensity to precipitate frank convulsions is exhibited in various laboratory test systems; for example, in mice, THC lowers the convulsive threshold in the 60-Hz-electroshock threshold and pentylenetetrazol minimal-seizure tests (19), and it also augments the development of electrically and pentylenetetrazol-caused kindling (4). Furthermore, THC produces frank convulsions in cobalt and iron epileptic rats (5,6), in epileptic beagles (7), and in a special strain of rabbits (8). The convulsive properties of THC are well-documented and, accordingly, are potentially important toxicologically.

The purpose of the present work is to identify possible electrphysiological mechanisms of action of the cannabinoid's convulsive effects to further the understanding of its pharmacological properties. The results of electrophysiological investigations carried out at various levels of the central nervous system, ranging from the cerebral cortex to the spinal cord, demonstrate that THC's excitatory effects are discernible at every level studied, even at individual synapses.

---

*Supported by NIDA grant DA-00346.

ISBN 0-12-044620-0

II. METHODS

The techniques used in the present work have been previously described: cobalt epilepsy by Chiu et al. (5); kindled limbic seizures by Smiley et al. (9); monosynaptic spinal reflexes by Esplin (10) and Tramposch et al. (11); cortical evoked responses by Turkanis and Karler (12); and synaptic potentials at spinal motoneurons by Weakly (13) and Kuno and Weakly (14). Spinal-cord studies were carried out with 2.4-3.6 kg male and female cats with their spinal cords severed at the atlanto-occipital junction and their brains destroyed ischemically (10); in all other studies, conscious, unrestrained male Sprague-Dawley rats with electrodes chronically implanted in their brains were used. The drug was prepared by previously published procedures (15) and was given intraperitoneally to rats and intravenously to cats.

III. RESULTS

In conscious rats, THC produces numerous excitatory electrophysiological effects that appear to contribute to its convulsive properties: For instance, the cannabinoid exacerbates a pre-existing epileptic phenomenon; that is, the drug causes a dose-related increase in spontaneously-firing, cortical, focal epileptiform potentials in cobalt epileptic rats (Fig. 1); it is important to note that this excitatory effect occurs

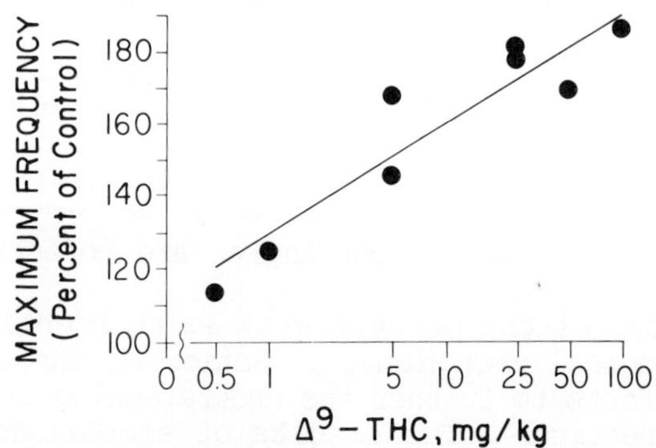

FIGURE 1. Influence of THC on the frequency of spontaneous-firing, focal epileptic potentials at a cobalt focus in the left cortex. Electrocorticographic recordings were made in rats with chronically implanted brain electrodes from a focus in the left parietal cortex. Each point represents the results from a different rat and is the maximum frequency expressed as a percentage of predrug control obtained in each experiment. The line was calculated by least squares regression. Adapted from Ref. 9.

with doses as small as 0.5 mg/kg. Furthermore, the increase in focal epileptiform activity results in the precipitation of convulsions. The drug also enhances neurotransmission between the cerebral cortices, as evidenced by an increase in the amplitude of the electrically caused transcallosal evoked response (Fig. 2). The augmentation of neurotransmission in the corpus callosum, which is important for the transfer of epileptic phenomena (16), may also contribute to the manifestation of the cannabinoid's convulsive effects (12).

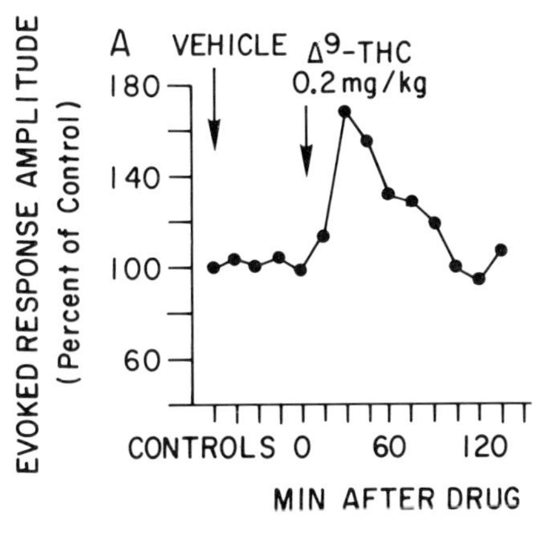

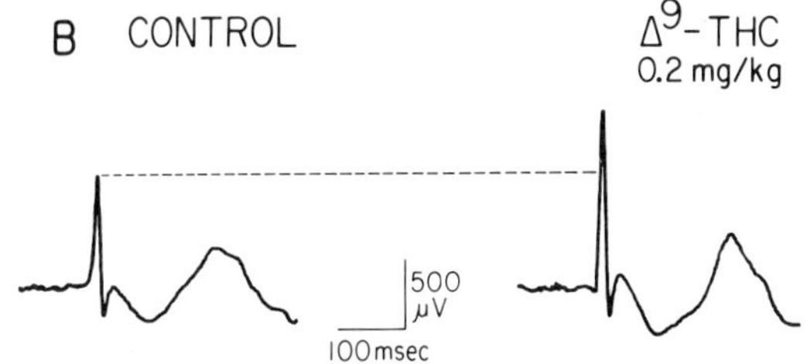

FIGURE 2. Influence of THC on the amplitude of the electrically-caused, transcallosal cortical evoked response. A, the time course represents the results from a rat. The data are amplitudes of the initial phase of averaged evoked responses, and the arrows indicate the time of vehicle or drug administration. Each response is an electronically obtained average of four consecutive potentials obtained 5 sec apart, while the rat was in a sitting position. B, ave. response from a rat before and 30 min after drug. In six rats, THC (0.1-1.0 mg/kg) increased the mean amplitude and its range to 153 (127-208) percent of controls (obtained at the beginning of each experiment). Comparable vehicle values from six rats were 101 (88-111) percent of controls. The two values are statistically different by Mann-Whitney U statistic ($p < 0.05$) (25).

The results of the kindled limbic rat seizure studies show the effects of THC on the after discharge (AD), which is the elecrical manifestation of a seizure (17). In low doses (0.1-1 mg/kg), the cannabinoid prolongs the duration of the AD in the hippocampus and the cerebral cortex but not at the site of focal electrical stimulation in the subiculum (Table I). These data suggest that the drug increases the propagation of the AD selectively in different brain areas. At higher doses (5-15 mg/kg) this selectivity disappears because the AD is markedly prolonged at all three recording sites (Fig. 3). The behavioral consequence of a prolongation of the AD is an increase in the duration of the convulsion. In addition to these effects on electrically induced ADs, THC (0.5-100 mg/kg) produces AD-like bursts of potentials in the cortices of cobalt epileptic rats (Fig. 4); similar results were seen in iron epileptic and control rats (6). Despite the fact that the relationship between drug-induced AD-like bursts and convulsions is unknown, it is possible that the bursts may also contribute to the precipitation of convulsions.

The findings of the spinal reflex investigations with cats are consistent with the cortical and limbic findings: First, THC (0.05-0.15 mg/kg) in the cat increases the amplitude of

TABLE I. Delta-9-THC's Effects on AD Duration of Conscious Rats With Kindled Limbic Seizures

Recording Site	Means and Ranges of Maximum Effects[a]
Left subiculum	96 (75-107)
Right dorsal hippocampus	113 (106-134)[b]
Rigth cerebral cortex	115 (104-119)[b]

[a]Values expressed as percentage of internal vehicle control obtained in each experiment; five experiments were carried out with 0.1-1 mg/kg delta-9-THC. In these studies, the rats had chronically implanted electrodes in their brains; the left subiculum was the site of focal electrical stimulation, and ADs were recorded simultaeously from the subiculum, the hippocampus and the cerebral cortex.

[b]Value is significantly different from that obtained from the left subiculum, as determined by the many-one rank statistic ($p < 0.05$) (26). The mean vehicle control values and their ranges for the hippocampus and cerebral cortex were 92 (86-112) and 93 (86-112), respectively (Ref., Smiley, Turkanis and Karler, unpublised).

the monosynaptic reflex (Fig. 5). Such results support our cortical evoked data indicating that THC increases neurotransmission; furthermore, they implicate the synapse as a site of drug action. Secondly, the drug markedly enhanced posttetanic potentiation (Fig. 6), which is purported to be a mechanism by which seizures spread throughout the CNS (10).

Because the spinal-reflex data suggest that the synapse is a probable site of drug action, the effects of the cannabinoid on synaptic transmission at individual cat spinal motoneurons were also assessed. In this test system, the cannabinoid (0.01-0.1 mg/kg) elicits a consistent excitatory effect; that is, it evokes motoneuron action potentials (Fig. 7). Subsequent experiments demonstrated that in the same dosage range the cannabinoid increases the amplitude of the EPSP (Fig. 8), an effect which could, at least partially, account for the facilitation of the production of motoneuron action potentials. In addition, within the identical dosage range THC partially suppresses inhibitory postsynaptic potentials

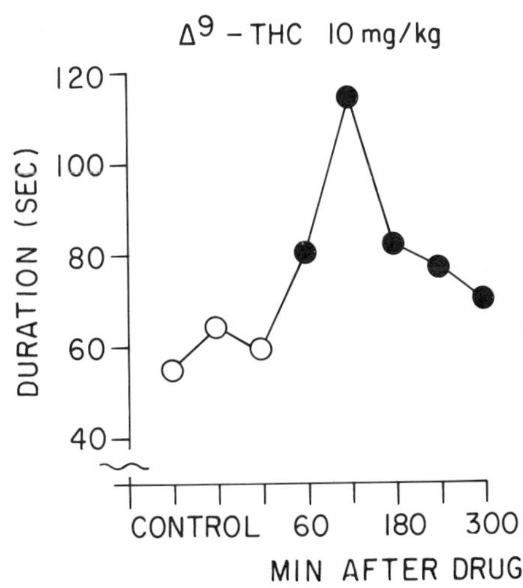

FIGURE 3. Influence of THC on limbic AD duration in a rat with kindled seizures. AD was evoked and recorded from left subiculum of a rat with chronically implanted electrodes. Open circles represent responses after vehicle; closed circles, responses after drug. Nine experiments were carried out with both vehicle and drug: the mean AD duration and its range after vehicle treatment was 93 (85-112) percent of control and after THC (5-15 mg/kg) was 174 (120-344) percent of control. Drug value is significantly different from control as determined by Mann-Whitney U statistic ($p < 0.05$) (25). Adaped from Ref. 3.

(IPSPs); it has, however, a limited efficacy because a 10 mg/kg dose is no more effective than is 0.1 mg/kg (Fig. 9). In short, the drug at a spinal synapse elicits excitation by two different mechanisms; that is, by enhancing EPSPs and by suppressing IPSPs. Since there is a possibility that the effects on these potentials result from a change in the afferent input (18), dorsal root action potentials were recorded extracellularly at the point where they enter the spinal cord. The findings of the experiments indicate that THC does not alter the afferent input; therefore, the results on synaptic potentials must be due to other causes. In fact, doses as

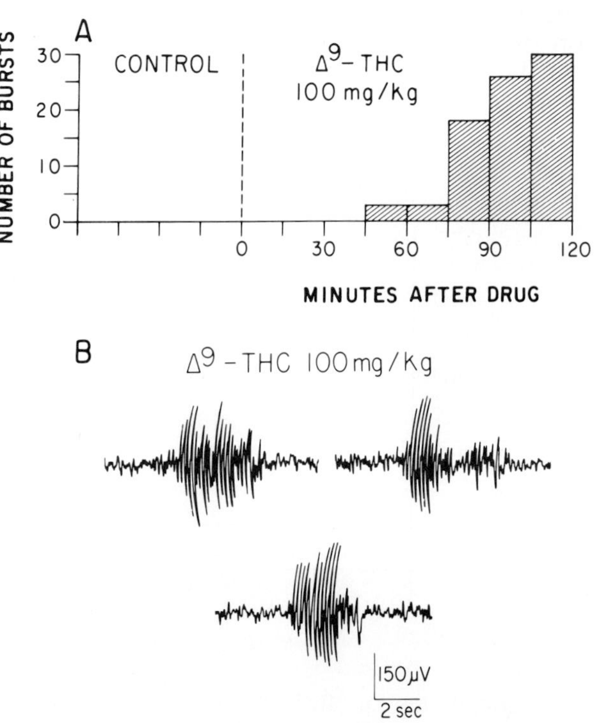

FIGURE 4. Spontaneous AD-bursts produced by THC in a cobalt epileptic rat. Bursts were recorded from the cerebral cortex at a site away from the epileptic focus. A, time course of AD-like bursts from a conscious rat Vehicle was given 15 min after the beginning of the control period; drug, at the beginning of 120-min test period. B, AD-like bursts occurring 81-90 min after THC. Similar results were observed in seven additional animals. Adapted from Ref. 5.

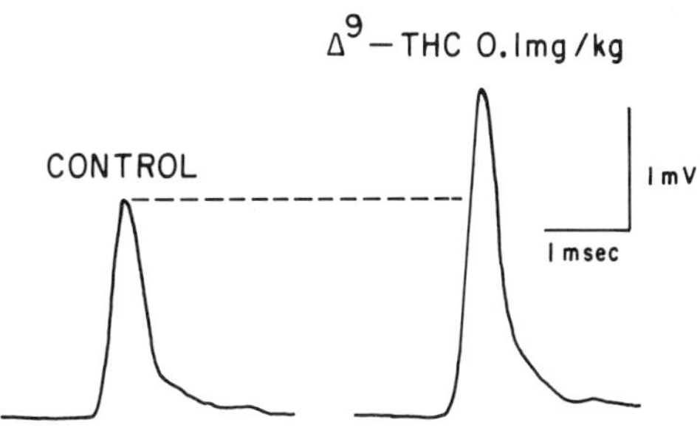

FIGURE 5. Influence of THC on the cat spinal monosynaptic reflex. The reflex was elicited by stimulating L7 dorsal roots and was recorded extracellularly from L7 ventral roots. Each response is an electronically obtained average of 16 consecutive responses recorded 5 sec apart. A, the control response 30 min after vehicle; B, response 30 min after THC. THC was studied in six cats; vehicle, five. The mean monosynaptic reflex amplitude and its range after vehicle was 98 (89-112) percent of control and after THC (0.01-0.1 mg/kg), 152 (126-185) percent of control. These values are significantly different as determined by a Mann-Whitney U statistic ($p < 0.05$) (25).

high as 10 mg/kg have no effect on the dorsal root action potential, whereas doses as low as 0.01-0.1 mg/kg elicit synaptic effects. These findings make it clear that the synapse is more sensitive to the cannabinoid than the axon.

IV. DISCUSSION

There is considerable evidence that THC can cause CNS excitation as well as the more generally recognized depression (1-3,19). The drug's excitatory character appears to manifest itself most dramatically by precipitating convulsions, especially in epileptic animals (5-7). Whether marijuana or THC will similarly affect human epilepsies must await detailed clinical assessment. The interaction with human epilepsies may, however, be very complicated because THC, like the well established antiepileptics, phenytoin and phenobarbital, elicits both anticonvulsant and convulsant effects in various laboratory tests (19); consequently, the clinical effects of the cannabinoids are likely to be as complex as are those of the antiepileptics, which exacerbate some types of epilepsies and suppress others (20). Nevertheless, when evaluating the pharmacological properties of any cannabinoid, central excitatory effects, including the precipitation of convulsions, must be considered.

The data reported here indicate that THC produces electrophysiological manifestations of central excitation, which may contribute to its propensity to cause convulsions. First, the drug raises the firing rate of an epileptic focus resulting in the precipitation of convulsions. Secondly, it increases the duration of the AD, which represents the electrical aspect of

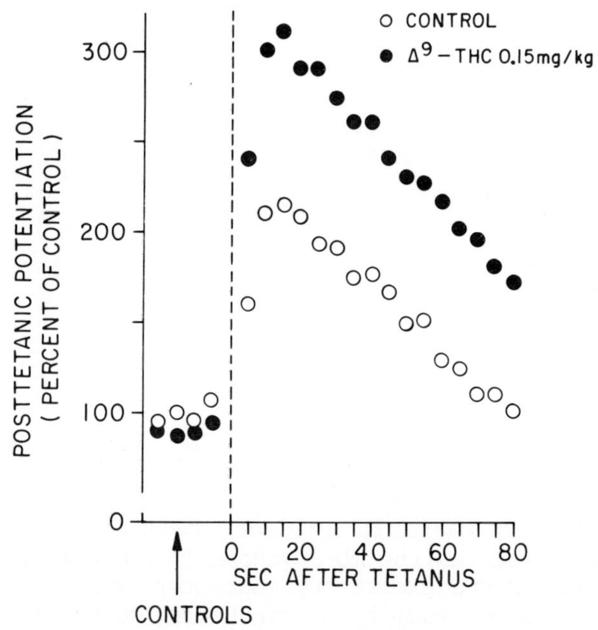

FIGURE 6. Influence of THC on posttetanic potentiation of a cat spinal monosynaptic reflex. Posttetanic potentiation is the amplitude of the posttetanic response expressed as a percentage of the pretetanic response. The responses were evoked by stimulating L7 dorsal root and were recorded from the corresponding ventral root. Similar results were observed in four additional cats.

the seizure (17), and results in a marked prolongation of the convulsion (4). This enhancement of AD duration is significant for another reason; that is, it suggests that the cannabinoid increases susceptibility to seizures (21). Thirdly, the drug promotes neurotransmission in pathways known to be important for the spread of epileptiform phenomena and the precipitation of convulsions. Lastly, the cannabinoid enhances posttetanic potentiation, which is reported to be the mechanism of action for the spread of epileptiform potentials throughout the CNS (10). Altogether, THC produces a multitude of excitatory effects on neurotransmission, and all of them may contribute to the mechanisms of the drug's convulsive actions.

Although THC clearly alters central neurotransmission, the results indicate that it does not affect axonal conduction. Our failure to observe a depression of the dorsal root action potential, however, appears to contradict the findings of Byck and Ritchie, who repored that in vitro the cannabinoid decreased the size of the compound action potential of the rabbit vagus nerve (22). The discrepancy in results may be

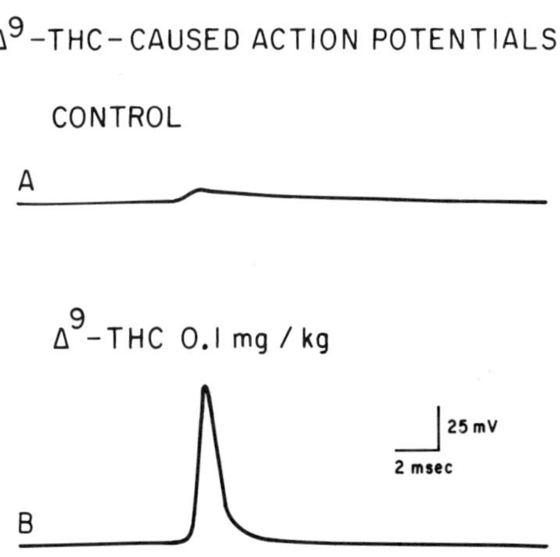

FIGURE 7. Enhancement of the production of action potentials of spinal motoneurons by THC. Intracellular recordings were made with glass microelectrodes from a cat triceps surea motoneuron. Each response is an electronically obtained average of 16 consecutive potentials obtained 5 sec apart. A, electronically averaged control EPSP 15 min after vehicle. B, electronically averaged motoneuron action potential 15 min after THC. Similar results observed in three additional experiments.

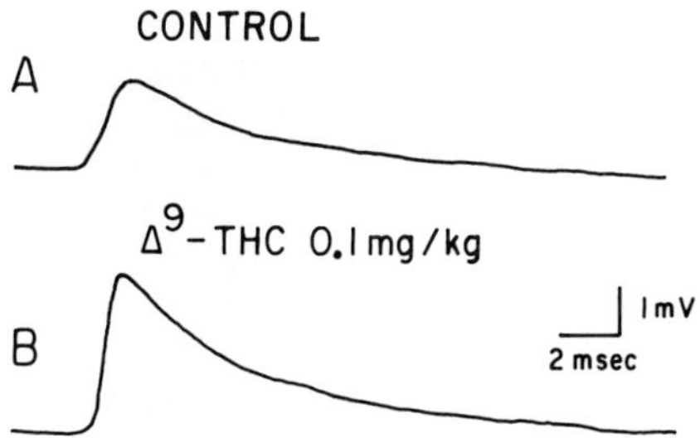

FIGURE 8. Influence of THC on EPSPs. EPSPs were recorded intracellularly from a cat triceps surea spinal motoneuron, and each response is an electronically obtained average of 16 consecutive potentials obtained 5 sec apart. A, control 15 min after vehicle; B, response 5 min after drug. In four cats, the mean EPSP amplitude and its standard deviation after THC (0.01-0.1 mg/kg) was 188 +/- 29 percent of control, which was significantly different from initial vehicle controls obtained in each experiment as determined by a t-test ($p < 0.05$) (27).

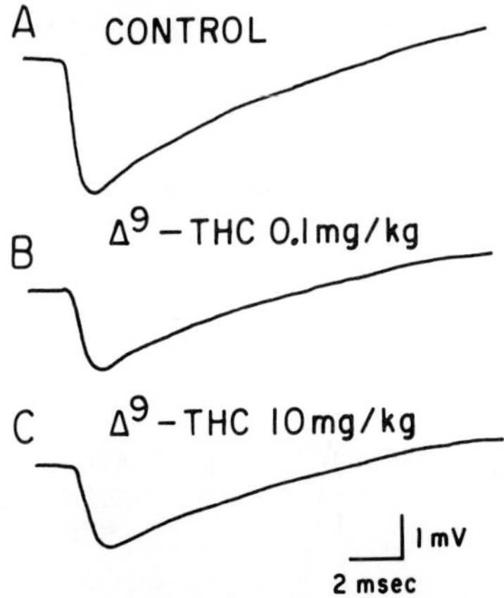

FIGURE 9. Influence of THC on IPSPs. IPSPs were recorded from a cat biceps-semitendinous spinal motoneuron, and each response is an electronically obtained average of 16 consecutive potentials obtained 5 sec apart. A, control 15 min after vehicle; B, response 15 min after drug; C, response 15 min after drug. In four cats, the mean IPSP amplitude and its standard deviation after THC (0.01-0.1 mg/kg) was 65 +/- 3.1 percent of control, which was significantly different from initial vehicle controls obtained in each experiment as determined by a t-test ($p < 0.05$) (27).

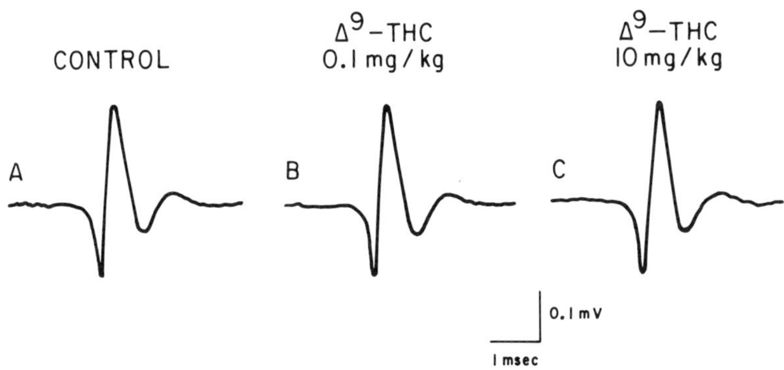

FIGURE 10. Influence of THC on afferent input. Traces were dorsal root action potentials recorded just prior to their entry into the cat spinal cord, and each response is an electronically obtained average of 16 consecutive potentials obtained 5 sec apart. A, control 15 min after vehicle; B, response 15 min after drug; C, response 15 min after drug. In four cats, the mean amplitude of the dorsal root action potential and its standard deviation after THC (0.01-0.1 mg/kg) was 101 +/- 9.0 percent of control, which was not significantly different from initial vehicle controls obtained in each experiment as determined by a t-test ($p < 0.05$) (27).

due to differences in experimental conditions: For instance, because cannabinoids have a very high partition coefficient, they will concentrate in tissues in vitro (2,9,23); consequently, the tissue concentrations in vitro may, in fact, be orders of magnitude higher than that of the bathing medium or that achievable by in vivo administration (2,9). Another possiblity is that different neurons may have different sensitivities to THC, for Brady and Carbone failed to detect any cannabinoid effect in vitro on squid-axon action potentials (24). Regardless of the reason for these discrepancies, our findings suggest that cat synapses are more sensitive to the effects of THC than are axons and, therefore, are probable sites of drug action.

The results of the spinal motoneuron experiments, in fact, point to possiible synaptic mechanisms for the cannabinoid's convulsive action; that is, the drug elicits excitation by increasing the amplitude of the EPSP and partially reducing the amplitude of the IPSP. The limited effect on IPSPs may explain why the cannabinoid is not a strychnine-like convulsant and why its convulsive responses only occur in subjects with a propensity towards convulsions, such as the epileptic rats described here, epileptic beagles (7) and a special strain of rabbits (8). Nevertheless, if the spinal motoneuron findings are applicable to higher centers, they provide feasible synaptic mechanisms for THC's convulsive properties.

ACKNOWLEDGMENT

The authors are grateful to Dr. Monique C. Braude, Division of Research, NIDA, for supplying the cannabinoids and for her continuing advice and encouragement.

REFERENCES

1. Truitt, E. B., Jr., and Braude, M. C., Preclinical pharmacology of marihuana, in "Research Advances in Alcohol and Drug Problem" (R. J. Gibbins, V. Israel, H. Kalant, R. E. Popham, W. Schmidt, and R. G. Smart, eds.), Vol. 1, pp. 199-242. John Wiley and Sons, New York, 1974.
2. Paton, W. D. M. Pharmacology of marijuana, Ann. Rev. Pharmacol. 15:191-220 (1975).
3. Turkanis, S. a., and Karler, R., Electrophysiologic properties of the cannabinoids, J. Clin. Pharmacol. 21:449S-463S (1981).
4. Karler, R., and Turkanis, unpublished results.
5. Chiu, P., Olsen, D. M., Borys, H. K., Karler, R., and Turkanis, S. A., The influence of delta-9-tetrahydrocannabinol on cobalt epilepsy in rats, Epilepsia 20:365-375 (1979).
6. Turkanis, S. A., and Karler, R., Central excitatory properties of delta-9-tetrahydrocannabinol and its metabolites in iron-induced epileptic rats, Neuropharmacol. 21:7-13 (1982).
7. Feeney, D. M., Spiker, M., and Weiss, G. K., Marihuana and epilepsy: Activation of symptoms by delta-9-THC, in "The Therapeutic Potential of Marihuana" (S. Cohen and R. C. Stillman, eds.), pp. 343-362. Plenum Publishing Corp., New York, 1976.
8. Consroe, P., Jones, B., Laird, H., II, and Reinking, J., Anticonvulsant-convulsant effects of delta-9-tetrahydrocannabinol, in "The Therapeutic Potential of Marihuana" (S. Cohen and R. C. Stillman, eds.), pp. 363-382. Plenum Publishing Corp., New York, 1976.

9. Smiley, K. A., Karler, R., and Turkanis, S. A., Effects of cannabinoids on the perfused rat heart, Res. Commun. Chem. Pathol. Pharmacol. 14:659-675 (1976).
10. Esplin, D. W., Synaptic system models, in "Experimental Models of Epilepsy" (D. P. Purpurs, J. K. Penry, D. B. Tower, D. M. Woodbury, and R. D. Walter, eds.), pp. 223-248. Raven Press, New York, 1972.
11. Tramposch, A., Sangdee, C., Franz, D. N., Karler, R., and Turkanis, S. A., Cannabinoid-induced enhancement and depression of cat monosynaptiic reflexes, Neuropharmacol. 20:617-621 (1981).
12. Turkanis, S. a., and Karler, R., Excitatory and depressant effects of delta-9-tetrahydrocannabinol and cannabidiol on cortical evoked responses in the conscious rat, Psychopharmacol. 75:294-298 (1981).
13. Weakly, J. N., Effects of barbiturates on 'quantal' synaptic transmission in spinal motoneurones, J. Physiol. (Lond.) 204:63-77 (1969).
14. Kuno, M., and Weakly, J. N., Quantal components of the inhibitory sybnaptic potential in spinal motoneurones of the cat, J. Physiol. (Lond.) 224:287-303 (1972).
15. Turkanis, S. A., Cely, W., Olsen, D. M., and Karler, R., Anticonvulsant properties of cannabidiol, Res. Commun. Chem. Pathol. Pharmacol. 8:231-246 (1974).
16. Morell, F., Secondary epileptogenic lesions, Epilepsia 1:538-560 (1959).
17. Racine, R., Kindling: The first decade, Neurosurgery 3:234-252 (1978).
18. Eccles, J. C., "The Understanding of the Brain". McGraw-Hill Book Co., New York, 1973.
19. Karler, R., and Turkanis, S. A., The cannabinoids as potential antiepileptics, J. Clin. Pharmacol. 21:437S-448S (1981).
20. Rall, T. W., and Schleifer, L. S., Drugs effective in the therapy of the epilepsies, in "The Pharmacological Basis of Therapeutics", 6th ed. (A. G. Gilman, L. S. Goodman, and A. Gilman, eds.), pp. 448-474. Macmillan Publishing Co., New York, 1980.
21. Ajmone Marsan, C., Focal electrical stimulation in "Experimental Models of Epilepsy" (D. P. Purpura, J. K. Penry, D. B. Tower, D. M. Woodbury, and R. D. Walter, eds.), pp. 147-172. Raven Press, New York, 1972.
22. Byck, R., and Ritchie, J. M., Delta-9-tetrahydrocannabinol: Effects on mammalian nonmyelinated nerve fibers, Science 180:84-85 (1973).
23. Egan, S. M., Graham, J. D. P., and Lewis, M. J., The uptake of tritiated delta-9-tetrahydrocannabinol by the isolated vas deferens of the rat, Br. J. Pharmacol. 56:413-416 (1976).

24. Brady, R. O., and Carbone, E., Comparison of the effects of delta-9-tetrahydrocannabinol, 11-hydroxy-delta-9-tetrahydrocannabinol, and ethanol on the electrophysiological activity of the giant axon of the squid, Neuropharmacol. 12:601-605 (1973).
25. Snedecor, G. W., and Cochran, W. G., "Statistical Methods," 6th ed. Iowa State University Press, Ames, 1967.
26. Steel, R. G. D., A multiple comparison rank sum test: Treatment versus control, Biometrics 15:560-572 (1959).
27. Steel, R. G. D., and Torrie, J. H., "Principles and Procedures of Statistics," 2nd ed. McGraw-Hill Book Company, New York, 1980.

ANTIEMETIC PROPERTIES AND PLASMA CONCENTRATIONS OF DELTA-9-TETRAHYDROCANNABINOL AGAINST CISPLATIN VOMITING IN CATS*

Lawrence E. McCarthy

Department of Pharmacology
Dartmouth Medical School
Hanover, New Hamshire

Karl P. Flora, B. Rao Vishnuvajjala

Pharmaceutical Resources Branch
Developmental Therapeutics Program
Division of Cancer Treatment
National Cancer Institute
Bethesda, Maryland

I. INTRODUCTION

Current interest in the therapeutic potential of the cannabinoids, especially delta-9-tetrahydrocannabinol (THC), has focused largely on the possible use of these agents for preventing the vomiting associated with cancer chemotherapy. The severity of the problem and the progress made in clinical trials have been well reviewed recently by Seigel and Longo (1) and by Davignon (2). It seems clear that some cannabinoids do indeed possess antiemetic activity, but it is not certain whether the limitations in the therapeutic efficacy of these agents stem from differences in patient populations, the variety of emetogenic chemotherapeutic regimens used, bioavailability of the cannabinoids or from other factors.

The present study investigates the antiemetic properties of THC against an anticancer agent of defined emetic liabil-

*Supported in part by NIH grant CA-25190.

ISBN 0-12-044620-0

ity. It compares plasma concentration and antiemetic efficacy of THC in cats following oral, intramuscular and intravenous administration. In addition, THC and its primary metabolite, 11-hydroxy-delta-9-THC, are compared for relative antiemetic activity and associated behavioral concomitants.

II. METHODS

This study incorporated a total of 57 adult cats, undiscriminated as to sex. Animals were conditioned to the laboratory and prepared for recording of emetic activity as described previously (3). The unique pressures which herald emesis were recorded oscillographically by means of central venous catheters, which were advanced into the chest by way of the jugular vein. Sterile, operative techniques were employed to implant the catheters and to exteriorize them for recording purposes. At least 72 hrs were allowed for recovery from surgery prior to testing. Animals were housed in cages especially prepared for recording and were monitored for the occurrence of vomiting for at least 8 hrs after the administration of the emetic substance. Blood samples were obtained by means of the same indwelling venous catheters. Following centrifugation the plasma was stored frozen for later analysis. In the present study blood was collected from animals in the i.v. series at selected times for up to 8 hours after giving THC and for 24 or more hours from those in the oral and intramuscular groups. Those animals scheduled to receive THC by the i.v. route were provided with a second jugular catheter to void contamination of blood samples by the catheter used for injection.

The anticancer agent cisplatin was used as the emetic challenge in this series. Vomiting to this substance had been characterized in cats during a preliminary study (4). A dose of 7.5 mg/kg of cisplatin produced vomiting in all cats tested. Animals responded with the shortest latency and the greatest number of emetic episodes at this dose, which was therefore selected as our standard emetic challenge. We judged the antiemetic activity of the cannabinoids by the degree to which they could modify this emetic response to cisplatin.

Cannabinoid treatment varied with the route of administration and consisted of 3 dose regimens. THC was given orally in the sesame oil capsules as provided by the National Institute on Drug Abuse (NIDA) or intramuscularly in a 5% ethanol-emulphor vehicle. When given by these routes, injections were made between 60 and 90 min before the administration of the cisplatin challenge. Alternately, THC was given intravenously, also in a 5% ethanol-emulphor vehicle, 60 min prior to cisplatin. The intravenous dose schedule included supplemental injections of THC,50 mcg/kg, given hourly for 6 to 7 hrs after the initial priming dose. The 11-hydroxy-delta-9-THC was given intramuscularly in the same vehicle as THC.

Cat plasma samples were assayed for delta-9-THC using a radioimmunoassay (RIA) procedure, which employed a delta-9-THC selective antiserum and [^{3}H]-delta-8-THC. The RIA kits, which were intended for the measurement of THC in human plasma, were supplied by the Research Triangle Institute, Research Triangle Park, NC (NIDA Contract No. 271-79-3621). The kit was adapted for application to cat plasma samples in our laboratory. Generally, the assay was performed according to the instructions supplied with the kits. However, some minor modifications were necessary. Instead of 0.1 ml plasma samples, 0.025 ml samples were assayed. This was necessary due to the relatively high doses of drugs used in this study. Standards were prepared using pooled, blank cat plasma at 200, 100, 40, 20 and 10 ng/ml. Since only 0.025 ml was used for assay, the total amounts of delta-9-THC for each standard were the same as those provided with the RIA kit (50, 25, 10, 5 and 2.5 ng/ml of delta-9-THC in human plasma). Standard curves constructed from samples prepared in cat plasma produced slopes and intercepts similar to those seen using the standards supplied with the kits.

Plasma samples from two cats receiving THC (2 mg/kg) orally were assayed by GC-MS at the Research Triangle Institute, Research Triangle Park, NC. Surprisingly, no significant amounts of 11-hydroxy-delta-9-THC metabolite were detected in samples collected 0.5 to 8 hours after administration. This result impacts directly on the specificity of the RIA method. Since 11-hydroxy-delta-9-THC cross-reacts significantly with the antisera employed, assay results obtained from samples collected after oral administration of drug must be carefully interpreted. However, in the absence of this metabolite the RIA method becomes rather specific for the parent delta-9-THC.

III. RESULTS

A. Antiemetic Activity of THC

The cannabinoid THC exhibited considerable antiemetic activity against cisplatin induced vomiting in the cat model. Antiemetic activity was detected at doses ranging from 100 mcg/kg to 4 mg/kg depending upon the route of administration. The dose-response relationships obtained following the intravenous, intramuscular and oral administration of THC are illustrated in Figure 1. In these cases the criterion of protection was the complete absence of emetic behavior for the entire 8 hour period of observation.

The figure illustrates that at doses between 100 and 800 mcg/kg, given intravenously, the dose-response relationships were remarkably flat. Complete protection in all of the animals of the group was never achieved at the doses tested by this route nor was the average emetic latency or number of emetic responses statistically altered (Table I). Marked behavioral effects evident at the 800 mcg dose discouraged further testing at higher levels by this route.

THC had a more predictable antiemetic action when the agent was given either orally or intramuscularly as evidenced in part by steeper dose-response relationships obtained by these routes. Vomiting was not entirely blocked in any of the 6 animals pretreated with THC at 2 mg/kg regardless of the

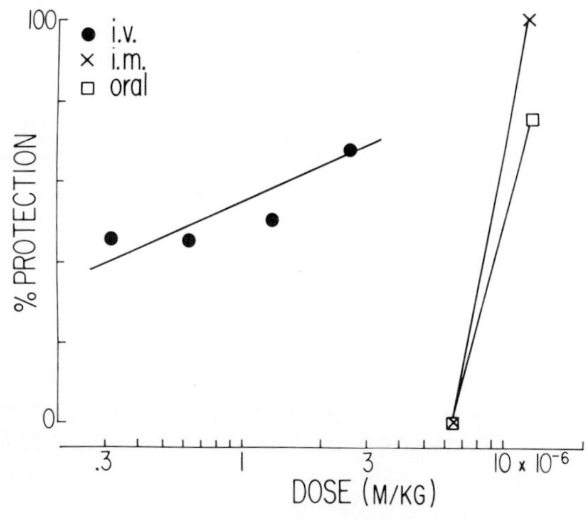

FIGURE 1. Dose response relationships for antiemetic activity of delta-9-THC against cisplatin-induced vomiting. Protection in this test consisted of the complete absence of emetic activity as recorded oscillographically during the 8 hr observation period following the i.v. administration of 7.5 mg/kg of cisplatin to cats. Oral and i.m. regimens were single doses administered 30 to 60 min prior to cisplatin. The i.v. schedule consisted of the priming dose, as plotted, followed by 6 to 7 supplemental doses of 50 mcg/kg each, given hourly.

TABLE I. Effect of Intravenous Delta-9-THC on Cisplatin-induced Emesis

Dose* (mcg/kg)	Responded /Tested	Mean Latency (min)	Mean No. of Episodes
100	4/7	95 +/- 43	2.0 +/- 1.4
200	4/7	97 +/- 28	2.7 +/- 2.1
400	3/6	107 +/- 30	3.7 +/- 2.3
800	1/3	103	1.0
CONTROL	7/7	71 +/- 18	3.8 +/- 2.3

*All initial doses of THC were supplemented with additional doses of 50 mcg/kg/hour for 6 to 8 hours after cisplatin.

route of administration (Figure 1). However, 4 out of 4 animals were completely protected by the intramuscular administration of 4 mg/kg, and 3 out of 4 were protected following the oral administration of the same dose.

As judged by the all-or-none endpoint of emesis/no emesis, THC appeared to be essentially equally effective by the oral and intramuscular routes in blocking cisplatin-induced vomiting in cats. Closer inspection of the emetic response to cisplatin following pretreatment with 2 mg/kg of THC indicates an apparent advantage of the i.m. over the oral route in moderating this response. As noted above, all animals tested at this dose of THC did vomit regardless of the route of administration. Nonetheless, those receiving the cannabinoid by the i.m. route exhibited both an increase in the emetic latency and reduction in the number of emetic episodes recorded during the observation period (Table II). By contrast, those animals receiving this same dose by the oral route failed to demonstrate any changes in these measures when compared to controls.

B. Plasma Concentrations of THC

Analysis of plasma THC levels revealed marked differences in plasma-time course which varied with the route of drug administration (Fig. 2 and 3). RIA determination of plasma THC concentrations showed a characteristic high peak as early as 5 minutes following its intravenous administration. The dose regimen employed in this series consisted of an initial

TABLE II. Effects of Oral and Intramuscular Delta-9-THC on Cisplatin-induced Emesis

Dose (mg/kg)	Route	N	Vomited /Tested	Latency (min)	$\bar{X}$ Emetic Episodes
CONTROL	--	7	7/7	71 +/- 18	3.67
2	oral	3	3/3	104 +/- 33	3.0
2	i.m.	3	3/3	121 +/- 21[b]	1.67[b]
4	oral	4	1/4[a]	164	1
4	i.m.	4	0/4[a]	---	---

[a]Statistically different from control $p < 0.01$.
[b]Statistically different from control $p < 0.05$.

priming dose of from 100 to 800 mcg/kg followed by 6 or more hourly supplements of 50 mcg/kg each, all given intravenously. Nonetheless, this procedure failed to sustain plasma levels which rapidly fell during the early period of observation.

When THC was given by the oral or intramuscular routes, analysis of plasma samples showed that peak concentrations were not achieved until approximately 1 to 2 hours after drug administration. In addition, plasma levels were sustained for much greater periods of time (Fig. 2). The mean plasma concentrations in animals receiving the 4 mg/kg dose of THC were remarkably similar in the oral and i.m. groups for the first four hours. Subsequently, the plasma concentrations declined in such a way that they appeared to be more sustained in those animals receiving the drug intramuscularly. The figure shows that 24 hours after dosing the mean plasma concentration of THC in the i.m. group was maintained at approximately double those receiving the drug orally.

The animals receiving the 2 mg/kg dose of THC by the oral and i.m. routes showed marked differences in mean plasma levels during the early period after administration (Fig. 3). Plasma concentrations peaked between 1 and 2 hours for both groups, but they fell off more rapidly in those animals of the oral group. By contrast, plasma THC concentrations in the animals of the i.m. group were well sustained for several hours. It was noted above that all animals receiving this dose of THC had positive emetic responses to cisplatin regardless of the route of administration. However, the increased latency and reduced number of emetic episodes seen in the i.m. group were associated with the more sustained plasma concentrations.

C. Antiemetic Action of 11-Hydroxy-delta-9-THC

A limited amount of the THC metabolite 11-hydroxy-delta-9-THC was available for testing of antiemetic activity in this model. A total of 4 animals were pretreated with either 3 or 4 mg/kg prior to challenging with cisplatin. The effects of this cannabinoid on the incidence, latency and recurrence of cisplatin induced vomiting are shown in Table III.

The intramuscular administration of 4 mg/kg of 11-hydroxy-delta-9-THC completely protected 1 out of 3 animals from cisplatin vomiting. In addition, the mean emetic latency of the 2 responding animals was 189 min compared with 71 min for the control group. Additionally, each of these animals responded only once during the 8 hr observation period. These observations should be compared with the finding seen after 4 mg/kg of THC also given intramuscularly. Statistical tests indicate that this group had less vomiting than the control group but that protection from cisplatin vomiting was not as marked as that seen following THC at this dose.

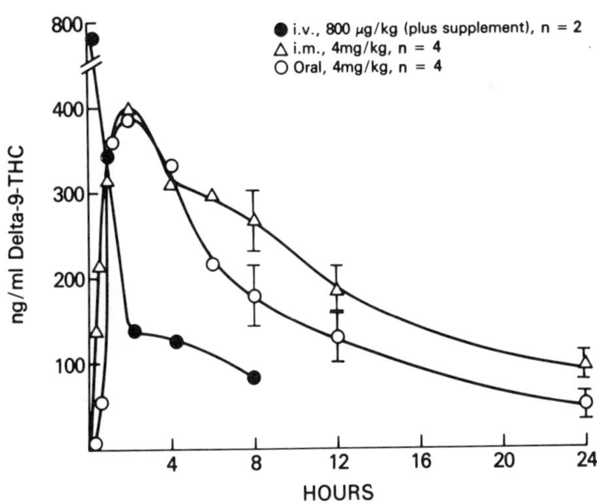

FIGURE 2. Time course of mean plasma THC levels following i.v., oral and i.m. administration to cats. Vertical bars are standard errors. Solid circles: i.v., 800 mcg/kg (plus supplement), n = 2; open circles: oral, 4 mg/kg, n = 4; open triangles: i.m., n = 4.

D. Behavioral Effects of Cannabinoids

The antiemetic actions of THC were manifested at doses which also modified behavioral activity in unanesthetized cats. The time of onset of these effects, their severity and duration of action varied considerably with route of administration and were not strictly related to the degree of antiemetic activity seen. These behavioral effects are summarized in Tables IV and V.

The intravenous administration of THC at doses ranging from 100 to 800 mcg/kg produced effects which were qualitatively similar at all doses but which varied primarily in severity. The onset of eyesigns and ataxia occurred very rapidly by this route. Reversal of drug effects were dependent upon the total amount of drug given. Thus, the larger the dose, the more long lasting were the drug effects. Behavioral effects produced by the larger doses, such as 800 mcg/kg, persisted for several hours. However, even at this dose drug action could be seen to be lessening by 1.5 to 2 hrs after injection. The most notable behavioral effect of THC following the i.v. administration of the large dose was the

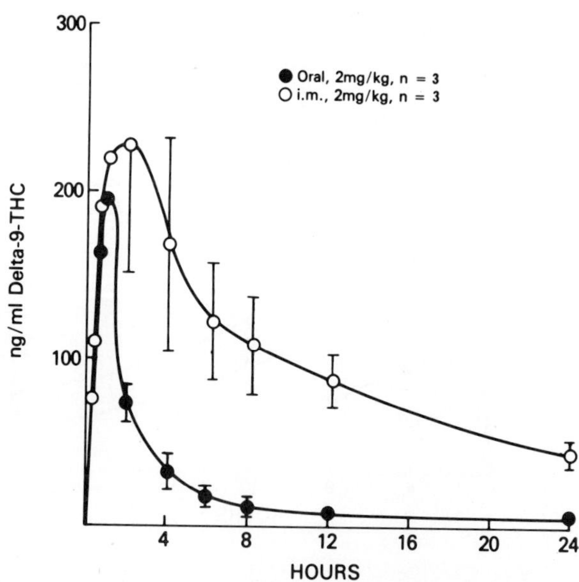

FIGURE 3. Comparison of mean plasma THC levels following the oral and i.m. injection of 2 mg/kg. Vertical bars are standard errors. Solid circles: oral, 2 mg/kg, n = 3; open circles: i.m., 2 mg/kg, n = 3.

pronounced excitement which it produced. This excitement was manifested as vocalization, startle behavior and enhanced locomotor activity. These effects were evident at lower doses by this route than by any other route tested.

The behavioral effects of THC seen after oral or intramuscular administration occurred later than those following i.v. injection. Slight but unmistakable ataxia and relaxation of the nictitating membranes were first detected 30 to 60 minutes after THC when it was given by either of these routes. Behavioral effects progressed in severity over the ensuing hour to a maximum and gradually reversed. The waning of drug action was generally evident at an earlier time in the animals receiving the 2 mg/kg dose than in those of the 4 mg group. The most notable difference in behavioral effects seen following the oral and i.m. administration of THC was the tendency for more excitement to be evident in the former group and to be rarely evident in the latter (Table IV).

With regard to the behavioral effects of 11-hydroxy-delta-9-THC given intramuscularly, they differed from those produced by THC in two respects. Firstly, it appeared that the onset of drug effects were evident much earlier than after THC, being apparent in as little as 5 to 10 minutes compared with 30 to 60 minutes for the latter. Secondly, the predominent behavioral feature of the 11-hydroxy compound was excitement as manifested by vocalization, and hyperstartle activity (Table V).

As noted in the Methods section above, GC-MS analysis of plasma samples from cats treated with THC failed to detect appreciable concentrations of 11-hydroxy-delta-9-THC. These observations, made from samples containing a large amount of THC, suggest that the cat does not metabolize THC along the 11-hydroxy pathway or rapidly converts it to other metabolites. In view of this, the occurrence of differential behavioral and antiemetic actions of these two compounds is not unexpected.

TABLE III. Effect of Intramuscular 11-OH-delta-9-THC on Cisplatin Emesis

Dose (mg/kg)	Responded /Tested	Mean Latency	Mean No. of Episodes
3	1/1	45	2
4	2/3	189 +/- 63	1 +/- 0
CONTROL	7/7	71 +/- 18	3.8 +/- 2.3

TABLE IV. Comparison of Oral, Intramuscular and Intravenous Delta-9-THC on Cat Behavior

2 mg/kg oral -	onset 30-60 min.; relaxation of nict. memb.; sl. ataxia; startle to external cues; sl. depressed affect; waning by 3 hrs.
i.m. -	onset 30-60 min.; relaxation of nict. memb.; sl. depressed affect; sl. to moderate ataxia; some startle behavior; waning by 4 hrs.
4 mg/kg oral -	onset by 60 min.; effects variable ranging from mild to marked; sl. to moderate ataxia; eye signs; some dozing; effects reversing by 6 hrs.
i.m. -	sl. to moderate effects; onset 30-60 min.; ataxia; eye signs; some dozing; effects reversing by 6 hrs.
800 mcg/kg i.v. + suppl. -	onset within 1 min.; labile then dilated pupils; severe ataxia; vocalization; pronounced startle behavior; excitement; startle behavior reversed by 1.5-2 hrs., then quiet and subdued.

IV. DISCUSSION

The emetic response to the anticancer agent cisplatin has been objectively quantified in an animal model and characterized as to latency of onset, incidence and severity. The antiemetic activity of THC has been assessed in this test following its intravenous, oral and intramuscular administration. Analysis of circulating plasma levels of THC by RIA techniques, has provided rational bases for apparent differences in antiemetic activity by these various routes. The intravenous administration of a priming dose of as little as 100 mcg/kg of THC provided significant protection fromcisplatin-induced emesis. Surprisingly, 800 mcg/kg was only slightly more effective. Plasma concentrations of THC following its intravenous administration attained extremely high levels immediately after injection. These subsequently fell to low levels within 1 to 2 hours after administration at a time

TABLE V. Behavioral Effects of 11-OH-delta-9-THC in Cats (4 mg/kg i.m.; N = 3)

- Early onset: 5 - 10 minutes; ataxia; vocalization; startle behavior.
- 15 minutes: severe ataxia, broad based; marked spontaneous startle activity.
- 30 to 60 minutes: overt but mild excitement; persistent vocalization.
- 4 hours: startle behavior gone but depressed affect remaining.

when, based upon findings in control animals, cisplatin emesis was most likely to occur.

THC, by the oral and intramuscular routes, exhibited a steeper dose-response relationship for antiemetic activity than that seen following its intravenous administration. Larger doses were required by these routes but plasma levels were found to build more gradually and achieve lower peak values. Plasma concentrations were sustained longer by these routes than after intravenous administration and THC wasstill detectable in plasma 24 hours after administration. Overt excitement and hyperstartle behavior were prominent signs in animals receiving the high intravenous dose of THC. These effects were also observed in animals treated with the high oral dose but they were either absent or only minimally evident when THC was given intramuscularly. A dissociation of antiemetic action and behavioral effects was most apparent in those animals given 11-hydroxy-delta-9-THC. Excitement, startle behavior and vocalization were prominent aspects of this agent's actions at a dose which gave minimal evidence of antiemetic action compared with THC itself. While these observations are, in part, subjective in nature, they do suggest that the antiemetic actions of the cannabinoids may be separable from their untoward behavioral effects.

ACKNOWLEDGMENTS

THC and 11-hydroxy-delta-9-THC used in this study were provided by the Research Technology Branch, National Institute on Drug Abuse, Rockville, MD.

REFERENCES

1. Seigel, L. J., and Longo, D. L., The control of chemotherapy-induced emesis, Ann. Int. Med. 95:352-359 (1981).
2. Davignon, J., Delta-9-tetrahydrocannabinol: Comments on Antiemetic trials, Front. Radiat. Therap. Oncol. 15:148-156 (1981).
3. McCarthy, L. E., Fetting, J. H., Daubenspeck, J. A., and Borison, H. L., Noninvasive documentation of emesis in cats, Cancer Treat. Rep. 66:363-368 (1982).
4. McCarthy, L. E, and Borison, H. L., Antiemetic activity of N-methyllevonantradol and nabilone in cisplatin-treated cats, J. Clin. Pharmacol. 21:30S-37S (1981).

CANNABINOIDS IN GLAUCOMA III: THE EFFECTS OF DIFFERENT CANNABINOIDS ON INTRAOCULAR PRESSURE IN THE MONKEY*

C. W. Waller, D. A. Benigni
E. C. Harland, J. A. Bedford
J. C. Murphy, M. A. ElSohly

The Research Institute of Pharmaceutical Sciences
School of Pharmacy
University of Mississippi
University, Mississippi

I. INTRODUCTION

The use of the constituents of *Cannabis sativa* as therapeutic agents in glaucoma was initiated by Hepler et al., who observed the lowering of intraocular pressure in normal and glaucomatous subjects when marijuana was smoked and when delta-9-tetrahydrocannabinol (THC) was given (1,2). The ocular effects of the cannabinoids were reviewed in 1979 by Green (3) and more recently in the Institute of Medicine's report "Marijuana and Health" (4). The extensive literature on marijuana was annotated by Waller et al. (5,6).

In previous communications we reported on a screening procedure using the rabbit for the lowering of intraocular pressure (IOP) by certain constituents of *Cannabis sativa* (7,8). Since there is no ideal methodology for the screening of compounds for IOP lowering effects in animals that simulate the pathological condition of glaucoma, a second animal model was deemed necessary. The monkey has been used in glaucoma research. Green and Kim (9) used five juvenile (3 kg) rhesus monkeys which were immobilized with ketamine and averaged the results from the group. Our experience with ketamine-immobi

---

*Supported in part by National Eye Institute grant EY-03353 and the Research Institute of Pharmaceutical Sciences.

ISBN 0-12-044620-0

lized rhesus monkeys (unpublished obervations) showed that it was difficult to control the degree of anesthesia during the time of IOP measurements. Excessive intersubject variability in baseline readings were observed.

Thus it was necessary to develop the use of conscious monkeys (M. arctoides) to validate the rabbit data for the testing of cannabinoids for IOP lowering effects.

II. METHODS

A. Animals

Groups of six stumptailed macaque (M. arctoides) monkeys (3 males and 3 females) were used. The animals wre maintained in individual cages with free access to water. They were given monkey chow (Purina) twice daily and each animal was given a multiple vitamin tablet daily. On the day preceding testing, each animal was anesthetized with ketamine, weighed and placed in a restraint chair (Plas. Labs). During the test day, intraocular pressure readings were taken in the conscious animals using a Digilab R 30 instrument preceded by one drop of 0.5% proparacaine HCl solution in each eye.

A period of 4 to 6 weeks was spent in adapting the animals to IOP measuring procedures. A positive reward of banana pellets or fruit was given to encourage cooperation. The goal of the procedure was to use as little restraint as possible in obtaining IOP readings.

Compounds were tested by obtaining IOP readings as follows: At least two baseline readings separated by more than 30 minutes were taken. Following a uniform baseline reading, a dose of the drug was given orally by intubation. Readings were taken hourly for up to 6 hours.

B. Compounds

The major cannabinoids (THC, delta-8-THC and CBD) were obtained through the National Institute on Drug Abuse. The epoxides of delta-8-THC and the epoxide of delta-9-THC were prepared by literature procedures (10,11). Their structures are shown on the opposite page. Dosage forms were prepared as previously described (7).

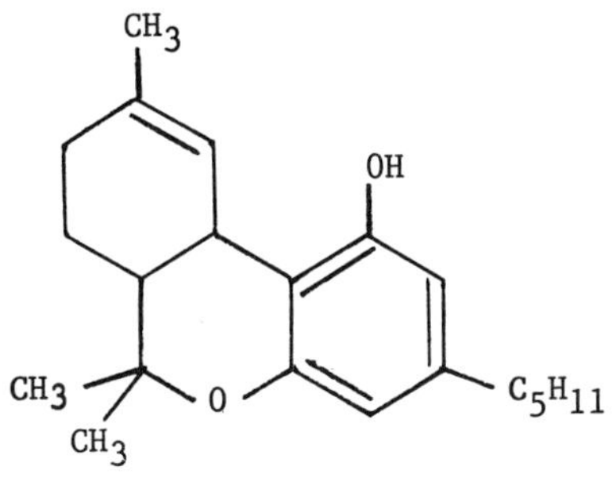

Δ^9-Tetrahydrocannabinol
Δ^9-THC

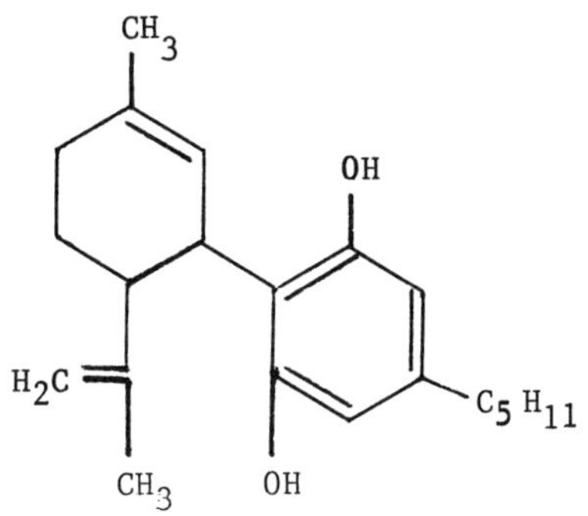

Cannabidiol
CBD

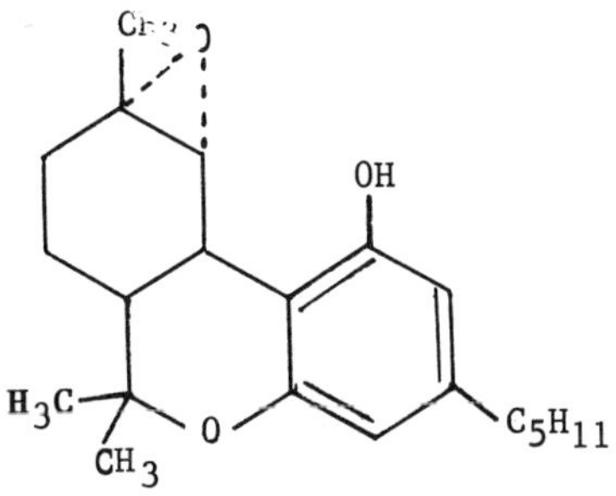

$9\alpha,10\alpha$ - epoxyhexahydrocannabinol
$9\alpha,10\alpha$ - EHHC

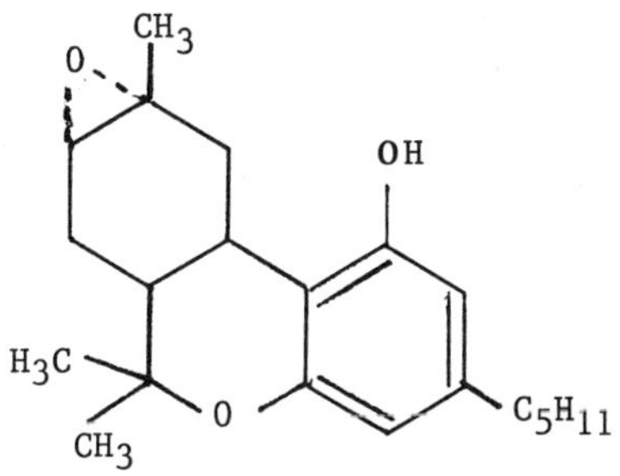

$8\alpha,9\alpha$ - Epoxyhexahydrocannabinol
$8\alpha,9\alpha$ - EHHC

C. Analysis of the Data

Data were converted to mean percent of control by the following formula:

$$\text{Mean \% of control} = \text{Sigma}(n)\ \frac{(IOP_{(t)D}/IOP_C \times 100)}{n}$$

where $IOP_{(t)D}$ is the $IOP_R + IOP_L/2$ at time t, IOP_C is the $IOP_R + IOP_L/2$ at time 0, IOP_R and IOP_L are the IOP readings for the right and left eye, respectively, and n is the number of animals used (6 in this case).

Statistical comparisons were accomplished via the Wilcoxon Matched-Pairs Signed Ranks (12).

III. RESULTS

When THC was given orally, IOP was reduced for 1 to 4 hours post dosage. A dose of 3 mg/kg of THC lowered IOP from 20.3 to 15.9 mm of mercury or 22% in 2 hours (Fig. 1). Figure 2 shows the dose response curves for THC dosage range of 0.25 - 3.0 mg/kg.

The epoxide of THC (9alpha,10alpha-EHHC) was found to be active orally in the conscious monkeys. Figure 3 shows the effect of 3 mg/kg dose in absolute IOP values in mm of mercury while Figure 4 shows the dose response curves at doses of 0.25 - 3.0 mg/kg.

The epoxide 8alpha,9alpha-EHHC was tested in this model at 1 mg/kg and found to have slight activity at this dose (Figure 5). Cannabidiol was found to be inactive at a dose of 10 mg/kg orally.

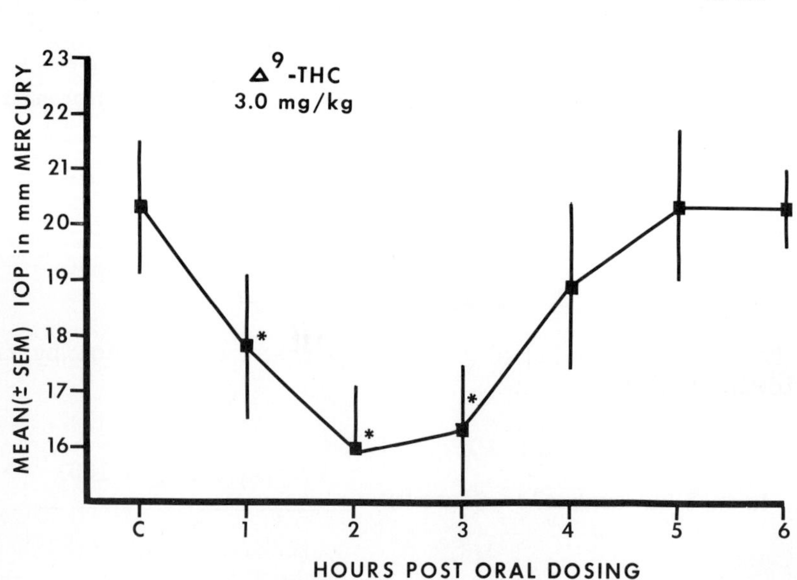

FIGURE 1. Effects on IOP in mm of mercury of 3 mg/kg of THC given orally to 6 conscious Macaque monkeys. (*$p < 0.05$)

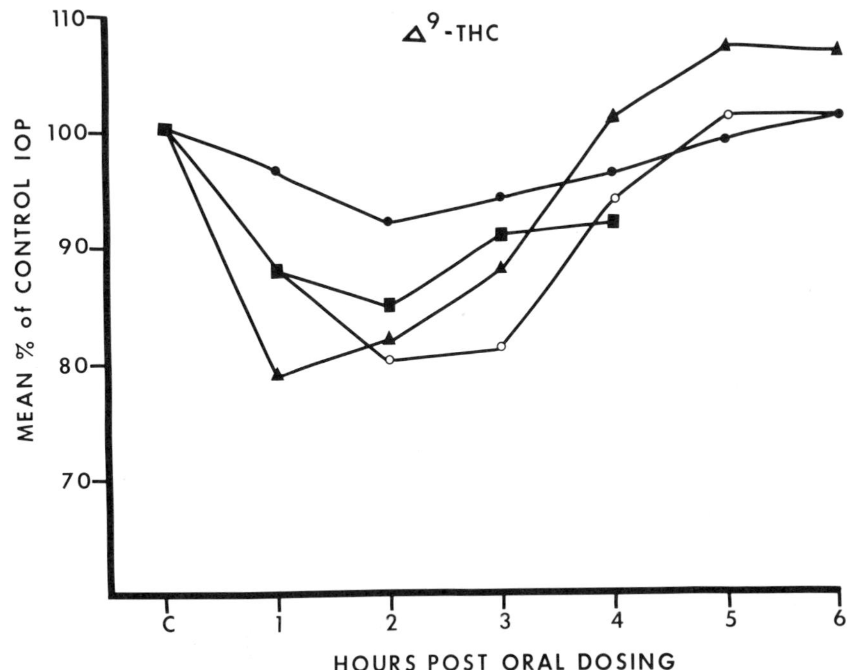

FIGURE 2. The dose response effects of THC on IOP when given orrally to conscious Macaque monkeys: (●) 0.25 mg/kg; (■) 1.0 mg/kg; (▲) 2.0 mg/kg; (O) 3.0 mg/kg.

IV. DISCUSSION

Cannabis and its constituents have evolved as a lead for the development of new and hopefully useful chemotherapeutic agents for the treatment of wide angle glaucoma. In one respect, it is an ideal lead since its major constituent, THC, has been shown to lower IOP in glaucomatous patients. Yet, it is a difficult problem to execute since there is no good laboratory animal or biological system to follow the chemical progress through a stepwise determination of the structure to activity relationships. The use of the rabbit as a test animal for screening compounds for their effects on IOP has been reported by several investigators. Green publised several reports on the effects of cannabinoids on IOP. However, Green's methodology using the rabbit as an animal model was deficient in that cannabidiol (CBD), which he reported as active, was found to be inactive in both rabbits (7) and in humans (13). Perez-Reyes et al., compared several cannabinoids (including CBD) in normal humans as to their psychoactivity, effects on heart rate and IOP lowering when given by intravenous infusion (13). They suggested that CBD was inactive in all of these parameters and it could be used as a placebo drug.

We have reported on a refined methodology using the rabbit for primary screening of cannabinoids for their ability to lower IOP (7) with the following conclusions (8):

1. THC is active by the IV route.
2. The IOP effects appear to parallel the psychoactivity.
3. Most compounds related to THC that have psychoactivity show lowering effects on IOP.
4. The activity appears to be biphasic.
5. Topical activity is erratic and both eyes are affected even when the drug is applied to only one eye.
6. The activity needs to be confirmed in other animal species.

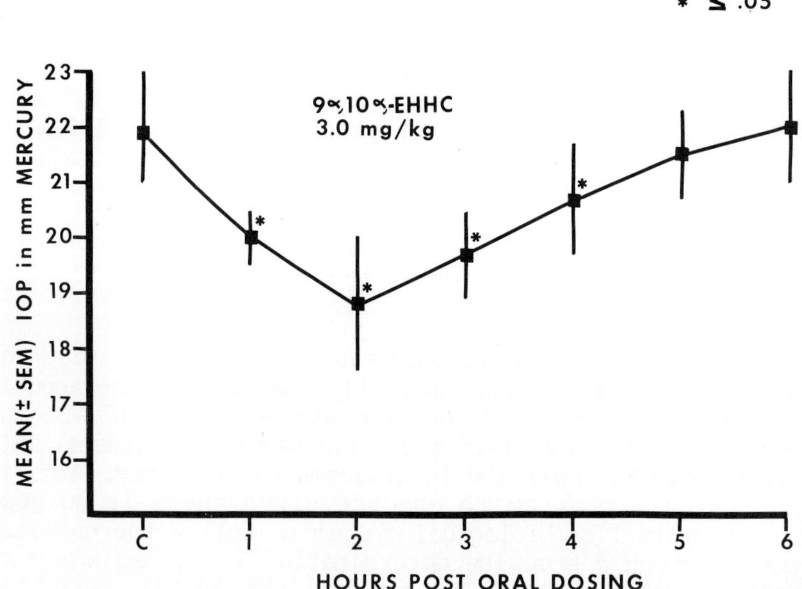

FIGURE 3. Effects on IOP in 6 conscious monkeys when 3 mg/kg of 9alpha,10alpha-EHHC was given as a single dose orally. (*$p < 0.05$)

The use of the monkey as a second animal model was investigated. The anesthetized rhesus monkey was unacceptable because of the inter-subject variability in the IOP baseline readings. It was decided to attempt to train monkeys to accept IOP measurements while conscious.

The stumptailed macaque was chose over the rhesus macaque because this species is generally more docile. The oral route of administration was selected over i.v. since the i.v. route is impractical.

The compounds used in this investigation were previously tested in rabbits and in rhesus monkeys by the i.v. route. All compounds that showed activity in these models were found to be active in the present model. Cannabidiol was found to be inactive in this investigation as it was in other studies.

Examination of Figure 2 shows the biphasic nature of the activity of THC which is in agreement with our previous observations (7,8). The 9alpha,10alpha-epoxyhexahydrocannabinol appeared to have a longer duration of action than did THC.

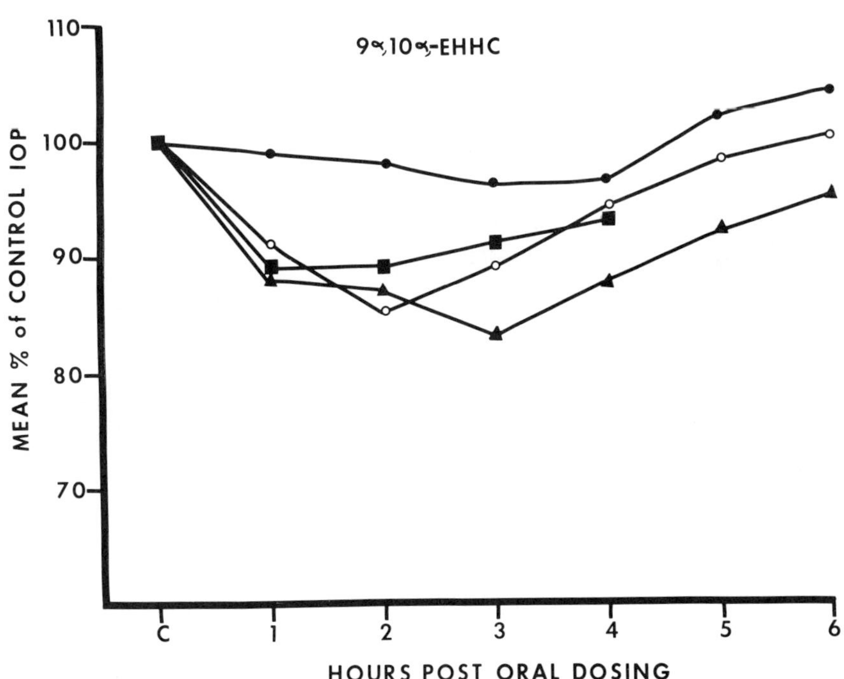

FIGURE 4. Average percentage change of IOP in 6 conscious Macaque monkeys/group when given 9alpha,10alpha-EHHC orally at (●) 0.25 mg/kg; (■) 1.0 mg/kg; (▲) 2.0 mg/kg; (O) 3.0 mg/kg.

IV. CONCLUSION

The data in both rabbits and monkeys confirm that THC is an active agent for the lowering of IOP in these normal laboratory animal models as has been reported for humans.

The 9alpha,10alpha-epoxyhexahydrocannabinol is a minor metabolite of THC and it has pharmacological properties very similar to THC (14) and delta-8-THC (15). The data reported herein and by ElSohly et al. (8) show that 9alpha,10alpha-EHHC is an active agent in lowering IOP in both the rabbit and monkey models.

The rabbit and the monkey models will be used in our laboratories to continue the search for useful agents to treat glaucoma in humans. Within this program is a search for methodology with suitable dosage forms to affect IOP when the drug is given topically.

ACKNOWLEDGMENT

The authors thank the National Institute on Drug Abuse for all the cannabinoids used in this work. Special thanks go to

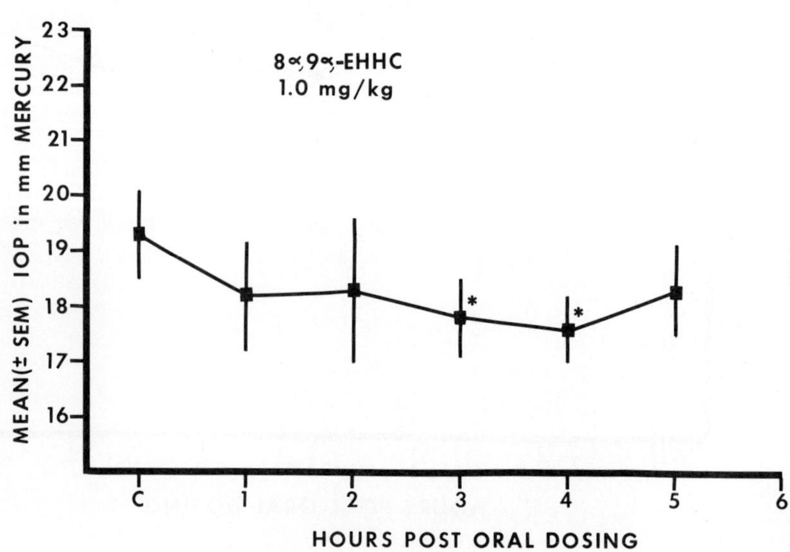

FIGURE 5. Effects on IOP of 8alpha,9alpha-EHHC at 1 mg/kg orally in 6 conscious Macaque monkeys. (*$p < 0.05$)

Dr. Carlton E. Turner for continued assistance and to Dr. Theodore Krupin, Department of Opthalmology, Washington University School of Medicine, for consulting with us on the screening procedures.

REFERENCES

1. Hepler, R. S., Frank, I. M., Marijuana smoking and intraocular pressure, J. Amer. Med. Assoc. 217:1392 (1971).
2. Hepler, R. S., and Petrus, R. J., Experiences with administraton of marijuana to glaucoma patients, in "The Therapeutic Potential of Marijuana" (S. Cohen and R. Stillman, eds.), pp. 63-75. Plenum Medial Book Co., New York, 1976.
3. Green, K., Current status of basic and clinical marijuana research in Opthalmology, in "Offprints from Symposium on Ocular Therapy", Vol. II (I. H. Leopold and R. P. Burns, eds.), pp. 37-49. Wiley, New York, 1979.
4. Marijuana and Health", (A. S. Relman, Chairman), pp. 140-142. Institute of Medicine, National Academy Press, Washington, D. C., 1982.
5. Waller, C. W.., Johnson, J. J., Buelke, J., and Turner, C. E., "Marijuana - An Annotated Bibliography", Vol. I. Macmillan, Riverside, N. J., 1976.
6. Waller, C. W., Nair, R. S., McAllister, A. F., Urbanek, B., and Turner, C. E, "Marijuana - An Annotated Bibliography", Vol. II. Macmillan, Riverside, N. J., 1982.
7. ElSohly, M. A., Harland, E., Murphy, J. C., Wirth, P., and Waller, C. W., Cannabinoids in glaucoma: A primary screening procedure, J. Clin. Pharm. 21:472S-478S (1981).
8. ElSohly, M. A., Harland, E., Murphy, J. C., Wirth, P., and Waller C. W., Cannabinoids in glaucoma II: The effects of different cannabinoids on intraocular pressure, A. Ph. A., Academy of Pharmaceutical Sciences 128th Annual Meeting, March 31, 1982.
9. Green, K., and Kim, K., Acute response of intraocular pressure to topical and oral cannabinoids, Proc. Soc. Exp. Biol. Med. 154:228-231 (1977).
10. Yamamoto, I., Narimatsu, S., Watanabe, K., and Yoshimura, H., Synthesis of 8alpha,9alpha- and 8beta,9beta-epoxyhexahydrocannabinols, Chem. Pharm. Bull. 29:3378-3381 (1981).
11. Mechoulam, R., Ben Zvi, Z., Varconi, H., and Samuelov Y., Cannabinoids rearrangements. Synthesis of delta-5-tetrahydrocannabinol, Tetrahedron 29:1615-19a (1973).
12. Siegal, S., "Nonparametric Statistics for the Behavioral Sciences". McGraw-Hill, New York, 1956.

13. Perez-Reyes, M., Wagner, D., Wall, M. E., and Davis K. H., Intravenous administration of cannabinoids and intraocular pressure, in "The Pharmacology of Marijuana" (M. C. Braude and S. Szara, eds.) pp. 829-832. Raven Press, New York, 1976.
14. Mechoulam, R., and Edery, H., Structure - activity relationship in the cannabinoids series, in "Marijuana, Chemistry, Pharmacology, Metabolism and Clinical Effects" (R. Mechoulam, ed.), pp. 101-136. Academic Press, New York, 1973.
15. Ohlsson, A., Widman, M., Carlsson, S., Ryman, T., and Strid, C., Plasma and brain levels of delta-6-THC and seven monooxygenated metabolites correlated to the cataleptic effect in the mouse, Acta Pharmacol. et Toxicol. 47:308-17 (1980).

ANTIGLAUCOMA EFFECTS OF TOPICALLY AND ORALLY ADMINISTERED CANNABINOIDS

John F. Howes

SISA Pharmaceutical Laboratories Inc.
Cambridge, Massachusetts

I. INTRODUCTION

The studies by Hepler and Frank in 1971 (1), led to the discovery of marijuana as an agent capable of lowering intraocular pressure (IOP) in humans and thereby indicating a therapeutic use for this material in the treatment of glaucoma.

Although, delta-9-tetrahydrocannabinol (THC) is clearly effective at lowering IOP in humans when smoked (1), given intravenously (2), or orally (3), results with topical formulations have been disappointing (4). This is surprising in view of the reported significant lowering in IOP in experimental animals following topical administration of THC (5,6).

Similarly, pirnabine (Fig. 1) was studied by us in 1977 and shown to be ineffective when administered topically to humans in spite of reported IOP lowering in animals (7).

Using the normotensive rabbit as a model we have reinvestigated the effects of topically applied drugs on the IOP. The data are summarized in Table I. The results of these studies failed to confirm the previously reported animal data for cannabinoids, but seemed to parallel the results in human studies with THC and pirnabine. Using the oral route of administration, THC, nabilone and nabitan all caused statistically significant lowering of IOP in normotensive rabbits.

Nabitan was also as effective in lowering IOP of human ocular hypertensives (8), when administered orally, but suffered from cardiovascular side effects at effective doses.

Naboctate was developed at SISA Incorporated as an oral antiglaucoma agent. It will lower IOP when administered orally to the normotensive rabbit (9) or to normal human volunteers (10). The incidence of cardiovascular side effects is markedly reduced with this compound and doses which signifi-

The Cannabinoids: Chemical,
Pharmacologic, and Therapeutic Aspects

ISBN 0-12-044620-0

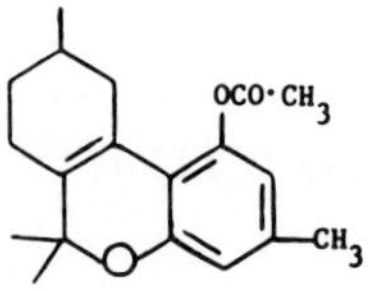

PIRNABINE

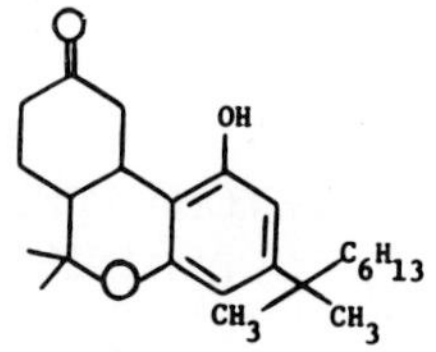

NABILONE

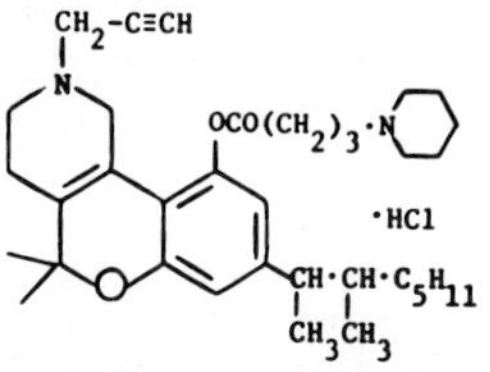

NABITAN

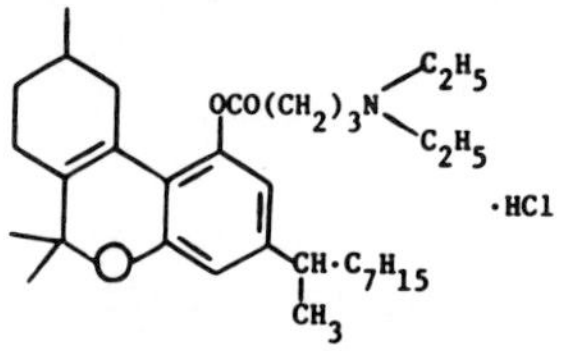

NABOCTATE

FIGURE 1. Structures of cannabinoids discussed in text.

TABLE I. Summary of effects of topically administered drugs on the intra-ocular pressure of the normotensive rabbit

Compound	Vehicle	Effect on IOP
Epinephrine	Water	Dose relatedfall: long duration
Pilocarpine	Water	Small transient fall
Timolol	Water	Small transient fall
THC	Lt. min. oil	No effect
Pirnabine	Lt. min. oil	No effect
Nabilone	PEG. 200	No effect
Nabitan	Water	Weak, erratic effect: irritation

cantly reduce IOP in normal human volunteers were below the lowest dose causing subjective CNS effects.

In the normotensive rabbit, naboctate administered topically gave a weak ocular hypotensive response (Fig. 2).

By temporarily elevating the IOP of the rabbit using the water loading procedure described by Vareilles et al. (11), we have been able to demonstrate an ocular hypotensive action to topically administered naboctate. Table II is a flow diagram of the protocol used for these studies.

Figures 3, 4, 5 and 6 show the results obtained with aqueous naboctate at 0.2%, 0.5% and 1% and with timolol at 0.25% respectively. In this model naboctate shows a dose related response on the intra-ocular pressure. The results with timolol confirm the data generated by Vareilles et al. (11). The choice of an aqueous vehicle for naboctate was important since even at concentrations of up to and including 2% in light mineral oil naboctate was ineffective in lowering IOP in this model. Nabilone was also ineffective when administered topically in light mineral oil, whereas THC did produce a weak ocular hypotensive response (Fig. 7).

These studies demonstrate the importance of the vehicle for delivering drug. Studies with naboctate in the normal

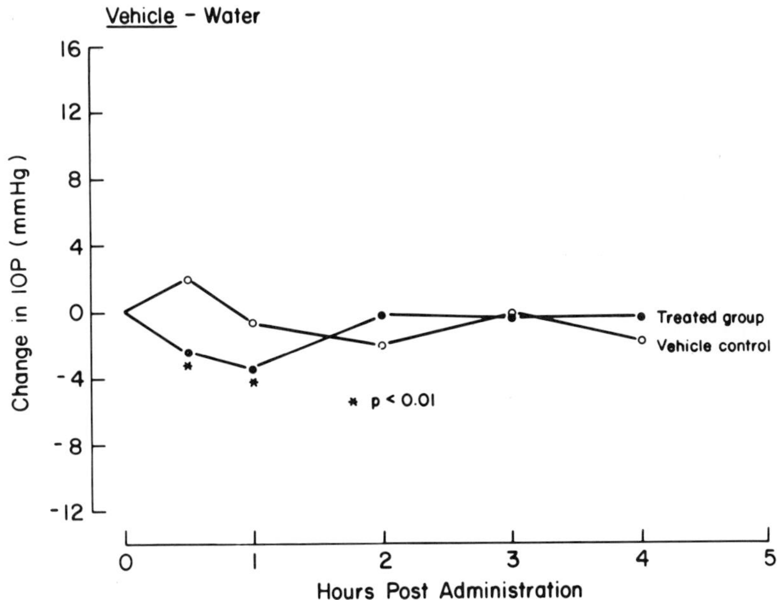

FIGURE 2. Effect of naboctate (0.8% topically) on the IOP of normal rabbits. Vehicle: water. ● = Treated group; o = vehicle control; *p < 0.01.

TABLE II. Protocol for Studying Topical Drugs in the Temporarily Ocular Hypertensive Rabbit

Day	Group I (N = 4)	Group II (N = 4)
1	a. 2 control IOP readings b. 100 ml/kg water by stomach tube c. 0.05 ml test drug solution to both eyes d. determine IOP at 1/3, 1, 2, 3 & 4 hours	a. 2 control IOP readings b. 100 ml/kg water by stomach tube c. 0.05 ml control vehicle to both eyes d. determine IOP at 1/3, 1, 2, 3 & 4 hours
2,3	No studies	No studies
4	a. Same as day 1 b. Same as day 1 c. 0.05 ml control vehicle to both eyes d. Same as day 1	a. Same as day 1 b. Same as day 1 c. 0.05 ml test drug solution to both eyes d. Same as day 1

rabbit (without water loading) demonstrated that an oral dose of 20 mg/Kg naboctate was an effective ocular hypotensive when the vehicle was water, less so when sesame seed oil was used and was inactive when light mineral oil was used as the vehicle (see Figures 8, 9 and 10). THC administered orally in light mineral oil was shown to be active (Fig. 11).

II. Conclusions

Cannabinoid drugs clearly lower intra-ocular pressure in humans. Whether this is best achieved by oral administration of drugs or by topical administration, is still open to question. Topically applied cannabinoids have so far been disappointing, probably due to the use of non-aqueous formulations. Water soluble compounds such as naboctate show promise of being useful topically but stable formulations of these materials have to be developed.

While there is little doubt that cannabinoids will be effective orally, there are other problems to be faced when using this route of administration. Although side effects with naboctate do not appear to be a problem, at the proposed dosages, there is only a small margin between these and doses

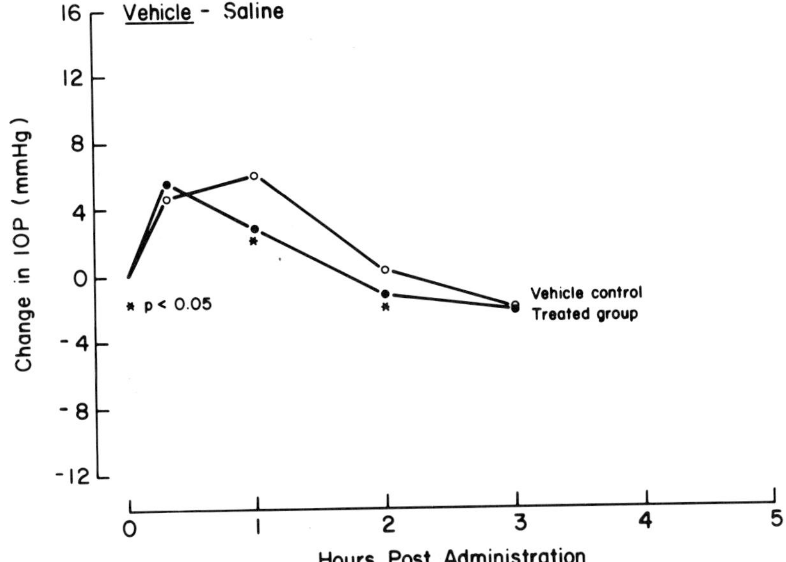

FIGURE 3. Effect of naboctate (0.2% topically) on the IOP of water loaded rabbits. Vehicle: saline. ● = Treated group; o = vehicle control; *$p < 0.05$.

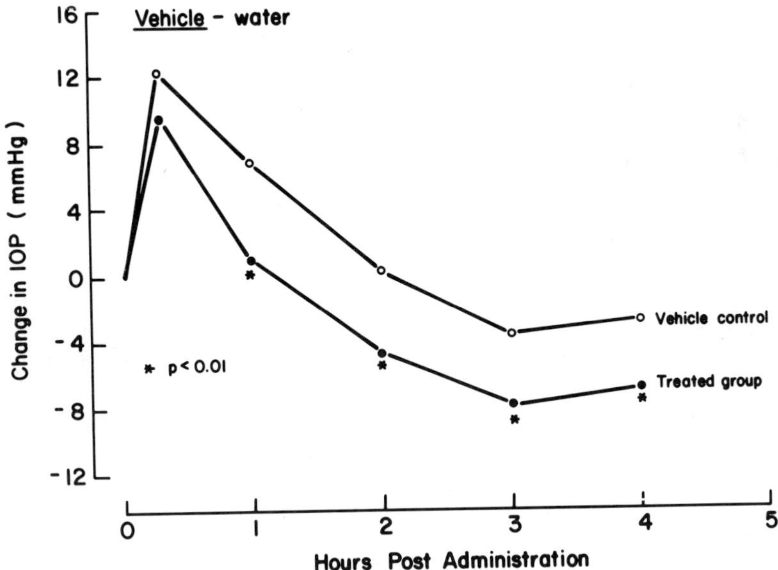

FIGURE 4. Effect of naboctate (0.5% topically) on the IOP of water loaded rabbits. Vehicle: water. ● = Treated group, o = vehicle control; *$p < 0.01$.

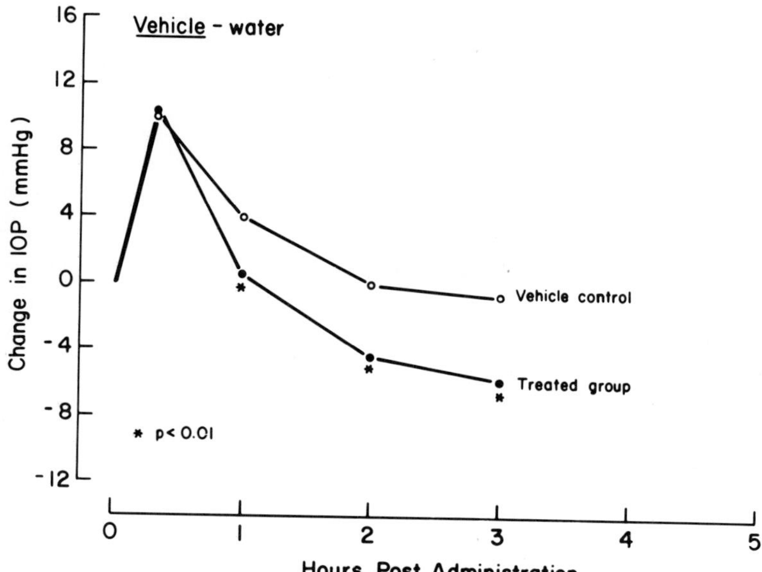

FIGURE 5. Effect of naboctate (1.0% topically) on the IOP of water loaded rabbits. Vehicle: water. ● = Treated group, o = vehicle control; *p < 0.01.

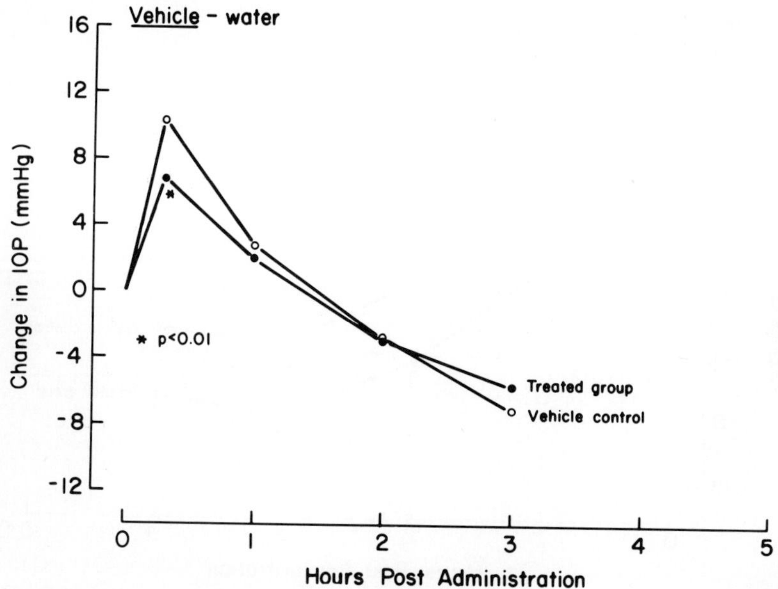

FIGURE 6. Effect of timoptic (0.25% topically) on the IOP of water loaded rabbits. Vehicle: water. ● = Treated group; o = vehicle control; *p < 0.01.

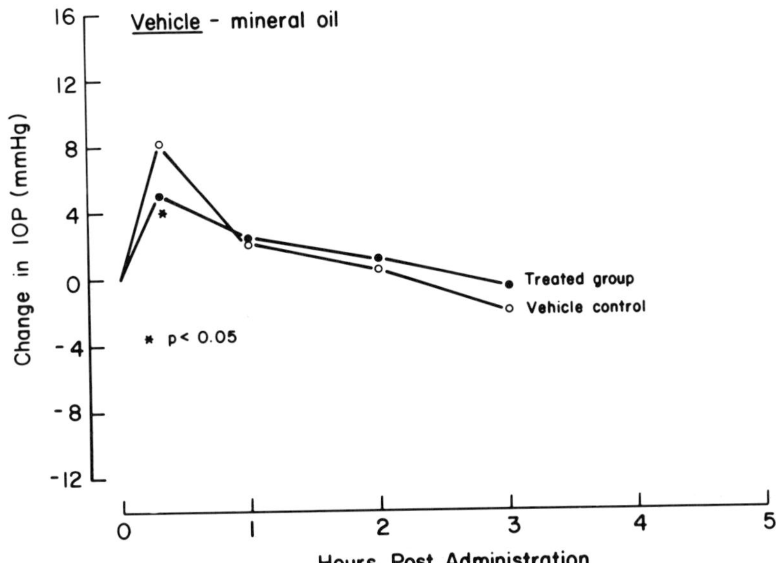

FIGURE 7. Effect of THC (1.0% topically) on the IOP of water loaded rabbits. Vehicle: mineral oil. ● = Treated group; o = vehicle control; $^*p < 0.05$.

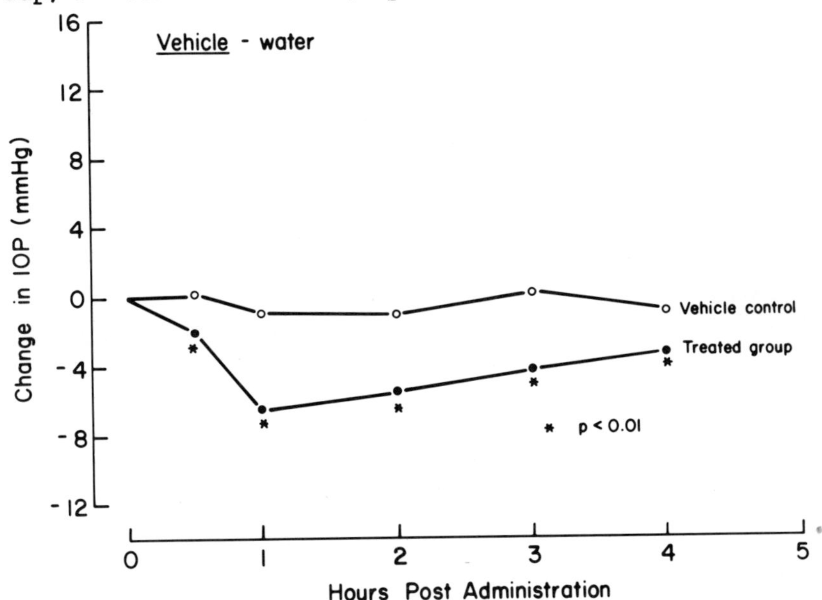

FIGURE 8. Effect of naboctate hydrochloride (20 mg/kg p.o.) on the IOP of normal rabbits. Vehicle: water. ● = Treated group; o = vehicle control; $^*p < 0.01$.

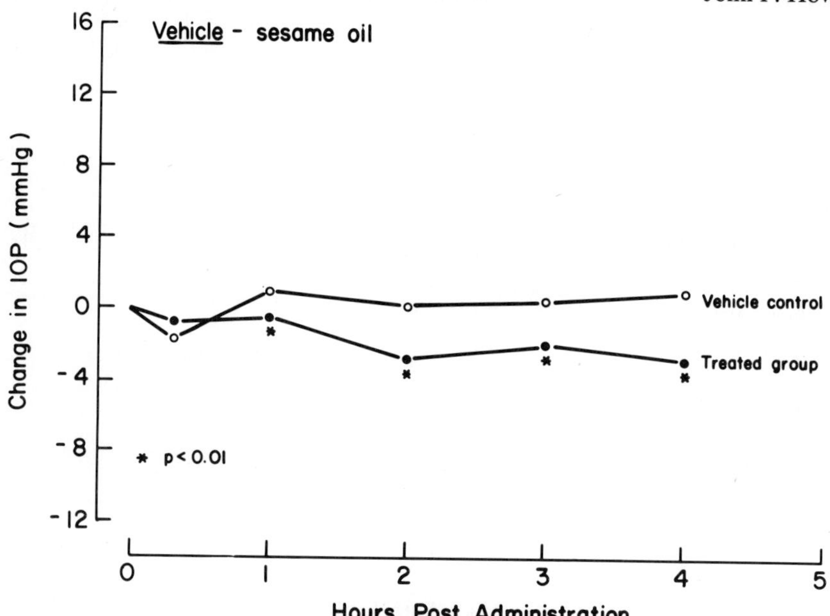

FIGURE 9. Effect of naboctate free base (20 mg/kg p.o.) on the IOP of normal rabbits. Vehicle: sesame oil. ● = Treated group; o = vehicle control; *p < 0.01.

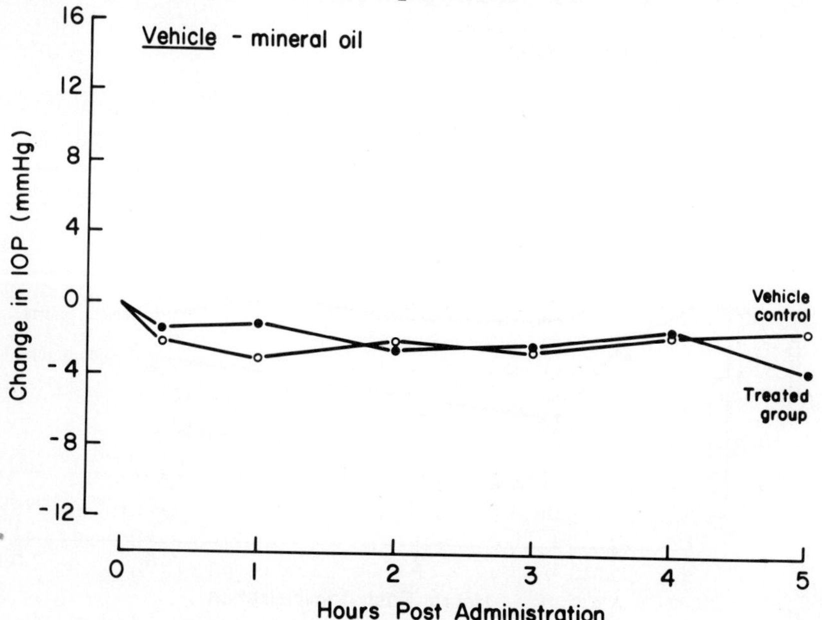

FIGURE 10. Effect of naboctate free base (20 mg/kg p.o.) on the IOP of normal rabbits. Vehicle: mineral oil. ● = Treated group; o = vehicle control.

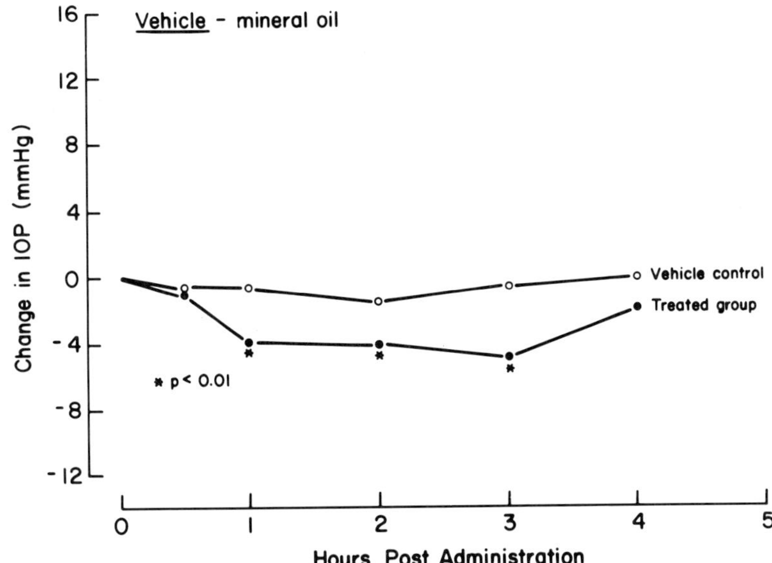

FIGURE 11. Effect of THC (20 mg/kg p.o.) on the IOP of normal rabbits. Vehicle: mineral oil. ● = Treated group; o = vehicle control; *$p < 0.01$.

producing side effects. Furthermore, an oral formulation is more likely to be diverted for abuse.

There are not yet adequate data available to allow one to speculate on the place that the cannabinoids will occupy in the therapy of glaucoma. Primarily, subjects refractory to other drugs, particularly timolol, would be candidates. A lot more work in humans must be carried out before this class of compound finds a niche in glaucoma therapy.

REFERENCES

1. Hepler, R. S., and Frank, I. M., Marijuana Smoking and intraocular pressure, J. Am. Med Assoc. 217:1392 (1971).
2. Perez-Reyes, M., Wagner, D., Wall, M. E., and Davis, K. H., Intravenous administration of cannabinoids and intraocular pressure, in "The Pharmacology of Marijuana", (M. C. Braude and S. Szara, eds.), Raven Press, New York, 1976.
3. Merritt, J. C., McKinnon, S. M., Armstrong, J. R., Hatem, G, and Reid, L. A., Oral delta-9-tetrahydrocannabinol

in heterogenous glaucomas, Ann. Ophthalmol. 12:947 (1980).

4. Merritt, J. C., Perru, D. D., Russell, D. N., and Jones, B. F., Topical delta-9-tetrahydrocannabinol and aqueous dynamics in glaucoma, J. Clin. Pharmacol. 21:4675 (1981).
5. Cool, S. J., Kaye, S. and Cullen, A. P., Topical and intravenous dosage of delta-9-THC. Effects on blood pressure and intraocular pressure. Presented at National Association for Research in Vision and Ophthalmology Meeting, Sarasota, Florida, 1974.
6. Green, K., and Bowman, K., Effect of Marijuana and derivatives on aqueous tumor dynamics in the rabbit, in "The Pharmacology of Marijuana". (M. C. Braude and S. Szara, eds.), Raven Press, New York, 1976.
7. Green, K., Unpublished data.
8. Tiedman, J., Shields, M. B., Weber, P. A., Crow, J. A., Cochetto, D., Harris, W. A. and Howes, J. F., Effects of synthetic cannabinoids on elevated intraocular pressure, Ophthalmology 88:270 (1981).
9. Razdan, R. K., and Howes, J. F., Naboctate, A novel cannabinoid with antiglaucoma activity, Fed. Proc. 40:278 (1981).
10. Razdan, R. K., Pars, H. G., and Howes J. F., Development of orally active cannabinoids for the treatment of glaucoma. Presented at the 44th Annual Scientific Meeting of the Committee on Problems of Drug Dependence, Toronto Ontario, 1982.
11. Vareilles, P., Silverston, D., Plazonnet, B., LeDonarec, J. C., Seens, M. L. and Stone, C. A., Comparison of the effects of timolol and other adrenergic agents on intraocular pressure in the rabbit, Invest. Ophthalmol. 16:987 (1977).

DELTA-9-TETRAHYDROCANNABINOL AND HERPES SIMPLEX VIRUS REPLICATION

R. Dean Blevins
Michael P. Dumic

Department of Biological Sciences
Health Science Division
East Tennessee State University
Johnson City, Tennessee

I. INTRODUCTION

Herpes simplex virus (HSV) is a frequent infectious agent in man with degrees of severity ranging from mild cutaneous lesions to severe, even life-threatening infections (1,3,4,16-18,20). The rising incidence of herpes genitalis (15) and the epidemiological association of HSV-2 infections with the development of cervical cancer in humans further underscores the need for the development of more effective chemotherapeutic agents to treat these infections.

The genetic material of HSV consists of double-stranded DNA which is present in the interior of the virion. Previous work by Blevins and Regan (6) has shown that delta-9-tetrahydrocannabinol (THC), the principal psychoactive compound extractable from marijuana, depressed DNA, RNA and protein synthesis in human skin fibroblasts and in both human and mouse neuroblastoma cells in culture. Similar observations have been reported in HeLa cells (5). Harris et al. (14) reported that mice, given oral doses of this drug, showed a 75% reduction in Lewis lung carcinoma DNA synthesis. These observations stimulated this research in which the effects of various concentrations of THC on the replication of HSV-1 and HSV-2 were observed in human and monkey tissue culture cells.

The Cannabinoids: Chemical, Pharmacologic, and Therapeutic Aspects

ISBN 0-12-044620-0

II. METHODS

A. Celland Virus Culture

The primary human skin fibroblast cells-HSBP-(18); SV-40 virus transformed human embryonic lung (WI-38, VA13) cells (American Type Culture Collection-ATCC-No. CCL-75.1; Rockville, MD.); and the African monkey kidney Vero cells (ATCC No. CCL-81; Rockville, MD.) used throughout this study,were grown to confluence in 75 cm^2 flasks (Falcon Plastics, Oxnard, CA.) using standard tissue culture procedures (10). Cells were grown in either Leibovitz L-15 medium or Eagle's minimum essential medium (MEM) (Grand Island Biological Company; Grand Island, NY.) supplemented with 10% fetal bovine serum. Herpes simplex virus type 1 and HSV-2 (kindly supplied by Dr. Thomas F. Smith, Department of Laboratory Medicine, Mayo Clinic; Rochester, MN.) were passaged four times on both confluent HSBP cells and confluent WI-38 cells, resulting inspecific HSV-1 and HSV-2 virus stock for each cell type. Virus passages were carried out at 37°C with 15 ml of serum-free (Leibovitz) medium in each culture flask. The resultant virus suspensions in this serum-free medium were harvested when virus-specific cytopathic effect was complete (100%), after 3 to 4 days of incubation. Centrifugation (900 X g for 15 minutes) removed the cellular debris, and viral stocks containing 8 X 10^8 PFU/ml of either HSV-1 or HSV-2 were stored at -70°C in sealed ampules. These stocks were quantitated by conducting plaque-titrations of infectious virus stock of HSV in Verocells grown to near confluency in 5 cm plastic dishes containing MEM as previously described (8).

B. Treatment of Cells and Virus with THC

Before use in any of the procedures described in the remainder of this report, the contents of each viral stock (ampule) were thawed and diluted with serum-free Leibovitz medium (pH 7.6) to a concentration of 1 X 10^8 PFU/ml for HSV-1 and 3 X 10^7 PFU/ml for HSV-2. Confluent cell cultures(HSBP and WI-38) with 2 X 10^6 cell/flask containing 15 ml of serum-free Leibovitz medium were inoculated in triplicate withan infectivity of 5-10 PFU/cell of HSV-1 or HSV-2 suspension plus 10 mcl of stock THC solution (lot SSC 69057, National Institute on Drug Abuse) containing 2 mg of THC/ml of absolute ethanol. Thus, each flask contained 1.3 mg of THC/ml of serum-free Leibovitz medium. HSBP and WI-38 cell viability under these conditions was determined to be >90% by the dye exclusion test as described previously (5,6). All cultures were

TABLE I. Virus Cytopathic Effect In Primary Human Epithelium (HSBP) Cells After Inoculation With THC Pretreated Herpes Simplex Virus (HSV) Types 1 and 2[a].

Concentration of THC in mcg/ml of HSV-containing medium	Number of days post inoculation				
	2	4	6	12	21
200	-	-	-	-	-
100	-	-	-	-	-
40	-	+[b]	+	+	+
20	-	+[b]	+	+	+
0	-	+	+	+	+
Control[c]	-	+	+	+	+

[a]THC pretreated HSV types 1 and 2 containing an infectivity of 5-10 PFU/cell tested in both HSBP and WI-38 cells with the data being identical for both cell lines - each datum represents the consistent results of a minimum of 12 determinations.

[b]These flasks had reduced cytopathic effect (less than 25% of cells affected).

[c]Absolute ethanol, the solvent for THC, controls at the concentrations utilized in collecting the experimental data.

Symbols: - = no virus cytopathic effect visible;
+ = cytopathic effect with 75 to 100% of cells affected or sloughed.

microscopically examined for 6 consecutive days for the appearance of virus-specific cytopathic effect or any other changes.

Direct exposure of HSV types 1 and 2 to THC was evaluated at 0, 20, 40, 100, and 200 mcg/ml concentrations of serum-free Leibovitz medium containing HSV. The control virus suspensions received the same amounts of absolute ethanol minus the THC. All virus suspensions were incubated in wide-mouth tubes at 22°C for one hour with vortex mixing at 10 minute intervals. After this incubation, aliquots containing an infectivity of 5-10 PFU/cell were carefully inoculated in triplicate from the tubes into flasks (containing 2 X 10^6 cells) of confluent cells (HSBP and WI-38). Before inoculation, the growth medium in each culture flask of HSBPand WI-38 cells was replaced with 20 ml of the serum-free Leibovitz medium (pH 7.6). The cell cultures were microscopically examined for 21 consecutive days for any signs of residual infectivity marked

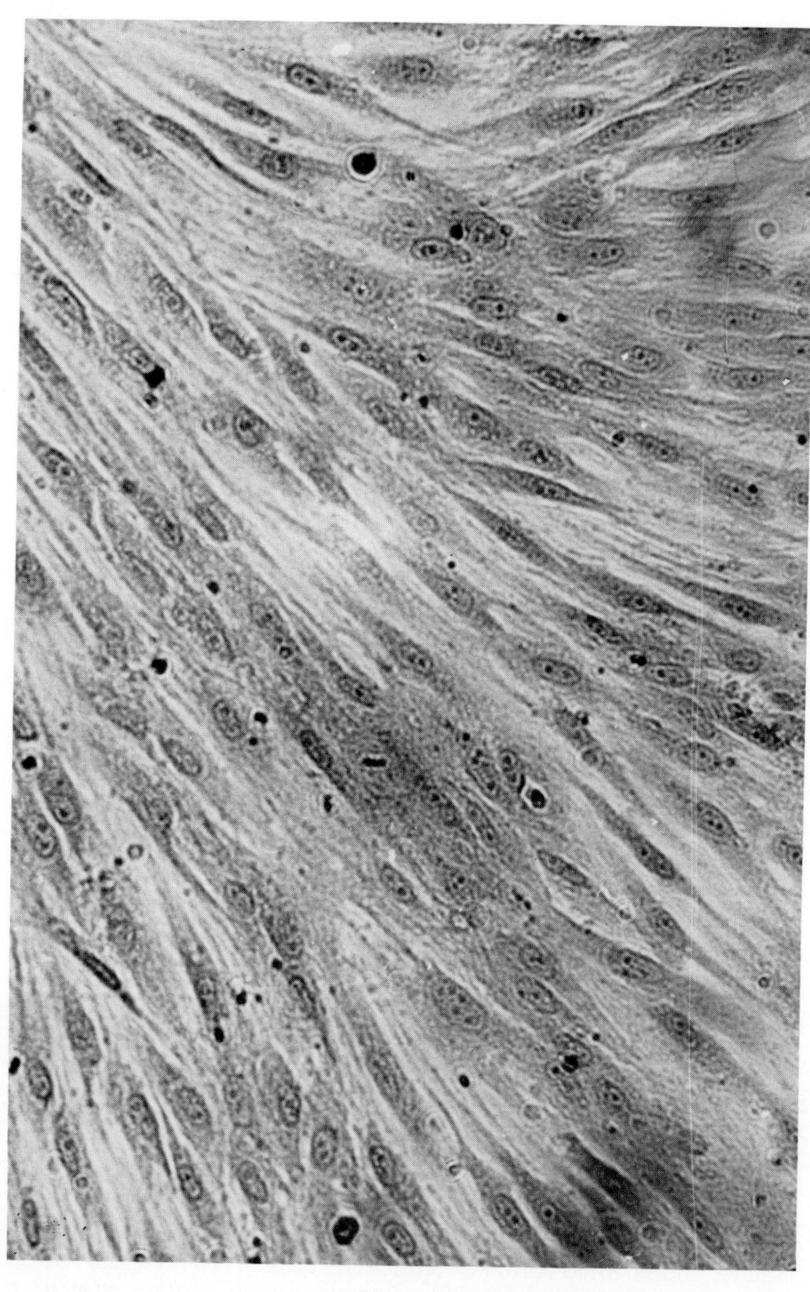

by the appearance of cytopathic effect. Every 7 days 15 ml of the 20 ml serum-free medium containing no additional THC was changed in order to maintain these cells.

C. Virus Infection of Cells for Plaque Titration withTHC

Human skin (HSBP) and human embryonic lung (WI-38)cell cultures (2 X 10^6 cells/ml) were pretreated for 8 hrs with THC at 0, 20, 40, 100, and 200 mcg/ml of serum-free MEM. The cell cultures were then infected with 3-5 PFU/cell of either HSV-1 or HSV-2 in 2 ml MEM. After 1 hr absorption at 37°C in serum-free MEM, the cells were washed 3 times with colorless Hank's solution and then incubated for 24 hr in fresh serum-free MEM containing no additional virus. The THC was again added to the MEM at 0, 20, 40, 100, and 200 mcg/ml MEM. At 24 hr post-infection the cells were scraped into the medium with a rubber policeman and disrupted by freezing (-70°C), thawing and sonication. The presence of infectious virus was assayed as previously described (8,9) utilizing Vero cells grown to near confluency in 5 cm plastic dishes containing MEM with 10% calf serum.

III. RESULTS

Simultaneous exposure of HSBP or WI-38 cells to THC (1.3 mcg/ml medium) and virus (HSV-1 or HSV-2 at 5-10 PFU/cell)resulted in at least a 75% retardation of observable cytopathic effects compared to controls for the 6 consecutive day period. Any viral cytopathic effect of the experimental culture was minimal and appeared at least 24 hr later than that of the controls. These same results occurred when the THC was added either 8 hr before or 8 hr after virus inoculation. The THC in the absence of virus had no observable effect at this concentration on either of the cell lines used. The inclusion of 10% fetal bovine serum into the medium, however, blocked the inhibition of virus cytopathic effect by the THC as well as prevented cytopathic effects caused by higher concentrations of THC. The observation that THC has a high affinity for serum lipoproteins (21) probably accounts for this effect.

FIGURE 1. A 96 hr culture of HSBP cells inoculated with 100mcg or 200 mcg of THC/ml of pretreated HSV-1containing medium (an infectivity of 5-10 PFU/cell); these cells are identical to the non-treated THC, non-HSV-1 control. Eosin, 100 X.

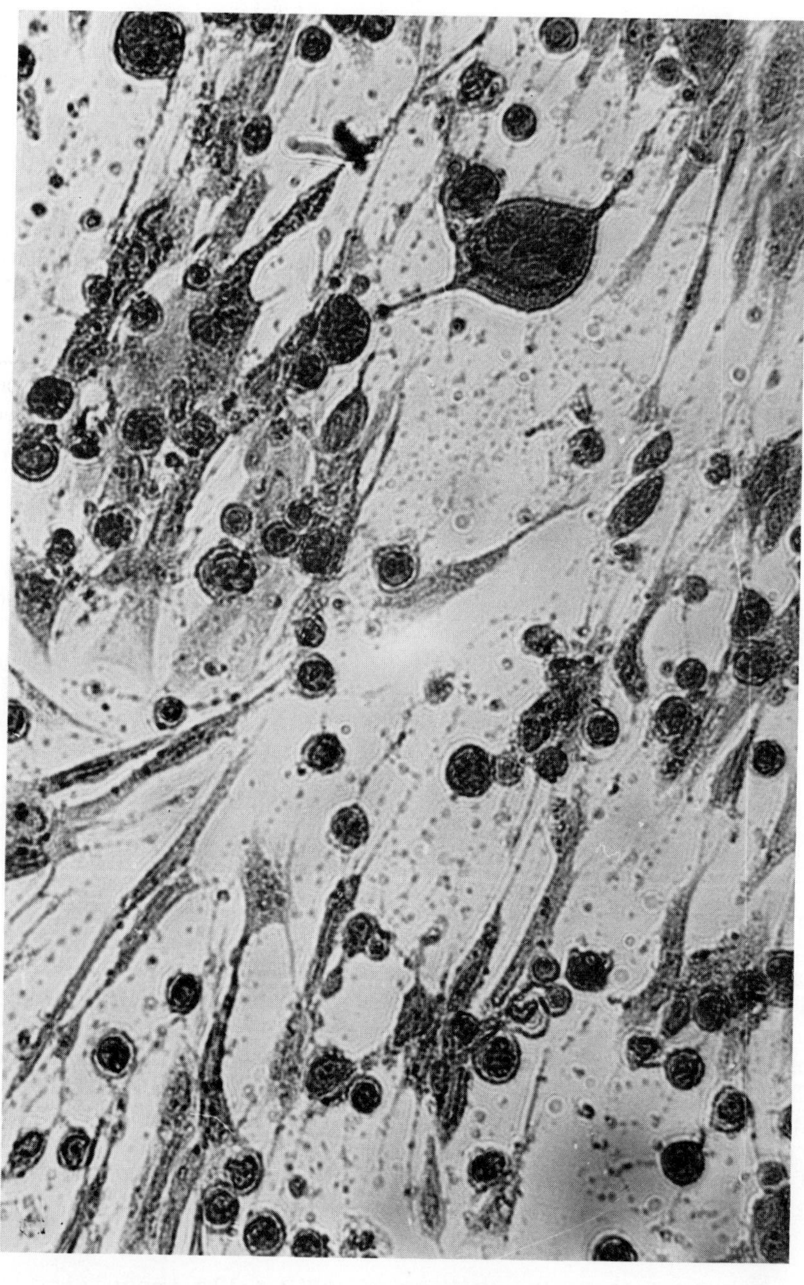

The effects of pretreatment of HSV-1 and HSV-2 with THC are summarized in Table I. Antiviral effect with human skin fibroblasts was very evident (Figure 1) at concentrations of 100 and 200 mcg of THC/ml of media containing HSV (5-10 PFU/cell). In the absence of THC (Figure 2) the virus caused marked cytopathic effects to parallel cultures. Ethanol alone, the solvent used for THC, had no antiviral effect at the concentrations utilized in these experiments (Table I and Figure 2).

HSV-1 and HSV-2 were equally sensitive to THC at allconcentrations used (200, 100, 40 and 20 mcg/ml of serum-free medium) showing no plaque formation in the Vero cells. In the presence of 20 mcg THC/ml, no PFU were seen at a 1:1 dilution of HSV; whereas, control virus preparations untreated with THC had 20 PFU at a dilution of 2^6.

IV. DISCUSSION

THC administered to cell cultures 8 hr before, simultaneously with, or 8 hr following infection with either HSV-1 or HSV-2 resulted in inhibition of cytopathic effects of the virus. A standard plaque forming assay confirmed these results indicating that THC can decrease HSV replication and/or infectivity in human cells. This effect could be mediated with the cells or by a direct effect on the virus. We have shown (5,6) that THC reduces DNA synthesis in human and other mammalian cells; and since HSV is a DNA containing virus, the drug could be blocking the replication of viral DNA. This notion is supported by the observation that THC is effective in preventing cytopathic effects in cell cultures when added 8 hr after viral inoculation, and that maximal DNA synthesis in the host cell occurs 8 hr post inoculation by HSV-2 in human cells (7).

A direct effect of THC on the virus cannot be ruled out at this time. Recently Gill (13) reported that lipophilic cannabinoids (THC) and other compounds with central nervous system activity cause molecular disorder of artificial membranes (liposomes). The comparison of a host-cell plasma membrane to the envelope surrounding the HSV capsid reportedly reveals a similar phospholipid composition and physicalconfiguration

FIGURE 2. Extensive cytopathic effect in a 96 hr culture of HSBP cells inoculated only with absolute ethanol (the solvent of THC) pretreated HSV-1-containing medium (an infectivity of 5-10 PFU/cell. Eosin, 100 X.

(2,11). In addition, agents which damage or remove this envelope are know, and they can greatly reduce the infectivity of the virion (12). Thus, the direct antiviral activity of THC that we report could involve structural changes in the lipid matrix of the HSV envelope. This possibility is being investigated presently using isotopically labeled cannabinoids.

The potential possibility of using THC as a therapeutic antiviral agent is probably limited to topical application due to the affinity of the drug for adsorption to serum lipoproteins. The need for such an agent, however, should stimulate research to determine the effectiveness of the drug for pharmaceutical use.

REFERENCES

1. Adam, E., et al., Seroepidemiologic studies of herpes virus type 2 and carcinoma of the cervix, III, Amer. J. of Epidemiol. 96:427-442 (1972).
2. Asher, Y., Heller,M., and Becker, Y., Incorporation of lipids into herpes simplex virus particles, J. of Gen. Virology 4:65-76 (1969).
3. Aurelian, L., Possible role of herpes virus Hominis type 2, inhuman cervical cancer, Fed. Proc. 31:1651 (1972).
4. Aurelian, L., Royston, I., and Davis, H. J., Antibody to genital herpes simplex virus: association with cervical atypia and carcinoma _in situ_, J. Nat. Cancer Inst. 45: 455-464 (1970).
5. Blevins, R. D., and Sholes, T. E., Response of HeLa cells toselected commercial pesticides and hallucinogens, Growth 42:478-485 (1978).
6. Blevins, R. D., and Regan, J. D., Delta-9-tetrahydrocannabinol: effect on macromolecular synthesis in human and other mammalian cells, Arch. Toxicol. 35:127-135 (1976).
7. Cheng, Y., Goz, B., and Prusoff,W. H., Deoxyribonucleotide metabolism in herpes simplex infected HeLa cells, Biochim. Biophys. Acta 390:253-263 (1975).
8. Courtney, R. J., McCombs, R. M., and Benyesh-Melnick, M., Antigen specified by herpes viruses. I. Effect of arginine deprivation on antigen synthesis, Virology 40:379-386 (1970).
9. Courtney, R. J., Steiner, S. M., and Benyesh-Melnick, M., Effects of 2-deoxy-d-glucose on herpes simplex replication, Virology 52:447-455 (1973).
10. Eagle, H., Amino acid metabolism in mammalian cell cultures, Science 130:432-437 (1959).

11. Epstein, M. A., Observations on the fine structure of mature herpes simplex virus and on the composition of its nucleotide, J. Exper. Med. 115:1-11 (1962).
12. Gentry, G. A., and Randall, C. C., The physical and chemical properties of the herpes viruses, in "The Herpes Viruses", (A. S. Kaplan, ed.), pp. 45-87. Academic Press, New York, 1973.
13. Gill, E. W., The effects of cannabinoids and other CNS depressants on cell membrane models, Ann. N. Y. Acad. Sci. 281:151-161 (1976).
14. Harris, L. S., et al., Retardation of tumor growth by delta-9-tetrahydrocannabinol, Pharmacologist 16:259-262 (1974).
15. Kalinyak, J. E., Fleagle, G., and Docherty, J. J., Incidence and distribution of herpes simplex virus type 1 and 2 from genital lesions in college women, J. Med. Virology 1:175-181 (1977).
16. Melnick, J. L., and Rawls, W. E., Herpes virus type 2 and cervical carcinoma, Ann. N. Y. Acad. Sci. 174:993-998 (1970).
17. Nahmias, A. J., et al., Antibodies to herpes virus Hominis type 1 and 2 in humans. II. Women with cervical cancer, Amer. J. Epidemiol. 91:547-552 (1970).
18. Rawls, W. E., Tompkins, W. A. F., and Melnick, J. L., Association of herpes virus type 2 and carcinoma of the uterine cervix, Amer. J. Epidemiol. 89:547-554 (1969).
19. Regan, J. E., Setlow, J. D , and Ley, R. D., Normal and defective repair of damaged DNA in human cells: a sensitive assay utilizing the photolysis of bromodeoxyuridine, Proc. National Acad. Sci. (U.S.A.) 68:708-712 (1971).
20. Sprecher-Goldberger, S., et al., Increasing antibody titer to herpes simplex virus type 2 during follow-up of women with cervical dysplasia, Amer. J. Epidemiol. 97:103-110 (1973).
21. Wahlquist, M., et al., Binding of delta-9-tetrahydrocannabinol to human plasma proteins, Biochem. Pharmacol. 19: 2579-2584 (1971).

INDEX

D

L

M

N

O

P

R

S

T

U

V

W